IMAGING AND INTERVENTION IN CARDIOLOGY

Developments in
Cardiovascular Medicine

VOLUME 173

Imaging and Intervention in Cardiology

Edited by

CHRISTOPH A. NIENABER
Department of Cardiology, University Hospital Eppendorf, Hamburg, Germany

and

UDO SECHTEM
Klinik III für Innere Medizin, University of Cologne, Cologne, Germany

Kluwer Academic Publishers

Dordrecht / Boston / London

Library of Congress Cataloging-in-Publication Data

Imaging and intervention in cardiology / edited by Christoph A.
  Nienaber and Udo Sechtem
      p.   cm. -- (Developments in cardiovascular medicine ; v. 173)
   Includes indexes.
   ISBN-13: 978-94-010-6538-2
   1. Myocardial infarction--Radionuclide imaging. 2. Myocardial
revascularization. 3. Radiology, Interventional. 4. Thrombolytic
therapy.   I. Nienaber, Christoph A.   II. Sechtem, Udo.
III. Series.
   [DNLM: 1. Myocardial Ischemia--diagnosis. 2. Diagnostic Imaging-
-methods. 3. Myocardial Revascularization.   W1 DE997VME v.173 1995
/ WG 300 I31 1995]
RC685.I6I46 1995
616.1'237'0754--dc20
DNLM/DLC
for Library of Congress   95-34054

ISBN-13: 978-94-010-6538-2   e-ISBN-13: 978-94-009-0115-5
DOI: 10.1007/978-94-009-0115-5

Published by Kluwer Academic Publishers,
P.O. Box 17, 3300 AA Dordrecht, The Netherlands.

Kluwer Academic Publishers incorporates
the publishing programmes of
D. Reidel, Martinus Nijhoff, Dr W. Junk and MTP Press.

Sold and distributed in the U.S.A. and Canada
by Kluwer Academic Publishers,
101 Philip Drive, Norwell, MA 02061, U.S.A.

In all other countries, sold and distributed
by Kluwer Academic Publishers Group
P.O. Box 322, 3300 AH Dordrecht, The Netherlands.

Printed on acid-free paper

Table of contents

Foreword

Less than 18 years have passed since the first coronary balloon angioplasty was performed in September 1977 by Andreas Gruntzig. In 1993, 185700 coronary angioplasties were performed in Europe and in many European countries, percutaneous transluminal coronary angioplasty is the most common method of myocardial revascularization, well ahead of coronary bypass surgery. This explosive growth of interventional cardiology results from major technological advances. The balloons have been markedly improved with a better profile, excellent trackability, and good pushability. The steerable guide wires are excellent and can reach the most difficult and the most distal parts of the coronary tree. The guiding catheters offer excellent support and good back-up in the ostium. Meanwhile, new tools have been proposed and designed for a "lesion specific" approach. Coronary stenting which is the "second wind" of angioplasty has dethroned most of the so-called new tools and stents are currently implanted in 30–60% of cases. Similar developments have occurred in the field of mitral valvuloplasty, ablative techniques in electrophysiology, and in the field of interventions in congenital heart disease.

However, these advances would not have been possible without the concomitant development of cardiac imaging. For many interventions, cardiac imaging is an necessary pre-requisite:

1. Imaging is mandatory to identify the lesions needing an intervention. Coronary bypass surgery or angioplasty cannot be performed without prior coronary angiography. However, scintigraphic stress testing is also needed to identify perfusion defects in the area supplied by the diseased artery.
2. Imaging is necessary to guide the interventions. This includes not only coronary angiography but also the new techniques like intracoronary ultrasound or angioscopy. The first technique is especially useful to identify the atherosclerotic mass but also the composition of the plaque and the dissections resulting from balloon dilatation. Angioscopy is the only tool able to adequately identify thrombus, a problem with which the interventional cardiologists has to deal more and more frequently. Finally,

intracoronary Doppler can assess the immediate results in determining coronary flow reserve.

3. Imaging is finally useful to asses the short and long term results of the various interventions. This includes a broad array of procedures from angiography to intracoronary ultrasound but also stress echocardiography, perfusion scintigraphy or positron emission tomography.

Whilst technological advances have rapidly improved interventional techniques, imaging technology has also undergone extraordinary development. Nobody can imagine a new catheterization laboratory without digital imaging. Digital storage of the data has been harmonized and the DICOM standard will allow us shortly to exchange digitised data not only by sending floppy disks or compact disks but even by transferring the images directly via information highways.

In nuclear medicine camera design has been improved and new tracers are available. New miniaturised imaging catheters provide cross-sectional ultrasound images of the coronary wall. Small guide wires are new tools to measure coronary blood flow velocity using the Doppler technique.

Promising advances have also been achieved with other non-invasive techniques such as the CT-scanners which are helpful to diagnose pulmonary embolism, and with magnetic resonance imaging. The interest in latter technique, which is well established in aortic imaging or depiction of complex congenital heart disease, has now been extended to the field of coronary arteries with the challenging goal of identifying the coronary lesions.

No field in medicine has proliferated and developed as extensively as imaging. This book is aimed at helping general cardiologists to get abreast of the latest developments in cardiac imaging. Obviously, each technique more or less competes with another one. This book will not and cannot provide the final answer to which technique is the best one. This is evident when reading the section on stress imaging before interventions. However, this book will provide an excellent opportunity of getting up-to-date with the most recent developments and forging a personal judgement.

The reader will discover that there is no longer competition between the cardiac imaging community and interventional cardiologists but, in contrast, a mutual interest to contribute to a better understanding and management of cardiovascular disease.

Michel E. Bertrand, M.D.
Professor of Medicine
Head Department of Cardiology
University Cardiological Hospital Lille
France

Preface

Interventional cardiology and cardiac imaging are closely inter-related subjects. Since the early days of catheter-based cardiovascular interventions,
imaging techniques have been used to define the necessity of and aid in the
performance of interventions, as well as assessing the results of this form of
therapy. Within the last 20 years, cardiac imaging as well as interventional
catheterization have come a long way.

Although imaging is often defined as noninvasive imaging, invasive x-ray
imaging continues to be the most important tool of the interventionalist.
Fluoroscopy remains the 'mother of all interventions' and coronary angiography is still the basis of all coronary procedures. X-ray imaging has wit-
nessed immense progress towards higher image quality at lower radiation
exposure. Today, radiation exposure from thallium scintigraphy is higher
than that of a state-of-the-art diagnostic cardiac catheterization including
coronary angiography using digital image acquisition technology.

On the other hand, noninvasive techniques have matured from imperfect
substitutes for invasive diagnosis into high quality imaging tools in their own
right, often replacing invasive procedures or adding information which cannot
be obtained invasively. Echocardiography has probably seen the most striking
progress: beginning with the M-mode technique, two- and three-dimensional
reconstructions of cardiac anatomy, Doppler assessment of functional parameters, and stress imaging as well as the transesophageal approach have
been developed. Radionuclide imaging has progressed from planar to tomographic imaging and attenuation correction is now undergoing clinical studies.
New imaging modalities such as positron emission tomography (PET) or
ultrafast computed tomography have entered the clinical arena. More recently, magnetic resonance imaging has established itself as an important new
tool for the anatomic diagnosis and functional assessment of cardiovascular
disease. Even from within the coronary arteries, new forms of imaging have
become available such as intracoronary ultrasound or Doppler measurements
of intracoronary flow velocities.

Parallel to this breath-taking speed of development in the imaging field,
numerous new cardiac interventions have been introduced and more and

more complex procedures are now possible for diseases which, only a few years ago, were thought to be the exclusive battle-ground of cardiac surgery. Thrombolytic therapy is now firmly established as a means of significantly decreasing infarct mortality and a multitude of catheter-based coronary interventions including balloon angioplasty and stenting, among others, have proved useful to ameliorate anginal symptoms in patients with coronary disease. Although balloon valvuloplasty has not yielded improved outcome in aortic stenosis, it has proved to be as successful as surgical procedures in mitral and pulmonic stenosis. The recent development of catheter-based curative interventions in congenital heart disease now offers an alternative to surgery or a means of avoiding repeated surgery in a significant number of children or adult patients with congenital heart disease.

What makes imaging such an integral part of all types of interventions? The patient's complaints and a straightforward clinical examination are rarely sufficient to justify an immediate intervention. In our opinion, some form of functional noninvasive cardiac imaging is crucial in many patients to more objectively define the need for an intervention. Undoubtedly, some patients require some form of intervention on an emergency basis solely based on clinical symptoms and others have such impressive abnormalities in their stress ECG that further evaluation would simply be a waste of time and money. However, in current practice these patients constitute only an – albeit sizeable – minority. The majority of coronary patients will profit from some form of noninvasive stress imaging in order to clearly define the need for invasive investigation and intervention. It may, however, be advisable not to have the same physician interpret the results of imaging stress studies and perform the intervention to avoid 'self referral bias'. An objective functional assessment of myocardial perfusion or wall motion during stress should counteract the dreaded 'oculo-stenotic' reflex. Managing patients in this way will have a positive impact on the quality of care and at the same time help to contain costs in this era of incessant increase in health-care expenditure.

Today, imaging in the form of angiography is still indispensable in guiding coronary interventions. Recently, new imaging tools such as intracoronary ultrasound or blood flow measurements by Doppler guidewires have become available to the interventionalist and provide additional information for on-line guidance of procedures. Although these new tools may ultimately result in less reliance on noninvasive stress imaging studies, the interventionalist often collaborates with an imaging oriented specialist in the catheterization laboratory for optimal interpretation of images and on-line measurements of luminal areas or flow velocities. Another good example of close collaboration between interventionalist and imaging specialist during an intervention is balloon dilatation of cardiac valves guided by transthoracic or transesophageal echocardiography.

Objective documentation of the success or failure of an intervention beyond the angiographic depiction of the immediate result requires the use of invasive or noninvasive imaging techniques. Again, intracoronary ultrasound may be helpful for the interventionalist in deciding whether the lumen enlargement achieved by the procedure is indeed satisfactory even though the ultrasound image is the less forgiving modality of incomplete dilatation as compared to the angiogram. However, postinterventional imaging stress tests or Doppler assessment of intracoronary blood flow may remain abnormal for some time to become only normal at follow-up angiography weeks to months later. Thus, some caveats remain with respect to the role of postinterventional stress imaging.

Imaging and intervention belong together and it is important that specialists in each field understand the concepts and the potential, the capabilities and the shortcomings of the other field. However, the increasing complexity of a multitude of new developments makes it increasingly difficult for the individual physician to keep pace and gain or retain sufficient knowledge in both fields. Therefore, the intention of this book is to provide clinical cardiologists and interventionalists with an up to the minute overview on the use of cardiac imaging techniques in combination with modern interventional procedures such as thrombolysis, nonsurgical coronary revascularization, valvuloplasty, and interventions in congenital heart disease. Each section of the book contains several chapters describing how imaging techniques can be used before, during, and after intervention to select the optimal interventional strategy including the choice of simply continuing medical therapy. However, imaging can also be helpful to understand the interaction between disease and interventional therapy, and this aspect is also reflected in the book.

Some readers may miss certain topics such as the role of electron beam CT in the diagnosis and prognostic assessment of coronary artery disease. However, the idea of the book was to select a number of frequently used interventions and imaging techniques rather than producing an encyclopedia which would combine all possible imaging modalities with every type of cardiac intervention. Unavoidably, there will be some bias in some chapters written by recognized and enthusiastic experts in the topic. The competition between nuclear cardiologists and stress echocardiography proponents is likely to exist even between the staff members in many cardiology departments and to some extent merely reflects the positive experiences each investigator has made with his favourite imaging tool. "Imaging and intervention" will provide the reader with an opportunity to study the competing techniques in detail and develop his or her own personal preference on how to use the various options most efficiently. For the interventional cardiologist, this book will be useful to learn more about the many ways cardiac imaging can be of assistance to him in the catheterization laboratory. It cannot be overemphasized that the exclusive reliance on good old coronary angiography may result in suboptimal treatment and an unnecessary risk to the patient.

The book is structured around a number of interventional procedures with special emphasis on the clinically relevant problems. For instance, imaging in conjunction with thrombolysis is focused on the assessment of the risk zone, on the evidence of postinfarct viability, and on prognostic evaluation. This structure should help the reader to quickly find the information pertaining to a given clinical problem. Since the main focus of the book is on imaging, there is a large number of carefully selected colour and black and white figures illustrating the key points of each chapter to the reader. The bibliographies contain up-to-date references as well as the classic quotations on the topic. Therefore, we hope that this book may also be useful for the reader who would like to study certain aspects in more detail.

We gratefully acknowledge the excellent work of the many contributors to the book who helped us to capture the dynamic developments in both fields. Nettie Dekker, Monique Pagels, and Helen Liepman at Kluwer deserve our grateful recognition for their patience and support during the planning and the production phase of the project. We are also obliged to many friends and colleagues at our institutions for all their constructive criticism.

Christoph Nienaber
Udo Sechtem

List of contributors

FRANK M. BAER
  Klinik III für Innere Medizin, University of Cologne, Joseph-Stelz-
  mannstrasse 9, D-50924 Cologne, Germany
  Co-author: Hans J. Deutsch

GEORGE A. BELLER
  Cardiovascular Division, P.O. Box 158, Univerisity of Virginia, Health
  Sciences Center, Charlottesville, VA 22908, USA
  Co-author: Lawrence W. Gimple

MORTEN BØTTCHER
  Positron Emission Tomography Center (PET), Building 10 (10C), Aarhus
  Kommunehospital, DK-8080 Aarhus C, Denmark
  Co-authors: Johannes Czernin and Heinrich R. Schelbert

CHUNGUANG CHEN
  Echocardiography Laboratory, Division of Cardiology, Hartford Hospital,
  80 Seymour Street, Hartford, CT 06102, USA
  Co-authors: Lianglong Chen, Linda Gillam and Raymond McKay

TIMOTHY F. CHRISTIAN
  Cardiovascular Diseases and Internal Medicine, Mayo Clinic, 200 1st Street
  SW, Rochester, MN 55905, USA

JAN H. CORNEL
  Thoraxcenter, Ba 350, Erasmus University, P.O. Box 1738, 3000 DR
  Rotterdam, The Netherlands
  Co-authors: Ambroos E.M. Reijs, Joyce Postma-Tjoa and Paolo M.
  Fioretti

FRANZ FOBBE
   Department of Radiology, Klinikum Steglitz, Free University Berlin, Hindenburgdamm 30, D-12200 Berlin 45, Germany

DAVID P. FOLEY
   Thorax Center, Bd 416, Erasmus University, P.O. Box 1738, 3000 DR Rotterdam, The Netherlands
   Co-author: Patrick W. Serruys

STEVEN A. GOLDSTEIN
   Noninvasive Cardiology, Washington Hospital Center, 110 Irving St. NW, Suite 4B-14, Washington, DC 20010-2975, USA

MICHAEL HAUDE
   Cardiology Department, University of Essen, Hufelandstrasse 55, D-45122 Essen, Germany
   Co-authors: Dietrich Baumgart, Guido Caspari, Junbo Ge and Raimund Erbel

GERD HAUSDORF
   Charité, Department of Pediatric Cardiology, Humboldt-University Berlin, Schumannstrasse 20-21, D-10117 Berlin, Germany

DIRK HAUSMANN
   Department of Cardiology, Hannover Medical School, Konstanty-Gutschow-Strasse 8, D-30625 Hannover, Germany
   Co-authors: Peter J. Fitzgerald and Paul G. Yock

GUNNAR K. LUND
   Department of Cardiology, University Hospital Eppendorf, Martinistrasse 52, D-20246 Hamburg, Germany
   Co-author: Christoph A. Nienaber

WARREN J. MANNING
   Cardiovascular Division, Beth Israel Hospital, 330 Brookline Avenue, Boston, MA 02215, USA
   Co-author: Robert R. Edelman

JACQUES A. MELIN
   Department of Nuclear Medicine, University of Louvain Medical School, Avenue Hippocrate 10/2580, B-1200 Brussels, Belgium
   Co-authors: Jean-Louis Vanoverschelde, Bernhard Gerber and William Wijns

CHRISTOPH A. NIENABER
Department of Cardiology, University Hospital Eppendorf, Martinistrasse 52, D-20246 Hamburg, Germany
Co-author: Gunnar K. Lund

LEONARD M. NUMEROW
c/o Foothills Hospital, Department of Radiology, 1403 29 Street NW, Calgary, Alberta, Canada
Co-authors: Michael F. Wendland, Maythem Saeed and Charles B. Higgins

DUDLEY J. PENNELL
Magnetic Resonance Unit, Royal Brompton Hospital, Sydney Street, London SW3 6NP, UK

LUC A. PIERARD
Service de Cardiologie, CHU du Sart-Tilman, B-4000 Liege, Belgium

ELIZABETH PRVULOVICH
Institute of Nuclear Medicine, Middlesex Hospital, Mortimer St., London W1N 8AA, UK
Co-author: Richard Underwood

PATRICIA J. RUBIN
Cardiovascular Division, Washington University School of Medicine, P.O. Box 8086, 660 S. Euclid Ave., St. Louis, MO 63110, USA
Co-author: Steven R. Bergman

UDO SECHTEM
Klinik III für Innere Medizin, University of Cologne, Joseph-Stelzmannstrasse 9, D-50924 Cologne, Germany
Co-authors Chapter 14: Frank M. Baer, Eberhard Voth, Peter Theissen, Christian Schneider and Harald Schicha
Co-authors Chapter 25: Hans-Wilhelm Höpp and Dirk Rudolph

CHRISTIAN SEILER
Department of Internal Medicine, University Hospital Bern, Freiburgstrasse, CH-3010 Bern, Switzerland

RÜDIGER SIMON
Klinik für Kardiologie, I. Medizinische Universitäts-Klinik, Christian-Albrechts-University Kiel, Schittenhelmstrasse 12, D-24105 Kiel, Germany

OLIVER STÜMPER
Heart Unit, Birmingham Childrens Hospital, Ladywood Middleway, Birmingham B16 8ET, UK

MICHAEL J. TYNAN
Department of Paediatric Cardiology, 11th Floor Guy's Tower-Guy's Hospital, St. Thomas' Street, London SE1 9RT, UK
Co-author: Gunter Fischer

ALBERT VARGA
2nd Department of Medicine, Albert Szent-Gyorgyi University Medical School, P.O. Box 480, 6701 Szeged, Hungary
Co-author: Eugenio Picano

EDNA H.G. VENNEKER
Department of Cardiology, University Hospital Leiden, Building 1, C5-P25, Rijnsburgerweg 10, 2333 AA Leiden, The Netherlands
Co-authors: Berthe L.F. van Eck-Smit and Ernst E. van der Wall

FRANS J. TH. WACKERS
Department of Diagnostic Radiology and Medicine, Yale University School of Medicine, 333 Cedar Street, TE-2, P.O. Box 208042, New Haven, CT 06510-8042, USA

1. Serial myocardial perfusion imaging with Tc-99m-labeled myocardial perfusion imaging agents in patients receiving thrombolytic therapy for acute myocardial infarction

FRANS J. Th. WACKERS

Introduction

Numerous studies have shown the beneficial effect of thrombolytic therapy early in the course of acute myocardial infarction. Long term mortality of patients with acute infarction treated with thrombolytic therapy is dramatically lower than that of patients receiving conventional therapy [1]. Nevertheless, reocclusion of the infarct artery may occur in approximately 30% of patients. Interestingly, reocclusion may be silent and not associated with recurrent myocardial infarction [2]. Reocclusion without reinfarction may result in ongoing hibernating myocardium. This condition may be associated with unfavorable outcome. Accordingly, substantial effort has been directed toward "fine tuning" appropriate adjunctive therapy with antithrombotic agents to enhance permanent infarct artery patency. However, since mortality is low, and since reocclusion of infarct artery may be silent, it may be difficult to definitively assess improved comparative efficacy of a novel treatment strategies. Very large numbers of patients would need to be enrolled in trials to demonstrate statistically significant differences in outcome.

The single most important, and direct effect of thrombolytic therapy is that of restoration of blood flow in the infarct artery. This will generally result in salvage of myocardium, and consequently preservation of global left ventricular function. Indeed, the majority of patients presently treated in thrombolytic trials have, in spite of sustained acute myocardial infarction, preserved normal global left ventricular function at hospital discharge. However, in the *individual* patient it is generally impossible to know how much myocardium was initially at jeopardy, and how much true benefit was gained by thrombolytic therapy.

Early after acute myocardial infarction therapeutic efforts should be directed toward administering thrombolytic therapy (or performing primary coronary angioplasty) as soon as possible after onset of chest pain. No time should be wasted in these early hours, when every minute counts, on diagnostic procedures.

C.A. Nienaber and U. Sechtem (eds): Imaging and Intervention in Cardiology, 1–12.
© 1996 *Kluwer Academic Publishers.*

Concept of serial myocardial perfusion imaging

The new technetium-99m(Tc-99m) labeled myocardial perfusion imaging agents provide the unique possibility to assess noninvasively the efficacy of new strategies in thrombolytic therapy utilizing the one characteristic that these agents share: *absence of significant redistribution* after injection [3, 4]. Regional myocardial accumulation of these radiotracers reflects the distribution of regional myocardial blood flow *at the time of injection*. In other words, the pattern of myocardial blood flow can be "frozen over time". This makes it feasible to assess noninvasively the extent of myocardium at risk without delaying therapy. This can be achieved with myocardial perfusion imaging as follows. As soon as a patient with acute chest pain arrives in the emergency depeartment a Tc-99m-labeled agent, for instance Tc-99m-Sestamibi, is injected (Figure 1). If the patient meets appropriate criteria, thrombolytic therapy or revascularization can be initiated at the earliest possible time. The actual area of myocardium at risk can be assessed noninvasively by myocardial perfusion imaging *at later time*, convenient for medical staff and patient. A subsequent repeat injection of Sestamibi allows assessment of the amount of apparent myocardial salvage. In this manner the patient serves as his, or her, own control (Figures 2–4). Using change in myocardial perfusion defect as an end point, considerable fewer patients may need to be enrolled in studies that evaluate potential benefit effects of new treatment strategies, than when other end points are used.

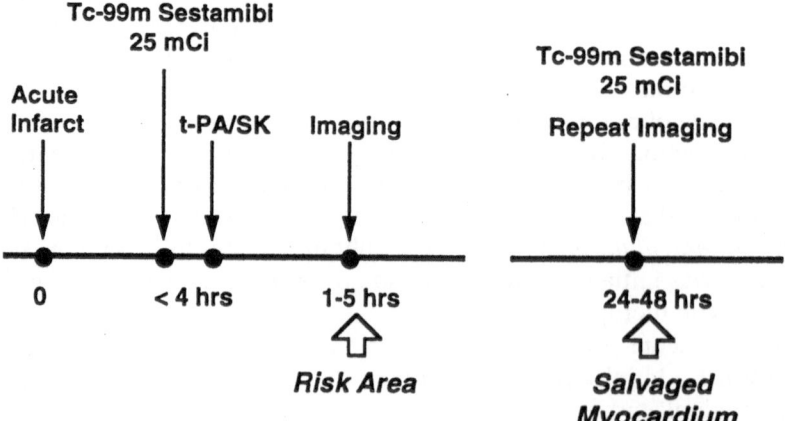

Figure 1. Diagram of myocardial perfusion imaging protocol in setting of trombolytic therapy for acute myocardial infarction. Abbreviations: t-PA = tissue-type plasminogen activator; SK = streptokinase.

THROMBOLYSIS

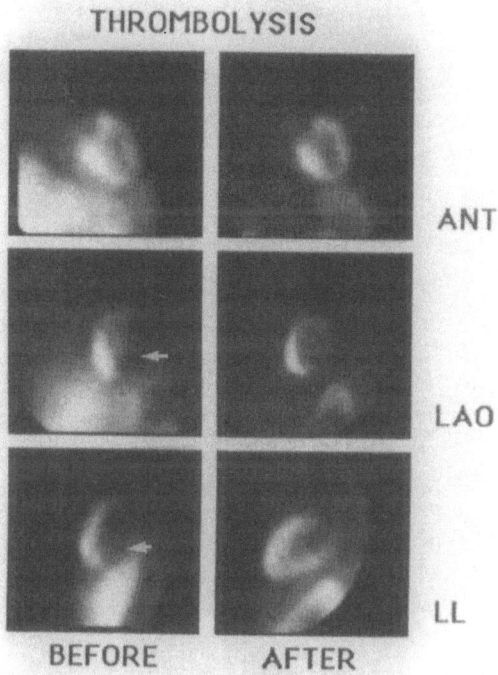

ANT

LAO

LL

BEFORE   AFTER

Figure 2. Planar myocardial perfusion imaging with Tc-99m-Sestamibi before and after successful thrombolytic therapy for acute inferior wall myocardial infarction. The images on the left
were obtained after radiotracer injection in the emergency department prior to initiation of
thrombolytic therapy. The images were acquired 2 hours later at the patient's bed side. The
area at risk for infarction is in the inferoposterior and lateral wall (arrows). The images on the
right were obtained one day later after a repeat injection with Tc-99m-Sestamibi. Improved
visualization of the inferoposterior wall (LL view) due to successful reperfusion of the infarct
artery can be appreciated. On the LAO view the residual posterolateral infarct is visualized.
Quantitatively 42% of the initial risk area was salvaged by thrombolytic therapy. Abbreviations:
ANT = anterior view; LAO = left anterior oblique view; LL = left lateral view. (Reproduced
with permission from [3].)

Imaging protocol

Depending on the initial dose (10–30 mCi) of Tc-99m-Sestamibi administered
in the emergency department, good quality images can be obtained up to 5
hours after administration of radiotracer. Imaging can be performed either
at the patient's bedside using a mobile planar gamma camera, or if the
patient is relatively stable, in the nuclear medicine laboratory using tomographic imaging equipment. The latter obviously requires careful monitoring
and close physician supervision. Wackers et al. [3] and Gibbons et al. [4]
were first to demonstrate the feasibility of this approach. Subsequently,
numerous reports have confirmed that patients with acute infarction can be

THROMBOLYSIS

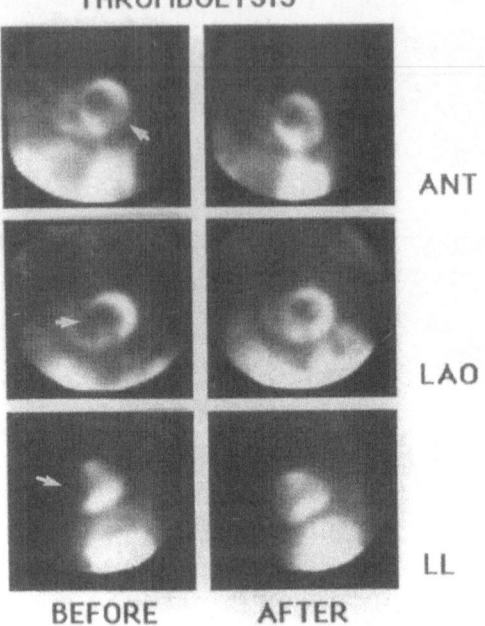

BEFORE   AFTER

Figure 3. Planar myocardial perfusion imaging with Tc-99m-Sestamibi before and after successful thrombolytic therapy for acute anteroseptal myocardial infarction. Same imaging protocol
as in Figure 2. The risk area prior to thrombolytic therapy is in the anteroseptal walls (arrows).
After thrombolytic therapy improved radiotracer uptake is noted consistent with successful
reperfusion of the infarct artery. Quantitatively 33% of the initial risk area was salvaged by
thrombolytic therapy. (Reproduced with permission from [3].)

safely subjected to nuclear imaging [5–10]. A second injection of T-99m-
Sestamibi can be administered either on the same day or on another day.

For serial imaging on the same day 10 mCi and 25 mCi is administered
with a time interval of approximately 3 hours. For serial imaging on different
days 25–30 mCi can be administered for each injection.

Insights in pathophysiology of acute infarction

Myocardial perfusion studies in patients with acute myocardial infarction
have provided useful insight into the human pathophysiology of acute myocardial infarction. Similar to what was demonstrated previously in experimental animals, patients with acute infarction may have extremely variable
myocardial areas at risk, ranging from small to very large [3, 4]. The extent
of the area at risk cannot be predicted from the clinical presentation or from
the angiographic site of coronary occlusion. Patients with acute anterior wall
myocardial infarction, have in general a larger area at risk than patients with

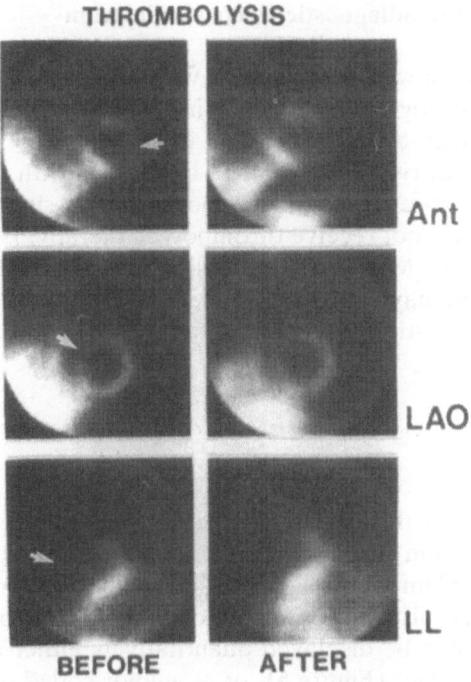

Figure 4. Planar myocardial perfusion imaging with Tc-99m-Sestamibi before and after failed thrombolytic therapy for large acute anteroseptal myocardial infarction. Same imaging protocol as in Figure 2. The left ventricle is dilated. The risk area prior to thrombolytic therapy is in the anteroseptal walls (arrows). After thrombolytic therapy radiotracer uptake is not improved, consistent with failure to reperfuse the infarct artery. This is confirmed by quantification of defect sizes. The defect size prior to thrombolytic therapy was 61 and 59 after thrombolytic therapy (insignificant 3% difference). Angiographically there was persistent occlusion of the infarct artery. (Reproduced with permission from [3].)

acute inferior wall myocardial infarction. However, there is considerable overlap between groups. An intriguing and clinically relevant observation is that patients with large area at risk and patients with small area at risk may have a similar clinical presentation. Obviously it would be preferable to identify patients with small risk area early, before they are exposed to the risk and cost of aggressive treatment of acute myocardial infarction. This can be achieved by sestamibi imaging in the emergency department.

The underlying cause for the wide variation in area at risk is not immediately clear, but is conceivably related to individual variation of coronary anatomy and the presence or absence of collateral circulation [11].

Acute infarction and nondiagnostic electrocardiogram

Christian et al. [12] showed that patients with acute chest pain, but without diagnostic electrocardiograms for acute infarction, who later had enzyme releases consistent with acute myocardial infarction, may have a substantial area of myocardium at risk, not less than in patients with diagnostic electro-cardiograms. These observations are important. The single most important reason why patients do not receive thrombolytic therapy, is *the nondiagnostic electrocardiogram* [13]. Myocardial perfusion imaging in the acute phase of myocardial infarction may be helpful to identify patients at an increased risk, despite of a nondiagnostic electrocardiogram.

Quantification

In order to determine the extent of myocardium at risk and the amount of salvaged myocardium accurately, quantification of myocardial perfusion images is necessary. Computer quantification can be performed by comparing the patient's regional distribution of radiotracer uptake to that of a normal database [14]. This can be displayed quantitatively either as circumferential count distribution profiles (Figure 5), or as a color-coded polar map or bull's eye. The size of an infarct can be measured as a percentage of the total left ventricle.

Myocardial perfusion defect size at hospital discharge represents the ulti-mate size of infarction. The extent of the myocardial perfusion deficit at hospital discharge has been shown to correlate inversely with global left ventricular function [15]. However, in some individual patients, improvement of ejection fraction may occur over time, suggesting recovery of stunned myocardium. Thus myocardial perfusion defect is a better measurement of infarct size than left ventricular ejection fraction. The final myocardial per-fusion defect size correlates also with enzymatic infarct size.

An intriguing observation in patients who had successful reperfusion of the infarct artery, is that defect size in some patients may *continue to decrease* during subsequent days after thrombolytic therapy has been completed [16] (Figure 6). This may be due to recovery of stunned myocardium and dimin-ishing partial volume effect. Figure 7 shows an extreme example of resolution of an apparent myocardial perfusion defect as result of recovery of stunned regional function.

In the TIMI IV and V trials decrease of myocardial perfusion defects after thrombolysis occurred in approximately 40% of patients [17]. Patients with anterior wall infarcts, who had such late improvement of perfusion defect size after thrombolysis, had significantly higher left ventricular ejection frac-tion than patients who had no change in defect size. In patients with inferior infarction, no such difference was observed.

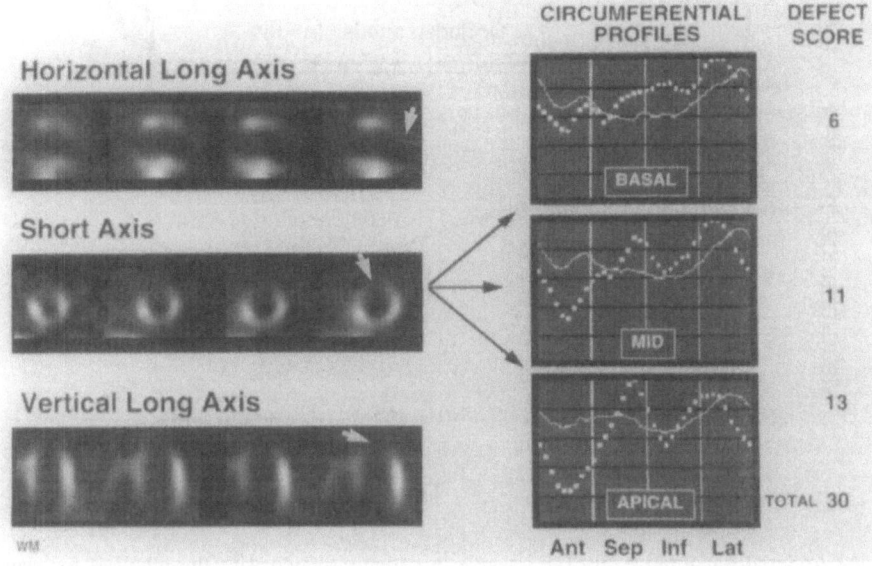

Figure 5. Quantitative single photon emission tomography in a patient with acute anteroseptal myocardial infarction. Selected reconstructed horizontal long axis, short axis and vertical long axis slices are shown. An extensive anteroseptal myocardial perfusion defect (arrows) is present. Quantification of the perfusion defect relative to a normal data base is shown on the right for representative basal (top), mid-ventricular (middle) and apical (bottom) short axis slices. The patient's relative distribution of radiotracer uptake is shown as circumferential profiles (square dots). The lower limit of normal tracer distribution is shown as a continuous curve. Total defect size involves 30% of left ventricle.

Clinical usefulness of serial imaging in thrombolytic therapy

Research tool

Serial myocardial perfusion imaging as described above can be used as a research tool in clinical trials, aimed to assess efficacy of new agents for thrombolytic or adjunctive antithrombotic therapy. Since patients serve as their own control, considerable fewer patients may be required to prove treatment efficacy. Thus, serial myocardial perfusion imaging constitutes a potentially powerful research tool. Gibbons et al. [18] demonstrated this in evaluating the outcome of primary angioplasty for acute infarction. Using sestamibi myocardial perfusion imaging, it was demonstrated that two randomly assigned patient groups were comparable as far as area at risk was concerned.

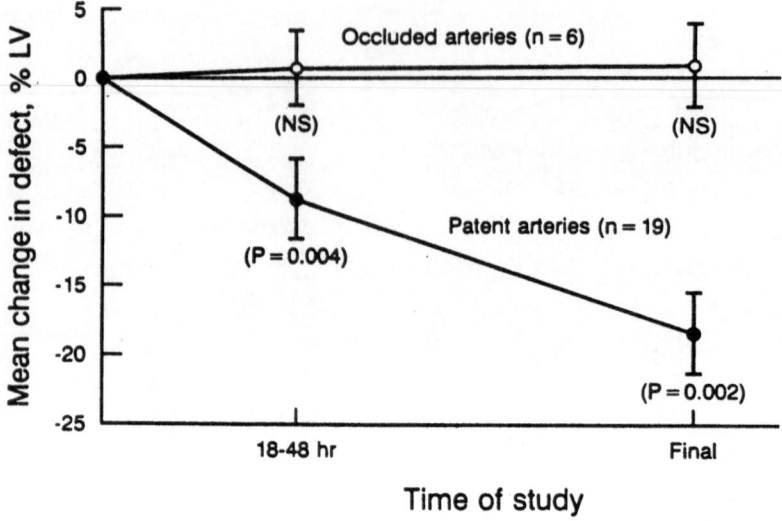

Figure 6. Serial quantitative SPECT imaging in patients treated with thrombolysis for acute myocardial infarction. In patients with occluded infarct arteries no change in mycardial perfusion defect size occurred. In contrast in patients with successful reperfusion of the infarct arteries significant decrease in perfusion defect size was measured. Interestingly, defect size continued to decrease during the days after thrombolytic therapy was completed. (Reproduced with permission from [16].)

Selection of individual patients for thrombolytic therapy

As mentioned above, myocardial perfusion imaging may be useful to identify candidates for thrombolytic therapy who otherwise would not be considered eligible: patients with non diagnostic electrocardiogram and acute chest pain suggestive of acute infarction. Myocardial perfusion imaging may provide objective evidence of the presence, extent and location of regional myocardial hypoperfusion. In patients with nonspecific electrocardiograms and large perfusion defects, initiation of thrombolytic therapy may be justified.

Management decisions in individual patients

Serial myocardial perfusion imaging in patients who had thrombolytic therapy, may be useful for patient management. Numerous studies have shown that a significant decrease in myocardial perfusion defect size on serial imaging predicts patency of the infarct artery [19]. In patients who received thrombolytic therapy, it is clinically important to assess noninvasively whether the infarct artery was successfully reperfused. If reperfusion therapy failed an aggressive intervention attitude is warranted [20]. Although *serial pre and post thrombolysis myocardial perfusion imaging* provides unequivocal

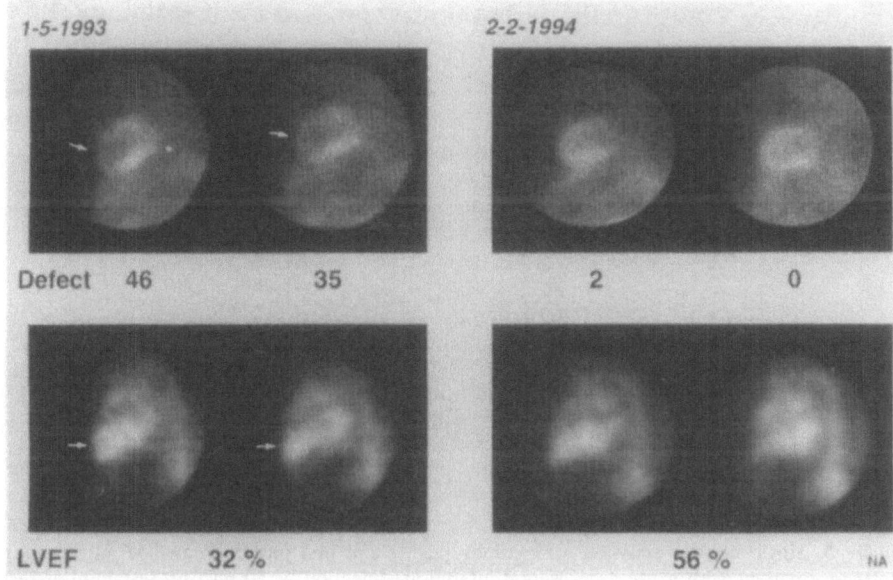

Figure 7. Example of apparent anteroapical myocardial perfusion defect due to partial volume effect in a patient with myocardial stunningin the infarct area. The patient was treated successfully with thrombolytic therapy for acute anterior wall myocardial infarction on 12-28-1992. Reperfusion of the infarct artery was documented angiographically . At hospital discharge (1-5-1993) exercise myocardial perfusion imaging with thallium-201 was performed prior to discharge (top). The images (exercise-left; delayed-right) show a large predominantly fixed anteroapical defect (perfusion defect size 46 and 35). Equilibrium radionuclide ventriculography (bottom) shows anteroapical akinesis (arrows) and depressed left ventricular ejection fraction (32%). The patient returned one year later on 2-2-1994 for follow-up. He had been well and was asymptomatic. Left ventricular ejection fraction had improved markedly to 56%, with near normal anteroapical wall motion. Thallium-201 exercise imaging was repeated and was essentially normal. This patient had stunning of the reperfused anteroapical wall on 1-5-1993. The apparently fixed anteroapical defect was artifactual and most likely caused by partial volume effect.

information on efficacy of treatment, clinically useful information can potentially also be derived from *single imaging after thrombolytic therapy*. After thrombolytic therapy, a wide range of myocardial perfusion defect sizes can be expected. We propose that clinically meaningful decisions can be made on the basis of quantified defect size in two extreme situations: in patients with small and in patients with large perfusion defects. If the defect is small, thrombolytic therapy was probably successful and "watchful waiting" is justified, i.e. the patient can be observed until recurrence of ischemia or other complications occur. If, on the other hand, the perfusion defect is large, either reperfusion failed or very little salvage occurred. In the latter situation, the patient prognosis is unfavorable (Figure 8). Early aggressive interventional therapy may be warranted in these patients. In patients with moderate

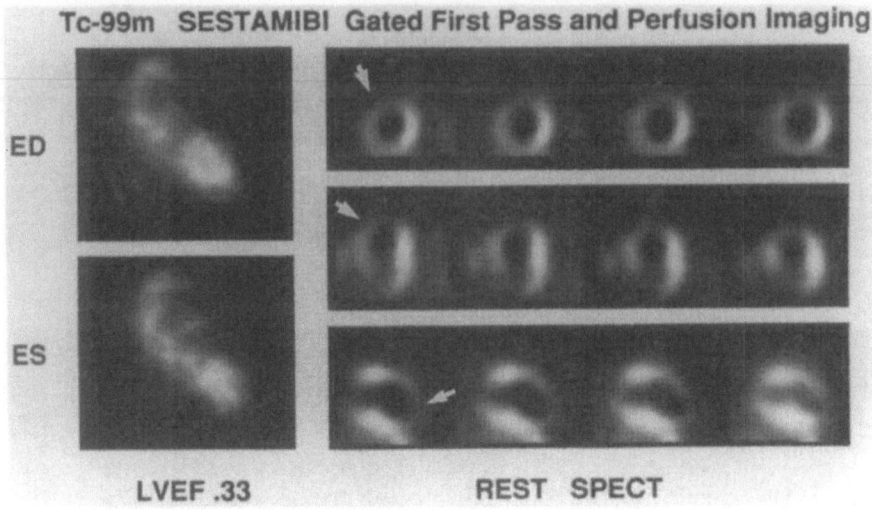

Figure 8. Single photon emission tomography (right) and first pass radionuclide angiography (left) in a patient with acute anteroseptal infarction. Injection of 20 mCi of Sestamibi at rest was uitized for first pass radionuclide angiography. Left ventricular ejection fraction (LVEF) is depressed (33%) with anteroapical akinesis. SPECT myocardial perfusion images (short axis: top; horizontal long axis: middle; vertical long axis: bottom) show an extensive anteroapical and septal myocardial perfusion defect (arrows). The new Tc-99m-labeled myocardial perfusion agents make it possbile to obtain both myocardial perfusion and function in one single study.

size defects, only serial imaging is helpful for assessing the effect of thrombolytic therapy. Reocclusion of the infarct artery can be monitored by serial imaging after completion of thrombolytic therapy.

Other imaging agents for assessment of the effect of reperfusion therapy

Several Tc-99m-labeled myocardial perfusion imaging agents are now available. Although the most clinical experience is based on the use of Tc-99m-Sestamibi, similar results can be expected with other Tc-99m-labeled non-distributing agents (Tc-99m-Tetrofosmin [21] and Tc-99m-Furifosmin [22]). Images obtained with Sestamibi, Tetrofosmin and Furifosmin are generally of comparable quality. Sestamibi has the disadvantage of slow liver clearance and rest imaging has to be delayed for 45–60 minutes after injection. Tetrofosmin and Furifosmin clear faster from the liver and rest imaging is feasible 15 minutes after injection. Teboroxime is another Tc-99m-labeled agent with entirely different characteristics [23]. Teboroxime accumulates rapidly in the myocardium according to regional myocardial blood flow and then clears very rapidly from the myocardium within 5 minutes. Consequently, imaging has to be performed immediately and rapidly after injection. Good quality diagnostic imaging is a substantial challenge. Teboroxime can be used conceivably in combination with Sestamibi. For example, Teboroxime could be used immediately prior to, or during, the first minutes of thrombolytic therapy to assess rapidly the myocardial area at risk, Sestamibi can then be used later to assess reperfusion of the infarct artery.

Summary

Serial myocardial perfusion imaging in patients who received thrombolytic therapy for acute myocardial infarction, has provided new insights in the pathophysiology of human acute myocardial infarction. The area at risk for infarction can be assessed and quantified. The amount of myocardial salvage can be assessed and reperfusion of the infarct artery can be predicted. This information may be useful in the clinical management of individual patients with acute infarction. (See also Chapters 2–4).

References

1. Simoons ML, Vos J, Tijssen JGP et al. Long-term benefit of early thrombolytic therapy in patients with acute myocardial infarction: 5 year follow-up of a trial conducted by the Interuniversity Cardiology Institute of the Netherlands. J Am Coll Cardiol 1989; 14: 1609–15.
2. Meijer A, Verheugt FWA, van Eenige MJ et al. Left ventricular function at 3 months after successful thrombolysis: Impact of reocclusion without reinfarction on ejection fraction, regional function, and remodeling. Circulation 1994; 90: 1706–14.
3. Wackers FJTh, Gibbons RJ, Verani MS et al. Serial quantitative planar technetium-99m-isonitrile imaging in acute myocardial infarction: Efficacy for noninvasive assessment of thrombolytic therapy. J Am Coll Cardiol 1989; 14: 861–73.
4. Gibbons RJ, Verani MS, Behrenbeck T et al. Feasibility of tomographic ^{99m}Tc-hexakis-2–methoxy-2–methylpropyl-isonitrile imaging for the assessment of myocardia area at risk and the effect of treatment in acute myocardial infarction. Circulation 1989; 80: 1278–1286.
5. Faraggi M, Assayag P, Messian et al. Early isonitrile SPECT in acute myocardial infarction: Feasibility and results before and after fibrinolysis. Nucl Med Commun 1989; 10: 539–49.
6. Santoro GM, Bisi G, Sciagra R et al. Single photon emission computed tomography with technetium-99m-hexakis-2–methoxyisobutyl isonitrile in acute myocardial infarction before and after thrombolytic treatment: Assessment of salvaged myocardium and prediction of late functional recovery. J Am Coll Cardiol 1990; 15: 301–14.
7. DeCoster PM, Wijns W, Cauwe F et al. Area at risk determination by technetium-99m-hexakis-2–methoxyisobutyl isonitrile in experimental reperfused myocardial infarction. Circulation 1990; 82: 2152–62.
8. Bisi G, Sciagra R, Santoro GM et al. Comparison of tomography and planar imaging for the evaluation of thrombolytic therapy in acute myocardial infarction using pre- and post-treatment myocardial scintigraphy with technetium-99m sestamibi. Am Heart J 1991; 122: 13–22.
9. Bostrom PA, Diemer H, Freitag M et al. Myocardial perfusion minthrombolysis: A Tc-99m-Sestamibi SPECT study in patients with acute myocardial infarction. Clin Physiol 1992; 12: 679–84.
10. Gibson W, Christian TF, Pellikka PA, Behrenbeck T, Gibbons RJ. Serial tomographic

imaging with technetium-99m-sestamibi for the assessment of infarct-related arterial patency following reperfusion therapy. J Nucl Med 1992; 33: 2080–5.

11. Christian TF, Schwartz RS, Gibbons RJ. Determinants of infarct size in reperfusion therapy for acute myocardial infarction. Circulation 1992; 86: 81–90.

12. Christian TF, Clements IP, Gibbons RJ. Noninvasive identification of myocardium at risk in patients with acute myocardial infarction and nondiagnostic electrocardiograms with Technetium-99m-sestamibi. Circulation 1991; 83: 1615–20.

13. Karlson BW, Herlitz J, Edvarsson N et al. Eligibility for intravenous thrombolysis in suspected acute myocardial infarction. Circulation 1990; 82: 1140–6.

14. Wackers FJTh. Science, art and artifacts: How important is quantification for the processing physician interpreting myocardial perfusion studies. J Nucl Cardiol 1994; 109S–17S.

15. Christian TF, Behrenbeck T, Pellikka PA et al. Mismatch of left ventricular function and infarct size demonstrated by technetium-99m isonitrile imaging after reperfusion therapy for acute myocardial infarction: Identification of myocardial stunning and hyperkinesia. J Am Coll Cardiol 1990; 16: 1632–8.

16. Pellika PA, Behrenbeck T, Verani MS et al. Serial changes in myocardial perfusion using tomographic technetium-99m-hexakis-2–methoxypropyl-isonitrile imaging following reperfusion therapy of myocardial infarction. J Nucl Med 1990; 31: 1269–75.

17. Barr SA, Zaret BL, Cannon CP, Wackers FJTh. Does decreasing defect size on serial quantitative planar Tc-99m-sestamibi imaging following thrombolytic therapy for acute myocardial infarction correlate with improved left ventricular function? Circulation (Suppl) 1993; 88: I–486.

18. Gibbons RJ, Holmes DR, Reeder GS et al. Immediate angioplasty compared with the administration of a thrombolytic agent followed by conservative treatment for myocardial infarction. N Engl J Med 1993; 328: 685–91.

19. Gibbons RJ. Technetium-99m-sestamibi in the assessment of aucte myocardial infarction. Semin Nucl Med 1991; 21: 213–22.

20. Wackers FJ. Thrombolytic therapy for myocardial infarction: Assesment of efficacy by myocardial perfusion imaging with Tc-99m-Sestamibi. Am J Card 1990; 66: 36E–41E.

21. Jain D, Wackers FJTh, Mattera J et al. Biokinetics of Tc-99m-tetrofosmin, a new myocardial perfusion imaging agent: Implications for a one day imaging protocol. J Nucl Med 1993; 34: 1254–9.

22. Gerson MC, Millard RW, Roszell NJ et al. Kinetic properties of Tc-99m-Q12 in canine myocardium. Circulation 1994; 89: 1291–300.

23. Hendel RC, McSherry B, Karimeddini M, Leppo JA. Diagnostic value of a new myocardial perfusion agent, teboroxime (SQ30,217), utilizing a rapid planar imaging protocol: Preliminary results. J Am Coll Cardiol 1990; 16: 855–61.

Corresponding Author: Dr Frans J. Th. Wackers, Yale University School of Medicine, Cardiovascular Nuclear Imaging Laboratory, 333 Cedar Street, TE-2, P.O. Box 208042, New Haven, CT 06520–8042, USA.

2. Contraction-perfusion matching in reperfused acute myocardial infarction

TIMOTHY F. CHRISTIAN

Introduction

Prior to the commonplace use of acute reperfusion therapy, estimates of resting left ventricular function in the early days following acute myocardial infarction were found to be highly predictive of long-term survival. The Multicenter Post Infarction Research Group showed that one-year survival was exponentially related to left ventricular ejection fraction prior to discharge with mortality at one year approaching 50% for patients with a left ventricular ejection fraction of 15% [1]. This study was conducted in the prethrombolytic era. With the use of acute reperfusion therapy during acute myocardial infarction, it became apparent that mechanical estimates of left ventricular function could be inaccurate during the acute hospitalization [2–6]. Specifically these studies documented that left ventricular ejection fraction and regional wall motion could improve significantly in the weeks following thrombolytic therapy or direct coronary angioplasty. Consequently, to obtain a reliable estimate of infarct size from mechanical measures of left ventricular function, acquisition should be delayed at least several weeks [7, 8].

Delayed recovery in myocardial contractility in the setting of normal resting coronary blood flow is caused by myocardial stunning. This phenomenon was first popularized in a brief review article by Braunwald and Kloner [9]. Since that time, myocardial stunning has been clearly reproduced in the animal laboratory [10–13]. Yet actual demonstration of the phenomenon in the clinical setting (simultaneous demonstration of normal blood flow and depressed but reversible myocardial contractile function), is actually quite scant in the literature. This is remarkable given the vast amount of attention this phenomenon has received. This chapter will present potential mechanisms of myocardial stunning, why radionuclide approaches to imaging should be relatively unaffected by myocardial stunning, and present the radionuclide data which exists on the topic at the present time.

C.A. Nienaber and U. Sechtem (eds): Imaging and Intervention in Cardiology, 13–27.
© 1996 Kluwer Academic Publishers.

Mechanisms of myocardial stunning

A number of metabolic conditions have been postulated as possible explanations for the delayed recovery of myocardial function in the presence of adequate blood flow following reperfusion but none have been conclusive. Potential mechanisms include 1) inadequate adenosine triphosphate nucleotide synthesis [14], 2) impairment of sympathetic neural activity [15], 3) damage to the extra cellular collagen matrix [16], 4) intracellular calcium overload [17], 5) sarcoplasmic reticulum dysfunction [18], 6) generation of oxygen free radicals [19, 20]. Clearly, some of these mechanisms, if operative, have implications regarding the uptake of perfusion tracers, whereas other mechanisms can be expected to have minimal effect on tracer uptake.

ATP levels have been shown to be depressed in myocytes following reperfusion and only recover after several weeks paralleling the recovery in contractile function [14]. Thus, it is an attractive mechanism to account for myocardial stunning. Thallium-201 is partially dependent on the ATP driven Na^+/K^+ pump for cellular uptake. If ATP depletion is the cause of myocardial stunning, then thallium-201 uptake should be impaired due to inactivation of this pump. However, restoration of normal ATP levels does not result in resolution of contractile dysfunction, and therefore, is unlikely to be the primary mechanism [21].

Several studies have implicated that cellular levels of calcium are elevated following coronary reperfusion [20]. Interventions which reduce calcium levels appear to attenuate myocardial stunning [22], but the exact mechanism of how increased calcium inhibits myocardial contractile function is unknown. A potentially related mechanism is transient dysfunction of the sarcoplasmic reticulum [18]. This cellular organelle actively takes up cellular calcium during diastole and releases a bolus of calcium to the myofibrils during electrical depolarization to trigger mechanical systole. The consequences of impaired active uptake of calcium by the sarcoplasmic reticulum is a rise in calcium within the cytosol and less calcium delivered to the contractile proteins during systole.

With therapeutic reperfusion the reintroduction of oxygen-rich blood into ischemic myocardium can produce oxygen free radicals via reactions of oxygen with enzymes (xanthine oxidase), decreased levels of free-radical scavengers, and production of free radicals by neutrophils which accumulate during reperfusion [19]. Several animal studies have demonstrated that introduction of oxygen derived free radicals depress cardiac contractility [19]. However, free radicals are not specific in which cellular function they can alter. Consequently, the precise mechanism by which they bring about myocardial stunning is uncertain. One attractive and unifying hypothesis is that these radicals inhibit calcium-stimulated ATP in the sacrolemma, thereby disrupting calcium homeostasis and transport within the myocyte [23]. This scenario links the observations of calcium overload in the cystosol which have been experimentally observed to the oxygen-derived free radical hypothesis.

It is evident from the preceding discussion that the mechanisms by which myocardial stunning can be produced are, as yet, still to be defined and may be multifactorial. It is important to establish which is known, and to determine whether it is reasonable to assume that the myocardial uptake of perfusion tracers can be expected to be independent of stunning. The next section will deal briefly with the mechanism of cellular uptake of two commonly used perfusion tracers: thallium-201 and Tc-99m-sestamibi. (See also Chapters 1, 3, 5, 14–18.)

Radionuclide kinetics in reperfused myocardium

The transport from the capillaries into the myocardial cell and subsequent retention are different for thallium-201 and Tc-99m-sestamibi during resting conditions with normal blood flow [24]. Thallium-201 can exit the capillary vessel significantly faster than Tc-99m-sestamibi, but its uptake into the myocyte is partially dependent on active transport via the Na/K^+ ATPase pump which slows overall net extraction. The dependence on ATP for uptake has significant implications if ATP levels are, indeed, depressed in the setting of myocardial stunning. Tc-99m-sestamibi leaves the circulation at a considerably slower rate than thallium-201, likely due to the large size of the molecule [24, 25]. However, due to the high lipophilicity of the isonitrile complex, it crosses the myocyte membrane readily without the necessity of active transport [26].

The net result of the divergent kinetics is that the net extraction of the two tracers under resting conditions is fairly similar despite different mechanisms of cellular uptake. Consequently, in the setting of reperfusion and myocardial stunning, myocardial uptake of the tracers may be selectively altered; particularly if ATP depletion is responsible for myocardial stunning following reperfusion. Piwnica-Worms et al. demonstrated divergent kinetics of thallium-201 and Tc-99m-sestamibi in cultured chick myocytes where the production of ATP was blocked [27]. Thallium-201 uptake into the myocytes declined in proportion to the degree inhibition of the Na/K^+ ATPase pump as ATP levels fell. Conversely, Tc-99m-sestamibi uptake actually increased during the early phases of ATP depletion, perhaps, reflecting hyperpolarization of the cell membrane (sestamibi is retained largely by the negative intracellular charge) [27]. However, evidence that ATP depletion is the primary cause of myocardial stunning in the animal literature is scant.

Divergent uptake characteristics of thallium-201 and Tc-99m sestamibi have also been reported during reperfusion following 30 to 60 minutes of coronary occlusion in rabbit hearts [28]. The net extraction of sestamibi was one third lower than thallium under resting conditions but had increased to 90% above extraction levels for thallium at one hour following reperfusion [28]. Thus, the potential exists of these tracers to behave differently in the setting of coronary reperfusion and myocardial stunning. The next section

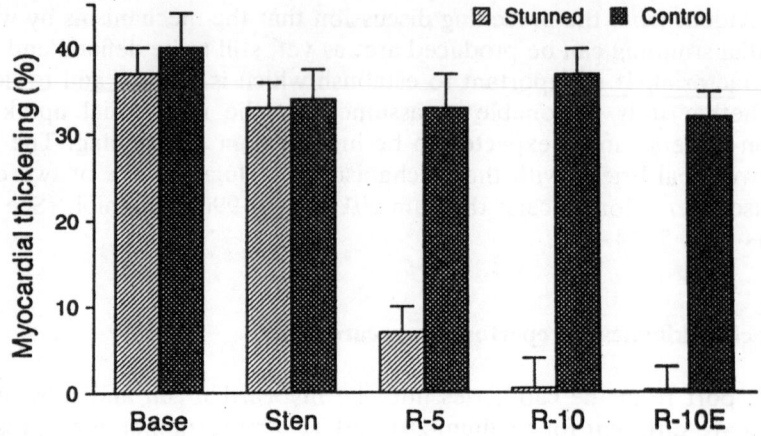

Figure 1. Comparison of regional wall motion by myocardial thickening for control dogs and dogs subjected to repetitive occlusion and reperfusion of the left anterior descending artery. The region supplied by the left anterior descending artery was rendered akinetic by this method. Base = baseline, sten = initial stensosis, R-5 = wall motion after 5 cycles of occlusion, R-10 = 10 cycles of occlusion, R-10E = wall motion 40 minutes after the 10th cycle of occlusion and reperfusion. From Moore et al. Circulation 1990; 81: 1622–32 [13].

will explore animal models of stunning, and whether there is evidence that radionuclides may behave differently in this setting.

Animal studies of myocardial stunning and radionuclide imaging

In an elegant series of experiments, Moore et al. demonstrated conclusively that thallium-201 scintigraphy could identify myocardial stunning by providing a visual mismatch of myocardial perfusion and ventricular function [13]. The investigators repetitively occluded the left anterior descending artery of a dog for 10 minutes and allowed 5 minutes of reperfusion. After approximately 10 series of occlusion cycles, regional wall motion in the supplied territory became akinetic (Figure 1). However, thallium activity in the akinetic zone paralleled myocardial blood flow and remained normal and no area of infarction could be identified at pathology (Figure 2) [13]. This landmark study established that myocardial stunning could be identified invivo by establishing the existence of normal perfusion and viability via thallium-201 scintigraphy in the setting of significant ventricular contractile dysfunction but no infarction. Thus, the concept of mismatch of flow and function was firmly established. It also provided strong evidence that disorders of the Na/K$^+$ ATPase pump are not present in the setting of myocardial stunning as thallium uptake was normal.

The findings above were replicated by Sinusas et al. who found that

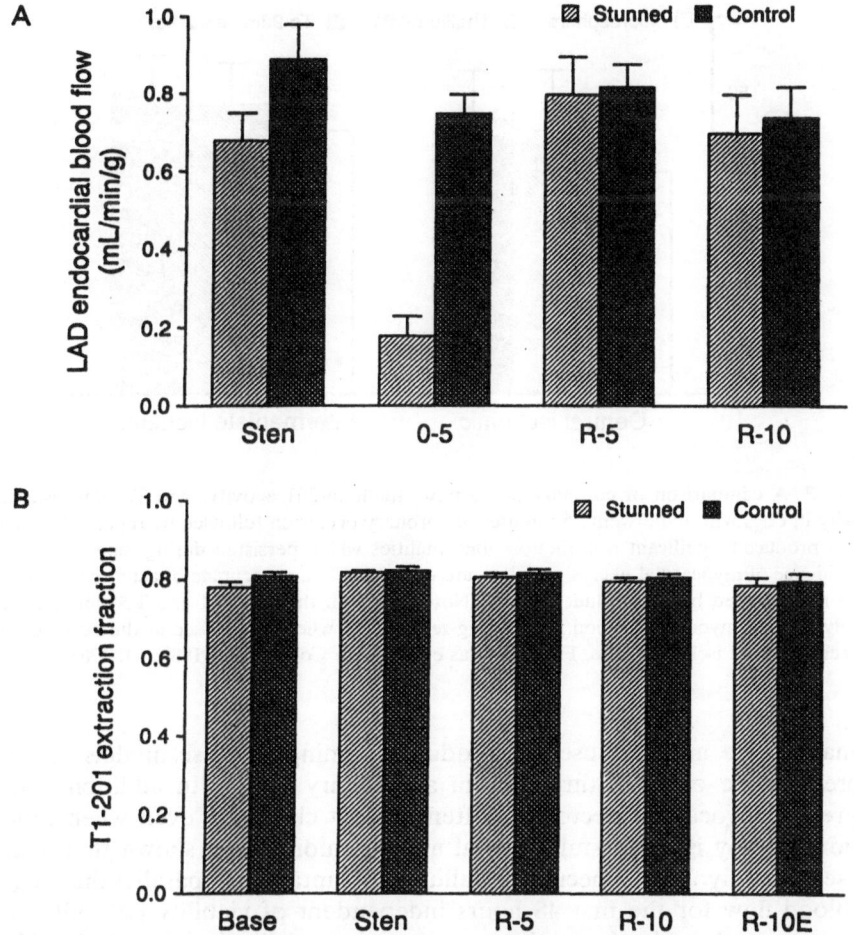

Figure 2. (A) Myocardial blood flow in the left anterior descending artery zone as measured by radiolabelled microspheres for control and stunned dogs. Note that blood flow following the 10th cycle of occlusion and reperfusion was not significantly different from baseline despite marked impairment of systolic function (Figure 1, Moore et al. [13]). (B) First pass thallium extraction fraction for control and stunned dogs in the left anterior descending territory. Thallium extraction is normal in stunned dogs despite marked systolic function abnormalities. No area of infarction was found at pathology (Figure 1, Moore et al. [13]).

thallium-201 uptake closely paralleled reperfusion blood flow measured by radiolabelled microspheres in the setting of transient ventricular dysfunction produced by 15 minutes of coronary occlusion in an animal model. Following reperfusion, significant wall motion abnormalities were evident but both blood flow and thallium uptake were in the normal range, and there was no evidence of myocardial necrosis at pathology (Figure 3) [12]. However, some caution should be taken when extrapolating these studies to a clinical

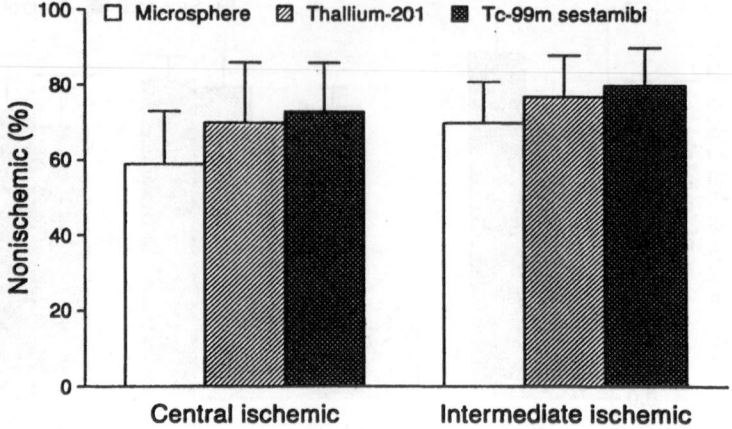

Figure 3. A comparison of coronary blood flow, thallium-201 activity, and Tc-99m-sestamibi activity in dogs who underwent 15 minutes of coronary occlusion followed by reperfusion. This model produced significant wall motion abnormalities which persisted during reperfusion, but no evidence of myocardial necrosis. Values are expressed as a percentage of activity in myocardium not supplied by the occluded artery. Note that both thallium-201 and Tc-99m-sestamibi closely parallel myocardial blood flow during reperfusion whether assessed at the periphery or the center of the ischemic zone. From Sinusas et al. J Am Coll Cardiol 1989; 14: 1785–93 [12].

scenario. The methods used to produce stunning in these models are not representative of lysed thrombus in a coronary artery. In addition, some degree of myocardial necrosis is often present clinically, even when reperfusion therapy is successful. Several animal studies have shown that in the presence of myocardial necrosis, thallium-201 uptake will parallel the degree of blood flow for the first 48 hours independent of viability [29, 30]. This phenomenon has also been observed in patients following reperfusion [31]. This suggests that early thallium uptake and contractile dysfunction may not reflect stunning, but rather an overestimation of myocardial viability by thallium-201. Hence, contractile dysfunction may not be reversible despite a normal thallium scan if performed too early.

Myocardial uptake of Tc-99m-sestamibi is linearly related to myocardial blood flow up to approximately 2 ml/min/gram. However, in the absence of an intact cellular membrane or mitochondrial function, myocytes will not accumulate the tracer despite adequate blood flow [32]. In a canine model, Sinusas et al. demonstrated that early following reperfusion, Tc-99m-sestamibi uptake did not occur when myocardial necrosis was present despite adequate coronary flow measured by radiolabelled microspheres (Figure 4) [33]. Thus, Tc-99m-sestamibi should be an ideal agent to identify myocardial stunning, even early on in the time period following successful reperfusion, as uptake appears to be both flow and viability dependent.

Sinusas et al. demonstrated (in the same canine model previously de-

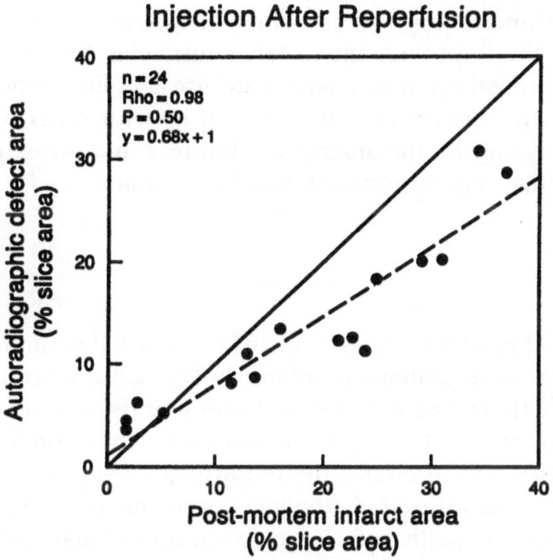

Injection After Reperfusion

Figure 4. Comparison of infarct size at pathology versus Tc-99m-sestamibi defect size by autora-diographs of myocardial slices when sestamibi was injected after release of coronary occlusion in a dog model. Despite adequate blood flow, sestamibi was not taken up in areas of necrosis, although, it did slightly underestimate infarct size. From Sinusas et al. Circulation 1990; 82: 1424–37 [33].

scribed [12] with thallium-201 where 15 minutes of coronary occlusion was followed by reperfusion) that persistent contractile dysfunction could be produced without myocardial infarction. Myocardial uptake of Tc-99m-sesta-mibi following intravenous injection closely correlated with myocardial blood flow assessed by microspheres (Figure 3). This occurred despite marked contractile dysfunction monitored by ultrasonic epicardial crystals [12]. Consequently, sestamibi appears to be able to identify stunned myocardium in an animal model similar to thallium-201.

Clinical studies of myocardial stunning

As stated earlier, true clinical examples of myocardial stunning are rare in the literature. A true example is defined by a simultaneous measure of adequate blood flow and depressed myocardial contractility (in the same vascular territory) which subsequently improves with time. There are a number of reports which infer the existence of myocardial stunning by a temporal resolution in myocardial dysfunction, but most of these studies lack a measure of myocardial perfusion [2–5]. Thus, the influence of collateral development or recanalization of the infarct related artery relieving chronically ischemic (hibernating) myocardium cannot be excluded as a possible explanation for the improvement in left ventricular function. Angiography alone cannot be relied upon as a surrogate for adequate blood flow because of the no-reflow phenomenon which can occur with reperfusion. This phenomenon of plugging of the microvasculature can resolve over time, and hence, contractility may improve on that basis alone.

Thallium-201

One of the first clinical demonstrations of myocardial stunning was by Maddahi et al. using intracoronary thallium during acute myocardial infarction in five patients [34]. The extent of myocardium at risk was assessed by planar thallium scintigraphy following an intravenous injection of thallium-201. After identification of the infarct-related artery by angiography, intracoronary streptokinase was infused. Following successful recanalization, an intracoronary injection of thallium-201 was given and planar imaging was repeated. Left ventricular ejection fraction was determined four hours later by gated radionuclide ventriculography and repeated 10 and 100 days after the procedure. Two patients showed evidence of myocardial stunning with significantly improved perfusion images immediately in the catheterization laboratory but delayed recovery in left ventricular function. Three other patients had no improvement in perfusion or subsequent left ventricular function consistent with minimal myocardial salvage [34].

Identification of myocardial stunning following myocardial infarction implies that myocardial salvage has occurred. Myocardial salvage can be defined as the difference between myocardium at risk and final infarct size. Thallium-201 is not an ideal agent to assess salvage, due to two factors. As discussed previously, there is evidence in the literature to suggest that early after reperfusion, thallium-201 largely tracks flow and not viability [29–31]. Consequently, myocardial salvage can be overestimated in the setting of reperfusion into necrotic myocardium when injected early. Secondly, due to the property of redistribution, imaging should be done soon after injection to assess myocardium at risk prior to reperfusion. This may lead to delays in therapy which are unacceptable in the setting of coronary occlusion.

Tc-99m-sestamibi

In contrast to thallium-201, Tc-99m-sestamibi is not taken up by necrotic myocardium in the setting of hyperemic reperfusion flow and redistributes minimally when injected at rest [33, 35, 36]. Therefore, it can be given prior to reperfusion therapy and still accurately reflect the extent of myocardium at risk if imaged after such therapy. This property makes Tc-99m-sestamibi a convenient agent for measurement of myocardial salvage. The physical properties of Tc-99m-sestamibi allow for better count statistics for perfusion defect quantification. These two properties facilitate the clinical identification of myocardial stunning.

In a report by the author, 32 patients were injected with Tc-99m-sestamibi at the time of hospital discharge following acute reperfusion therapy for myocardial infarction and underwent tomographic imaging. Perfusion defect size was quantified as a measure of infarct size [8]. Patients underwent gated radionuclide ventriculography the following day and six weeks later. Based upon a previous regression equation derived from a comparison of left ventricular ejection fraction to infarct size in a small series of patients using sestamibi, a predicted ejection fraction was generated for each patient in the subsequent study based upon their discharge perfusion defect [predicted EF = 62.3-(0.61 × perfusion defect size)] (Figures 5A and 5B) [8]. For example, a patient with an infarct size of 20% of the left ventricle would be predicted to have an ejection fraction of 50%.

Patients whose actual measured ejection fractions were significantly less than predicted were classified as having stunning, and consequently, were predicted to demonstrate marked improvement when the assessment of left ventricular was repeated at six weeks. Conversely, those patients with inappropriately high ejection fraction for infarct size (compensatory hyperkinesia) were expected to show a decline at six weeks [8].

Table 1 classifies the patients in this study by their changed ejection fraction from discharge to six weeks. 15% of patients demonstrated a significant improvement in left ventricular function. At discharge, the ejection fractions of these patients were significantly lower than predicted based on the size of the discharge perfusion defect. At six weeks, the mean ejection fraction for these patients was near predicted with a slight overshoot. A similar return to the predicted ejection fraction values were found in patients with inappropriately high left ventricular function for infarct size. The individual data points for the study group are shown in Figure 5 with patients coded by the change in ejection fraction over the six-week period.

The line of investigation from this laboratory has been extended. Gitter et al. [37] prospectively predicted ejection fraction for 84 patients based upon the regression equation produced from Figure 5B in the prior study by Christian et al. [8]. A similar percentage of patients (14%) was prospectively predicted to have stunning because their discharge ejection fraction fell significantly below predicted values based on their infarct size (Table 2). This group classified as having stunning, subsequently, showed an overall improvement in ejection fraction of six percentage points. As before, those with inappropriately high ejection fractions had a significant fall in ejection fraction (6 percentage points), whereas those with values close to predicted values showed no change [37].

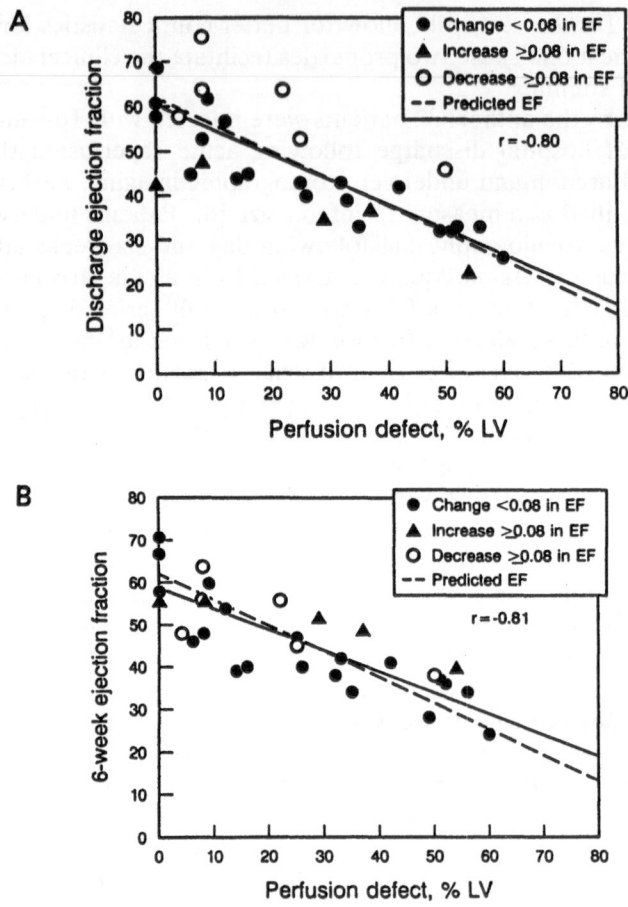

Figure 5. (A) The relationship between infarct size measured by tomographic Tc-99m-sestamibi imaging and left ventricular ejection fraction by radionuclide ventriculography at discharge. Patients are coded by their subsequent change in ejection fraction at six weeks. The dashed line represents the predicted ejection fraction based upon perfusion defect size. Note that patients who improved more than 8 points had ejection fractions at discharge which were less than predicted. From Christian et al. J Am Coll Cardiol 1990; 16: 1632–8 [8]. (B) The relationship between infarct size at discharge and ejection fraction measured six weeks later. Note that patients with significant improvement or decline fell near the value predicted by the size of the perfusion defect by Tc-99m-sestamibi at hospital discharge (dashed line). From Christian et al. J Am Coll Cardiol 1990; 16: 1632–8 [8].

Implications for clinical testing

The animal-based literature has extensively investigated the time course of resolution of myocardial stunning. Ellis et al. carefully documented the resolution of contractile dysfunction and metabolic abnormalities in a canine

Table 1. Actual versus predicted ejection fraction[a] [8].

Change in EF	No. of patients	Ejection fraction			p value	
		Discharge	Predicted	Six weeks	Discharge vs six weeks	Six weeks vs predicted
Increase ≥8%	5 (15%)	37 ± 9%	47 ± 9%	51 ± 7%	0.002	NS
No change	21 (67%)	46 ± 13%	45 ± 12%	47 ± 13%	NS	NS
Decrease ≥8%	6 (18%)	60 ± 10%	50 ± 10%	51 ± 9%	<0.0001	NS

[a]Predicted EF based upon discharge perfusion defect size. Predicted EF = 62.3 −[0.61 (perfusion defect size)].

Table 2. Prospective identification of myocardial stunning [8].

Acute ejection fraction vs ejection fraction predicted from infarct size[a]	No. of patients	Infarct size	Change in EF	P (discharge vs six weeks)
Inappropriately low (stunned)	21	13 ± 16% LV	+6 ± 8%	<0.001
Approapriate	45	13 ± 15% LV	0 ± 6%	NS
Inappropriately high (hypokinetic)	15	14 ± 15% LV	−6 ± 6%	<0.001

[a] Predicted EF = (From Table 4B) = 58.2−(0.47 × perfusion defect size).

model of two hours of total coronary occlusion followed by prolonged reperfusion. It was evident from this study that contractile function did not recover until approximately 14 days following occlusion and reperfusion [38]. Ito et al. studied 21 patients with anterior myocardial infarction reperfused within six hours from the onset of symptoms [39]. Serial echocardiography was performed over the ensuing four weeks. Improvement in regional wall motion plateaued at 14 days in agreement with the animal data of Ellis et al. [38].

Most likely, the duration of myocardial stunning is proportional to the duration of coronary occlusion, the degree of collateral flow to the risk zone during occlusion and the metabolic demand of the tissue during the occlusion period. Although logical, such factors are difficult to precisely measure in the clinical setting, and therefore, this relationship remains speculative. On the basis of the above data, it is reasonable to presume that myocardial stunning may be identified as far as two weeks post-infarction but is likely to be resolved by six weeks.

Decisions regarding clinical care for post-myocardial infarction patients often need to be made at hospital dismissal and such decisions are dependent on left ventricular function, at least in part. Clearly, these measurements can be misleading following reperfusion therapy. Should mechanical estimates of left ventricular function be abandoned in the thrombolytic era following myocardial infarction? Perhaps, but there are three factors which argue against this: 1) Despite much literature describing myocardial stunning, the actual phenomenon is not common at hospital discharge. In the two largest series examining perfusion and function simultaneously, the prevalence of mismatch of perfusion and function at discharge was only 15% [8, 37]. There were many patients in these series with marked myocardial salvage and no evidence of stunning, 2) left ventricular ejection fraction has remained a powerful prognosticator at discharge in trials utilizing acute reperfusion therapy [40], and 3) the phenomenon of hibernating myocardium.

Hibernating myocardium is a clinical term to describe a "match" in hypoperfusion and hypocontractility which is reversible upon restoration of normal levels of resting blood flow. This may reflect down regulation of the myocytes due to limited energy stores from chronic ischemia [41, 42]. No clear mechanism has been established, and there is no animal model to study the phenomenon. Several excellent reviews of the subject have been recently written [41–44], and since it is usually observed in the setting of chronic coronary artery disease, it will only be dealt with briefly in this chapter.

Tc-99m-sestamibi, for reasons outlined previously, is the preferable radionuclide in conjunction with a measure of left ventricular function to identify patients with stunned myocardium. The possible simultaneous acquisition of a first-pass ejection fraction during injection with this tracer is a factor that will likely be utilized in the future for exactly this purpose. However, Tc-99m-sestamibi cannot reliably identify hibernating myocardium. This is because the tracer does not redistribute significantly over time. Hibernating myocardium, by definition, means ischemia at rest. Thallium-201 when injected at rest [45] or with reinjection protocol [46] will initially show a perfusion defect in the hypofused territory but will redistribute into hypocontractile but viable myocardium given enough time, thus, distinguishing wall motion abnormalities which are due to myocardial fibrosis from those due to viable but severely ischemic tissue. Positron emission tomography is also very useful in this regard and can be considered the gold standard for viability. Tc-99m-sestamibi, however, has no properties which allow accurate identification of ischemia at rest. The isotope is largely sequestered within mitochondria and decays over time. Therefore, patients with hibernating myocardium following acute infarction due to a severe reduction in residual blood flow will be missed by this technique. The prevalence of hibernating myocardium following myocardial infarction, and thus, the importance of the limitation, is unknown. (See also Chapters 14–18.)

Conclusions

The mechanism of myocardial stunning remains uncertain but from the data currently available, it does not appear to involve the cellular functions necessary for the uptake and retention of the most commonly used radionuclides. This permits an accurate assessment of infarct size by myocardial perfusion techniques independent of the confounding influences of post-reperfusion contractile dysfunction. It also provides a means to prospectively identify patients at the time of hospital dismissal who likely have some degree of stunning and in whom left ventricular function should improve over the following weeks.

Because of superior quantitative properties and lack of an influence of reperfusion flow on distribution, Tc-99m-sestamibi is the preferable radionuclide to identify stunning. The possibility of simultaneous acquisition of perfusion and function with this agent is particularly attractive. However, myocardial stunning at the time of hospital discharge is not common and detection of hibernating myocardium is forfeited with this approach. Thus, because stunning resolves with no intervention necessary on the clinicians' part, it is probably not cost effective to screen all post infarction patients using this or any similar approach.

References

1. The Multicenter Postinfarction Research Group. Risk stratification and survival after myocardial infarction. N Engl J Med 1983; 309: 331–6.
2. Stack, RS, Phillips HR III, Grierson DS et al. Functional improvement of jeopardized myocardium following intracoronary streptokinase infusion in acute myocardial infarction. J Clin Invest 1983; 72: 84–95.
3. Reduto LA, Freund GC, Gaeta JM et al. Coronary artery reperfusion in acute myocardial infarction: Beneficial effects of intracoronary streptokinase on left ventricular salvage and performance. Am Heart J 1981; 102: 1168–77.
4. Topol EJ, Weiss JL, Brinker JA et al. Regional wall motion improvement after coronary thrombolysis with recombinant tissue plasminogen activator: Importance of coronary angioplasty. J Am Coll Cardiol 1985; 6: 426–33.
5. Grines CL, O'Neill WW, Anselmo EG et al. Comparison of left ventricular function and contractile reserve after successful recanalization by thrombolysis versus rescue percutaneous transluminal coronary angioplasty for acute myocardial infarction. Am J Cardiol 1988; 62: 352–7.
6. Satler LF, Kent KM, Fox LM et al. The assessment of contractile reserve after thrombolytic therapy for acute myocardial infarction. Am Heart J 1986; 111: 821–5.
7. White HD, Norris RM, Brown MA et al. Effect of intravenous streptokinase on left ventricular function and early survival after acute myocardial infarction. N Engl J Med 1987; 317: 850–5.
8. Christian TF, Behrenbeck T, Pellikka, PA, Huber KC, Chesebro JH, Gibbons RJ. Mismatch of left ventricular function and infarct size demonstrated by technetium-99m-isonitrile imaging after reperfusion therapy for acute myocardial infarction: Identification of myocardial stunning and hyperkinesia. J Am Coll Cardiol 1990; 16: 1632–8.
9. Braunwald E, Kloner RA. The stunned myocardium: Prolonged, postischemic ventricular dysfunction. Circulation 1982; 66: 1146–9.
10. Heyndrickx GR, Millard RW, McRitchie RJ et al. Regional myocardial functional and electrophysiological alterations after brief coronary artery occlusion in conscious dogs. J Clin Invest 1975; 56: 978–85.
11. Charlat ML, O'Neill PG, Hartley CJ et al. Prolonged abnormalities of left ventricular diastolic thinning in the "stunned" myocardium in conscious dogs: Time-course and relation to systolic function. J Am Coll Cardiol 1989; 13: 185–94.
12. Sinusas AJ, Watson DD, Cannon JR Jr, Beller GA. Effect of ischemia and post-ischemic

dysfunction on myocardial uptake of technetium 99 m labeled methoxyisobutyl isonitrile and thallium-201. J Am Coll Cardiol 1989; 14: 1785–93.

13. Moore CA, Cannon J, Watson DD et al. Thallium-201 kinetics in stunned myocardium characterized by severe post ischemic systolic dysfunction. Circulation 1990; 81: 1622–32.

14. Ellis SG, Henschke CI, Sandor T et al. Time course of functional and biochemical recovery of myocardium salvaged by reperfusion. J Am Coll Cardiol 1983; 1: 1047–55.

15. Ciuffo AA, Ouyang P, Becker LC, Levin L, Weisfeldt ML. Reduction of sympathetic inotropic response after ischemia in dogs: Contributor to stunned myocardium. J Clin Invest 1985; 75: 1504–9.

16. Zhao M, Zang H, Robinson TF et al. Profound structural alterations of the extracellular collagen matrix in post-ischemic dysfunctional ("stunned") but viable myocardium. J Am Coll Cardiol 1987; 10: 1322–34.

17. Marban E. Myocardial stunning and hibernation: The physiology behind the colloquialisms. Circulation 1991; 83: 681–8.

18. Krause SM, Jacobus WE, Becker LC. Alterations in cardiac sarcoplasmic reticulum calcium transport in the postischemic "stunned" myocardium. Circ Res 1989; 65: 526–30.

19. Goldhaber JI, Weiss JN. Oxygen free radicals and cardiac reperfusion abnormalities. Hypertension 1992; 20: 118–27.

20. Bolli R. Mechanism of myocardial stunning. Circulation 1990; 82: 723–38.

21. Ambrosio G, Jacobus WE, Mithcell MC et al. Effects of ATP precursors on ATP and free ADP content and functional recovery of postischemic hearts. Am J Physiol 1989; 256: 560H–6H.

22. Kusuoka H, Porterfield JK, Weisman HF et al. Pathophysiology and pathogenesis of stunned myocardium: Depressed calcium activation of contraction as a consequence of reperfusion-induced cellular calcium overload in ferret hearts. J Clin Invest 1987; 79: 950–61.

23. Corretti MC, Koretsure Y, Kusuoka H et al. Glycolytic inhibition and calcium overload as consequences of exogenously-generated free radicals in rabbit hearts. J Clin Invest 1991; 88: 1014–25.

24. Leppo JA, Meerdink DJ. Comparison of the myocardial uptake of a technetium-labelled isonitrile analogue and thallium. Circ Res 1989; 65: 632–9.

25. Meerdink DJ, Leppo JA. Experimental studies of the physiologic properties of technetium-99m agents: Myocardial transport of perfusion imaging agents. Am J Cardiol 1990; 66: 9E–15E.

26. Meerdink DJ, Leppo JA. Comparison of hypoxia and oubain effects on the myocardial uptake kinetics of technetium-99m hexakis-2-methoxy-isobutyl isonitrile and thallium-201. J Nucl Med 1989; 30: 1500–6.

27. Piwnica-Worms D, Chiu ML, Kronauge JF. Divergent kinetics of thallium-201 and Tc-99m-sestamibi in cultured chick ventricular myocytes during ATP depletion. Circulation 1992; 85: 1531–41.

28. Meerdink DJ, Leppo JA. Myocardial transport of hexakis (2-methoxy isobutyl isonitrile) and thallium before and after coronary reperfusion. Circ Res 1990; 66: 1738–46.

29. Okada RD, Pohost GM. The use of preintervention and postintervention thallium imaging for assessing the early and late effects of experimental coronary arterial reperfusion in dogs. Circulation 1984; 69: 1153–60.

30. Forman R, Kirk ES. Thallium-201 accumulation during reperfusion of ischemic myocardium: Dependence on regional blood flow rather than viability. Am J Cardiol 1984; 54: 659–63.

31. Melin JA, Becker LC, Bulkley BH. Differences in thallium-201 uptake in reperfused and nonreperfused myocardial infarction. Circ Res 1983: 53: 414–9.

32. Beanlands RSB, Dawood F, Wen WH et al. Are the kinetics of technetium-99m-methoxy-isobutyl-isonitrile affected by cell metabolism and viability? Circulation 1990; 82: 1802–14.

33. Sinusas AJ, Trautman KA, Bergin JD et al. Quantification of "area at risk" during coronary occlusion and degree of myocardial salvage after reperfusion with technetium-99m-methoxy-isobutyl-isonitrile. Circulation 1990; 82: 1424–37.

34. Maddahi J, Ganz W, Ninomiya K et al. Myocardial salvage by intracoronary thrombolysis in evolving acute myocardial infarction: Evaluation using intracoronary injection of thallium-201. Am Heart J 102: 664–74.
35. DeCoster PM, Wijns W, Cauwe F et al. Area at risk determination by technetium-99m-hexakis-2-methoxy-isobutyl-isonitrile in experimental reperfused myocardial infarction. Circulation 1990; 82: 2151–62.
36. Okada RD, Glover D, Gaffney T, William S. Myocardial kinetics of technetium-99m-hexakis-2-methoxy-2-isonitrile. Circulation 1988; 77: 491–98.
37. Gitter MJ, Christian TF, Gibbons RJ. Technetium-99m sestamibi distinguishes stunned from infarcted myocardium and predicts 6 week left ventricular ejection fraction after acute myocardial infarction. J Am Coll Cardiol 1994, 476A (Abstr).
38. Ellis SG, Henschke CI, Sandor T et al. Time course of functional and biochemical recovery of myocardium salvaged by reperfusion. J Am Coll Cardiol 1983; 1: 1047–55.
39. Ito H, Tomooka T, Sakai N et al. Time course of functional improvement in stunned myocardium in risk area in patients with reperfused anterior infarction. Circulation 1993; .87: 356–62.
40. Simoons ML, Vos J, Tjissen JG et al. Long term benefit of early thrombolytic therapy in patients with acute myocardial infarction: 5 year followup of a trial conducted by the interuniversity cardiology institute of the Netherlands. J Am Coll Cardiol 1989; 14: 1609–15.
41. Rahimtoola SH. A perspective on the three large multicenter randomized clinical trials of coronary bypass surgery for chronic stable angina. Circulation 1985; 72 (Suppl V): V123–35.
42. Ross J Jr. Myocardial perfusion-contraction matching: Implications for coronary heart disease and hibernation. Circulation 1991; 83: 1076–82.
43. Dilsizian V, Bonow RO. Current diagnostic techniques of assessing myocardial viability in patients with hibernating and stunned myocardium. Circulation 1993; 87: 1–20.
44. Hendel RC, Bonow RO. Disparity in coronary perfusion and regional wall motion: Effect on clinical assessment of viability. Coron Artery Dis 1993; 4: 512–20.
45. Iskandrian AS, Hakki AH, Kane SA et al. Restand redistribution thallium-201 myocardial scintigraphy to predict improvement in left ventricular function after coronary arterial bypass grafting. Am J Cardiol 1983; 51: 1312–16.
46. Dilsizian V, Rocco TP, Freedman NM et al. Enhanced detection of ischemic but viable myocardium by the reinjection of thallium after stress-redistribution imaging. N Engl J Med 1990; 323: 141–6.

Corresponding Author: Dr Timothy F. Christian, Mayo Clinic and Mayo Foundation, 200 First Street, SW, Rochester, MN 55905, USA

3. Metabolic characteristics of the infarct zone: PET findings

MORTEN BØTTCHER, JOHANNES CZERNIN and HEINRICH R. SCHELBERT

Introduction

A sudden reduction in luminal diameter or a complete occlusion of a coronary artery triggers a cascade of metabolic events leading to myocardial ischemia. These events may differ from the slowly progressing narrowing of the coronary lumen due to developing atherosclerosis which allows for formation of collateral vessels. Yet, both situations are interrelated. They lead to an impairment of contractile function and to metabolic changes in the dependent myocardium. Considerable research has focused on elucidating mechanisms underlying the ischemia related changes in metabolism. Yet, the study of metabolism, especially in humans, has been limited. Tissue sampling for measurements of metabolites is highly invasive and provides only very regional information. Alternatively, collection of blood draining from the coronary sinus provides information on only average but not regional changes.

Positron Emission Tomography (PET) affords the noninvasive evaluation of regional functional processes. Myocardial blood flow is evaluated with N-13 ammonia, O-15 water and Rb-82 [1–6]. Oxidative metabolism can be quantified with C-11 acetate [7–10]. The rate of release of the tracer label in the form of C-11 CO_2 from the myocardium corresponds to the tricarboxylic acid cycle activity, which in turn is coupled to oxidative phosphorylation and thus affords a measure of regional myocardial oxygen consumption (MVO_2) [11, 12]. The biexponential clearance of C-11 palmitate from the myocardium reflects the distribution of free fatty acid between an endogenous pool of lipids and immediate oxidation [13–15]. The relative size of the rapid clearance curve component and its slope serve as indices of the fraction of fatty acid entering the mitochondria and their rate of oxidation [15, 16]. Lastly, F-18 deoxyglucose traces the initial transmembranous exchange of glucose and its hexokinase mediated phosphorylation [17–19]. Concentrations of F-18 activity in the myocardium therefore correspond to regional rates of exogenous glucose utilization.

This chapter describes findings with PET in patients with acute and suba-

C.A. Nienaber and U. Sechtem (eds): *Imaging and Intervention in Cardiology*, 29–42.
© 1996 *Kluwer Academic Publishers*.

cute myocardial infarction, discusses possible underlying mechanisms and proposes diagnostic and therapeutic opportunities.

Patterns of blood flow and metabolism in human myocardial infarction

Early PET investigations noted invariably regional reductions in myocardial blood flow [20, 21] corresponding to the electrocardiographic site of the acute myocardial infarction or the site of abnormal wall motion. An early study already delineated the extent of an acute myocardial infarction with C-11 palmitate and reported a statistically significant correlation between the tomographically measured and the enzymatically determined infarct size [22]. Serial PET imaging of the initial regional uptake of C-11 palmitate and its subsequent clearance from the myocardium demonstrated regionally prolonged retention of tracer in the infarct zone, consistent with an impairment of fatty acid oxidation (Figure 1) [20]. Also, F-18 deoxyglucose uptake was found to be segmentally increased in some patients [20, 23]. This increase was either relative to the regionally decreased blood flow or relative to the uptake of tracer in remote and presumably normal myocardium or both (Figures 2 and 3). The augmented F-18 deoxyglucose uptake was attributed to a shift in substrate utilization in the infarct zone, reflecting increased glucose oxidation and/or glycolysis. Increased glycolysis would be consistent with findings in acute experimental myocardial ischemia with enhanced glucose utilization, increased lactate release, diminished MVO_2 and reduced fatty acid oxidation [24–27]. The augmented F-18 deoxyglucose uptake in acutely infarcted myocardium associated with reduced blood flow became subsequently known by its operational term as "blood flow-metabolism mismatch", whereas a concordant reduction in F-18 deoxyglucose and regional blood flow was defined as a "blood flow-metabolism match" [28]. Serial evaluations of regional systolic wall motion shed some light on the possible significance of these flow metabolism patterns. Because wall motion failed to recover in "match" segments, this early pattern after an acute myocardial infarction implied the presence of irreversible injury (necrosis and scar tissue) [20]. Conversely, because regional wall motion recovered spontaneously in segments with early post-infarction "mismatches", they were referred to as "ischemic" to indicate that tissue had been injured only reversibly. (See also Chapters 3, 5, 21 and 22.)

Improved spatial and temporal resolution of PET together with newly developed tracer kinetic models permitted the quantification of regional functional processes and their interdependency. These processes included the measurement of regional myocardial blood flow with either O-15 water or N-13 ammonia [3, 4, 29, 30], of regional MVO_2 with C-11 acetate [7, 8, 11], and of exogenous glucose utilization with F-18 deoxyglucose [18, 19]. In 22 patients studied at 3.6 ± 1.6 days after onset of acute symptoms, quantitative image analysis [31] found in 20 patients regionally reduced blood

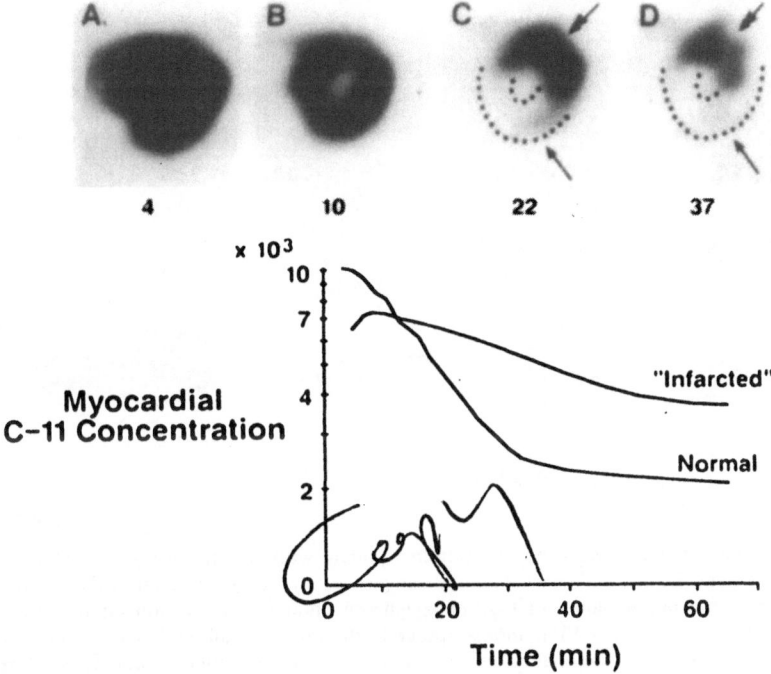

Figure 1. Serially acquired images of the myocardial uptake of C-11 palmitate and its subsequent clearance. Note on the initial image the tracer activity in both, blood pool and myocardium. After C-11 palmitate has cleared from the blood pool, the myocardium becomes visible and reveals a modest reduction in uptake in the infarct territory located in the anterior wall. The serial images reveal prompt clearance of C-11 acetate from remote myocardium but tracer retention in the infarcted territory. The corresponding time activity curves are shown in the lower panel; the delayed clearance of C-11 activity from the infarct territory is consistent with an impairment of fatty acid metabolism.

flow in the infarct territory as defined by electrocardiographic criteria and/or wall motion abnormalities [32]. Of these 51 flow defects, 29 revealed "mismatches" (57%) on F-18 deoxyglucose imaging whereas the remainder (43%) exhibited "matches". The absence of flow defects in 2 patients was attributed to early revascularization either by thrombolysis or direct percutaneous coronary angioplasty (PTCA).

In remote myocardium, blood flow averaged 0.83 ± 0.20 ml min^{-1} g^{-1} and thus was similar to those in normal volunteers [33]. Also, the C-11 acetate clearance rate, referred to as k_{mono}, as in index of MVO$_2$, averaged 0.063 ± 0.012 min^{-1} which again was comparable to that in normal volunteers [8]. Both parameters correlated with overall cardiac work as defined by the

Myocardial Blood Flow

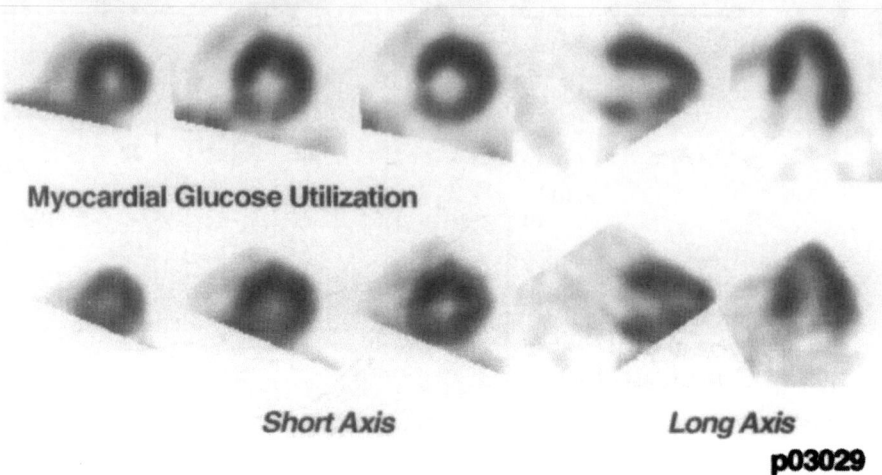

Myocardial Glucose Utilization

                     Short Axis   *Long Axis*
                                                                p03029

Figure 2. Blood flow and glucose utilization in a patient with an inferior myocardial infarction. Short axis and horizontal and vertical long axis images of myocardial blood flow (N-13 ammonia) are shown in the upper panel, of F-18 deoxyglucose uptake (glucose utilization in the lower panel). Note the reduced N-13 ammonia uptake in the inferior wall while glucose utilization is entirely preserved. This discrepancy between flow and F-18 deoxyglucose uptake is referred to as "blood flow-metabolism mismatch".

rate pressure product. However, exogenous glucose utilization in remote myocardium varied considerably between patients. Although all patients received glucose orally in order to stimulate insulin secretion and to enhance myocardial glucose uptake, elevated circulating free fatty acid and catecholamine levels, known to be present during the early post-infarction period [34] may have interfered with myocardial glucose utilization to varying degrees.

In infarct myocardium, blood flow was reduced to 0.57 ± 0.2 ml min^{-1} g^{-1} in "mismatch" and to 0.32 ± 0.12 ml min^{-1} g^{-1} in "match" regions. While this difference was statistically significant, there was considerable overlap of individual flow values (e.g., range from 0.27 to 0.89 ml min^{-1} g^{-1} in "mismatch" and from 0.11 to 0.61 ml min^{-1} g^{-1} in "match" regions. Oxidative metabolism was significantly correlated with myocardial blood flow, yet unexpectedly, in a biphasic rather than direct linear fashion. As illustrated in Figure 4, for mild to modest flow reductions, the C-11 acetate clearance rate k_{mono} declined disproportionately less. However, once flows decreased below 0.56 ml min^{-1} g^{-1}, oxidative metabolism declined steeply. (See also Chapters 2, 3 and 5.)

MVO_2 is thought to be correlated linearly with coronary blood flow [35]. Yet, more recent observations agree with the observed biphasic correlation

Myocardial Blood Flow

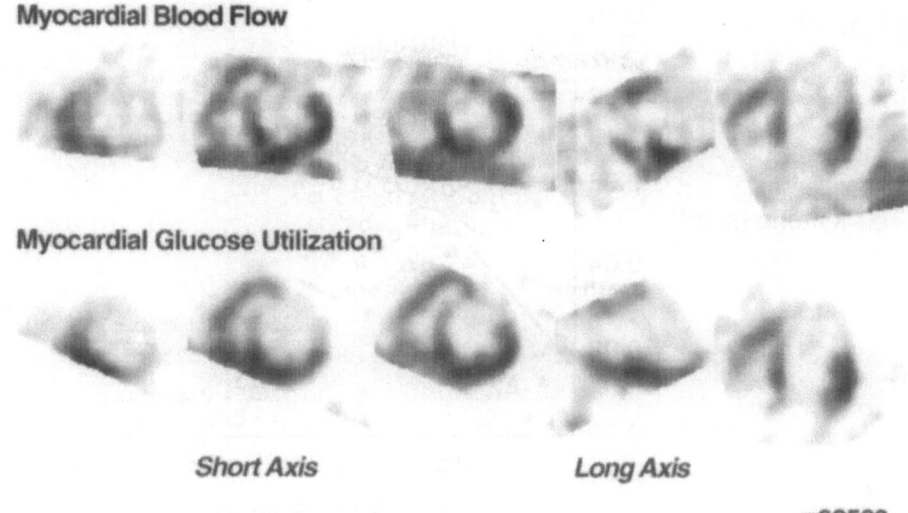

Myocardial Glucose Utilization

Short Axis   Long Axis

p02533

Figure 3. Myocardial blood flow and glucose metabolism in a patient with an acute extensive anterior and anteroseptal myocardial infarction. The image display is the same as in Figure 2. Note the extensive blood flow defect in the anterior wall extending into the anterior septum and the lateral wall. As shown in the lower panel, glucose utilization is decreased in proportion to blood flow "blood flow-metabolism match".

[36]. Modeling the interrelationships between coronary blood flow and pressure, O_2 saturation and extraction, the resulting biphasic correlation was attributed to a progressive increase in O_2 extraction. If one assumes an average O_2 extraction of 62%, as determined with the coronary sinus catheter technique in coronary artery disease patients [37] and if k_{mono} is converted to actual values of MVO_2 [8, 11, 37], then the O_2 extraction increases to a maximum of 93% at flows of $0.56 \, ml \, min^{-1} \, g^{-1}$. Unlike MVO_2, exogenous glucose utilization in the 22 patients [32] failed to correlate with myocardial blood flow. As mentioned above, the lack of a correlation most likely resulted from the interpatient variability in glucose utilization in normal myocardium. However, normalization of regional rates of glucose utilization in "infarcted" to that in remote myocardium (Figure 5) revealed a linear correlation between relative glucose utilization and relative myocardial blood flow for "match" regions yet increased glucose utilization for "mismatch" regions. The latter implies regional increases in the extraction of glucose.

The increases in extraction of both, O_2 and glucose, could be considered as compensatory mechanisms under conditions of limited blood flow and, hence, oxygen delivery. Enhanced glucose extraction might represent a shift to a more oxygen efficient substrate because for the same amount of oxygen, about 10 to 15% more ATP can be generated by oxidating glucose instead

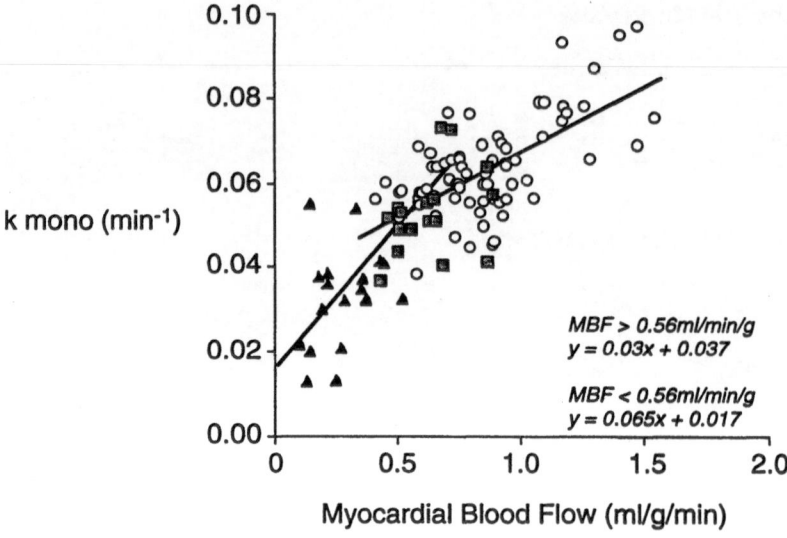

Figure 4. Correlation between oxidative metabolism and myocardial blood flow in patients studied during the early post-infarction period. Oxidative metabolism was determined from the clearance rate (k_{mono}) of C-11 acetate from the myocardium. Note the biphasic relationship between blood flow and oxidative metabolism. The open circles represent measurements in remote myocardium, the rectangles measurements in regions with "blood flow metabolism mismatches" and the solid triangles measurements in regions with "blood flow-metabolism matches". Note the biphasic relationship between oxidative metabolism and myocardial blood flow. (Reproduced with permission of the American Heart Association from Czernin et al. [32].)

of free fatty acid [38]. Additionally, the enhanced glucose utilization might reflect increased glycolysis as a key metabolic event during acute myocardial ischemia [24, 25]. Glycolytically generated ATP, located strategically in the proximity of the sarcolemmal membranes, has been suggested to be critical to cell survival and for prevention of ischemic contracture [39].

Abnormal states – patterns of blood flow and metabolism

Regardless of the underlying mechanisms, the flow metabolism patterns as observed on PET may be relevant for the clinical characterization of an acute myocardial infarction and its management. For example, in patients studied with C-11 acetate at an average of six days after an acute myocardial infarction, oxidative metabolism in infarct regions that improved contractile function following revascularization were reduced only modestly relative to those in remote myocardium (by about 26%) [40]. Conversely, in segments without an improvement in contractile function after revascularization, oxidative metabolism was reduced more severely (by about 55%). Importantly, flow

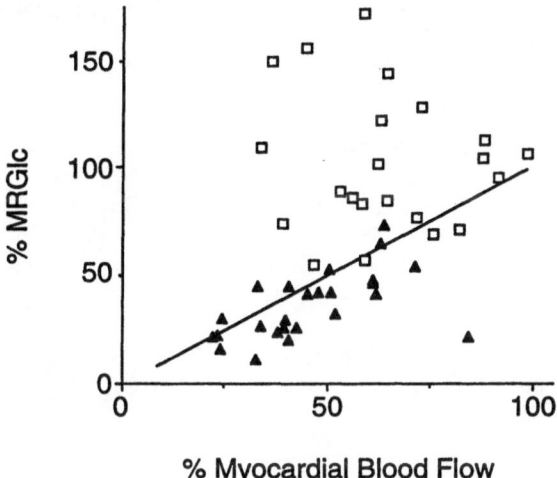

% Myocardial Blood Flow

Figure 5. Comparison of the relative of F-18 deoxyglucose uptake to relative myocardial blood flow in "infarct territories". Note the nearly linear relationship between flow and glucose metabolism in "match segments" (solid triangles) and the enhanced glucose utilization in "mismatch" segments (open rectangles). (Reproduced with permission of the American Heart Association from Czernin et al. [32].)

reductions were found to be similar in both types of segments. Further, enhanced glucose utilization during the early post-infarction period was associated with a long-term improvement in contractile function either spontaneously [20] or after interventional revascularization [40, 41]. Thus, blood flow metabolism patterns on PET may represent distinct "altered states" in acutely infarcted myocardium that are clinically relevant:

Pattern A: Obviously, normal regional blood flow and metabolism might represent myocardium that has recovered fully from the ischemic episode, relieved either by a spontaneous restoration of blood flow, by early thrombolysis or direct coronary angioplasty or both. A residual wall motion abnormality in this situation might represent resolving "stunning".

Pattern B: An only modest reduction in blood flow, normal MVO_2 and enhanced glucose utilization may reflect "myocardial stunning". Depending on the infarct vessel, this condition may resolve spontaneously if the stenosis is minimal and non-flow limiting. Conversely, the presence of a residual flow limiting stenosis might lead to "repetitive stunning" [42], a condition that can be characterized further with PET by quantifying blood flow responses to pharmacologically induced hyperemia. An absent or markedly impaired regional flow reserve would be consistent with "repetitive stunning".

INITIAL STUDY   FOLLOW-UP STUDY

MBF   Glucose   MBF   Glucose

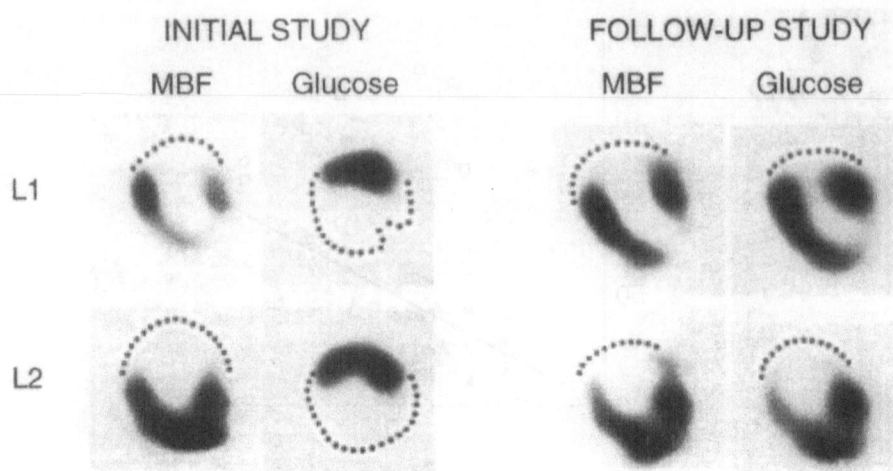

Figure 6. Follow-up blood flow and glucose metabolism study in a patient who exhibited early after the acute myocardial infarction a "blood flow metabolism mismatch". Two contiguous transaxial images through the mid-left ventricle are shown. On the N-13 ammonia blood flow images, an extensive defect is noted in the anterior wall associated with a selectively increased uptake of F-18 deoxyglucose. When studied six weeks later, the N-13 ammonia images again reveal the same perfusion defect in the anterior wall yet F-18 deoxyglucose uptake is reduced in proportion to blood flow. Hence, the initially present "blood flow-metabolism mismatch" pattern converted to a "match" pattern, presumably as a result of progression of ischemia to necrosis and scar tissue formation.

Pattern C: Less certain is the significance of a more severe reduction in regional myocardial blood flow associated with increased glucose utilization. It may represent on-going ischemia. Myocardium has survived the initial ischemic insult. Yet, as blood flow remains inadequate, ischemia progresses to necrosis and scar tissue formation. Early investigations demonstrated the conversion of an early post-infarction "mismatch" to a late "match" (Figure 6) [20]. Alternatively, if blood flow is sufficient for maintaining tissue viable, the affected myocardium may enter a chronic state of "hibernation". In fact, this pattern can persist for weeks to months [28, 43].

Pattern D: Lastly, concordant reductions in blood flow, glucose utilization and oxidative metabolism most likely represent truly infarcted or necrotic myocardium and thus, an irreversible tissue injury [20, 41]. It should be noted, however, that in some instances (about 10 to 15% in our experience; unpublished data) an even severe flow metabolism "match" may, when re-examined several weeks to months later, convert to a "blood flow metabolism mismatch" with a possible, long term improvement in contractile function.

Although this condition occurs only rarely, it may result from a very severe though non-fatal ischemic insult.

PET thus demonstrates several patterns, distinct and unique or at times confluent and complex, which nevertheless reveal myocardium that has survived the initial ischemic assault. The presence of such patterns offer an opportunity for salvage of compromised myocardium or of myocardium destined to succumb to the ischemic process. (See also Chapters 14–18.)

Comparison of PET to conventional diagnostic techniques

Clinical investigations indicated a limited accuracy of conventional diagnostic criteria for identifying surviving and potentially salvageable myocardium.

On electrocardiography, Q-waves correlated poorly with the blood flow metabolism patterns on PET. In 13 patients studied within 72 hours of onset of symptoms, 12 patients exhibited Q-waves. Six of the "Q-wave regions" were associated with "mismatches" and six with "matches" [20]. In another series of 22 patients studied with PET at an average of 3.6 days after onset of acute symptoms, Q-waves similarly failed to correlate with "match" and "mismatch" patterns [44]. Even in 15 patients studied during the subacute phase (2.9 weeks after the acute event), Q-waves correlated only poorly with "matches". [28]. The latter study did however demonstrate a significant correlation between post-infarction angina and/or electrocardiographic evidence of acute ischemia and the presence of "blood flow metabolism mismatches".

The three above investigations failed to observe also significant differences in the severity of wall motion abnormalities between "match" and "mismatch" regions [20, 28, 32]. In fact, the wall motion scores were similar for "match" and for "mismatch regions".

Regional flow reductions discriminated poorly between "match" and "mismatch" segments. While one study observed significantly more severe flow reductions in "match" than in "mismatch regions" [32], other studies found virtually identical or at least similar flow reductions [20, 40, 43]. Despite the different mean values in the one study, regional flow varied considerably and widely overlapped between both groups.

Preliminary data further suggests that Tl-201 rest-redistribution studies correlated only poorly with blood flow metabolism patterns and PET [45]. For example, half of all fixed defects on planar rest-redistribution Tl-201 scintigraphy at day one after the acute event were associated with a "mismatch" on PET performed on day 33. Conversely, six of the redistributing defects revealed "mismatches" on PET. It is also of note that in 12 patients studied during the subacute phase, only 4 patients or one-third revealed resolving stress induced defects on planar redistribution scintigraphy while nearly half of all patients exhibited "mismatches" on PET [43].

Thus, conventional techniques like electrocardiography, wall motion assessment, evaluation of regional blood flow as well as conventional Tl-201 scintigraphy fail to distinguish accurately and reliably between irreversibly injured and potentially salvageable myocardium. (See also Chapters 2, 4, 5, 6 and 15–18.)

Implications for revascularization

Of note, in earlier observations, a functional improvement was found in only half of the segments with early post-infarctions "mismatches" [20]. Because these patients did not undergo any revascularization procedure, these findings suggest that revascularization should be instituted early because as shown in this study, "mismatch" can convert to "matches," suggesting that ischemia progressed to necrosis.

While revascularization of infarct territories with blood flow metabolism "mismatches" appears to lead to an improvement or recovery of regional systolic wall motion, regional flow and metabolism abnormalities may persist for some time. In 15 patients with a first acute myocardial infarction and prompt thrombolysis (within 207 ± 183 minutes after onset of chest pain), Q-waves developed in all. Coronary angiography performed 20 ± 18 days after the acute event revealed patent infarct vessels although the residual diameter stenosis averaged $80 \pm 11\%$ [43]. Studied with PET at 42 ± 25 days after the acute myocardial infarction, all patients exhibited persistent flow defects in the infarct territory. Seven of the 15 patients or nearly half revealed "mismatches". Regional flow reductions in "match" and "mismatch" regions were nearly identical ($60 \pm 10\%$ in "match" and $61 \pm 14\%$ in "mismatch segments"). Both types of segments revealed similar degrees of impairment in regional contractile function. Further, there was a linear correlation between blood flow and MVO_2. Because no immediate post-infarction PET studies were available, it remains uncertain whether there were more "mismatches" early after the acute event but had already converted to "matches" when studied later. Significant residual stenoses of the infarct vessels may have resulted in "repetitive stunning" [42] or "hibernating" myocardium. This then raises the question whether relief of the residual stenosis by coronary angioplasty in addition to the initial thrombolytic treatment would have reduced the number of flow defects and, by inference, improved regional wall motion in these patients examined during the subacute post-infarction period.

Nevertheless, these findings imply that there is a time window during which interventional revascularization may lead to an improvement in contractile function. This possibility is indeed supported by findings in several investigations. (See Chapters 3–5 and 14–18.)

In 11 patients studied with C-11 acetate and F-18 deoxyglucose at an average of six days following the acute infarction, subsequent coronary angioplasty led to a significant improvement in contractile function as well as normalization of blood flow in 19 segments with an initially mild (about 26%) decrease in oxidative metabolism [40]. In contrast, a more recent study in 18 patients examined with C-11 acetate and PET at an average of 14 ± 2 days after the acute infarction reported lower predictive accuracies [46]. The authors point to disparities between flow and oxidative metabolism in their patients. Further, they infer that the high predictive accuracy in the earlier investigation may have been due to the fact that all patients were submitted to coronary angioplasty after the PET study. Conversely, in 12 segments with a significant, about 55% decrease in oxidative metabolism, contractile function remained impaired. Similarly, preservation of glucose utilization or a "mismatch" was 84% accurate in predicting a post-revascularization improvement in contractile function. Conversely, function failed to improve in 70% of segments with "matches". In a somewhat more heterogeneous population of 15 post-infarction patients, blood flow and MVO_2 normalized in "mismatch" regions and contractile function improved when re-examined three months later. In contrast, blood flow, MVO_2 and contractile function remained impaired in "match regions". In this preliminary study, two "matches" converted to "mismatches" on follow-up without a change in wall motion [41].

Summary and conclusions

Investigations with tracers of blood flow and metabolism and PET have uncovered distinct patterns of flow, oxidative metabolism and glucose utilization. These patterns likely represent various altered states such as stunning, hibernation and progressive ischemia and have considerable predictive power for the functional outcome after revascularization. PET appears diagnostically superior to conventional techniques for identifying surviving and potentially salvageable tissue in infarcted myocardium. While the mechanisms underlying the patterns noted on PET remain understood only incompletely, future studies with PET exploring protein synthesis, adrenergic neuronal activity and β-receptor activity might provide additional insights.

Acknowledgements

The authors wish to thank Diane Martin for preparing the illustrations and Eileen Rosenfeld for her assistance in preparing this manuscript.

References

1. Schelbert HR, Phelps ME, Huang SC et al. N-13 ammonia as an indicator of myocardial blood flow. Circulation 1981; 63: 1259–72.

2. Schelbert HR, Phelps ME, Hoffman EJ et al. Regional myocardial perfusion assessed with N-13 labeled ammonia and positron emission computerized axial tomography. Am J Cardiol 1979; 43: 209–18.
3. Bergmann SR, Herrero P, Markham J et al. Noninvasive quantitation of myocardial blood flow in human subjects with oxygen-15-labeled water and positron emission tomography. J Am Coll Cardiol 1989; 14: 639–52.
4. Araujo L, Lammertsma A, Rhodes C et al. Noninvasive quantification of regional myocardial blood flow in coronary artery disease with oxygen-15-labeled carbon dioxide inhalation and positron emission tomography. Circulation 1991; 83: 875–85.
5. Budinger TF, Yano Y, Moyer B et al. Myocardial extraction of Rb-82 vs. flow determined by positron emission tomography. J Nucl Med 1983; 68: III–81.
6. Gould KL, Goldstein RA, Mullani NA et al. Noninvasive assessment of coronary stenoses by myocardial perfusion imaging during pharmacologic coronary vasodilation. VIII. Clinical feasibility of positron cardiac imaging without a cyclotron using generator-produced rubidium-82. J Am Coll Cardiol 1986; 7: 775–89.
7. Henes CG, S.R. B, Walsh MN et al. Assessment of myocardial oxidative metabolic reserve with positron emission tomography and carbon-11 acetate. J Nucl Med 1989; 30: 1489–99.
8. Armbrecht JJ, Buxton DB, Brunken RC et al. Regional myocardial oxygen consumption determined noninvasively in humans with [1-^{11}C] acetate and dynamic positron tomography. Circulation 1989; 80: 863–72.
9. Buxton DB, Schwaiger M, Nguyen A et al. Radiolabeled acetate as a tracer of myocardial tricarboxylic acid cycle flux. Circ Res 1988; 63: 628–34.
10. Brown M, Marshall DR, Burton BS et al. Delineation of myocardial oxygen utilization with carbon-11-labeled acetate. Circulation 1987; 76: 687–96.
11. Buxton DB, Nienaber CA, Luxen A et al. Noninvasive quantitation of regional myocardial oxygen consumption in vivo with [1-^{11}C] acetate and dynamic positron emission tomography. Circulation 1989; 79: 134–42.
12. Brown MA, Myears DW, Bergmann SR. Noninvasive assessment of canine myocardial oxidative metabolism with ^{11}C-acetate and positron emission tomography. J Am Coll Cardiol 1988; 12: 1054–63.
13. Schön HR, Schelbert HR, Najafi A et al. C-11 labeled palmitic acid for the noninvasive evaluation of regional myocardial fatty acid metabolism with positron computed tomography. I. Kinetics of C-11 palmitic acid in normal myocardium. Am Heart J 1982; 103: 532–47.
14. Schelbert HR, Henze E, Schön HR et al. C-11 palmitate for the noninvasive evaluation of regional myocardial fatty acid metabolism with positron computed tomography. III. In vivo demonstration of the effects of substrate availability on myocardial metabolism. Am Heart J 1983; 105: 492–504.
15. Rosamond TL, Abendschein DR, Sobel BE et al. Metabolic fate of radiolabeled palmitate in ischemic canine myocardium: Implications for positron emission tomography. J Nucl Med 1987; 28: 1322–9.
16. Schelbert HR, Henze E, Sochor H et al. Effects of substrate availability on myocardial C-11 palmitate kinetics by positron emission tomography in normal subjects and patients with ventricular dysfunction. Am Heart J 1986; 111: 1055–64.
17. Phelps ME, Hoffman EJ, Selin CE et al. Investigation of [18F] 2-fluoro-2-deoxyglucose for the measure of myocardial glucose metabolism. J Nucl Med 1978; 19: 1311–9.
18. Ratib O, Phelps ME, Huang SC et al. Positron tomography with deoxyglucose for estimating local myocardial glucose metabolism. J Nucl Med 1982; 23: 577–86.
19. Gambhir SS, Schwaiger M, Huang SC et al. Simple noninvasive quantification method for measuring myocardial glucose utilization in humans employing positron emission tomography and Fluorine-18 deoxyglucose. J Nucl Med 1989; 30: 359–66.
20. Schwaiger M, Brunken R, Grover-McKay M et al. Regional myocardial metabolism in patients with acute myocardial infarction assessed by positron emission tomography. J Am Coll Cardiol 1986; 8: 800–8.

21. Schwaiger M, Brunken R, Krivokapich J et al. Beneficial effect of residual antegrade flow on tissue viability as assessed by positron emission tomography in patients with myocardial infarction. Eur Heart J 1987; 8: 981–988.
22. Sobel BE, Breshahan GF, Shell WE et al. Estimation of infarct size in man and its relation to prognosis. Circulation 1972; 46: 640–8.
23. Pierard L, De Landsheere C, Berthe C et al. Identification of viable myocardium by echocardiography during dobutamine infusion in patients with myocardial infarction after thrombolytic therapy: Comparison with positron emission tomography. J Am Coll Cardiol 1990; 15: 1021–31.
24. Liedtke AJ. Alterations of carbohydrate and lipid metabolism in the acutely ischemic heart. Progr Cardiovasc Dis 1981; 23: 321–36.
25. Opie LH, Owen P, Riemersma RA. Relative rates of oxidation of glucose and free fatty acids by ischemic and non-ischemic myocardium after coronary artery ligation in the dog. Eur J Clin Invest 1973; 3: 419–35.
26. Schelbert HR, Phelps ME, Selin C et al. Regional myocardial ischemia assessed by 18Fluoro-2-deoxyglucose and positron emission computed tomography. In: Schelbert HR, Neely JR., Phelps ME and Heiss HW (eds.) Advances in clinical cardiology (Vol I): Quantification of myocardial ischemia. New York: Gehard Witzstrock, 1988: 437–47.
27. Schön HR, Schelbert HR, Najafi A et al. C-11 labeled palmitic acid for the noninvasive evaluation of regional myocardial fatty acid metabolism with positron computed tomography. II. Kinetics of C-11 palmitic acid in acutely ischemic myocardium. Am Heart J 1982; 103: 548–61.
28. Marshall RC, Tillisch JH, Phelps ME et al. Identification and differentiation of resting myocardial ischemia and infarction in man with positron computed tomography 18F-labeled fluorodeoxyglucose and N-13 ammonia. Circulation 1983; 67: 766–78.
29. Kuhle W, Porenta G, Huang S-C et al. Quantification of regional myocardial blood flow using 13N-ammonia and reoriented dynamic positron emission tomographic imaging. Circulation 1992; 86: 1004–17.
30. Krivokapich J, Smith GT, Huang SC et al. N-13 ammonia myocardial imaging at rest and with exercise in normal volunteers: Quantification of absolute myocardial perfusion with dynamic positron emission tomography. Circulation 1989; 80: 1328–37.
31. Porenta G, Kuhle W, Czernin J et al. Semiquantitative assessment of myocardial viability and perfusion utilizing polar map displays of cardiac PET images. J Nucl Med 1992; 33: 1623–31.
32. Czernin J, Porenta G, Brunken R et al. Regional blood flow, oxidative metabolism, and glucose utilization in patients with recent myocardial infarction. Circulation 1993; 88: 884–95.
33. Czernin J, Müller P, Chan S et al. Influence of age and hemodynamics on myocardial blood flow and flow reserve. Circulation 1993; 88: 62–9.
34. Mueller H, Ayres S. Metabolic response of the heart in acute myocardial infarction in man. Am J Cardiol 1978; 42: 363–71.
35. Berne R, Rubio R. Coronary circulation. Hndbk Physiol 1979; I: 873–952.
36. Feigl E, Neat G, Huang A. Interrelations between coronary artery pressure, myocardial metabolism and coronary blood flow. J Mol Cell Cardiol 1990; 22: 375–90.
37. Holmberg S, Serzysko W, Varnauskas E. Coronary circulation during heavy exercise in control subjects and patients with coronary heart disease. Acta Med Scand 1971; 190: 465–80.
38. Buxton D. Myocardial metabolism. In: Schelbert HR, editor. Cardiac imaging: A companion to Braunwald's heart disease, Philadelphia: W.B. Saunders Company, 1991: 39–55.
39. Opie LH. Myocardial ischemia – metabolic pathways and implications of increased glycolysis. Cardiovasc Drugs Ther 1990; 4: 777–90.
40. Gropler R, Siegel B, Sampathkumaran K et al. Dependence of recovery of contractile function on maintenance of oxidative metabolism after myocardial infarction. J Am Coll Cardiol 1992; 19: 989–97.

41. Czernin J, Porenta G, Brunken R et al. Metabolic and functional fate of viable myocardium by PET early after acute infarction. J Am Coll Cardiol 1991; 17: 120A.
42. Vanoverschelde J-L, Wijns W, Depre C et al. Mechanisms of chronic regional postischemic dysfunction in humans: New insights from the study of noninfarcted collateral-dependent myocardium. Circulation 1993; 87: 1513–23.
43. Vanoverschelde J-LJ, Melin J, Bol A et al. Regional oxidative metabolism in patients after recovery from reperfused anterior myocardial infarction. Circulation 1992; 85: 9–21.
44. Czernin J, Barnard J, Sun K et al. Beneficial effect of cardiovascular conditioning on myocardial.blood flow and coronary vasodilator capacity. Circulation 1993; 88: I–51.
45. Kotler T, Nienaber C, Lew A et al. Early post-thrombolysis assessment of necrosis and viability with rest-redistribution thallium scintigraphy: Correlation with positron emission tomography (PET). J Am Coll Cardiol 1989; 13: 28A.
46. Hicks R, Melon P, Kalff V et al. Metabolic imaging by positron emission tomography early after myocardial infarction as a predictor of recovery of myocardial function after reperfusion. J Nucl Cardiol 1994; 1: 124–37.

Corresponding Author: Dr Heinrich R. Schelbert, Department of Molecular and Medical Pharmacology, UCLA School of Medicine, Los Angeles, CA 90024, USA

4. Assessment of myocardial viability with positron emission tomography after coronary thrombolysis

PATRICIA J. RUBIN and STEVEN R. BERGMANN

Introduction

Revascularization of occluded coronary arteries during evolving myocardial infarction with thrombolytic agents or by mechanical means has revolutionized the treatment of patients with acute myocardial ischemia. Clinical trials have shown conclusively that pharmacologically induced revascularization, especially when instituted early after acute ischemia, reduces morbidity and mortality [1].

Nonetheless, the ultimate fate of myocardium at risk and of left ventricular function is dependent on several factors in addition to the reestablishment of macrovascular coronary blood flow. These include the magnitude and duration of ischemia before reperfusion, the severity and eccentricity of residual stenoses, the occurrence of reocclusion, and the metabolic and structural damage induced by ischemia [2]. In addition, adjunctive therapy can be salutary to reperfused myocardium [3].

Patients frequently undergo coronary angiography and ventriculography early after initial treatment for evolving myocardial infarction to aid their physicians in planning of ongoing therapy. Although angiography provides critical details regarding vessel patency and the length, severity, and location of coronary stenoses, and ventriculography provides valuable data regarding function, neither provides complete information regarding the need for, and ultimate efficacy of, further therapeutic interventions. It is well established that the angiographically determined severity of stenosis does not correlate with the physiologic ability of the coronary vessel to deliver flow [4]. Similarly, reperfusion does not result in immediate, full recovery of contractile function in viable myocardium. This may take days, and perhaps weeks, after revascularization (a phenomenon termed myocardial stunning), and thus results of early functional studies can be ambiguous.

Positron emission tomography (PET) is a noninvasive approach for evaluation of myocardial perfusion and metabolism and can be used early after coronary thrombolysis or other revascularization procedures to assess myocardial viability [5–9]. PET provides a means to evaluate both regional

C.A. Nienaber and U. Sechtem (eds): Imaging and Intervention in Cardiology, 43–52.
© 1996 *Kluwer Academic Publishers*.

perfusion and the metabolic abnormalities that may be responsible for ventricular dysfunction after myocardial ischemia and reperfusion. Although not a primary modality for measurement of contractile capacity, functional assessments can be made as well [10, 11]. Labeling of physiologic substrates with positron-emitting agents provides a unique approach for sequential studies of regional perfusion and metabolism after thrombolytic therapy; the technique is especially useful in acutely ill patients in whom substantial alterations in the pattern of substrate use can occur over relatively short periods of time [12]. Recent studies have demonstrated that even when ventricular dysfunction due to myocardial stunning is present, the pattern of metabolism assessed with PET can predict ultimate functional recovery [3, 15–18].

Measurement of myocardial perfusion

Restoration of regional myocardial perfusion is crucial for salvage of ischemic myocardium [5]. A number of radiolabeled agents can be used to provide accurate estimates of regional myocardial perfusion using PET [14].

Although findings in experimental studies have suggested that acute occlusion followed by reperfusion is accompanied by a "no-reflow" phenomenon (diminished nutritive perfusion despite macrovascular patency) that can manifest itself either early or late after reperfusion, clinical studies do not seem to uniformly support this concept [6] in human subjects. This may be because reperfusion is established more slowly with thrombolytic agents in the clinical, as opposed to in the experimental setting, or because residual stenosis, frequent after revascularization, limits rapid total reperfusion, which can lead to cell swelling and extravascular compression. The Washington University has demonstrated that myocardial perfusion, assessed quantitatively with PET and $H_2^{15}O$, is reestablished promptly and completely in jeopardized zones after early treatment with tissue-type plasminogen activator (t-PA) (Figures 1 and 2) [6]. Flow in the reperfused zone was observed to be stable to the time of hospital discharge in these patients without symptoms of recurrent ischemia.

Similar findings were observed in 11 patients, five of whom received thrombolytic therapy early during the course of their evolving myocardial infarction; eventually all went on to bypass surgery or angioplasty [8]. Dysfunctional but viable myocardium (myocardium that showed improved contractile function after revascularization) exhibited slightly decreased levels of perfusion at the time of the initial PET study, which was performed an average of 6 days after symptom onset. Flow increased to nearly normal levels after revascularization. In contrast, nonviable myocardium exhibited significantly decreased levels of perfusion on the early studies. Nonetheless, because of the wide range of flows observed in these patients (most of whom did not undergo early reperfusion), viability could not be determined based

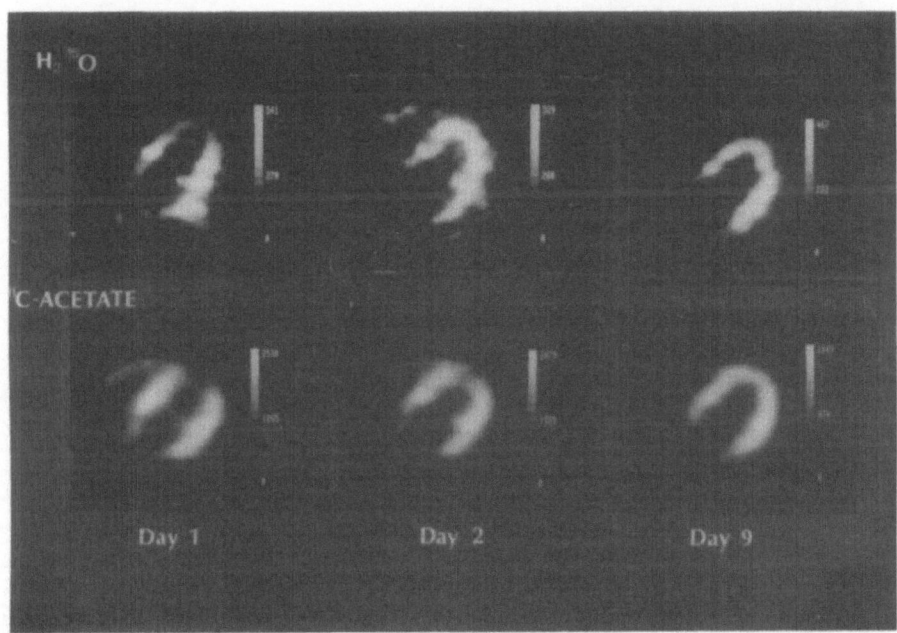

Figure 1. Midventricular PET reconstructions from a patient with anterior myocardial infarction studied 1, 2, and 9 days after acute anteroseptal myocardial infarction. The top row of images delineate relative myocardial perfusion after the administration of $H_2^{15}O$ and the bottom row show the myocardial accumulation of 1-^{11}C-acetate. These images demonstrate the rapid restoration of perfusion in the reperfused region and the slower recovery of accumulation of acetate. The top of each image corresponds to anterior and the left of each to the patient's right. (Reproduced, with permission, from Henes et al. [6].)

solely on estimates of perfusion. This suggests that factors other than restoration of perfusion are necessary for recovery of myocardial function. Experimental studies from our laboratory indicated that salvage of ischemic myocardium was achieved only when reperfusion was induced within 6 hours of the onset of acute ischemia. Reperfusion after 6 hours was observed to restore macrovascular patency and nutritive perfusion to tissue, but was not associated with restoration of uptake of fatty acids [5]. Similarly, large clinical studies have demonstrated that maximum benefit is achieved when reperfusion is established early, likely because the metabolic processes that underlie cell survival are unable to withstand prolonged durations of ischemia before reperfusion [1].

Recently, Iida and colleagues have suggested that an index of perfusable tissue, or PTI, can be used to differentiate viable from nonviable myocardium [15, 16]. Yamamoto et al. studied 11 patients with acute evolving myocardial infarction who received thrombolytic therapy and found higher levels of PTI in viable than in nonviable myocardium, with no overlap between the groups

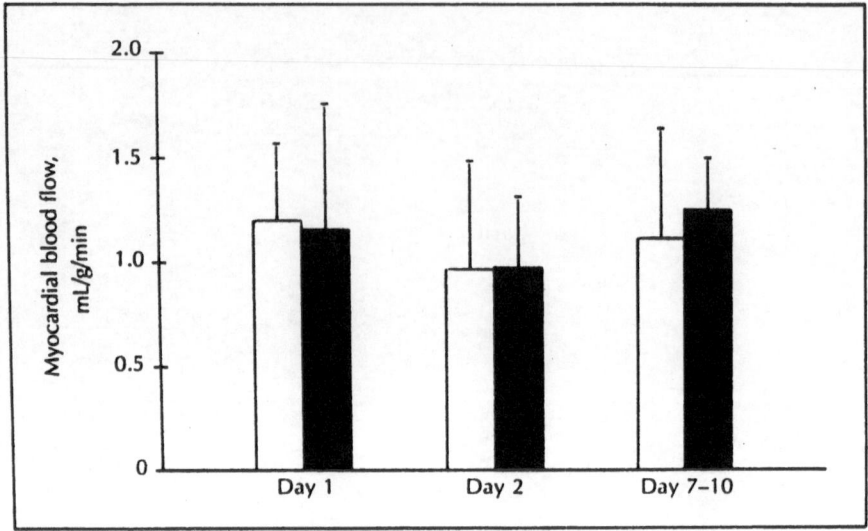

Figure 2. Regional myocardial nutritive perfusion in reperfused regions (solid bars) and remote normal zones (open bars) in eight patients with acute anterior myocardial infarction evaluated after administration of t-PA. The data demonstrate that nutritive myocardial perfusion, assessed with $H_2^{15}O$ and PET, is restored promptly and completely after t-PA and is maintained throughout the hospital period. (Reproduced, with permission, from Henes et al. [6].)

[16]. Preliminary studies from our laboratory have not been able to corroborate the lack of overlap in PTI values between viable and nonviable myocardium [17]. Although originally PTI was believed to reflect the ability of myocardium to exchange $H_2^{15}O$, recent studies from our laboratory suggest that PTI more likely reflects a complex relationship between tissue heterogeneity and flow [18]. Nonetheless, PTI can be determined with rapid scanning protocols, and further studies in larger numbers of patients are warranted to determine its utility for distinguishing viable from nonviable myocardium. (See also Chapters 2, 3, 11 and 14.)

Measurement of myocardial metabolism

The heart can be considered an aerobic organ that relies to a large extent on the oxidative metabolism of fatty acid for production of energy to fuel contraction, with lesser contributions from the use of glucose and lactate. Changes in myocardial metabolism occur rapidly during myocardial ischemia and after reperfusion [12]. Oxidation of fatty acids diminishes during ischemia and use of glucose is enhanced and remains elevated even after restoration of blood flow. The pattern of substrate and oxygen use during occlusion and after reperfusion has formed the basis for metabolic determinations of viability. (See also Chapters 4, 17 and 18.)

Use of labeled fatty acids

Since fatty acid oxidation is decreased rapidly after the onset of ischemia, studies evaluating the myocardial kinetics of 1-^{11}C-palmitate were the focus of initial studies. These investigations demonstrated that areas of infarction could be delineated accurately and quantitatively by the use of 1-^{11}C-palmitate [5, 19–22], and that restoration of myocardial perfusion, especially early after the onset of ischemia, could restore the uptake and utilization of fatty acids [5]. The ability of the myocardium to accumulate 1-^{11}C-palmitate early after reperfusion predicted ultimate recovery of metabolic function [23].

Sobel et al. studied 19 patients with evolving myocardial infarction treated with thrombolytic therapy. PET studies were performed on admission and again after 48 to 72 hours [22]. Accumulation of 1-^{11}C-palmitate increased by almost 30% in patients with successful thrombolysis, suggestive of metabolic salvage.

Metabolic imaging has also been used to demonstrate the utility of adjunctive therapies [24]. For example, when the calcium-channel blocker diltiazem was administered just before reperfusion, infarct size, delineated tomographically, was diminished to an even greater extent than that achievable with reperfusion alone. Benefits were corroborated by ex vivo analysis as well.

One difficulty with the use of 1-^{11}C-palmitate is the inability to distinguish oxidation from back-diffusion of nonmetabolized tracer by exponential clearance techniques under conditions of myocardial ischemia [25]. In addition, uptake and metabolism are dependent on arterial fatty acid concentration, fatty acid/albumin binding ratio, the neurohumoral environment and level of oxygenation among other factors [26]. Accordingly, the use of 1-^{11}C-palmitate for studies of myocardial ischemia has been abandoned.

Use of ^{18}F-fluorodeoxyglucose

Because glucose utilization is increased with myocardial ischemia, the use of ^{18}F-fluorodeoxyglucose (^{18}F-FDG), an analog of glucose that traces the initial uptake and phosphorylation (but not further metabolism) of glucose into the myocyte, has been proposed to delineate viable from nonviable myocardium. However, like 1-^{11}C-palmitate, the uptake of ^{18}F-FDG is dependent on arterial substrate concentrations as well as the pattern of substrate use and oxygenation of the myocardium [27].

^{18}F-FDG has been used extensively for the delineation of myocardial viability in patients with chronic coronary artery disease in whom a pattern of normal or decreased perfusion with enhanced ^{18}F-FDG uptake reflects viability of dysfunctional myocardium [28]. Unfortunately, the uptake of ^{18}F-FDG does not distinguish aerobic from anaerobic metabolism [29], and since

it is thought that anaerobic metabolism cannot support myocardial viability for prolonged periods of time, this differentiation may be crucial for the identification of jeopardized but viable myocardium under circumstances of acute myocardial ischemia. It is therefore not surprising that interpretation of uptake patterns of ^{18}F-FDG under conditions of early evolving myocardial infarction followed by reperfusion is complex [7–9, 28–30].

Seventeen patients with acute anterior myocardial infarction given a thrombolytic therapy within 3 hours of the onset of symptoms were studied [7]. Patients had PET scans an average of 9 days after admission. Eleven patients had increased glucose uptake in reperfused regions suggesting viable myocardium and five of these had normal perfusion and recovery of myocardial contractile function on late follow-up studies. Six of the 11 patients with increased glucose uptake had decreased perfusion, one of whom had recovery of contractile function at late follow-up. Six patients had decreased glucose uptake and perfusion (a matched defect, typically indicative of infarction) and in none of these did contractile function recover. Thus, PET with ^{18}F-FDG was able to accurately identify viability in only 11 of 17 patients after reperfusion therapy and was more accurate when flow and metabolism were diminished concordantly, which is indicative of nonviable myocardium. Similar results were reported by Schwaiger et al. [30]. It has been demonstrated that deoxyglucose may accumulate in necrotic myocardium [31], complicating interpretation of myocardial imaging with this tracer and explaining some of these discordant results. Thus, although use of ^{18}F-FDG to distinguish viable from nonviable myocardium in patients with chronic coronary artery disease is a useful approach, the utility of this agent for delineating viable from nonviable myocardium in the acute setting is more limited. (See also Chapters 4, 17 and 18.)

Use of 1-^{11}C-acetate

Because in the heart acetyl-CoA is the common pathway for catabolism of all substrates entering mitochondrial tricarboxylic acid (TCA) cycle metabolism, 1-^{11}C-acetate clearance has been advocated as an index of TCA cycle flux [32]. Since the TCA cycle is closely linked to oxidative metabolism, the clearance rate of ^{11}C-radioactivity from the heart, assessed with dynamic PET scanning and reflecting oxidation of acetate to [11]CO_2, correlates closely with directly measured myocardial oxygen consumption. Uptake and utilization of 1-^{11}C-acetate is relatively independent of both arterial substrate concentrations and the pattern of myocardial substrate use, making it a valuable tracer for studies of overall intermediary metabolism [32].

Walsh et al. evaluated patients with myocardial infarction treated conservatively and found that oxidative metabolism, assessed with 1-^{11}C-acetate, was markedly decreased in the center of the infarct zone compared with that in remote myocardium and did not improve before hospital discharge [33]. Henes et al. studied patients receiving thrombolytic therapy within 6 hours

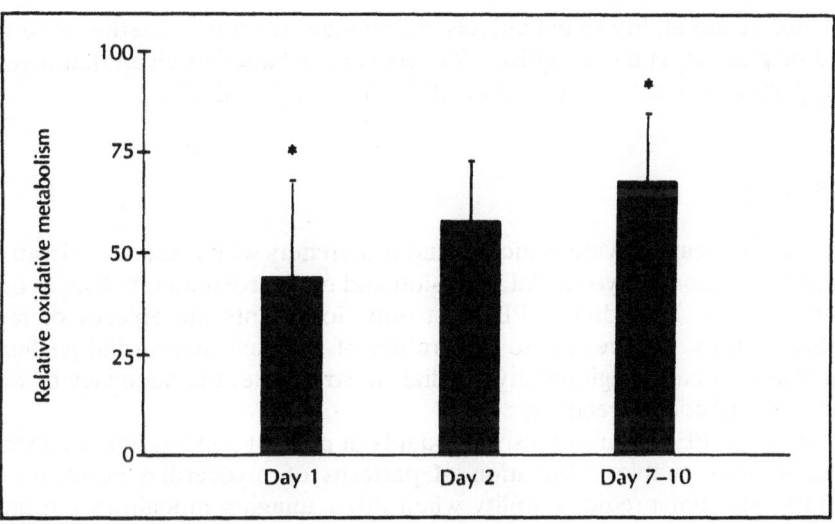

Figure 3. The mean rate of oxidative metabolism (assessed from delineation of myocardial clearance of extracted 1-^{11}C-acetate) in eight patients with acute myocardial infarction treated with t-PA. The rate is expressed as a percentage of that in remote, normal zones (calculated individually for each patient). The progressive improvement in relative oxidative metabolism was predictive of zones that recover contractile function. *p < 0.05 for the difference in metabolism between the initial and final studies. (Reproduced, with permission, from Henes et al. [6].)

of the onset of symptoms [6]. Oxidative metabolism (assessed with PET and 1-^{11}C-acetate) was $45 \pm 25\%$ of that observed in the remote segments 18 hours after reperfusion, had increased to $59 \pm 16\%$ at 48 hours, and before discharge it was $68 \pm 17\%$ (Figure 3). Recovery of wall motion was observed only in segments with restored perfusion and oxidative metabolism. Experimental studies have demonstrated that preservation of oxidative metabolism after myocardial ischemia followed by reperfusion is a prerequisite for recovery of metabolic function and therefore ultimately of mechanical function [13].

The above-mentioned study on 11 patients with acute myocardial infarction, including five who received thrombolytic therapy 6 days after hospital admission, viable regions (defined by sequential wall motion studies) demonstrated oxidative metabolism that was 74% of normal [8], whereas in nonviable myocardium, oxidative metabolism was 45% of that seen in remote, normal myocardium. These observations were recently extended to 21 patients with myocardial infarction, 11 of whom either received thrombolytic therapy or underwent primary angioplasty [9]. Estimates of myocardial oxidative metabolism with PET and 1-^{11}C-acetate had a better positive and negative predictive value for recovery of myocardial function (88 and 72%, respectively) than did estimates of glucose metabolism with ^{18}F-FDG (67 and 60%, respectively). These findings provide further evidence that maintenance of the ability to oxidatively metabolize substrate, whether it be fatty acid or glucose, is a prerequisite for recovery of function given that myocardial perfusion is maintained. (See also Chapters 4 and 17.)

Conclusions

Cardiac PET can provide clinicians and researchers with essential information regarding regional myocardial perfusion and myocardial metabolism in quantitative terms. In addition, PET not only documents the efficacy of reperfusion therapy with regard to restoration of regional myocardial perfusion, but also delineates regional myocardial substrate use, the adequacy of which underlies functional recovery.

Although PET is an expensive modality at present and has limited distribution, it does enable delineation of patterns of myocardial perfusion and metabolism that predict viability when other imaging modalities are inconclusive or ambiguous. Thus, PET should prove a particularly useful aid in planning therapeutic strategies for patients at high risk or in those in whom results of more conventional diagnostic procedures are equivocal.

Acknowledgements

The authors thank Becky Leonard for preparation of the typescript and Beth Engeszer for editorial assistance.

References

1. Tiefenbrunn AJ, Sobel BE. The impact of coronary thrombolysis on myocardial infarction. Fibrinolysis 1989; 3: 1–15.
2. Bergmann SR, Fox KAA, Ludbrook PA. Determinants of salvage of jeopardized myocardium after coronary thrombolysis. Cardiol Clin 1987; 5: 67–77.
3. Vanoverschelde JL, Bergmann SR. Myocardial reperfusion injury. Concepts, mechanisms, and therapeutic strategies. In: Sobel BE, Collen D, editors. Coronary thrombolysis in perspective. New York: Marcel Dekker, Inc., 1993: 271–301.
4. White CW, Wright CB, Doty DB et al. Does visual interpretation of the coronary arteriogram predict the physiologic importance of a coronary stenosis? N Engl J Med 1984; 310: 819–24.
5. Bergmann SR, Lerch RA, Fox KAA et al. Temporal dependence of beneficial effects of coronary thrombolysis characterized by positron tomography. Am J Med 1982; 73: 573–81.
6. Henes CG, Bergmann SR, Perez JE et al. The time course of restoration of nutritive perfusion, myocardial oxygen consumption, and regional function after coronary thrombolysis. Coron Artery Dis 1990; 1: 687–96.
7. Piérard LA, De Landsheere CM, Berthe C et al. Identification of viable myocardium by echocardiography during dobutamine infusion in patients with myocardial infarction after thrombolytic therapy: Comparison with positron emission tomography. J Am Coll Cardiol 1990; 15: 1021–31.

8. Gropler RJ, Siegel BA, Sampathkumaran K et al. Dependence of recovery of contractile function on maintenance of oxidative metabolism after myocardial infarction. J Am Coll Cardiol 1992; 19: 989–97.

9. Rubin PJ, Lee DS, Geltman EM et al. The superiority of PET with C-11 acetate compared with F-18 fluorodeoxyglucose for prediction of functional recovery early after myocardial infarction. J Nucl Med 1994; 35: 39P (Abstr).

10. Yamashita K, Tamaki N, Yonekura Y et al. Quantitative analysis of regional wall motion by gated myocardial positron emission tomography: Validation and comparison with left ventriculography. J Nucl Med 1989; 30: 1775–86.

11. Miller TR, Wallis JW, Landy BR et al. Measurement of global and regional left ventricular function by cardiac PET. J Nucl Med 1994; 35: 999–1005.

12. Myears DW, Sobel BE, Bergmann SR. Substrate use in ischemic and reperfused canine myocardium: Quantitative considerations. Am J Physiol: Heart Circ Physiol 1987; 253: 107H–14H.

13. Weinheimer CJ, Brown MA, Nohara R et al. Functional recovery after reperfusion is predicated on recovery of myocardial oxidative metabolism. Am Heart J 1993; 125: 939–49.

14. Bergmann SR. Quantification of myocardial perfusion with positron emission tomography. In: Bergmann SR, Sobel BE, editors. Positron emission tomography of the heart. New York: Futura Publishing, Inc., Mount Kisco, 1992: 97–127.

15. Iida H, Rhodes CG, de Silva R et al. Myocardial tissue fraction – correction for partial volume effects and measure of tissue viability. J Nucl Med 1991; 32: 2169–75.

16. Yamamoto Y, de Silva R, Rhodes CG et al. A new strategy for the assessment of viable myocardium and regional myocardial blood flow using ^{15}O-water and dynamic positron emission tomography. Circulation 1992; 86: 167–78.

17. Lee DS, Walsh JF, Herrero P et al. Superiority of estimates of myocardial oxidative metabolism compared to measurements of flow in predicting functional recovery after coronary revascularization. J Am Coll Cardiol (February Suppl) 1994: 116A (Abstr).

18. Herrero P, Staudenerz A, Walsh JF et al. Heterogeneity of myocardial perfusion provides the physiological basis of "perfusable tissue index". J Nucl Med 1995; 36: 320–7.

19. Lerch RA, Ambos HD, Bergmann SR et al. Localization of viable but ischemic myocardium by positron emission tomography (PET) with ^{11}C-palmitate. Circulation 1981; 64: 689–99.

20. Ter-Pogossian MM, Klein MS, Markham J et al. Regional assessment of myocardial metabolic integrity in vivo by positron-emission tomography with ^{11}C-labeled palmitate. Circulation 1980; 61: 242–55.

21. Schwaiger M, Schelbert HR, Keen R et al. Retention and clearance of C-11 palmitic acid in ischemic and reperfused canine myocardium. J Am Coll Cardiol 1985; 6: 311–20.

22. Sobel BE, Geltman EM, Tiefenbrunn AJ et al. Improvement of regional myocardial metabolism after coronary thrombolysis induced with tissue-type plasminogen activator or streptokinase. Circulation 1984; 69: 983–90.

23. Knabb RM, Bergmann SR, Fox KAA, Sobel BE. The temporal pattern of recovery of myocardial perfusion and metabolism delineated by positron emission tomography after coronary thrombolysis. J Nucl Med 1987; 28: 1563–70.

24. Knabb RM, Rosamond TL, Fox KAA et al. Enhancement of salvage of reperfused ischemic myocardium by diltiazem. J Am Coll Cardiol 1986; 8: 861–71.

25. Fox KAA, Abendschein D, Ambos HD et al. Efflux of metabolized and nonmetabolized fatty acid from canine myocardium. Implications for quantifying myocardial metabolism tomographically. Circ Res 1985; 57: 232–43.

26. Lerch RA, Bergmann SR, Sobel BE. Delineation of myocardial fatty acid metabolism with positron emission tomography. In: Bergmann SR, Sobel BE, editors. Positron emission tomography of the heart. New York: Futura Publishing, Inc., Mount Kisco, 1992: 129–52.

27. Gropler RJ, Siegel BA, Lee KJ et al. Nonuniformity in myocardial accumulation of fluorine-18-fluorodeoxyglucose in normal fasted humans. J Nucl Med 1990; 31: 1749–56.

28. Porenta G, Czernin J, Schelbert HR. Assessment of myocardial viability with tracers of

blood flow and metabolism of glucose. In: Bergmann SR, Sobel BE, editors. Positron emission tomography of the heart. New York: Futura Publishing, Inc., Mount Kisco, 1992: 185–207.

29. Schwaiger M, Neese RA, Araujo L et al. Sustained nonoxidative glucose utilization and depletion of glycogen in reperfused canine myocardium. J Am Coll Cardiol 1989; 13: 745–54.
30. Schwaiger M, Brunken R, Grover-McKay M et al. Regional myocardial metabolism in patients with acute myocardial infarction assessed by positron emission tomography. J Am Coll Cardiol 1986; 8: 800–8.
31. Sebree L, Bianco JA, Subramanian R et al. Discordance between accumulation of C-14 deoxyglucose and Tl-201 in reperfused myocardium. J Mol Cell Cardiol 1991; 23: 603–16.
32. Bergmann SR, Sobel BE. Quantification of regional myocardial oxidative utilization by positron emission tomography. In: Bergmann SR, Sobel BE, editors. Positron emission tomography of the heart. New York: Futura Publishing, Inc., Mount Kisco, 1992: 209–29.
33. Walsh MN, Geltman EM, Brown MA et al. Noninvasive estimation of regional myocardial oxygen consumption by positron emission tomography with carbon-11 acetate in patients with myocardial infarction. J Nucl Med 1989; 30: 1798–1808.

Corresponding Author: Dr Steven R. Bergmann, Cardiovascular Division, Washington University School of Medicine, Box 8086, 660 S. Euclid Ave., St. Louis, MO 63110, USA

5. Postthrombolysis noninvasive detection of myocardial ischemia and multivessel disease and the need for additional intervention

GEORGE A. BELLER and LAWRENCE W. GIMPLE

Introduction

Nuclear cardiology techniques have proven useful for determination of global and regional left ventricular function, regional myocardial perfusion, and myocardial viability in patients with acute myocardial infarction. Noninvasive stress imaging techniques with exercise or pharmacologic agents are capable of detecting residual ischemia within or remote from the infarct zone (with exercise or pharmacologic stress), sizing the extent of irreversible myocardial injury, and distinguishing viable from irreversible injury in regions of a-synergy. The perfusion imaging techniques are useful in the noninvasive assessment of myocardial salvage after reperfusion in patients who have received thrombolytic therapy or direct angioplasty during the acute phase of infarction. The information acquired from these techniques is valuable in risk stratification and decision-making with respect to the selection of stable postinfarction patients who would benefit from further invasive evaluation and revascularization.

Prognosis after acute myocardial infarction

Data from the prethrombolytic era suggest that prognosis in survivors of acute myocardial infarction is related to the degree of left ventricular dysfunction, the extent and severity of coronary artery disease (CAD), and the development of complex ventricular arrhythmias [1–4]. Recognition of prognostic factors derived from the clinical history, physical examination, and the chest X-ray should not be neglected. These include history of previous infarction, diabetes mellitus, advanced age, antecedent angina pectoris, peripheral or carotid vascular disease, symptoms and signs of congestive heart failure on admission, sinus tachycardia on entry, peak creatine kinase level, pulmonary congestion on admission chest X-ray, and persistence of resting ST-segment or T wave abnormalities on the electrocardiogram (ECG). The left ventricular ejection fraction (LVEF) measured at the time of discharge

C.A. Nienaber and U. Sechtem (eds): *Imaging and Intervention in Cardiology*. 53–73.
© 1996 *Kluwer Academic Publishers*.

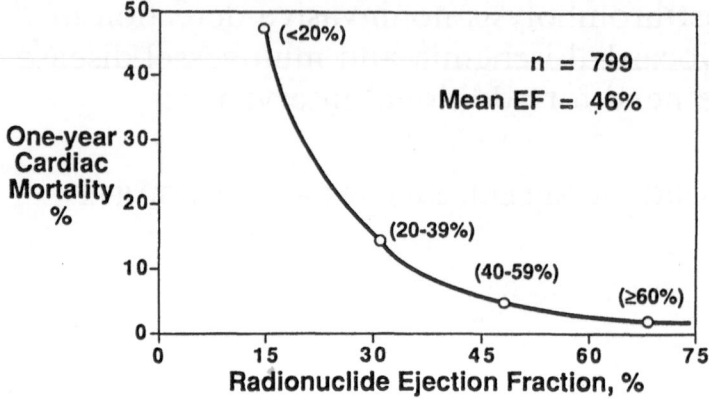

Figure 1. Relationship between left ventricular ejection fraction as determined by radionuclide ventriculography and 1-year cardiac mortality after acute myocardial infarction. (Reproduced with permission [1].)

is an important prognostic variable [1]. This variable is accurately measured by either first-pass or equilibrium-gated radionuclide ventriculography. In the report from the Multicenter Postinfarction Research Group of 866 infarct survivors, univariate analysis showed a progressive increase in cardiac mortality in the first year after discharge as the LVEF fell below 40% [1]. This relationship is depicted in Figure 1. Only four risk factors were independent predictors of mortality: a radionuclide LVEF below 40%, ventricular ectopy of 10 or more ventricular ectopic beats/hour, advanced New York Heart Association functional class before infarction, and rales detected in the upper two-thirds of the lung fields when the patient was in the coronary care unit. Various combinations of these four factors identified five risk subsets with 2-year mortality rates ranging from 3% (no factors) to 60% (all four factors present).

In patients who receive thrombolytic therapy for acute myocardial infarction, the LVEF is still an important prognostic variable [5]. However, such patients may have improved survival at any level of depressed LVEF compared to infarction patients treated in the prethrombolytic era [6]. Figure 2 demonstrates this enhanced 1-year survival for any given value of LVEF in the TIMI-II trial compared to the ejection fraction to mortality relationship derived in the prethrombolytic era from the Multicenter Postinfarction Trial [7]. Similarly, the GISSI-2 trial showed that mortality increased with an LVEF that fell below 40%. However, an LVEF of 30% was associated with only an 8% mortality (Figure 3) [8]. Simoons et al. [5] sought to determine the 5-year survival rates relative to LVEF quantitated during the hospitalization for acute infarction. As shown in Figure 4, patients with a resting LVEF of >40% had an excellent (>95%) 5-year survival. Patients with an LVEF between 30–39 had a 5-year survival rate of approximately 85%. In

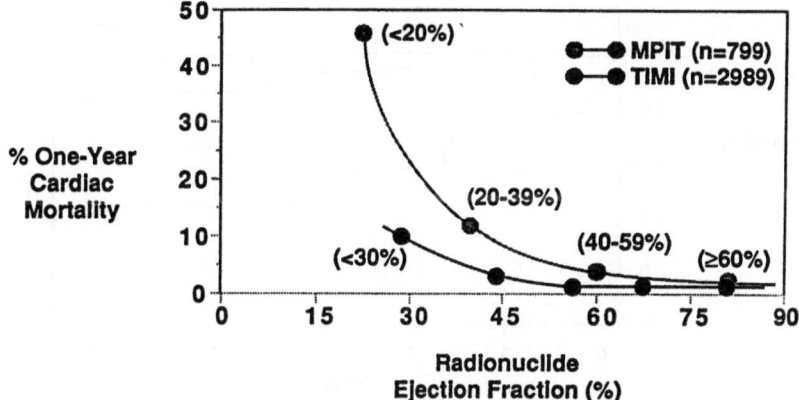

Figure 2. One-year cardiac mortality versus the resting radionuclide ejection fraction for patients in the Multicenter Postinfarction Trial (also depicted in Figure 1) compared to the same relationship for patients in the TIMI-II trial in which all patients received thrombolytic therapy. Note a lower mortality at any value of ejection fraction. (Reproduced with permission [7].)

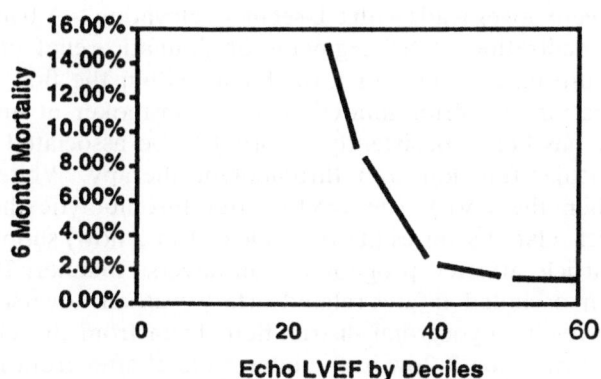

Figure 3. Six-month mortality versus left ventricular ejection fraction (LVEF) estimated by echocardiography in patients in the GISSI-2 trial. Mortality increases as the LVEF falls below 40%. However, mortality rates are lower for LVEF values between 20 and 40% compared to similar data derived in the prethrombolytic era (see Figure 1). (Reproduced with permission [8].)

contrast, patients with an LVEF of <30% had a <50% survival rate over 5 years. Thus, as in the prethrombolytic era, patients receiving thrombolytic therapy for acute myocardial infarction and having an LVEF of <30% have a high mortality rate during follow-up.

Rogers et al. [9] investigated the variables predictive of a good functional outcome following thrombolytic therapy in the Thrombolysis in Myocardial Infarction Phase II (TIMI-II) Pilot Study. In patients assigned to 18- to 48-

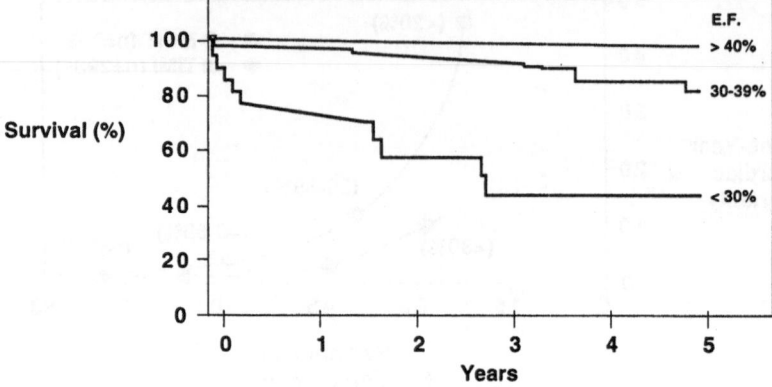

Figure 4. Five-year survival rates relative to left ventricular ejection fraction (E.F.) during hospitalization in patients receiving thrombolytic therapy for acute myocardial infarction in the Interuniversity Cardiology Institute of the Netherlands trial. (Reproduced with permission [5].)

hour angioplasty, variables independently predicting survival with a resting LVEF >50% were fewer leads with ST-segment elevation > 1.0 mV, younger age, rapid normalization of ST segments or dramatic relief of chest pain during rt-PA infusion, absence of arrhythmias within the first 24 hours of treatment initiation, no prior infarction, and nonsmoker at entry. Infarct artery patency has been consistently reported to be associated with better regional ventricular function after thrombolytic therapy. White et al. [10] found that when the LVEF was ≥50% after thrombolytic therapy, only occluded infarct-related arteries (TIMI grade 0, 1 or 2 flow) supplying >25% of the left ventricle affected prognosis in an adverse manner. If the LVEF was <50%, an occluded infarct-related artery was an adverse prognostic variable whatever its myocardial distribution. Data from the GUSTO trial indicate that TIMI grade 3 flow in the infarct vessel after front-loaded t-PA infusion results in a higher LVEF (61 ± 14%) compared to TIMI grade 0 flow and TIMI grade 1 flow (56 ± 14% and 54 ± 12%, respectively) [11]. Mortality at 30 days was 3.9% among patients with 90-minute LVEF values >45%, but 14.7% among those with an LVEF of ≤45%. In the TIMI Phase I trial, the regional ejection fraction was higher in the region subtended by the infarct-related artery in patients with sustained reperfusion [12]. In that study, a trend was noted toward a better average infarct region ejection fraction in patients treated with t-PA than in patients treated with streptokinase (0.40 vs 0.36; p < 0.06). In 542 patients reported by Harrison, patients with TIMI grade 0 flow were less likely to improve function than were patients with patent infarct-related arteries. Interestingly, the correlation between time to reperfusion and improvement in function was not strong [13]. Routine revascularization of patent but stenotic arteries, however, does not improve resting global ventricular function. In the TIMI study, LVEF 6 weeks postinfarction was comparable in patients randomized to a "conservative" strategy and compared with those randomized to an "invasive" strategy [14]. Grines and coworkers [15] showed that LVEF was comparable in patients randomized to direct angioplasty and patients randomized to t-PA (53% both). The 6-week exercise LVEF was also comparable (56% both).

Event-free survival after acute myocardial infarction is consistently correlated with the extent and severity of CAD. Schulman et al. [16] followed a cohort of 143 postinfarction patients in which 50% had three-vessel CAD but only 7% had a resting LVEF <29%. Multivariate analysis showed that right plus left anterior descending disease (p < 0.01), LVEF (p < 0.01), and number of risk segments (defined as areas of contracting segments on ventriculography supplied by stenotic vessels, p < 0.05) were significant predictors of outcome. The angiographic variables added significantly to the clinical variables for prediction of future cardiac events. A significant interaction exists between the LVEF and the extent of angiographic CAD with respect to prognosis after discharge after an uncomplicated myocardial infarction. De Feyter [17] reported a mortality rate of 22% in infarct survivors with an LVEF <30% or three-vessel CAD, and 1% in patients with an LVEF ≥30% and one- or two-vessel disease.

Extent of CAD persists as a major risk variable in postinfarction patients who have received thrombolytic therapy. Three-vessel CAD was a significant risk factor for cardiac mortality and recurrent myocardial infarction in patients who underwent coronary angioplasty in the TIMI-II trial [18]. Mortality rate was increased threefold during follow-up after angioplasty in 68 patients with three-vessel disease compared to the 921 patients with single-vessel CAD. Despite this difference, the survival rate was 90% in the three-vessel disease cohort. In a similar analysis, Muller et al. [19] reported correlations between angiographic findings and in-hospital outcome from 855 consecutively enrolled patients from the TAMI database. These investigators reported that patients with multivessel CAD had significantly increased mortality (11.4% vs 4.2%; p < 0.0001) which resulted largely from myocardial failure and shock. In a multivariate analysis, the number of diseased coronary arteries was the strongest predictor of in-hospital mortality, followed closely by the ejection fraction. Interestingly, the prognostic significance for mortality of one additional diseased coronary artery was equivalent to a reduction in ejection fraction of 16 percentage points. Fifty percent of the in-hospital deaths in the group with multivessel CAD occurred by the fourth hospital day. Data from the GUSTO trial [11] also demonstrate that patients with three-vessel CAD have a significant increase in early mortality rate compared to patients with one- or two-vessel CAD. Figure 5 shows that the mortality rate at 30 days was 11.2% for three-vessel disease patients, compared to 6.5% and 3.5% for one- and two-vessel disease patients, respectively. The role of stress testing with or without an imaging modality is to detect such high-risk patients with multivessel disease who do not manifest postinfarction angina.

Revascularization after thrombolytic therapy

Early investigations using thrombolytic therapy noted that severe coronary luminal obstruction typically remained 90 minutes after the onset of therapy. This led to several randomized trials seeking to define the role of early angioplasty after lytic therapy. Studies addressing the role of angioplasty immediately following thrombolytic therapy for stenotic infarct vessels showed no benefit or perhaps an increased complication rate in the angioplasty group compared with conservative management [20–22]. These increased complication rates resulted from additional bleeding and poor angioplasty results in recently recanalized, thrombotic lesions. Additionally, it was noted that many lesions which appeared severe on a 90-minute angiogram were not critical when reevaluated at later time points, presumably due to ongoing resolution of obstructive luminal thrombus [20]. In these studies, the role of angioplasty in patients with total coronary occlusion at 90 minutes (salvage angioplasty) was not studied, and the role of identifying and opening these arteries is, therefore, not known.

A "watchful waiting" approach was shown to be as effective as delayed revascularization after thrombolytic therapy with respect to outcomes. In the TIMI-IIB study [14], the cumulative 6-week mortality was 5.2% in the revascularization group compared with 4.7% in the group randomized to a conservative strategy. The latter entailed coronary angiography for spontaneous or stress-induced ischemia. Reinfarction was seen in 5.9% of the invasive group and 5.4% in the conservatively-treated group at 6 weeks. The discharge LVEF was also comparable (50.5% in the invasive and 49.9% in the conservative group). When follow-up was extended to 1 year postdischarge, mortality and reinfarction rates remained comparable between the two groups. Similarly, a 3-year follow-up of this patient cohort still showed no difference in cardiac mortality or reinfarction between the invasive (11.5%) and conservative (11.0%) groups [23]. The SWIFT trial showed a cumulative 1-year mortality of 5.8% in the intervention group, compared with 5.0% in the conservative groups, with reinfarction rates of 15.1% and 12.9%, respectively (difference not statistically significant) [24]. Ellis et al. [25] showed no functional or clinical benefit from routine predischarge coronary angioplasty after myocardial infarction in patients treated with thrombolytic agents who had no evidence for inducible ischemia by stress testing or stress radionuclide imaging prior to intervention. Actuarial 12-month infarct-free survival was 97.8% in the no-angioplasty group and 90.5% in the angioplasty group (p = 0.07). Thus, these studies indicate that neither immediate nor deferred routine angioplasty reduces mortality or morbidity or enhances left ventricular function following thrombolytic therapy in uncomplicated patients. Since "routine", rather than "selective", angioplasty after thrombolytic therapy does not appear to enhance survival or reduce the rate of reinfarction, patients who could potentially benefit from revascu-

larization might be adequately identified by noninvasive evaluation of resting
left ventricular function and a stress test to detect residual ischemia.

Coronary angiography after thrombolytic therapy

A significant number of patients treated with thrombolytic therapy will require early angiography. An aggressive invasive approach should be undertaken in patients suspected of experiencing sudden reocclusion of the infarct-
related artery or when spontaneous ischemia is recognized. Muller et al. [19]
reported that 26% of patients assigned to "conservative" therapy required
urgent cardiac catheterization within 4 days. Those patients who required
acute intervention could not be identified by baseline clinical characteristics.
Ellis et al. [26] reported a 14.9% in-hospital mortality rate in patients with
initially successful reperfusion who developed in-hospital evidence of recurrent ischemia, compared to a 2.0% mortality in patients who had successful
reperfusion and no recurrent ischemia. Early treatment of recurrent ischemia
in this setting was associated with improved survival. Unfortunately, although
several small series have reported angiographic correlates of abrupt closure,
the largest series of 174 patients reported no reliable angiographic predictors
of recurrent ischemia or infarction [27]. It is likely that thrombotic reocclusion results from complex interactions including coagulation, thrombosis,
ongoing thrombolysis, and arterial wall factors for which there are currently
no adequate models to predict reocclusion.

Angiography can be performed either "routinely" or "selectively" – that
is, only in the presence of a clear indication in clinically stable patients.
Certain patient groups are known to be at very high risk and may be good
candidates for routine angiography. These include patients with previous
myocardial infarction or poor ventricular function, or those presenting with
advanced Killip class [28]. Patients presenting with ST-segment elevation
who are treated with thrombolytic therapy and evolve non-Q wave infarctions
are also at increased risk of death or recurrent myocardial infarction [29].
Certainly, evidence of preserved viability in myocardial zones of asynergy
make such patients better candidates for angiography and subsequent revascularization [30]. In the study by Yamamoto et al. [30] regional ejection
fraction in the infarct zone did not improve after percutaneous transluminal
coronary angioplasty (PTCA) if the percent ^{201}Tl uptake on the preprocedure
delayed image was 50% or less. In contrast, regional ejection fraction increased from 39% to 47% in patients with >50% ^{201}Tl uptake in the infarct
zone.

Angiography has been advocated to identify certain patient subsets. These
include 15% of patients with minimal residual stenosis who can be reassured,
and the 5% of patients with important left main disease who require surgery;
it is also used to distinguish patients with single-vessel coronary disease from

those with multivessel disease who might benefit from more intensive medical therapy or surveillance. The Survival and Ventricular Enlargement (SAVE) study reported that 68% of postinfarction patients in the United States underwent coronary arteriography during admission, compared to 35% (p < 0.001) in Canadian hospitals [31]. Revascularization procedures were also more prevalent in the United States centers (31% vs 12%; p < 0.001). These differences were not associated with any difference in 42-month mortality (22% in Canada and 23% in the United States) or reinfarction (14% in Canada and 13% in the United States). More recently, McClellan et al. [32] analyzed the incremental benefit of catheterization and revascularization in the Medicare population and found that acute treatment shortly after acute infarction, rather than more aggressive use of invasive procedures, had the greatest impact on long-term mortality in the elderly. These data suggest that a strategy involving "routine" angiography does not confer benefit with respect to short-term outcome. Interestingly, Rogers et al. reported that 59% of patients assigned to "selective" angiography after infarction in the TIMI-IIA trial went on to develop an indication for angiography within 1 year [33].

Rationale for noninvasive approach to risk stratification

The main goal of predischarge risk stratification in patients who have survived an uncomplicated infarction is to distinguish high-risk patients who will benefit from early invasive evaluation and revascularization from patients with low risk for recurrent events medically treated. Decision-making algorithms using noninvasive testing for postinfarction risk stratification in the thrombolytic era have been used in several large clinical trials, and their usefulness is supported by the good clinical outcomes achieved with these strategies.

Exercise ECG stress testing for detection of residual ischemia

In the prethrombolytic era, certain ECG exercise stress test variables were found to be associated with an increased risk of future cardiac events [34]. These included exercise-induced ST-segment depression or further ST-segment elevation in leads exhibiting pathologic Q waves, attaining a workload of 4 METS or less, failure to adequately increase systolic blood pressure with increasing exercise workload, and exercise-induced ventricular arrhythmias such as nonsustained ventricular tachycardia. In one review, 29% of 3776 patients pooled from 17 series in the literature from the prethrombolytic era had exercise-induced ischemic ST-segment depression on submaximal testing [35]. The subsequent cardiac mortality rate was 15.6% in those patients manifesting ST-segment depression, compared to a 4.8% mortality rate in those without ST-segment depression during exercise. We previously reported a 29% prevalence of inducible ST-segment depression in 154 Q wave infarct patients and a 36% prevalence in 87 non-Q wave infarct patients on predischarge submaximal exercise testing [36]. As expected, those patients demonstrating ST-segment depression experienced an increased cardiac event rate during follow-up compared to those without ST-segment depression on the exercise ECG.

The prevalence of exercise-induced ST-segment depression after acute myocardial infarction is lower in patients treated with thrombolytic therapy. In the TIMI-IIB trial [14] 12.8% of the 1636 patients randomized to the invasive strategy had a positive exercise test at discharge compared to 17.7% of the 1626 patients in the conservative group. At 6 weeks, 16.8% of the invasive group and 19.4% of the conservative group had a positive exercise ECG stress test. These values are considerably lower than the 30% prevalence of a positive stress test in survivors of acute myocardial infarction undergoing testing in the prethrombolytic era [35]. Thus, it appears that patients in the thrombolytic trials are a lower risk group at the time of testing, with less inducible ischemia. However, as observed in the prethrombolytic era, 1-year mortality in the TIMI trial was greater in patients who did not perform the predischarge exercise test (7.7%) than those who did (1.8%) [37]. The GISSI investigators reported a 9.8% 6-month mortality rate in the 1037 patients who did not undergo predischarge exercise testing for cardiac reasons, compared to a 1.1% mortality rate for the 4661 patients with a negative stress test and a 1.7% mortality rate for patients with a positive test (Table 1) [8].

Tilkemeier [38] compared the prevalence of exercise-induced ST-segment depression on exercise ECG testing in postinfarction patients receiving thrombolytic therapy and/or angioplasty compared to those receiving no intervention during a comparable period of survey. In 64 patients receiving thrombolytic therapy, 15% had exercise ST-segment depression. This was substantially lower than the 35% prevalence of ST-segment depression in patients treated medically without any intervention. Haber et al. [39] from our institution showed only a 14% prevalence of inducible ST-segment depression on predischarge exercise testing in patients treated with a thrombolytic agent. This value is consistent with previous reports [14, 38] in comparable patient populations. White et al. [10] found that exercise duration

Table 1. Results of exercise testing on 6-month mortality rate in the GISSI-2 trial.

	No. patients	No. deaths	Odds ratio
Negative	4661	51 (1.1%)	1.0
Positive	1635	28 (1.7%)	1.64
Not done*	1037	102 (9.8%)	28.36

[a]For cardiac reasons: 15% had PTCA/CABG by 6 months.
From Volpi et al. Circulation 1993; 88: 416–29.

Table 2. Exercise test variables and outcome in patients receiving thrombolytic therapy.

Exercise test	Cardiac death (n = 18)	Alive (n = 287)	p value
Duration (min)	8.9 ± 3.4	11.1 ± 3.4	0.008
Percent with angina	27	21	0.49
Time to angina (min)	4.5 ± 3.2	6.8 ± 3.5	0.16

From White HD, Cross DB, Elliott JM et al. Long-term prognostic importance of patency of the infarct-related coronary artery after thrombolytic therapy for acute myocardial infarction. Circulation 1994; 89: 61–7.

was the only exercise test variable that distinguished those postinfarction patients receiving thrombolytic therapy who died during follow-up compared to those who were still alive (Table 2). The true prognostic implications of a positive ST-segment response in thrombolytic patients cannot be determined because patients with exercise-induced ST-segment depression are typically referred for angiography and, frequently, revascularization.

Froelicher et al. described limitations in the use of exercise ECG stress testing for assessing prognosis after acute myocardial infarction [34]. In a meta-analysis of various studies examining exercise test responses and prognosis after acute myocardial infarction, these authors found that only 11 of 24 institutions reported that an ischemic ST-segment response was associated with an increased risk of future cardiac events. Patients with an abnormal exercise blood pressure response or achieving a low workload were at higher risk for subsequent events than those with ≥ 1.0 mm ST-segment depression. Exercise-induced ST-segment depression was more predictive of increased risk of future events in patients with an inferior or posterior Q wave infarction than in patients with an anterior Q wave infarction. Interestingly, they found that submaximal testing had greater predictive power for prognostication than maximal testing. Similarly, the GISSI investigators reported that 50% of recurrent nonfatal infarctions occurred in patients without exercise test abnormalities [8]. Fortunately, although the mortality associated with reinfarction after thrombolytic therapy is high, the incidence of reinfarction is low. The GUSTO investigators reported a 4% in-hospital reinfarction rate [40] and the GISSI-2 investigators reported a 2.5% incidence of nonfatal reinfarction from hospital discharge to 6-month follow-up [41]. In this study, independent predictors of nonfatal infarction were cardiac ineligibility for an exercise test (relative risk 2.97), previous myocardial infarction (relative risk 1.70), and angina at follow-up (relative risk 1.5). Indicators of residual myocardial ischemia, such as early postinfarction angina and a positive exercise test, did not appear to be risk determinants. It should be pointed out that only 1.9% of patients had undergone PTCA and 4.1% bypass surgery in the first 6 months after discharge. This implies that early revascularization in patients with a positive stress test cannot be proposed as the sole explanation for failure of positive exercise test variables to predict reinfarction.

Exercise myocardial perfusion imaging

Detection of ischemia

Although clinical and ECG stress test variables are useful in separating high-from low-risk subgroups of survivors of acute myocardial infarction, variables derived from stress perfusion imaging using ^{201}Tl or one of the new ^{99m}Tc-labeled radiopharmaceuticals, provide additional prognostic information [36, 42–49]. Table 3 summarizes advantages of stress perfusion imaging compared to exercise ECG stress testing alone for risk stratification after uncomplicated acute myocardial infarction. The sensitivity of perfusion imaging for detecting ischemia is greater than that of ST-segment analysis or angina at submaximal exercise heart rates or workloads [50]. Perfusion imaging is superior to exercise ECG testing for localization of ischemia to specific coronary supply regions and can, therefore, better identify patients with underlying multivessel CAD who manifest ischemia in more than one vascular territory [51]. Increased lung ^{201}Tl uptake and transient left ventricular cavity dilation from the stress to the rest image are important supplementary prognostic variables. For patients who cannot exercise adequately, pharmacologic stress imaging with dipyridamole, adenosine, or dobutamine yield similar prognostic information as attained with exercise perfusion imaging [49, 52–54]. Another advantage of perfusion imaging is the ability to distinguish ischemic but viable myocardium from scar, which has important implications for management of patients with depressed left ventricular function after myocardial infarction.

In a prospective study of patients with uncomplicated myocardial infarction performed from our institution in the prethrombolytic era [42], approximately 50% who demonstrated either multiple ^{201}Tl defects in more than one coronary vascular region (multivessel CAD scan pattern), delayed ^{201}Tl redistribution within or remote from the infarct zone, or abnormal lung ^{201}Tl uptake experienced a subsequent cardiac event within 15 months (Figure 5). In contrast, the event rate was only 6% (2% mortality) in those postinfarction patients who had either a normal exercise scan or solely persistent ^{201}Tl defects confined to the infarct zone. Twenty-one of the 140 patients (15%) followed prospectively had multiple defects in >1 vascular supply region, redistribution, and increased lung ^{201}Tl uptake. This subgroup had an 86% recurrent cardiac event rate. As shown in Figure 6, exercise ^{201}Tl variables

Table 3. Advantages of myocardial perfusion imaging for risk stratification.

- ^{201}Tl redistribution is more prevalent than exercise ST-segment depression or inducible angina
- Ischemia can be localized to specific coronary supply regions
- Extent and severity of ischemia can be estimated by defect size
- Superior to exercise ECG in identifying multivessel ischemia
- Pharmacologic stress can be employed in patients unable to exercise
- Viability can be assessed on resting images

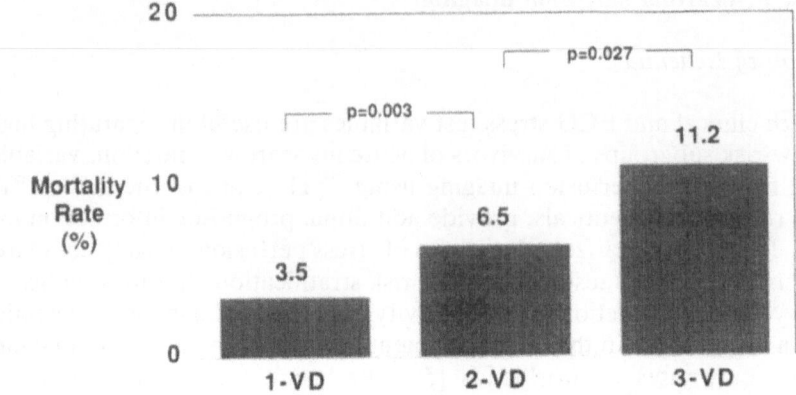

Figure 5. Mortality rate at 30 days relative to extent of coronary artery disease in patients enrolled in the GUSTO Angiographic Substudy. (Reproduced with permission [11].)

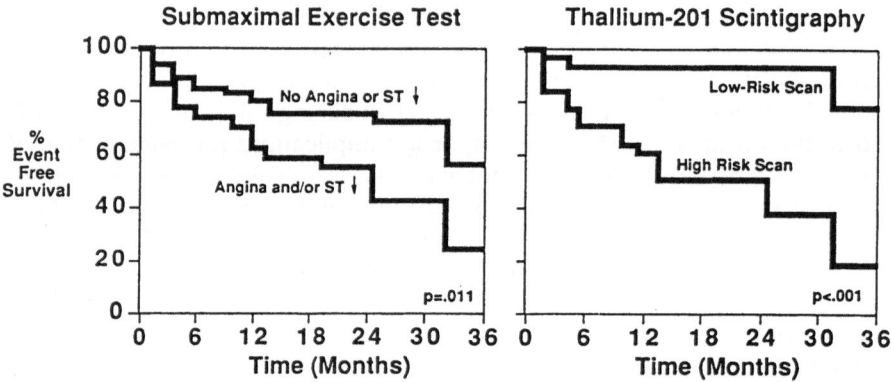

Figure 6. Event-free survival after uncomplicated myocardial infarction related to exercise ^{201}Tl data. (Adapted with permission [42].)

better separated high- and low-risk subsets than exercise-induced ST-segment depression or angina. In this study, ^{201}Tl redistribution was detected in 51% of postinfarction patients compared to 33% who exhibited inducible ST-segment depression. As expected, both ^{201}Tl redistribution and ST-segment depression are observed more frequently after non-Q wave infarction than after Q wave infarction.

In patients treated with thrombolytic therapy, ^{201}Tl redistribution is still more prevalent than ST-segment depression on stress testing (Figure 7). Tilkemeier et al. [38] reported a 42% prevalence of ^{201}Tl redistribution compared to 15% for ST-segment depression. Haber et al. [39] reported a 48% prevalence of ^{201}Tl redistribution, significantly higher than the 14%

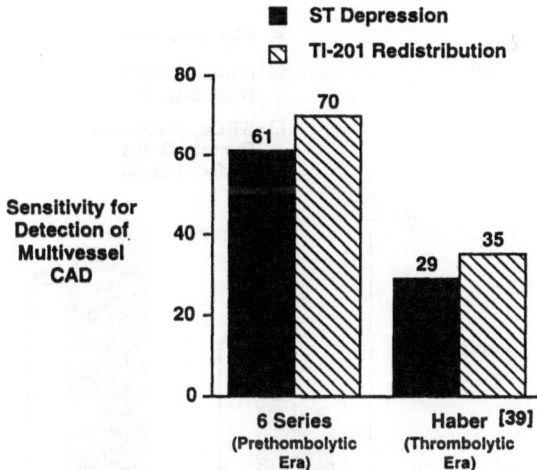

Figure 7. Prevalence of exercise-induced ST-segment depression and ^{201}Tl redistribution in patients treated with thrombolytic therapy for acute myocardial infarction at the Massachusetts General Hospital [38] and the University of Virginia [39]. (Adapted with permission [39].)

prevalence of ST-segment depression. Although exercise ^{201}Tl imaging was more sensitive than exercise ECG testing alone following thrombolytic therapy, the prevalence of reversible ^{201}Tl defects is less than observed in the prethrombolytic era. Figure 7 compares a prethrombolytic cohort [36] to a later thrombolytic cohort [39] at the University of Virginia. The prevalence of ST-segment depression decreased from 32% to 14%, and the prevalence of ^{201}Tl redistribution from 59% to 48%. Sutton et al. [55] evaluated postinfarction patients receiving thrombolytic therapy who had ≥70% residual stenosis of the infarct-related artery by angiography. They found only a 51% prevalence of ^{201}Tl redistribution on exercise testing using the single-photon emission computerized tomography (SPECT) imaging technique. This was presumably related, in part, to irreversible myocardial injury in the infarct zone distal to the stenotic infarct-related artery. Thus, as in the prethrombolytic era, detection of ischemia was better achieved with exercise perfusion imaging than the exercise ECG alone, although fewer ischemic responses by scintigraphic criteria are observed in patients who undergo reperfusion therapy.

Detection of multivessel coronary artery disease

As previously stated, multivessel CAD is one of the most important prognostic variables in patients surviving uncomplicated acute myocardial infarction, and one of the goals of predischarge noninvasive risk stratification is to identify those patients with functionally important multivessel CAD who might benefit from early coronary angiography and revascularization [11, 19,

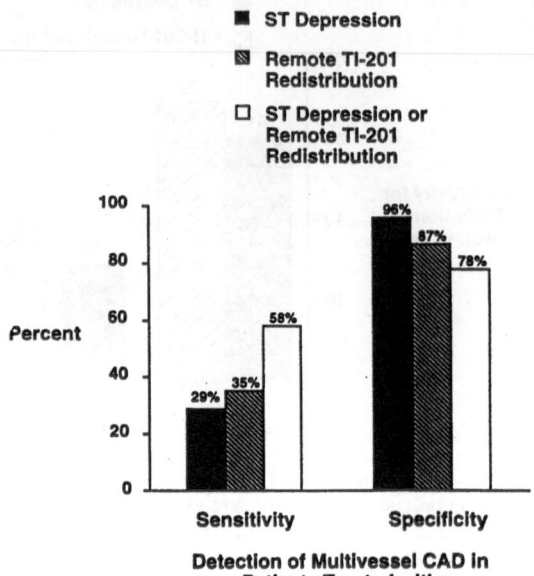

Figure 8. Sensitivity and specificity for detection of multivessel coronary artery disease of exercise-induced ST-segment depression (■), remote ^{201}Tl redistribution (▩), or both (□) in a cohort of patients treated with thrombolytic therapy for acute myocardial infarction. (Adapted with permission [39].)

42, 56]. Haber et al. [39] reported that 35% of patients treated with thrombolysis had multivessel CAD by coronary angiography (22% with two-vessel disease and 13% with three-vessel disease). A ^{201}Tl defect remote from the infarct zone was observed in only 35% of these patients (Figure 8). The sensitivity for detection of multivessel CAD by ^{201}Tl scintigraphy (35%) was slightly, but not significantly, higher than that of exercise-induced ST-segment depression (29%). However, if a remote ^{201}Tl defect and/or ischemic ST-segment depression was considered as a single variable for multivessel CAD detection, then 58% of those patients with significant angiographic multivessel CAD would have been identified. Using either ST-segment depression or a remote ^{201}Tl defect as a single variable decreased the specificity for multivessel CAD detection from 97% to 78%. The sensitivity of a remote ^{201}Tl defect for multivessel CAD detection in this study of patients receiving thrombolytic therapy was similar to that reported by Sutton and Topol [55] (35%) and Burns et al. [57] (40%).

Reports in the prethrombolytic era suggest a higher sensitivity of ^{201}Tl scintigraphy for detecting multivessel CAD. In a series of studies comprising 508 patients, there was a 72% sensitivity of a remote ^{201}Tl defect for detecting multivessel CAD associated with an 86% specificity [36, 43–45, 47]. In these

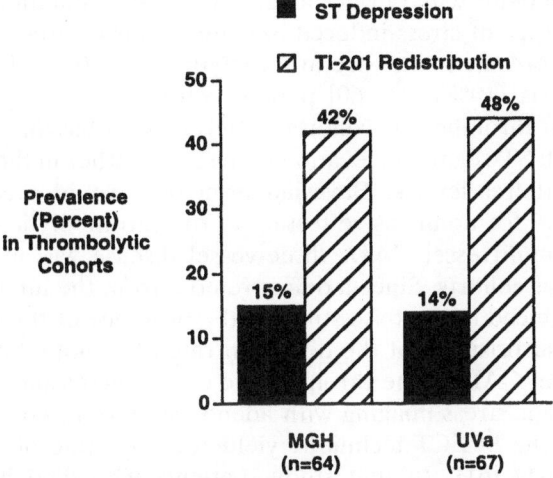

Figure 9. Comparison of sensitivity of exercise-induced ST-segment depression (■) versus remote ²⁰¹Tl redistribution (◪) for detection of multivessel coronary artery disease in patients
after infarction in a pooled analysis of six reports from the prethrombolytic era and in those
treated with thrombolytic therapy. (Adapted with permission [39].)

prior series, 59% of patients with multivessel CAD had ischemic ST-segment
depression. The positive predictive value of a remote ²⁰¹Tl defect for identifying multivessel CAD was significantly higher than the positive predictive
value of ST-segment depression for multivessel disease identification.

Remote ²⁰¹Tl defects following thrombolytic therapy are less common
(35%) in our laboratory than in the prethrombolytic era. Figure 9 shows the
differences in sensitivity of ST-segment depression and remote ²⁰¹Tl defects
for detection of multivessel CAD in pre- and postthrombolytic era cohorts.
In the prethrombolytic era, 61% of postinfarction patients with multivessel
CAD had exercise-induced ST-segment depression and 70% had remote
²⁰¹Tl defects compared to 29% and 35%, respectively, reported by Haber et
al. [39] in the thrombolytic era.

There are several possible explanations for the diminished sensitivity of
remote ²⁰¹Tl defects for multivessel CAD identification in the thrombolytic
era. First, the incidence of prior acute myocardial infarction is lower in the
thrombolytic era. In our study undertaken in the prethrombolytic era [36],
17% of patients had a prior acute myocardial infarction compared to 7% in
our thrombolysis cohort. A prior acute myocardial infarction remote from
the zone of new myocardial necrosis would be associated with a high prevalence of a remote defect. Second, non-Q wave infarctions were more common
in prethrombolysis cohorts because thrombolytic therapy is usually reserved
for patients presenting with ST-segment elevation. Patients with non-Q wave
acute myocardial infarction have a comparable angiographic extent of CAD

compared to patients with Q wave acute myocardial infarction, but they have a higher incidence of stress-induced ischemia. Third, three-vessel CAD was much more prevalent in prethrombolytic (30–50%) [58, 59] versus postthrombolysis (10%) [11, 60] patient cohorts. This may be due to the younger age in thrombolysis cohorts, differences in baseline characteristics, or patients with ST-segment elevation being seen earlier in the natural history of coronary atherosclerosis. Bayesian principles would predict diminished predictive value for noninvasive testing in the thrombolytic cohort. Among patients with multivessel CAD, three-vessel disease was more common in prethrombolysis cohorts. Since a defect remote from the infarct zone is more likely to be induced by exercise stress in the presence of three-vessel disease [51], it is not surprising that the detection rate of remote defects in patients with multivessel CAD in the thrombolytic era is decreasing.

Pharmacologic stress imaging with adenosine performed at 5 days postinfarction using the SPECT technique yielded a 70% rate of identification of multivessel CAD [61]. In that study, patients who died had significantly larger defects than patients who survived, and if >10% of the left ventricle showed reversibility indicative of ischemia, the prognosis was much worse than if <10% of the left ventricle was rendered ischemic. D'Urbano et al. [62] found that patients exhibiting dipyridamole-induced ^{201}Tl defects on stress imaging after acute myocardial infarction treated with thrombolysis had a significantly higher event rate during follow-up compared to those without redistribution (Figure 10).

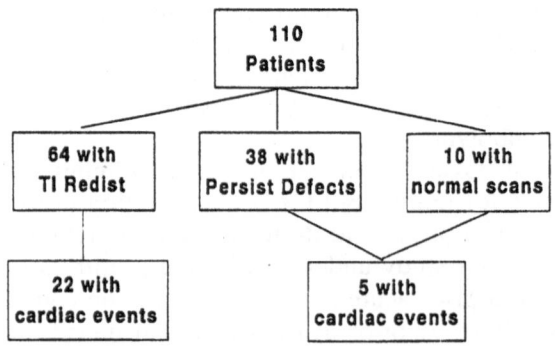

**DP TI-201 Imaging After
MI Treated with Thrombolysis**

110
Patients

64 with
TI Redist   38 with
Persist Defects   10 with
normal scans

22 with
cardiac events   5 with
cardiac events

Events: death, recurrent MI, unstable angina

Figure 10. Outcome of postinfarction patients who underwent dipyridamole (DP) thallium-201 (Tl-201) imaging prior to hospital discharge. The incidence of subsequent cardiac events was significantly higher in patients with redistribution defects compared to patients with persistent (Persist) defects or normal scans. (Reproduced with permission [62].)

Limitations of ^{201}Tl imaging

There are significant limitations to the use of ^{201}Tl as the perfusion agent for stress scintigraphy. The false-positive rate for detection of stenotic coronary arteries can be significant if attenuation artifacts are not appropriately identified. Quantitative image analysis is recommended to improve the accuracy of both planar and SPECT techniques. New ^{99m}Tc-labeled agents like sestamibi, teboroxime, and tetrofosmin are under investigation to determine their accuracy compared to ^{201}Tl for detection of ischemia, determining prognosis, and distinguishing viable from necrotic myocardium. Little data are available concerning the prognostic application of these new imaging agents in the postinfarction patient.

Summary

The physiologic approach to prognostication still appears to be valid in the evaluation of patients after uncomplicated acute myocardial infarction in the thrombolytic era. Because many patients with abnormal exercise tests are now routinely sent for angiography, there are no randomized trials or experimental confirmation that exercise test variables are still predictive of recurrent cardiac events in the thrombolytic era. Nevertheless, the excellent outcomes in patients treated with thrombolytic therapy and risk-stratified with noninvasive strategies provide strong empiric support for the continued use of noninvasive testing in the uncomplicated postinfarction patient after thrombolytic therapy. Patients with postinfarction angina either at rest or with exertion should be referred for coronary angiography, with revascularization undertaken if anatomy is appropriate. Patients with severely depressed left ventricular function or previous myocardial infarction should also be considered for early angiography, particularly when the prior myocardial infarction involves a separate vascular zone or is large, or viability is demonstrated in asynergic regions. Another group known to be at increased risk are patients presenting with ST-segment elevation who are treated with thrombolytic therapy and evolve non-Q wave infarctions. These patients often have evidence for preserved viability in zones of severe myocardial asynergy. Similarly, a small or modest rise in the creatine kinase MB fraction in the setting of marked regional dysfunction in a patient with a first infarction is an indicator of primarily ischemic dysfunction rather than irreversible myocardial injury. Interestingly, the prognosis of patients with non-Q wave infarction has improved with the advent of antithrombotic therapy [63]. In the TIMI-IIIB trial, the fatal and nonfatal reinfarction rate at 6 weeks in patients not given t-PA but managed with current conventional therapy was only 4.9%. Only 8.6% had a high-risk ^{201}Tl perfusion scan at hospital discharge.

Patients with no evidence of heart failure, postinfarction angina or complex ventricular arrhythmias are eligible for predischarge submaximal stress testing for risk stratification, preferably in conjunction with myocardial perfusion imaging. The addition of perfusion imaging will enhance the sensitivity for detection of ischemia within or remote from the infarct zone, while providing information regarding viability. Patients who are unable to exercise or those with poor exercise tolerance, an abnormal exercise blood pressure response, inducible ischemia, or nonsustained ventricular tachycardia are candidates for further invasive evaluation and consideration for coronary revascularization. With ^{201}Tl imaging, evidence for increased pulmonary uptake of the tracer is indicative of high risk and a high probability of an adverse outcome with medical therapy. Low-risk patients are those who achieve their target heart rate or workload without inducible angina, ST-segment depression, reversible perfusion abnormalities, or increased lung ^{201}Tl uptake. Defect size is reflective of infarct size, and patients with extensive areas of nonreversible hypoperfusion are also at high risk for future events, even in the absence of ischemia. Finally, pharmacologic stress imaging with dipyridamole, adenosine, or dobutamine imaging has been found to be safe when employed for stress testing soon after uncomplicated infarction. (See also Chapters 8–11, 15.)

References

1. Multicenter Post Infarction Research Group. Risk stratification and survival after myocardial infarction. N Engl J Med 1983; 309: 331–6.
2. Norris RM, Barnaby PF, Brandy PW et al. Prognosis after recovery from first acute myocardial infarction: Determinants of reinfarction and sudden death. Am J Cardiol 1984; 53: 408–13.
3. Taylor G, Humphries J, Mellitis D. Prediction of clinical course, coronary anatomy, and left ventricular function after recovery from acute myocardial infarction. Circulation 1980; 62: 960–70.
4. Moss AJ, Benhorin J. Prognosis and management after a first myocardial infarction. N Engl J Med 1990; 322: 743–53.
5. Simoons ML, Vos J, Tijssen JGP et al. Long-term benefit of early thrombolytic therapy in patients with acute myocardial infarction: 5 year follow-up of a trial conducted by the Interuniversity Cardiology Institute of the Netherlands. J Am Coll Cardiol 1989; 14: 1609–15.
6. Zaret BL, Wackers FJ, Terrin M et al. Does the left ventricular ejection fraction following thrombolytic therapy have the same prognostic impact described in the prethrombolytic era? Results of the TIMI-II trial (Abstr). J Am Coll Cardiol 1991; 17: 214A.
7. Bonow RO. Prognostic assessment in coronary artery disease: Role of radionuclide angiography. J Nucl Cardiol 1994; 1: 280–91.
8. Volpi A, DeVita C, Franzosi MG et al. Determinants of 6 months mortality in survivors of myocardial infarction after thrombolysis: Results of the GISSI-2 data base. Circulation 1993; 88: 416–29.
9. Rogers WJ, Bourge RC, Papapietro SE et al. Variables predictive of good functional outcome following thrombolytic therapy in the Thrombolysis in Myocardial Infarction phase II (TIMI II) pilot study. Am J Cardiol 1989; 63: 503–12.
10. White HD, Norris RM, Brown MA et al. Left ventricular end-systolic volume as the major

determinant of survival after recovery from myocardial infarction. Circulation 1987; 76: 44–51.

11. The GUSTO Angiographic Investigators. The effects of tissue plasminogen activator, streptokinase, or both on coronary-artery patency, ventricular function, and survival after acute myocardial infarction. N Engl J Med 1993; 329: 1615–22.

12. Wackers FJ, Terrin ML, Kayden DS et al. Quantitative radionuclide assessment of regional ventricular function after thrombolytic therapy for acute myocardial infarction: Results of phase I Thrombolysis in Myocardial Infarction (TIMI) trial. J Am Coll Cardiol 1989; 13: 998–1005.

13. Harrison JK, Califf RM, Woodlief LH et al. Systolic left ventricular function after reperfusion therapy for acute myocardial infarction: An analysis of determinants of improvement. Circulation 1993; 87: 1531–41.

14. The TIMI Study Group. Comparison of invasive and conservative strategies after treatment with intravenous tissue plasminogen activator in acute myocardial infarction. Results of the Thrombolysis in Myocardial Infarction (TIMI) phase II trial. N Engl J Med 1989; 320: 618–27.

15. Grines CL, Browne KF, Marco J et al. A comparison of immediate angioplasty with thrombolytic therapy for acute myocardial infarction. The Primary Angioplasty in Myocardial Infarction Study Group. N Engl J Med 1993; 328: 673–9.

16. Schulman SP, Achuff SC, Griffith LSC et al. Prognostic cardiac catheterization variables in survivors of acute myocardial infarction: A five year prospective study. J Am Coll Cardiol 1988; 11: 1164–72.

17. de Feyter PJ, van Eenige MJ, Dighton DH et al. Prognostic value of exercise testing, coronary angiography and left ventriculography 6–8 weeks after myocardial infarction. Circulation 1982; 66: 527–36.

18. Baim DS, Diver DJ, Feit F et al. Coronary angioplasty performed within the Thrombolysis in Myocardial Infarction II study. Circulation 1992; 85: 93–105.

19. Muller DW, Topol EJ, Ellis SG et al. Multivessel coronary artery disease: A key predictor of short-term prognosis after reperfusion therapy for acute myocardial infarction. Thrombolysis and Angioplasty in Myocardial Infarction (TAMI) Study Group. Am Heart J 1991; 121: 1042–9.

20. Topol EJ, Califf RM, George BS et al. A randomized trial of immediate versus delayed elective angioplasty after intravenous tissue plasminogen activator in acute myocardial infarction. N Engl J Med 1987; 317: 581–8.·

21. TIMI Research Group. Immediate versus delayed catheterization and angioplasty following thrombolytic therapy for acute myocardial infarction: TIMI IIA results. JAMA 1988; 260: 2849–58.

22. Simoons ML, Betriu A, Col J et al. Thrombolysis with tissue plasminogen activator in acute myocardial infarction: No additional benefit from immediate percutaneous coronary angioplasty (ECSG-5). Lancet 1988; 1: 197–202.

23. Terrin ML, Williams DO, Kleiman NS et al. Two- and three-year results of the Thrombolysis in Myocardial Infarction (TIMI) phase II clinical trial. J Am Coll Cardiol 1993; 22: 1763–72.

24. SWIFT (Should We Intervene Following Thrombolysis) Trial Study Group. Trial of delayed elective intervention versus conservative treatment after thrombolysis with anistreplase in acute myocardial infarction. Br Med J 1991; 302: 555–60.

25. Ellis SG, Mooney MR, George BS et al. Randomized trial of late elective angioplasty versus conservative management for patients with residual stenoses after thrombolytic treatment of myocardial infarction. Treatment of Post-Thrombolytic Stenoses (TOPS) Study Group. Circulation 1992; 86: 1400–6.

26. Ellis SG, Gallison L, Grines CL et al. Incidence and predictors of early recurrent ischemia after successful percutaneous transluminal coronary angioplasty for acute myocardial infarction. Am J Cardiol 1989; 63: 263–8.

27. Ellis SG, Topol EJ, George BS et al. Recurrent ischemia without warning: analysis of risk

factors for in-hospital ischemic events following successful thrombolysis with intravenous tissue plasminogen activator. Circulation 1989; 80: 1159–65.

28. Mueller HS, Cohen LS, Braunwald E et al. Predictors of early morbidity and mortality after thrombolytic therapy of acute myocardial infarction. Analyses of patient subgroups in the Thrombolysis in Myocardial Infarction (TIMI) trial. phase II. Circulation 1992; 85: 1254–64.

29. Tajer CD, Díaz R, Paolasso EA et al. Non-Q wave myocardial infarction after thrombolytic treatment predicts a high rate of reinfarction and death during the follow-up (Abstr). Circulation 1993; 88 (Suppl): I-490 (#2638).

30. Yamamoto K, Asada S, Masuyama T et al. Myocardial hibernation in the infarcted region cannot be assessed from the presence of stress-induced ischemia: Usefulness of delayed image of exercise thallium-201 scintigraphy. Am Heart J 1993; 125: 33–40.

31. Rouleau JL, Moye LA, Pfeffer MA et al. A comparison of management patterns after acute myocardial infarction in Canada and the United States. The SAVE investigators. N Engl J Med 1993; 328: 779–84.

32. McClellan M, McNeil BJ, Newhouse JP. Does more intensive treatment of acute myocardial infarction in the elderly reduce mortality? Analysis using instrumental variables. JAMA 1994; 272: 859–66.

33. Rogers WJ, Baim DS, Gore JM et al. Comparison of immediate invasive, delayed invasive, and conservative strategies after tissue-type plasminogen activator: Results of the Thrombolysis in Myocardial Infarction (TIMI) Phase II-A trial. Circulation 1990; 81: 1457–76.

34. Froelicher VF, Perdue S, Pewen W et al. Application of meta-analysis using an electronic spread sheet to exercise testing in patients after myocardial infarction. Am J Med 1987; 83: 1045–54.

35. Froelicher VF, Perdue ST, Atwood JE et al. Exercise testing of patients recovering from myocardial infarction. Curr Probl Cardiol 1986; 11: 370–444.

36. Gibson RS, Beller GA, Gheorghiade M et al. The prevalence and clinical significance of residual myocardial ischemia 2 weeks after uncomplicated non-Q wave infarction: A prospective natural history study. Circulation 1986; 73: 1186–98.

37. Chaitman BR, McMahon RP, Terrin M et al. Impact of treatment strategy on predischarge exercise test in the Thrombolysis in Myocardial Infarction (TIMI) II trial. Am J Cardiol 1993; 71: 131–8.

38. Tilkemeier PL, Guiney TE, LaRaia PJ et al. Prognostic value of predischarge low-level exercise thallium testing after thrombolytic treatment of acute myocardial infarction. Am J Cardiol 1990; 66: 1203–7.

39. Haber HL, Beller GA, Watson DD et al. Exercise thallium-201 scintigraphy after thrombolytic therapy with or without angioplasty for acute myocardial infarction. Am J Cardiol 1993; 71: 1257–61.

40. Ohman EM, Armstrong PW, Guerci AD et al. Reinfarction after thrombolytic therapy: Experience from the GUSTO trial (Abstr). Circulation 1993; 88 (Suppl): I-490 (#2636).

41. Ad Hoc Working Group of GISSI-2 Data Base: Volpi A, De Vita C, Franzosi MG et al. Predictors of nonfatal reinfarction in survivors of myocardial infarction after thrombolysis: Results of the Gruppo Italiano per lo Studio della Sopravvivenza nell'Infarto Miocardico (GISSI-2) data base. J Am Coll Cardiol 1994; 24: 608–15.

42. Gibson RS, Watson DD, Craddock GB et al. Prediction of cardiac events after uncomplicated myocardial infarction: A prospective study comparing predischarge exercise thallium-201 scintigraphy and coronary angiography. Circulation 1983; 68: 321–36.

43. Patterson RE, Horowitz SF, Eng C et al. Can noninvasive exercise test criteria identify patients with left main or 3-vessel coronary disease after a first myocardial infarction? Am J Cardiol 1983; 51: 361–72.

44. Dunn RF, Freedman B, Bailey IK et al. Noninvasive prediction of multivessel disease after myocardial infarction. Circulation 1980; 62: 726–34.

45. Brown KA, Weiss RM, Clements JP et al. Usefulness of residual ischemic myocardium

within prior infarct zone for identifying patients at high risk late after acute myocardial infarction. Am J Cardiol 1987; 60: 15-9.

46. Wilson WW, Gibson RS, Nygaard TW et al. Acute myocardial infarction associated with single vessel disease: An analysis of clinical outcome and the prognostic importance of vessel patency and residual ischemic myocardium. J Am Coll Cardiol 1988; 2: 223-34.

47. Abraham RD, Freedman SB, Dunn RF et al. Prediction of multivessel coronary artery disease and prognosis early after acute myocardial infarction by exercise electrocardiography and thallium-201 myocardial perfusion scintigraphy. Am J Cardiol 1986; 58: 423-7.

48. Moss AJ, Goldstein RE, Hall WJ et al. Detection and significance of myocardial ischemia in stable patients after recovery from an acute coronary event. Multicenter Myocardial Ischemia Research Group. JAMA 1993; 269: 2379-85.

49. Gimple LW, Beller GA. Assessing prognosis after acute myocardial infarction in the thrombolytic era. J Nucl Cardiol 1994; 1: 198-209.

50. Esquivel L, Pollock SG, Beller GA et al. Effect of the degree of effort on the sensitivity of the exercise thallium-201 stress test in symptomatic coronary artery disease. Am J Cardiol 1989; 63: 160-5.

51. Nygaard TW, Gibson RS, Ryan JM et al. Prevalence of high-risk thallium-201 scintigraphy findings in left main coronary artery stenosis: Comparison with patients with multiple- and single-vessel coronary artery disease. Am J Cardiol 1984; 53: 462-9.

52. Gimple LW, Hutter AJ, Guiney TE et al. Prognostic utility of predischarge dipyridamole-thallium imaging compared to predischarge submaximal exercise electrocardiography and maximal exercise thallium imaging after uncomplicated acute myocardial infarction. Am J Cardiol 1989; 64: 1243-8.

53. Leppo JA, O'Brien J, Rothendler JA et al. Dipyridamole-thallium-201 scintigraphy in the prediction of future cardiac events after acute myocardial infarction. N Engl J Med 1984; 310: 1014-8.

54. Brown KA, O'Meara J, Chambers CE et al. Ability of dipyridamole-thallium-201 imaging one to four days after acute myocardial infarction to predict in-hospital and late recurrent myocardial ischemic events. Am J Cardiol 1990; 65: 160-7.

55. Sutton JM, Topol EJ. Significance of a negative exercise thallium test in the presence of a critical residual stenosis after thrombolysis for acute myocardial infarction. Circulation 1991; 83: 1278-86.

56. Roubin GS, Harris PJ, Bernstein L et al. Coronary anatomy and prognosis after myocardial infarction in patients 60 years of age and younger. Circulation 1983; 67: 743-9.

57. Burns RJ, Freeman MR, Liu P et al. Limitation of exercise thallium single photon tomography early after myocardial infarction (Abstr). J Am Coll Cardiol 1989; 13: 125A.

58. Topol EJ, Holmes DR, Rogers WJ. Coronary angiography after thrombolytic therapy for acute myocardial infarction. Ann Intern Med 1991; 114: 877-85.

59. Nicod P, Gilpin EA, Dittrich H et al. Trends in use of coronary angiography in subacute phase of myocardial infarction. Circulation 1991; 84: 1004-15.

60. Rogers WJ, Babb JD, Baim DS et al. Selective versus routine predischarge coronary arteriography after therapy with recombinant tissue-type plasminogen activator, heparin and aspirin for acute myocardial infarction. TIMI II Investigators. J Am Coll Cardiol 1991; 17: 1007-16.

61. Verani MS. Exercise and pharmacologic stress testing for prognosis after acute myocardial infarction. J Nucl Med 1994; 35: 716-20.

62. D'Urbano M, Cafiero F, Cammelli F et al. Dipyridamole thallium-201 scintigraphy in uncomplicated acute myocardial infarction treated by thrombolysis: Diagnostic and prognostic value (Abstr). J Am Coll Cardiol 1994 Feb; 476A.

63. The TIMI IIIB Investigators: Effects of tissue plasminogen activator and a comparison of early invasive and conservative strategies in unstable angina and non-Q-wave myocardial infarction: Results of the TIMI IIIB trial. Circulation 1994; 89: 1545-56.

Corresponding Author: Dr George A. Beller, Cardiovascular Division, Box 158, University of Virginia Health Sciences Center, Charlottesville, VA 22908, USA

6. Imaging to justify no intervention

CHRISTOPH A. NIENABER and GUNNAR K. LUND

Introduction

"Words, words, words, I'm so sick of words", said Eliza Doolittle, which could well refer to the number of articles on the merits of *testing* by use of the electrocardiogram (rest, exercise and dynamic), Tl-201 and Tc-99m-MIBI perfusion scans, the rest and stress echocardiogram (transthoracic and transesophageal), arterial calcification etc., and reports on the various advantages of specific stress interventions (pacing, pharmacologic, psychologic) to uncover evidence of ischemia and other physiologic or anatomic abnormalities. A literature review gives the impression that initial reports are later superseded by newer reports claiming superiority in aspects such as diagnostic and prognostic evaluation, and shows that many "successful" testing options first enthusiastically reported, are later criticized, then abandoned or replaced by the latest "fashion" in diagnostics or risk stratification.

As a general rule the purposes of any clinical testing include, first, determination of the presence or absence of a disease; second, assessment of the severity of the disease and its relation to limitations and quality of a given patient's life; third, a prognosis under conditions of natural history, both in years of survival and in quality years (symptom free or reduced); and fourth, the assessment of the potential for benefit from various treatment options, including the option of doing nothing [1–6]. The traditional attitude in the medical community is to follow these steps either instinctively or in a structured manner. For the latter, however, little experience is availabe on how to deal with apparently persuasive statistical analyses such as the use of superior sensitivity/specificity, positive/negative predictive accuracy, incremental information content, classical statistics versus Bayesian analysis, prognostic models, demographic studies, clinical trials and so forth, when caring for the individual patient [2, 7–10]. However, the need for tests is indisputable considering that clinical evaluation will never be an exact and precise science [11–15].

Diagnostic and therapeutic decisions should rely on a profound philosophy of test interpretation. In regard to coronary artery disease as the most

C.A. Nienaber and U. Sechtem (eds): Imaging and Intervention in Cardiology. 75–92.
© 1996 *Kluwer Academic Publishers.*

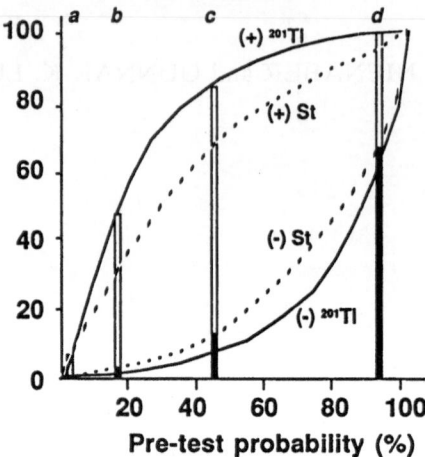

Post-test probability (%)

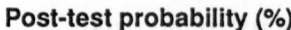

a 45 y/o M, asymptomatic, no risk factors;
b 45 y/o M, asymptomatic, HBP, chol. ↑, D.M.;
c 45 y/o M, atypical chest pain;
d 55 y/o M, typical angina

Figure 1. Demonstration of how to estimate the probability of significant coronary artery disease. Four typical clinical scenarios are depicted using patient examples (a, b, c, d); the solid vertical bars reflect the post-test probability of coronary artery disease both for a negative exercise ECG (-ST) and a normal thallium-201 scan (-Tl), whereas the open bars indicate the post-test probability in case of pathological stress ECG or thallium-201 perfusion studies. Note that the benefit from both – negative and positive testing is greatest in the intermediate range of pre-test probabilities (40–60%) and that the post-test probability after one test becomes the pre-test probability of a subsequent additional test. Modified and adopted, with permission from the American College of Cardiology, from: Patterson RE and Horowitz SF: Importance of epidemiology and biostatistics in deciding clinical strategies for using diagnostic test: A simplified approach using examples from coronary artery disease. JACC 13: 1653, 1989.

common condition referred for testing, a stepwise approach has proven useful. The first step includes medical history, physical exam, ECG, chest radiograph and, if appropriate, an ambulatory (electrocardiographic) exercise stress test. The second and any further step, such as stress testing by use of perfusion or wall motion imaging must be a consequence of the previous rather than an automatic component since additional testing is designed to provide incremental information to allow management decisions on a higher level of confidence [8, 16–19] as exemplified in Figure 1.

Crucial, indeed fundamental to the issue of diagnostic tests is a realistic estimate of the potential for treatment benefit in terms of survival and quality years. A typical example is how to use diagnostic tests to select patients for coronary revascularization [17, 20, 21]. Bypass surgery confers for survival benefit in some, but not all anatomic and functional subsets. On the other hand quality years survival, e.g. is clearly improved in symptomatic patients. However, with the exception of left main and proximal left anterior descending coronary artery lesions, survival of patients with single and double vessel coronary artery disease with mere medical treatment is also excellent (and similar to revascularization) mainly when ventricular function is unimpaired and symptoms benign [23–28]. With regard to revascularization procedures a particularly disturbing report on the use of angioplasty in cardiology practice (largely patients with single-vessel disease) indicated that only 27% had undergone a preangioplasty exercise stress test to estimate a potential benefit [29]. Thus, diagnostic tests must be directed at identifying patients belonging to subsets shown to derive maximal benefit from revascularization [8, 18, 30, 31]. No testing strategy makes a great deal of sense in the absence of either a concept of possible future benefit or an impact on the individual patient outcome [32–35]. This process is like chess; one has to anticipate the next move and an expert chess player has anticipated the possible options many moves ahead.

Concepts of testing

When does a test improve the chances of a correct answer to a relevant question? Most likely both empirical and statistical approaches contribute to that objective. Test results may be clearly positive (supporting a particular hypothesis), clearly negative (evidence against it) or equivocal and thus unhelpful, therefore requiring another discriminating measure (or test). The cardiologist must be aware of the limitations that pertain to reports of testing strategies in the literature. Dichotomization of results, arbitrary thresholds for positivity and exclusion of background characteristics limit the interpretation of group results. The academic life cycle of a noninvasive test depends on its ability to guide interventions and to predict outcome both in general and in the individual case [18, 36]. Both the positive and negative predictive values of a particular test are greatest at an a priori 50% (or intermediate) probability of the expected result. Prevalence of disease within a population is a principle determinant of sensitivity and specificity. Hence, for any test the predictive accuracy may vary between laboratories. But such limitations do not necessarily pertain to the assessment of test results in individual patients. A 4.0 mm ST segment depression is more impressive than one of 1.0 mm and a Bruce exercise time of 12 minutes in a 65-year-old male projects a more favorable outcome than the associated 1.5 mm ST segment depression in the inferior leads. One can have a higher level of "empirical" confidence in such a result than that conferred by analysis of the literature, and the clinician is not denied relevant background information and experience that can diminish or amplify the importance of a test result.

Table 1. Pre-test likelihood (%) of coronary artery disease in symptomatic patients.

Age	Nonanginal chest pain		Atypical angina		Typical angina	
	Men	Women	Men	Women	Men	Women
30–39	5.2	0.8	21.8	4.2	69.7	25.8
40–49	14.1	2.8	46.1	13.3	87.3	55.2
50–59	21.5	8.4	58.9	32.4	92.0	79.4
60–69	28.1	18.6	67.1	54.4	94.3	90.6

From Diamond and Forester [7] by permission of the New England Journal of Medicine. Numbers denote percent likelihood.

Pre-test (a priori) and revised (a posteriori) likelihoods

In accordance with the probability theory of Bayes the interpretation of a test result depends equally on two factors: first, the initial estimate of the likelihood that the disease is present in a given patient (pre-test likelihood) and second, the sensitivity and specifity of the applied test. If both factors are known the post-test or revised likelihood can be calculated [2, 7, 9, 11–13]. The pre-test likelihood can be derived from own experience, expert opinion (both are estimates made in advance of the test result) or from accumulated data from large series of patients in whom the clinical probability of conditions have been determined (Table 1).

After assessing a so-called a priori (or pre-test) likelihood (based on the distribution of a given disease or symptom) the specific information of a test result is implemented for the decision making process. For this, it is important to know how reliable a test result is, in other words, one has to know both sensitivity and specifity of the applied test. Sensitivity and specifity of various tests have been published and are summarized for different stress tests for detection of coronary heart disease (Tables 2 and 3).

The next step is to combine the a priori probability for the suspected disease with the sensitivity and specifity of the applied test to assess the

Table 2. Stress testing for detection of coronary artery disease in patients with chest pain.

	Sensitivity (%)	Specificity (%)
ST segment depression (≥1 mm) stress ECG [47, 48]	60–65	80–85
Exercise radionuclide angiography [49]	85–90	70–75
Visual 201-TI imaging [48]	80–85	75–85
Quantitative 201-TL imaging [50–54]	85–90	85–90
SPECT Tc-99m MIBI [46, 55]	85–93	75–85
Rb-82 PET [23, 56]	80–94	74–90
N-13 Ammonia PET [57]	95	100

In part from Beller by permission of the American Journal of Cardiology [54] and modified according to more recent literature [46, 55–57]. Ranges are approximate, as determined from a review of published studies.

Table 3. Sensitivity and specificity of exercise perfusion (Thallium-201) scintigraphy.

	Significant stenosis	Sensitivity	Specificity	Prevalence
Planar acquisition				
Qualitative [47, 48]	>50%	0.76	0.96	0.76
	>75%	0.93	0.92	0.63
	>50%	0.91	0.86	0.67
Quantitative [50, 51]	>50%	0.93	0.91	0.67
	>50%	0.88	0.90	0.65
Tomographic acquisition				
Qualitative SPECT [52]	>50%	0.90	0.91	0.69
Quantitative SPECT [53]	>50%	0.96	0.91	0.69

revised or a posteriori likelihood. The physician considers a set of 100 patients with the same clinical findings (of atypical angina and a negative ECG stress test below age-predicted maximal heart rate) as an hypothetical case. In such a scenario the estimated pretest likelihood is such that 60% have normal coronaries and 40% have one or more significant lesions. The sensitivity and specificy of the applied test is assumed 80% and 90%, respectively. In the 60 normal patients the physician can anticipate that the test will result in 54 true normals and 6 false positives or in a specificity of 90%. In the 40 patients with coronary heart disease the test will give a true positive result in 32 cases and a false normal test in 8 cases (sensitivity 80%). Based on this calculation the group of 100 patients provides 38 positive test results 32 of which stem from true positives and 6 from patients without significant lesions (false positives). Therefore, the revised likelihood of significant coronary artery disease in a patient with such a positive test result is 32/38 = 84% (TP/TP + FP) and 13% for a significant stenosis in presence of a normal test result (FN/FN + TN). These values represent the revised "a posteriori" likelihoods. The diagnostic likelihoods subsequently have been altered significantly by the test result, a dramatic change that a merely clinical approach will omit. Indeed, with the incorporation of a negative test result in the a priori likelihood of a suspected coronary heart disease has more than halved the chance for coronary artery disease or decreased by more than 100% and vice versa.

Value of a normal test

When a diagnostic test is reported as normal, the clinician uses it to rule out a suspected disease; however, a normal result may be of additional importance and help to differentiate among diagnoses that yield normal results with different frequencies [1, 8, 11]. A simple method allows the extraction of such information. The physician estimates the probability of various diagnoses and then combines these estimates with the anticipated frequency of negative results for each disease under consideration. Thus, the surface of a negative laboratory result may conceal information that helps to differentiate among possible diagnoses. Nevertheless, a negative test result offers insight into various important aspects of the diagnostic process:

1. Negative testing helps to identify and eliminate false positive results derived from clinical impression or from other tests with less predictive power;
2. Normal test results may exclude a specific disease in question and thus may help accelerate the process of differential diagnosis;
3. Negative test results on a specific issue may assess a benign prognosis and may avoid possibly dangerous, invasive procedures with questionable outcome;
4. May be very efficient in saving costs for unnecessary testing and procedures.

Serial testing

By combing the results of two diagnostic tests for the same disease the likelihood for the presence of the suspected disease can be markedley revised. By serial testing the a posteriori (post-test) likelihood of the first test becomes the a priori (pre-test) likelihood of the second test. Then, the revised a priori likelihood is combined with the sensitivity and specificy of the second test to calculate the new post-test likelihood. Table 4 shows three different patients in whom serial testing markedly revised the chance for suspected coronary heart disease and, thus, offers important additional information for further decisions in regards to coronary intervention.

Serial testing exemplified by perfusion imaging

A classic example of the value of likelihood analysis in the noninvasive diagnosis of coronary artery disease is adopted from pretest likelihood tables by Diamond and Forrester [7]. According to demographic information and risk factors a (model) 45-year-old man with nonanginal chest pain has a pretest likelihood of coronary artery disease of 15% (Figure 2). As a result of a positive ECG stress test his post-test likelihood increased to 32%, an intermediate value most likely to benefit from additional testing. Subsequently a wall motion stress test (revealing abnormalities) and fluoroscopic evidence of coronary calcifications were positive thereby increasing the likelihood of coronary artery disease to 82%. At this point a radionuclide perfusion study using either thallium-201 or Tc-99m Mibi would enhance the likelihood to 99% (when an abnormality is present), while a normal perfusion scan would decrease the likelihood to 46%.

Table 4. Calculations are based on an estimated sensitivity and specifity for exercise ECG (ST-segment depression ≥ 0.1 mV): 60% and 80%, respectively. For the perfusion scan sensitivity and specifity were both estimated as 85%.

	Pre-test likelihood	Exercise ECG ST $\downarrow \geq 0.1$ mV	Perfusion scan (^{201}TI, Tc-99m MIBI)
m, 58 yrs, nonanginal chest pain	21%	+ 43%	+ 80% / − 9%
		− 11%	+ 41% / − 2%
m, 45 yrs, atypical angina	46%	+ 75%	+ 94% / − 34%
		− 33%	+ 74% / − 8%
m, 33 yrs, typical angina	70%	+ 88%	+ 97% / − 56%
		− 54%	+ 87% / − 13%

The physician cannot only weigh up the cumulative impact of age, risk factors and discordant or concordant test results, but has to evaluate the cost effectiveness of various tests before using them. In this particular case, a positive radionuclide myocardial perfusion scan adds some information concerning the likelihood of coronary artery disease, whereas a negative perfusion scan brings one back again to a post-test probability in the intermediate range. Thus, the test would substantially increase costs as shown in a cost comparison of various non-invasive tests without having any impact on the decision to perform coronary angiography or not (Figure 3). In this particular patient, triple vessel disease was eventually documented angiographically. Although in this case perfusion imaging was not required to initiate angiography, it may, however, be of specific value after the diagnosis of coronary disease has been established to identify the culprit lesion (in the setting of multivessel disease) if an intervention such as angioplasty is considered for prognostic reasons. (See Chapters 9, 10 and 22.)

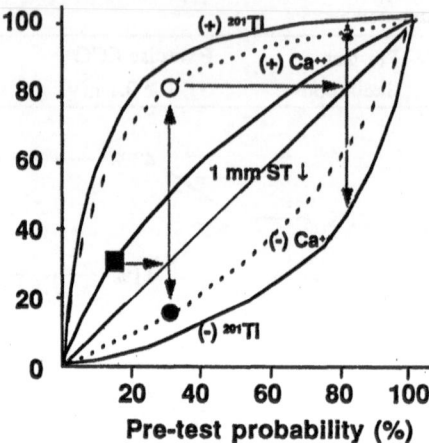

Figure 2. Illustration of the influence of serial testing with different diagnostic methods on the post-test likelihood of coronary artery disease. The closed circle represents a model patient with a pre-test likelihood of CAD of 15% and a 1.0 mm depression of the ST-segment with stress (heavy solid line) resulting in a post-test likelihood of 32%; the post-test likelihood would rise to 82% in presence of calcium (Ca^{2+}) on fluoroscopy and in absence of calcium fall to 14%. An additional positive (pathological) radionuclide (thallium) myocardial perfusion scan would enhance the post-test probability to 99%; in case of a negative (normal) perfusion scan the post-test probability of a significant (flow limiting) stenosis would be markedly decreased to 43% even with calcium present at fluoroscopy. (Modified and adopted, with permission from the New England Journal of Medicine, from: Diamond GA, Forrester JS. Analysis of probability as an aid in the clinical diagnosis of coronary artery disease. N Engl J Med 1979; 300: 1350–8.)

Alternative testing and cost considerations

Certain more specialized tests provide important information that may be vital in individual patients in whom there are unanswered questions, for example, on myocardial viability after a clinical infarction to be unambiguously addressed to the diagnostic expert. But still, as long as viability testing does not specifically relate to the question of benefit, such tests serve mainly for scientific objectives and still await broad acceptance as a clinical routine [5, 7, 10, 16, 17, 30]. Metabolic interrogation using PET and fluoro-18-deoxyglucose has been thought to represent the most accurate test for assessment of regional myocardial viability today. However, a preliminary comparison to thallium-201 reinjection SPECT and dobutamine echocardiography has suggested that stimulated wall motion, thallium-201 uptake and fluoro-18-deoxyglucose metabolism may have fewer discrepancies than anticipated. Thus, the proportion of patients who might benefit from analysis of myocardial viability using fluorine-18 fluorodeoxyglucose PET after thallium-201 reinjection studies remains open to question. More importantly, clinical stra-

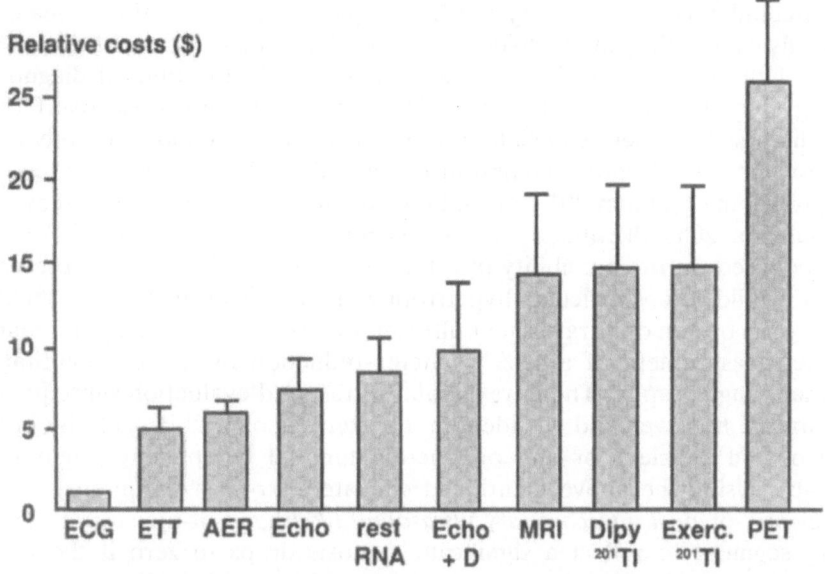

Figure 3. Relative costs of various non-invasive cardiovascular diagnostic tests calculated in relation to that of a resting electrocardiogram. ECG, electrocardiogram; ETT, exercise treadmill test; AER, ambulatory electrocardiographic recording; Echo, transthoracic echocardiography; PET, positron emission tomography; RNA, radionuclide angiography; D, Doppler ultrasound; MRI, magnetic resonance imaging; Dipy, dipyridamole. (Reproduced and modified with permission from O'Rourke, RA: Cost considerations. In: Pohost, GM, O'Rourke RA. Principles and Practice of Cardiovascular Imaging. Boston: Little & Brown, Inc., 1991.)

tegies that are not based on the potential of benefit may result in harm; to justify testing strategies, there must be the high likelihood that additional clinically relevant information is worth the additional costs (Figure 3). Quality control in medicine will be based quite properly on outcome research and thus demands a balanced assessment of the medical value as well as the cost of the various testing strategies.

The normal intravascular ultrasound scan

Another example is a 52-year-old employee with a history of atypical chest pain, past history of smoking and borderline arterial hypertension of 140/95 mm Hg. He is slightly obese and his 12 lead stress-ECG was not diagnostic and limited to 3 minutes of 75 watts due to a systolic arterial blood pressure of 210 mm Hg; at this stage no significant ST segment depression and no classic anginal symptoms were encountered. A thallium SPECT perfusion study after dipyridamole vasodilatory stress revealed a reversible defect confined to the lateral myocardium and suggestive of a stenosis of the circumflex coronary artery (CFX). Angiographic evaluation revealed a normally contracting, mildly hypertrophied left ventricle and a mid circumflex lesion with an estimated 70% diameter stenosis. At the time of diagnostic angiography the question of interventional therapy by use of elective PTCA was discussed. Expert clinicians estimated a 80% likelihood of the CFX stenosis to significantly comprovize lateral wall perfusion based on symptoms, the thallium-201 scan and the angiographic morphology; they also estimated a 20% likelihood of a nonsignificant obstruction to CFX flow mainly based on the possibility of a false positive thallium scan in presence of even mild left ventricular hypertrophy. In the clinical decision making process the option of intravascular ultrasound assessment came up stimulated by the measurement of a 45% diameter reduction by use of quantitative coronary angiography. The intravascular ultrasound evaluation subsequently performed, however, did not identify any stenosis or wall irregularity in the interrogated segment or any obstructing luminal component (Figures 4a and 4b). Using the above mentioned educated expert assumptions, the "a posteriori" or *post intracoronary ultrasound likelihood* of the suspected coronary segment to reflect a significant stenosis drops to zero if the IVUS study is accepted as the best standard for exclusion of significant coronary obstructions. The normal post-IVUS vessel diameter provides such a dramatic change in the quantitative lesion characterization that an angioplasty intervention appears not to be justified at this time.

This example of reassessing the significance of a given *angiographic* stenosis by an independent *intravascular ultrasound* evaluation is certainly sensitive to the input estimates of probability; however, irrespective of the actual likelihood figures, any superior method that has proven to be useful for quantitative characterization of any given morphological lesion will overrule the information provided by a less accurate technique. In the near future, it is conceivable that functional assessment using Doppler flow wires with high precision for vasodilator reserve or truly quantitative perfusion imaging with PET may shed even more light onto the vexing problem of imprecise assessment of lesion severity by angiography and may help to better reassess the true significance of a given lesion [27, 38, 39, 40].

Interestingly however, using a qualitative (visual) or semiquantitative approach, the superiority of PET compared to SPECT for lesion characterization has not yet been established. Demer et al. assessed dipyridamole PET using coronary flow reserve derived from quantitative coronary angiography to determine the presence of significant CAD in 193 patients, 69 of whom had prior myocardial infarction. If a coronary flow reserve ≥4 was considered normal, dipyridamole PET had a sensitivity of 94% and a specificity of 74% for detecting coronary artery disease; with flow reserve ≥3 considered as normal, dipyridamole PET had a sensitivity of 82% and a specificity of 95%. These values are strikingly similar to those observed with SPECT TI-201 or Tc-99m-Mibi imaging, respectively (Tables 2 and 3). These new techniques which are emerging as today's gold standards for the functional significance

A

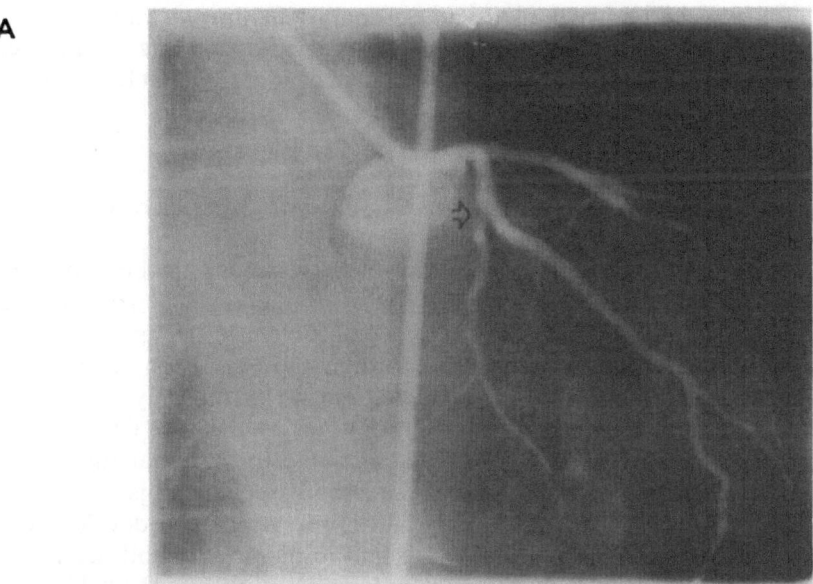

B

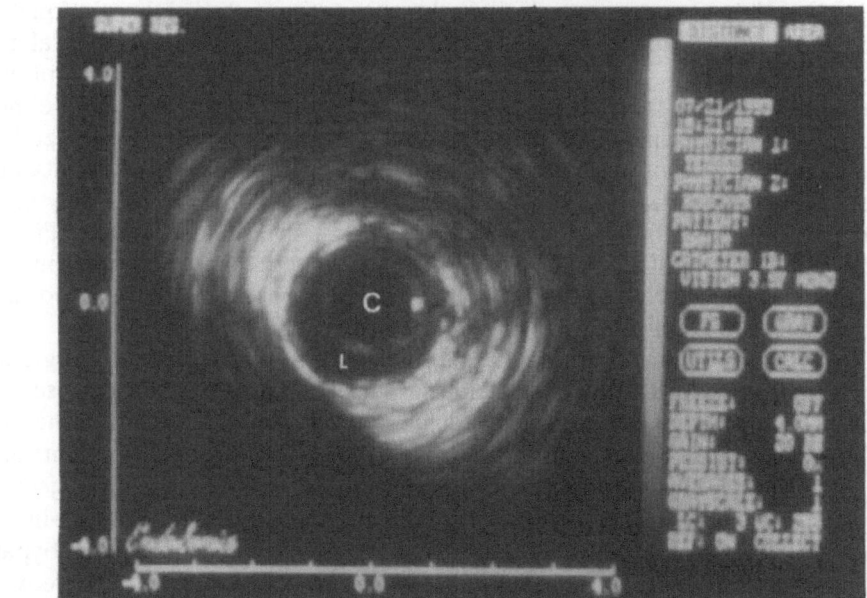

Figure 4. (a) Coronary angiogram in 30 degree RAO projection showing a proximal lesion in the left circumflex coronary artery of 70% diameter reduction consistent with a moderate reduction of calculated coronary flow reserve (arrow). This lesion was also documented in LAO projection. (b) The above depicted angiographic segment was subsequently interrogated by intravascular ultrasound using a 3.5 French diagnostic intravascular catheter (20 MHz) guided over a conventional PTCA guidewire. The CFX segment suspicious of a moderate stenosis on angiography showed an entirely normal lumen (L) by intravascular ultrasound and revealed consistantly an intraluminal diameter of 2.4 mm with no evidence of local atheroma, and normal intimal and media layers.

of a lesion are more likely to justify no coronary "*therapeutic*" intervention if the test result is negative, and thus may avoid unnecessary costs and protect patients from useless risks of interventional procedures unlikely to be of benefit (such as cosmetic or "prognostic" PTCA).

Stress testing in patients with asymptomatic coronary artery disease

Decision making in therapy is easiest when the treatment has been proved to be effective in achieving important goals for the patients and can be applied with low morbidity and mortality. The problem of the asymptomatic patient with a left anterior descending coronary artery lesion is one that occurs not infrequently in practice. When surgery was the only alternative to medical therapy, the decision was easier than today with PTCA. The uncertainties of definite benefit of revascularization in these patients, combined with the certain morbidity of a thoracotomy, weighed against bypass surgery and argued for medical therapy and observation. The development of PTCA with its high initial success rate and low mortality and morbidity makes the decision not to perform revascularization more difficult [24, 29, 40–43] mainly for two reasons, first, the temptation for the interventionalist for immediate action, and second, the vexing problem of self-referral for PTCA. There is no evidence in the literature that in absence of symptoms or silent ischemia, as defined by ST segment and changes in T wave either spontaneously occurring or precipitated by exercise, any revascularization procedure will be of any prognostic benefit for the individual patient. Conversely however, there is convincing evidence that silent ischemia may have prognostic significance similar to angina [24, 25, 32, 33] as depicted in Figure 5; thus regardless of coronary lesion morphology, especially in asymptomatic patients both negative and positive test results for ischemia have important impact on the recommended treatment strategy.

In practice, many angiographers consider the presence of a high-grade, proximal coronary arterial obstruction, especially in the left anterior descending coronary artery, an indication for angioplasty with or without ischemia. There is a certain temptation of treating angiograms rather than patients and a lingering "oculo-stenotic reflex" to perform angioplasty with no objective evidence of myocardial ischemia [30]. However, ignoring negative non-invasive tests may expose the patient to a cycle of early restenosis and bypass surgery sooner than the natural history would dictate [44, 45]. Moreover, there is objective evidence from the large randomized studies of surgical versus medical management, that revascularization of a single-vessel obstruction in symptomatic patients has no advantages over medical management, neither in survival nor in avoiding myocardial infarction [24, 25, 27, 28, 29, 38]. Although controversial, there is evidence that not all patients in the *single-vessel disease* category have the same prognosis and that symptomatic patients with high-grade proximal lesions of the left anterior descending

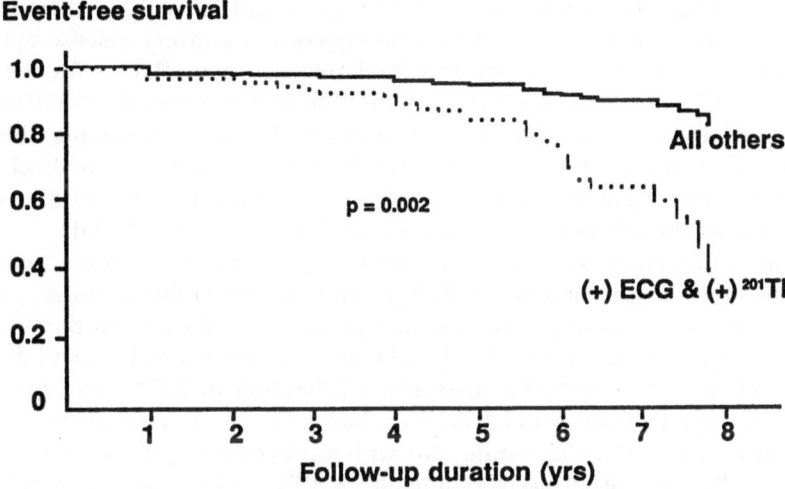

Figure 5. Relation between event-free survival and time of follow-up in 407 asymptomatic subjects stratified by the combination of a positive stress ECG and pathological thallium-201 scan as compared to all other test constellations associated with at least one negative finding (either ECG or perfusion imaging). The incidence of cardiac events was significantly lower in those who had either a normal thallium or ECG test – or both. By proportional hazard analysis, a concordant positive result predicted an 3.6 fold risk for a coronary event, independent of risk factors. Adopted from Fleg JL et al. Prevalence and prognostic significance of exercise-induced silent myocardial ischemia detected by thallium scintigraphy and ECG in asymptomatic volunteers. Circulation 1990; 81: 428. (Reproduced with permission from the American Heart Association, Inc.)

coronary artery are at higher risk than either those with more distal lesions of the left anterior descending coronary artery, or those with proximal right coronary artery or left circumflex coronary artery lesions. Califf and colleagues reported the annual mortality of patients with proximal left anterior descending coronary artery disease to be 2% per year compared with 0.4% per year mortality for patients with distal left anterior descending coronary artery lesions [28]. The mortality even in the patients with proximal lesions, syptomatic or silent, is low. There is some evidence, however, that selected patients with proximal left anterior descending coronary lesions can benefit from revascularization compared with those managed medically [24, 29]. With the use of the internal mammary artery as a bypass, long-term patency has proved to be excellent, and if it is accepted that the prognosis of asymptomatic patients with evidence of ischemia by noninvasive testing is similar to that of patients with angina, a case could be made for bypass surgery. There is, however, no randomized study in asymptomatic patients with left anterior descending coronary artery obstruction to demonstrate convincing benefit of surgical or interventional revascularization compared to medical therapy.

The unrandomized portion of the CASS study indicates that symptomatic patients with single left anterior descending coronary artery disease and left ventricular dysfunction do better with bypass surgery than with medical therapy. The only nonrandomized study with PTCA showed no difference in survival in patients with one- or two-vessel disease involving the left anterior descending artery, between PTCA (95% survival) and medical therapy (93% survival) at five years. On subgroup analysis patients with ejection fractions less than 50% had a better survival after PTCA [24, 25].

Against the background of these possible survival benefits of revascularization in symptomatic patients with left anterior descending coronary artery disease we have to consider the definite problems of PTCA. In the NHLBI registry the incidence of PTCA-related complications in single-vessel disease was death in 0.2%, nonfatal myocardial infarction in 3.5%, and need for emergency bypass surgery in 2.9%. The chance of one of these adverse events to occur is 5.5% [41]. Combining this with a procedural 3.9% occlusion rate and a 3.5% rate of prolonged angina, a 10% failure rate to achieve a satisfactory result, and a late restenosis rate of 25–35% of patients with some of these requiring second procedures or even bypass surgery, the attractiveness of the PTCA option for an asymptomatic patient diminishes markedly. Furthermore, if collateral vessels are present, there is probably a protective situation for the patient with a proximal left anterior descending lesion that would make extensive infarction less likely and, therefore, would mitigate against revascularization in the asymptomatic patient.

With all of these factors considered, a myocardial perfusion scan *negative* for inducible ischemia may justify no interventional action [44, 45]. With no evidence of a large volume of ischemic myocardium, such a patient is at no increased risk of an adverse event regardless of whether the subjective symptom of angina pectoris is present. Considering the benign prognosis to begin with, the indication for expensive and potentially dangerous interventions should be reviewed with great scrutiny. Conversely, in patients with evidence of redistribution (reversible perfusion defects) interventional revascularization may be justified (and beneficial) and is especially compelling in presence of reduced left ventricular function at rest or with exercise, indicative of both reduced contractile reserve and significant amount of ischemic myocardium.

As these cases suggest, normal findings may not only save costs by avoiding useless interventions, but are valuable in the differential diagnosis. Only when a normal test result occurs with nearly equal frequency among all the diseases being considered will a negative finding contribute little or nothing to the diagnostic process. Although most physicians will agree that the use of prevalence and likelihood analysis (including negative test results) should, in principle, contribute importantly to the process of differential diagnosis, many argue that its value is limited by the difficulty of choosing the appropriate probabilities. They are troubled, in particular, by the fact that data defining the incidence of normal findings are frequently difficult to obtain or, even when they are available, often quite imprecise [12, 26, 43, 46]. To deal with the inevitable uncertainties of estimates, however, the physician can estimate the errors in the likelihoods used, and recalculate the diagnostic profile from the extreme values. The range of diagnostic likelihoods obtained in this fashion establishes the limits of the revised probabilities. In many instances, the deviations from the physician's own best estimates will be relatively small and the range of likelihoods is consistent with the available data. Improved accuracy of differential diagnosis resulting from the more effective use of normal findings should improve patient care by aiding clinicians in the process of making sound decisions such as first, to avoid the invasive diagnostic intervention of coronary angiography in presence of a test result *negative* for an physiologically significant obstructive coronary lesion, and second, to justify no interventional or surgical revascularization procedure in *absence* of any potential for therapeutic or prognostic benefit.

Acknowledgements

The authors are endebted to Miss Jeanette Hoffmann for her expert secretarial assistance, to Miss Dörte Oestreich for the graphical support and to Dietmar H. Koschyk, M.D. for the intravascular ultrasound image.

References

1. Gorry GA, Pauker SG, Schwartz WB. The diagnostic importance of the normal finding. N Engl J Med 1978; 298: 486–9.
2. Rifkin RD, Hood WB Jr. Bayesian analysis of electrocardiographic exercise stress testing. N Engl J Med 1977; 297: 681–6.
3. Ladenheim ML, Kotler TS, Pollock BH et al. Incremental prognostic power of exercise electrocardiography and myocardial perfusion scintigraphy in suspected coronary artery disease. Am J Cardiol 1987; 59: 270–7.
4. Varetto T, Cantalupi D, Alberto Alteieri A, Orlandi C. Emergency room Technetium-99m Sestamibi imaging to rule out acute myocardial ischemic events in patients with nondiagnostic electrocardiograms. J Am Coll Cardiol 1993; 22: 1804–8.
5. Grayboys TB, Bieglson B, Lambert S et al. Results of a second opinion trial among patients recommended for coronary arteriography. J Am Med Assoc 1992; 268: 2537–40.
6. Fattah AA, Kamal AM, Pancholy S, Iskandrian AS. Prognostic implications of normal exercise tomographic thallium images in patients with angiographic evidence of significant coronary artery disease. Am J Cardiol 1994; 74:769–71.
7. Diamond GA, Forrester JS. Analysis of probability as an aid in the clinical diagnosis of coronary artery disease. N Engl J Med 1979; 300: 1350–8.
8. Fortuin NJ, Weiss JL. Reviews of contemporary laboratory methods. Circulation 1977; 56: 699–712.
9. Melin JA, Piret LJ, Vanbutsele RJM et al. Diagnostic value of exercise electrocardiography and thallium myocardial scintigraphy in patients without previous myocardial infarction: A Bayesian approach. Circulation 1981; 63: 1019–24.
10. Sivarajan Froelicher E. Usefulness of exercise testing shortly after acute myocardial infarction for predicting 10–year mortality. Am J Cardiol 1994; 74:318–23.

11. Brown KA, Boucher CA, Okada RD et al. Prognostic value of exercise thallium-201 imaging in patients presenting for evaluation of chest pain . JACC 1983; 1: 994–1001.
12. Schwartz WB, Gorry GA, Kassirer JP et al. Decision analysis and clinical judgment. Am J Med 1973; 55: 459–72.
13. Mc Neil BJ, Keeler E, Adelstein SJ. Primer on certain elements of medical decision making. N Engl J Med 1975; 293: 211–5.
14. Patton DD. Introduction to clinical decision making. Semin Nucl Med 1978; 8: 273–82.
15. Dixon J, Margolis J. Accuracy of exercise tests: Role of patient selection. Circulation 1976; 54 (Suppl): II-205.
16. Eagle KA, Coley CM, Newell JB et al. Combining clinical and thallium data optimizes preoperative assessment of cardiac risk before major vascular surgery. Ann Intern Med 1989; 110: 859–66.
17. Sox HC Jr, Littenberg B, Garber A. The Role of exercise testing in screening for coronary artery disease. Ann Intern Med 1989; 110: 456–69.
18. Weiner DA, Ryan TJ, McCabe CH et al. Exercise Stress Testing. Correlations among history of angina, ST-segment response and prevalence of coronary-artery-disease in the Coronary Artery Surgery Study (CASS). N Engl J Med 1979; 301: 230–5.
19. O'Rourke RA. Clinical decisions for post-myocardial infarction patients. Mod Concepts Cardiovasc Dis 1986; 55: 55–60.
20. The Multicenter Post-Infarction Research Group. Risk stratification and survival after myo-cardial infarction. N Engl J Med 1983; 309: 331–9.
21. Alderman EL, Bourassa MG, Cohen LS et al. Ten-year follow-up of survival and myocardial infarction in the Randomized Coronary Artery Surgery Study. Circulation 1990; 82: 1629–38.
22. Myers WO, Davis K, Foster ED et al. Surgical survival in the Coronary Artery Surgery Study (CASS) Registry. Ann Thorac Surg 1985; 40: 246–301.
23. Demer LL, Gould KL, Goldstein RA et al. Assessment of coronary artery disease severity by positron emission tomography: Comparison with quantitative arteriography in 193 pa-tients. Circulation 1989; 79: 825–34.
24. Parisi AF, Folland ED, Hartigan P. On behalf of the Veterans Affairs ACME Investigators. A comparison of angioplasty with medical therapy in the treatment of single-vessel coronary artery disease. N Engl J Med. 1992; 326:10–6.
25. Ellis SG, Fisher L, Dushman-Ellis S et al. Comparison of 3–5 year mortality and infarction rates after angioplasty (PTCA) or medical therapy for 1 or 2 vessel left anterior descending disease. Circulation 1987; 76: IV-392.
26. Little WC, Constantinescu M, Applegate RJ et al. Can coronary angiography predict the site of a subsequent myocardial infarction in patients with mild-to-moderate coronary artery disease? Circulation 1988; 78: 1157–63.
27. Brooks N, Cattall M, Jennings K et al. Isolated disease of left anterior descending coronary artery: Angiographic and clinical study of 218 patients. Br Heart J 1987; 47: 71–8.
28. Califf RM, Tomabechi Y, Lee K et al. Outcome in one vessel coronary artery disease. Circulation 1983; 67: 283–90.
29. Kouchoukas NT, Oberman O, Russell RO et al. Surgical versus medical treatment of occlusive disease compared to the left anterior descending coronary artery. Am J Cardiol 1975; 35: 836–43.
30. Topol EJ, Ellis SG, Cosgrove DM et al. Analysis of coronary angioplasty practice in the United States with an insurance claims data base. Circulation 1993; 87: 1489–97.
31. DeBusk RF. Specialized testing after recent acute myocardial infarction. Ann Intern Med 1989; 110: 470–81.
32. Chatterjee K. Ischemia: Silent or manifest – does it matter? J Am Coll Cardiol 1989; 13: 1503–6.
33. Villanueva FS, Smith WH, Watson DD, Beller GA. ST-segment depression during dipyrida-mole infusion, and its clinical, scintigraphic and hemodynamic correlates. Am J Cardiol 1992; 69: 445–8.

34. Leppo JA, O'Brien J, Rothendler JA et al. Dipyridamole-thallium-201 scintigraphy in the prediction of future cardiac events after acute myocardial infarction. N Engl J Med 1984; 310: 1014–8.

35. Boucher CA, Brewster DC, Darling RC et al. Determination of cardiac risk by dipyridamole-thallium imaging before peripheral vascular surgery. N Engl J Med 1985; 312; 389–94.

36. Bairey CN, Rozanski A, Maddahi J et al. Exercise Thallium-201 scintigraphy and prognosis in typical angina pectoris and negative exercise electrocardiography. Am J Cardiol 1989; 64: 282–7.

37. Pryor DB. The academic life cycle of a noninvasive test. Circulation 1990; 82: 302–4.

38. Folland ED, Vogel RA, Hartigan P et al. and the Veterans Affairs ACME Investigators. Relation between coronary artery stenosis assessed by visual, caliper, and computer methods and exercise capacity in patients with single-vessel coronary artery disease. Circulation 1994; 89: 2005–14.

39. Uren NG, Melin JA, De Bruyne B et al. Relation between myocardial blood flow and the severity of coronary artery stenosis. N Engl J Med 1994; 330: 1782–8.

40.. Miller DD, Donohue TJ, Younis LT et al. Correlation of pharmacological 99 mTC-sestamibi myocardial perfusion imaging with poststenotic coronary flow reserve in patients with angiographically intermediate coronary artery stenoses. Circulation 1994; 89: 2150–60.

41. Detre K, Holubkov R, Kelsery S et al. Percutaneous transluminal coronary angioplasty in 1985–1986 and 1977–1981: The National Heart, Lung and Blood Institute Registry. N Engl J Med 1988; 318: 256–61.

42. Bourassa MG, Noble J. Complication rate of coronary arteriography: A review of 5250 cases studied by a percutaneous femoral technique. Circulation 1976; 53: 106–11.

43. Ingelfinger FJ. Decision in medicine. N Engl J Med 1975; 293: 254–5.

44. Panter SG, Kopelman RI. Invasive interventions. N Engl J Med 1994; 331: 601–5.

45. Kern MJ, Bach RG. Clinical problem-solving: Invasive interventions (Letter). N Engl J Med 1995; 332: 125.

46. Kahn JK, McGhie I, Akers MS et al. Quantitative rotational tomography with Tl-201 and Tc-99m 2–methoxy-isobutyl-isonitrile: A direct comparison in normal individuals and patients with coronary artery disease. Circulation 1989; 79: 1282–93.

47. Ritchie JL, Trobaugh GB, Hamilton GW et al. Myocardial imaging with thallium-201 at rest and during exercise: Comparison with coronary arteriography and stress electrocardiography. Circulation 1977; 56: 6672.

48. Botvinick EH, Taradash MR, Shames DM et al. Thallium-201 myocardial perfusion scintigraphy for the clinical clarification of normal, abnormal, and equivocal electrocardiographic stress tests. Am J Cardiol 1978; 41: 43–9.

49. Borer JS, Bacharach SL, Green MV et al. Real-time radionuclide cineangiography in the noninvasive evaluation of global and regional left ventricular function at rest and during exercise in patients with coronary artery disease. N Engl J Med 1977; 296: 839.

50. Maddahi J, Garcia EV, Berman DS et al. Improved noninvasive assessment of coronary artery disease by quantitative analysis of regional stress myocardial distribution and washout of thallium-201. Circulation 1981; 64: 924–30.

51. Berger BC, Watson DD, Taylor GJ et al. Quantitative thallium-201 exercise scintigraphy for detection of coronary artery disease. J Nucl Med 1981; 22: 585–92.

52. Tamaki N, Yonekura Y, MukaiT et al. Stress thallium-201 transaxial emission computed tomography: Quantitative versus qualitative analysis for evaluation of coronary artery disease. J Am Coll Cardiol 1984; 4: 1213–9.

53. Garcia EV, Van Train K, Maddahi J et al. Quantification of rotational thallium-201 myocardial tomography. J Nucl Med 1985; 26: 17–24.

54. Beller GA. Role of nuclear cardiology in evaluating the total ischemic burden in coronary artery disease. Am J Cardiol 1987; 59, 31C.

55. Maddahi J, Kiat H, Van Train KF et al. Myocardial perfusion imaging with technetium-99m sestamibi SPECT in the evaluation of coronary artery disease. Am J Cardiol 1990; 66: 55E–62E.

56. Stewart R, Schwaiger M, Molina E et al. Comparison of rubidium-82 positron emission tomography and thallium-201 SPECT imaging for detection of coronary artery disease. Am J Cardiol 1991; 67: 1303–8.
57. Tamaki N, Yonekura Y, Senda M et al. Value and limitation of stress thallium-201 single photon emission computed tomography: Comparison with nitrogen-13 positron tomography. J Nucl Med 1988; 29: 1181–8.

Corresponding Author: Dr Christoph A. Nienaber, Department of Cardiology, University Hospital Eppendorf, Martinistrasse 52, D-20246, Hamburg, Germany

7. Interpretation of coronary angiograms prior to PTCA: Pitfalls and problems

RÜDIGER SIMON

Introduction

The indication for coronary angioplasty and related techniques has widened dramatically since its first application in 1977 [1]. Enhanced operator skills and improved technology have permitted an expanded use of interventional catheter methods in patients that were previously deemed too high risk or impossible candidates such as elderly patients, those with multiple or complex lesions, those with lesions at vessel origins, or patients with poor left ventricular function or prior bypass surgery [2].

A number of diagnostic procedures including exercise testing, scintigraphy, PET-scanning, and recently stress echocardiography have proven to be helpful in the decision for catheter-based coronary revascularization. Coronary angiography, however, has remained the cornerstone, since it not only outlines the anatomy and morphology of the coronary arteries, but it is also the basis for the selection of the strategy and technique to be used, the type and the size of the device for the procedure, as well for the estimation of procedural risk and potential side problems.

In addition to the fast development of interventional device technology, recent achievements in angiographic techniques have had a major role in the successfull expansion of angioplasty. The most important step in this field has been the advent of digital imaging to cardiac and coronary angiography. The improved quality of todays "on stage and on line" angiographic images in the cathlab prior to and during the procedure has significantly facilitated and accelerated interventional procedures [3, 4] In addition the routine use of multidirectional angulated views has proven very helpful in avoiding uncertainty in the interpretation of ambiguous situations.

Beside these improvements, however, there are still problems and pitfalls that can occur when interpreting angiograms prior to interventional procedures.

C.A. Nienaber and U. Sechtem (eds): Imaging and Intervention in Cardiology. 93–103.
© 1996 *Kluwer Academic Publishers.*

The submission angiogram

Anatomical problems

The coronary arterial circulation comprises straight as well as tortuous segments of the coronary arteries in a three dimensional space with multiple branching points, resulting in multiple overlapping and crossing parts of the vessels in the two-dimensional representation of angiography. Standard projections may fail to unveil the true degree of coronary disease. A typical example is shown in Figure 1. This 65-year-old patient was submitted for an angioplasty of his severely obstructed left circumflex artery: the other coronary vessels were described as non-obstructed by the submitting investigators. Control angiography immediately before angioplasty, however, demonstrated that the patient had double vessel disease with an additional significant obstruction in the mid part of the left anterior descending artery, that could only be detected by an extremely angulated cranial view, that was not performed at the original investigation. Obviously, the risk as well as the strategy had to be reconsidered in this case: the LAD lesion was dilated first, than followed by circumflex artery angioplasty.

Multiple experiences like this one have led us to perform a *full* preprocedure angiography of both the left as well as the right coronary artery in all patients prior to any intervention.

The recanalization of chronic total occlusions of coronary arteries is a demanding task. In experienced hands, up to 70% of the attempts can be successful [5]. Strategy and final outcome, however, are dependent on an optimal estimation of the occluded segment. An optimal antegrade delineation of the artery proximal to the occlusion as well as distal to the occlusion by a sufficient opacification of all collateral pathways is neccesary. Since diagnostic angiographers often are not aware of the needs of the interventional operator many diagnostic angiograms submitted for potential catheter revascularization do not fulfill these requirements. Even immediately before the procedure, the diagnostic "roadmap" angiogram will sometimes not delineate the occluded segment sufficiently when the angiogram is performed in the classic sequential way with right coronary angiography after left coronary angiography and vice versa. For this situation we have switched to simultaneous biplane and biarterial coronary angiography, injecting contrast material into the right and the left coronary artery through two catheters at the same time in order to outline the anatomy of the occlusion to be treated as optimally as possible.

Sizing

Sizing the lesion and the artery to be treated is important for the selection of strategy and device for the intervention. There is agreement between most "angioplasters" that revascularization of vessels smaller than 2 mm is

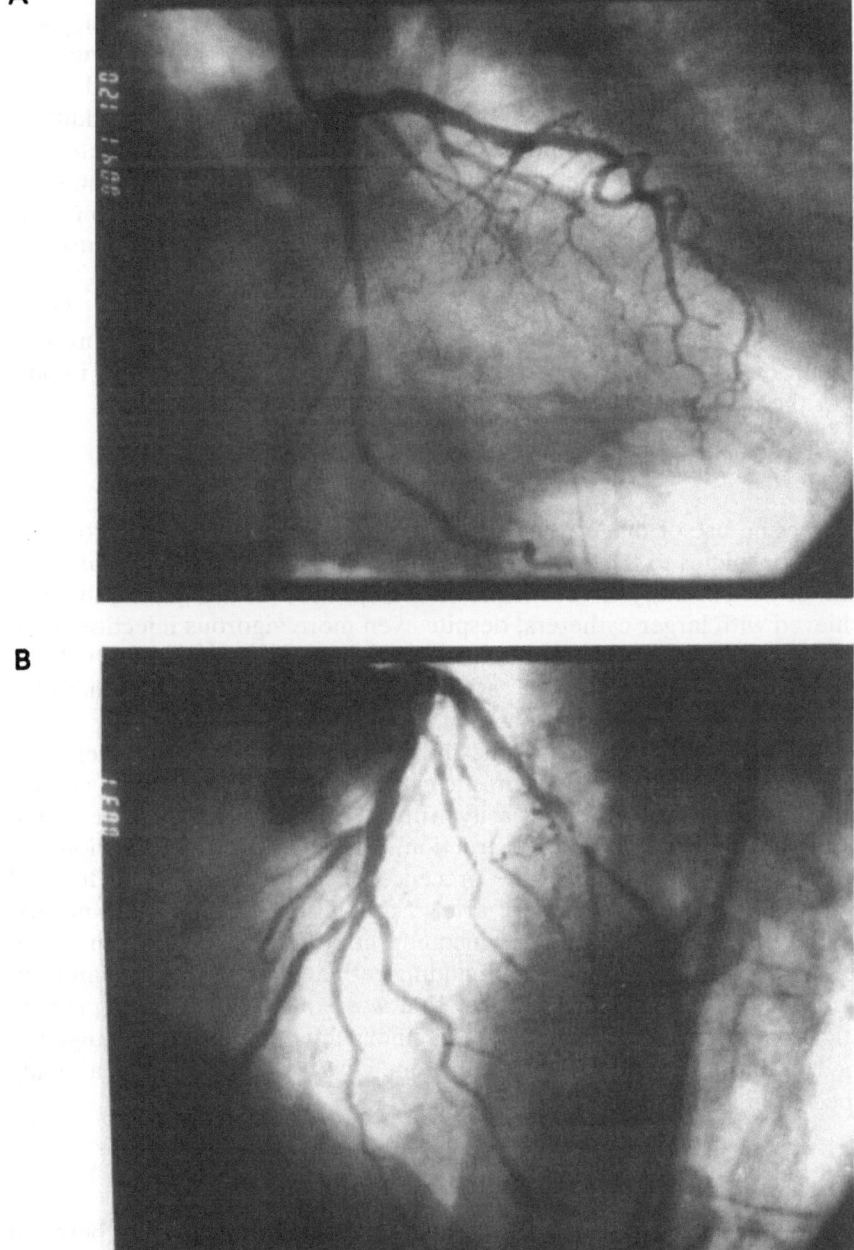

Figure 1. Sixty-five-year-old patient submitted for balloon angioplasty of a tight stenosis in the left circumflex artery (A). Control angiography immediately before the procedure disclosed an additional tight lesion in left anterior descending artery (B) in a cranial LAO-projection, that was not performed during the first diagnostic angiography.

associated with increasing complications and decreasing long term success rates. Sizing of the vessels and lesions under scrutinity from previous diagnostic angiograms, however, has become difficult with increasing use of multiple sizes and brands of diagnostic catheters. The size of the catheter used in the submission angiogram is often unknown to the "angioplaster". In addition, variations in X-ray density and variations in actual catheter diameters as compared to its claimed diameter may render estimations based on catheters as scaling factor erroneous [6]. Out-of-plane errors can further add to uncertainty, which may have particular importance with small catheters, since the error increases with a decreasing size of the scaling object.

Another problem arises from the fact that many angiograms are taken without vasodilation by nitrates or comparable drugs. Thus, the primary angiogram often does not allow an appropriate appreciation of the importance of the perfusion area distal to the lesion.

Problems with small catheters

The increasing use of diagnostic catheters of sizes below 6 F has introduced additional problems to the interpretation of angiograms. The degree of opacification of the coronary circulation is not comparable to the quality that can be achieved with larger catheters, despite even more vigorous injection force exerted by the investigator. This more vigorous injection may potentially be dangerous due to faster jet at the catheter tip with a smaller lumen that may set the stage for endothelial damage and/or dissection.

The use of these small catheters has introduced another new problem that we have not seen with larger diagnostic catheters. Due to the small catheter tip, the artery may be entered easily without any drop in pressure in the presence of a significant ostial obstruction. Vigorous contrast injection can lead to brisk backflow even in the precence of more than 70% of luminal narrowing in a left main coronary artery, thus displaying a pseudo-normal ostial look of the artery. We have encountered a number of cases in whom the first intubation with a 7 F or 8 F guiding catheter discovered a significant lesion of the left main coronary artery that was not detected at the primary investigation. (Figure 2). Obviously, this unexpected finding will change the planned dilatation of a mid LAD lesion from a low-risk procedure to a totally unexpected high-risk procedure.

Time factor

Due to limited capacity a considerable interval has to be allowed for between the primary diagnostic angiogram and angioplasty in many centers. Within this time, the aspect of the lesion to be treated may alter and may change the technical approach or the indication for any given procedure. In some patients, high grade lesions progress to total occlusions. These occlusions can most often be reopened easily, since the occlusion time has been short.

A

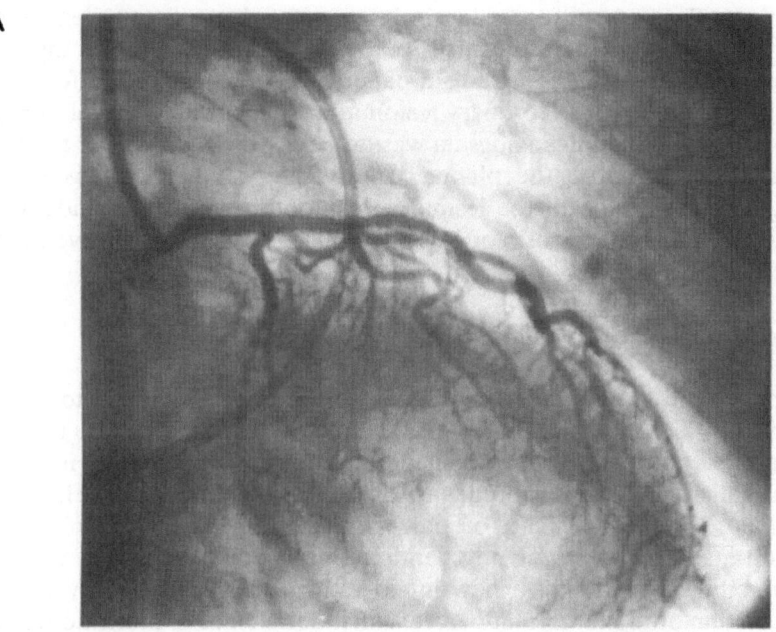

B

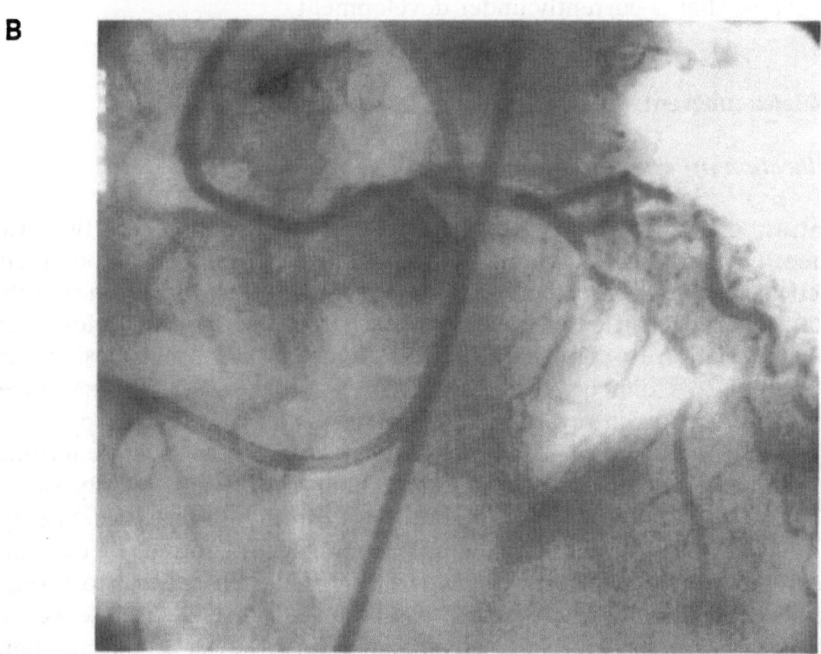

Figure 2. Sixty-seven-year-old female patient submitted for an angioplasty of a mid-LAD-lesion. Submission angiogram (A) displayed a normal aspect of the left main coronary artery. Control angiography immediately before the procedure unveiled a tight stenosis at the aortal orifice of the left main coronary artery (B).

Sometimes, however a regression in lesions severity and complexity can be observed, and this is particularly seen in patients early after myocardial infarction. Figure 3 demonstrates a patient who was submitted for atherectomy of a complex right coronary lesion after inferior myocardial infarction. The original submission angiogram was taken about 10 days after the infarct. The angiogram before the planned intervention, taken two weeks later, displayed a regression of the lesion with smoothing of the boundaries, and a residual diameter stenosis of less than 30%, so that an intervention was not felt to be necessary.

Filmless catheterization laboratory

Recently, a move towards the filmless catheterization laboratory can be observed in Europe as well as in the United States. Since so far there is no standard for the exchange of angiograms primarily acquired in a digital format, angiograms are stored and exchanged mainly on SVHS or VHS videotapes. The poor quality of many of these tapes is often prohibitive for decision-making concerning interventional procedures, so that in a considerable number of patients, a new angiogram of sufficient quality has to be taken on film or digital format before a final decision as to indication, strategy and device choice can be made [7, 8]. This undesirable dilemma will hopefully be solved, when a new standard for digital storage of coronary angiograms will evolve that is currently under development.

Problems inherent with angiography

Delineation of lesion morphology

Contrast angiography can only provide a "shadowgram" of the arterial lumen. Furthermore, only a limited number of projections can be taken for practical reasons. Since there is no available solution for an on-line three-dimensional reconstruction of the coronary tree, the operator is left with his own imagination to appreciate the full impact of a coronary lesion from a number of two dimensional projections. Comparison with other imaging techniques such as intravascular ultrasound (IVUS) or angioscopy have demonstrated, that significant differences may occur between these techniques and the angiographic aspect of a lesion comprising lesion severity and complexity as well as the presence or absence of thrombi, dissections, aneurysms or other features [9–11]. Angiography may suggest normal or only mildly diseased coronary arteries whereas IVUS – by design capable to reveal the thickness and composition of the vascular wall – may disclose advanced intimal hyperplasia, intimal plaque formation or even significant luminal obstructions [12]. It has therefore been questioned, whether angiography is an appropriate tool to estimate the degree of coronary artery disease. Recent

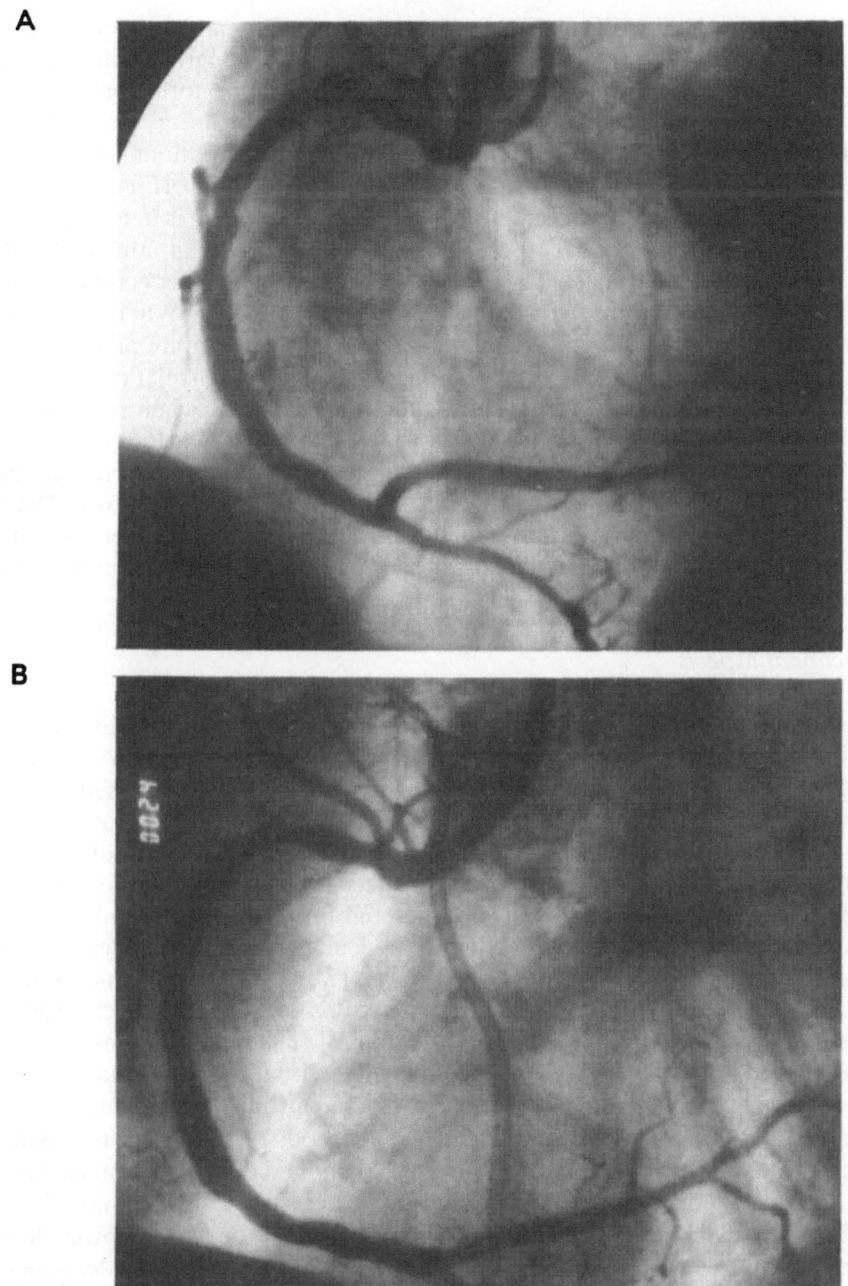

Figure 3. Regression of a complex lesion with time. (A) Complex aspect of a proximal RCA-obstruction early after myocardial infarction in a 61-year-old female patient submitted for directional atherectomy. (B) Lesion aspect in the same projection 5 weeks later, immediately before the intervention: lesion borders have smoothed, and quantitative analysis resulted in a 40% residual lesion, so that no intervention was performed.

thorough investigations including quantitative measurements of coronary lesions from calibrated simultaneous biplane coronary angiograms and simultaneous intravascular ultrasound registrations in our laboratories have shown that significant disagreements between angiography and intravascular ultrasound seem to occur primarily immediately after an interventional procedure, when the boundaries of the lesion are irregular and rough (Figure 4, midpanel). It is conceivable that under these conditions, a lesion is better appreciated by the "cross-sectional" IVUS display than the "longitudinal" angiographic display. Intimal flaps, local thrombi and dissections after interventional therapy may further add to the uncertainty. When untreated segments are compared, the correlation between angiography and IVUS is much better (Figure 4, upper panel). Interestingly, the correlation becomes better again at follow-up angiography 3 to 6 months later, when remodelling of the stenosis has led to smoother lesion borders (Figure 4, lower panel).

Finally it has to be mentioned, that discrepant results reported in the literature can be due to the fact that comparative measurements from IVUS and angiography registrations at exactly the same point in a vessel are not a trivial task, so that some of the differences could be due to non-identical measuring points.

Functional aspects

The functional impact of a coronary lesion is estimated traditionally from its angiographic appearance, that may visually be translated into a percentage obstruction of diameter and cross section by the operator, or assessed quantitatively by automatic detection methods (QCA). Although contrast density and run-off can be taken into consideration in addition to morphology, it is difficult to appreciate the physiologic impact of a coronary lesion from a subjective visual assessment of the angiogram. When "eyeballing" the stenosis, operators tend to overestimate the lesion before and underestimate the lesion after an interventional procedure. The application of quantitative coronary angiography (QCA) has improved this estimation process. QCA, primarily developed in animal experiments [13], has been demonstrated to be valid also in patients [14]. In uncomplicated situations, this analysis is in good agreement with other methods to assess the physiologic impact of a lesion on coronary hemodynamics. On-line methods for QCA are now available for most cathlab equipments, that can be applied during the intervention and provide the investigator with quantitative results within 2 minutes, thus enabling a rapid decision making process prior to and during the procedure. In more complex situations, however, with multiple sequential lesions or long complex lesions including vessel bending, QCA will be of limited value. In this situation, additional methods are necessary and available today: IVUS, angioscopy and Doppler-tipped catheters or guide wires have been used as an extension to angiography. These techniques, that should not be regarded as replacements but as complementary techniques to angiography,

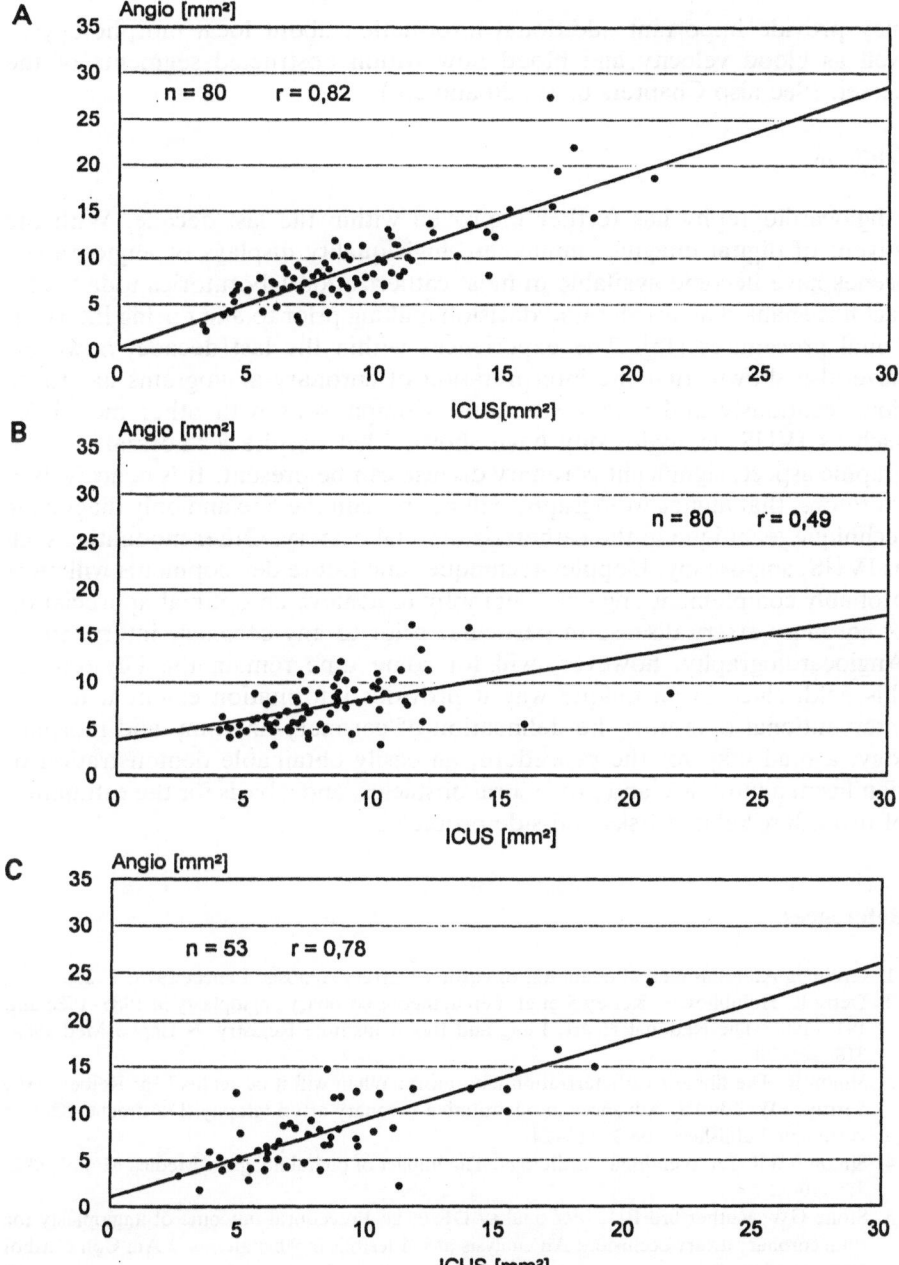

Figure 4. Comparison of minimal luminal area of a stenosed vessel assessed at the same site by intracoronary ultrasound (ICUS) and quantative biplane angiocardiography (angio) immediately and late after atherectomy. (A) Measurements of untreated segments distal to the lesion. (B) Measurements at the site of the directional atherectomy immediately after the intervention. (C) Measurements at the site of the directional atherectomy 3 to 6 months after the intervention. All assessments have been performed in the same patients.

may provide important additional information about local morphology as well as blood velocity and blood flow within obstructed segments of the vessel. (See also Chapters 6, 19, 20 and 25.)

Outlook

Angiocardiography has further improved within the last decade. With the advent of digital imaging, immediate high quality displays of angiographic scenes have become available in most catherization laboratories today. This fact has enabled an accelerated decision making prior to and during interventional procedures [15]. The experiences within the last decade, however, have also shown, that the interpretation of coronary angiograms has to be done cautiously and with restrictions. Comparisons with other modalities such as IVUS or angioscopy have shown, that despite a "normal" angiographic aspect, significant coronary disease can be present. It is conceivable, therefore, that angiocardiography will not remain the one and only diagnostic technique technique in the catheterization laboratory. Other modalities such as IVUS, angioscopy, Doppler-techniques and future developments will most probably complement angiocardiography to achieve an optimal appreciation of coronary artery disease in particular prior to any coronary intervention. Angiocardiography, however, will for some time remain the keystone in this field, since in an unique way it provides information essential for the interventional operator: the delineation of coronary anatomy and morphology, a road map for the procedure, an easily obtainable demonstration of significant anatomical and procedural obstacles, and a basis for the estimation of procedure related risks and side problems.

References

1. Grüntzig A. Transluminal dilatation of coronary-artery stenosis. Lancet 1978; 1: 263.
2. Detre K, Holubhov R, Kelsey S et al. Percutaneous coronary angioplasty in 1985–1986 and 1977–1981. The National Heart, Lung and Blood Institute Registry. N Engl J Med 1988; 318: 265–70.
3. Simon R. The filmless catheterization laboratory: When will it be reality? In: Reiber JHL, Serruys PW, editors. Advances in quantitative coronary arteriography. Dordrecht: Kluwer Academic Publishers, 1993: 113–24.
4. Simon RWR. Interventional cardiology: The impact of digital imaging. Medica Mundi 1992; 37: 110–4.
5. Stone GW, Rutherford BD, McConahay DR et al. Procedural outcome of angioplasty for total coronary artery occlusion: An analysis of 971 lesions in 905 patients. J Am Coll Cardiol 1990; 15: 849–56.
6. Reiber JHC, van der Zwet PMJ, von Land CD et al. Quantitative coronary arteriography: Equipment and technical requirements. In: Reiber JHC, Serruys PW, editors. Advances in quatitative coronary arteriography. Dordrecht: Kluwer Academic Publishers, 1993: 75–112.
7. Nissen SE, Pepine CJ, Bashore TM et al. Cardiac angiography without cinefilm: Erecting a "tower of Babel" in the cardiac catheterization laboratory – an ACC position statement. J Am Coll Cardiol 1994; 24: 834–7.

8. Simon R Brennecke R, Hess O et al. Report of the ESC Task Force on Digital Imaging in Angiocardiography. Eur Heart J 1994; 15: 1332–4.
9. Nissen SE, Gurley JC, Booth DC, Maria AN. Intravascular ultrasound of the coronary arteries: Current applications and future directions. Am J Cardiol 1992; 69: 18H–29H.
10. Hodgson JM, Reddy KG, Suneja R et al. Intracoronary ultrasound imaging: Correlation of plague morphology with angiography, clinical syndrome, and procedural results in patients undergoing coronary angioplasty. J Am Coll Cardiol 1993; 21: 35–44.
11. den Heijer P. Coronary angioscopy. Thesis. The Hague: Opmeer, 1994.
12. Porter TR, Sears T, Xie F et al. Intravascular ultrasound study of angiographically mildly diseased coronary arteries. J Am Coll Cardiol 1993; 22: 1858–65.
13. Gould KL, Kirkeeide RL, Buchi M. Coronary flow reserve as a physiologic measure of stenosis severity. J Am Coll Cardiol 1990; 15: 459–74.
14. Marcus ML, Harrison DG, White CW et al. Assessing the physiologic significance of coronary obstructions in patients: Importance of diffuse undetected atherosclerosis. Progr Cardiovasc Dis 1988; 31: 39–56.
15. Lund GK, Nienaber CA, Hamm CW et al. One-session cardiac catheterization and balloon dilatation ("prima vista"-PTCA): Results and risks. Dtsch Med Wschr 1994; 119: 169–74.

Corresponding Author: Dr Rüdiger Simon, Klinik für Kardiologie, I. Medizinische Universitäts-Klinik, Christian-Albrechts-Universität, Schittenhelmstrasse 12, D-24105, Kiel, Germany

8. Diagnostic accuracy of stress-echocardiography for the detection of significant coronary artery disease

FRANK M. BAER and HANS J. DEUTSCH

Introduction

Stress-echocardiography has been used for the detection of ischemia for more than a decade and was first reported to be a clinically feasible technique by Wann et al. [1]. Since then stress-echocardiography has become an increasingly popular non-invasive alternative method for the detection of coronary artery disease, which has a number of medical and economical advantages. A variety of stress modes has been applied to patients with suspected coronary artery disease to induce new wall motion abnormalities or to intensify preexisting wall motion abnormalities in the perfusion territory of a stenosed vessel. These wall motion abnormalities can be identified by 2D-echocardiography [2] and in experienced hands wall motion analysis based on stress-echocardiography has proved to be as sensitive and specific for the detection of coronary artery disease as myocardial scintigraphy [3, 4]. Moreover, stress echocardiography may be valuable to evaluate the functional relevance of coronary artery stenoses in patients with known coronary artery disease, which is often not reliably predicted by coronary angiography [5, 6].

This paper focuses on the review of stress echocardiography studies for the assessment of functionally significant coronary artery disease in patients with suspected and known coronary artery disease. Furthermore, the diagnostic reliability of different echocardiographic stress tests for the detection of stenosis is discussed and the diagnostic accuracy of stress echocardiography is compared to other imaging techniques currently used for the non-invasive detection of coronary artery disease.

Induction of wall motion abnormalities by different stress tests

Stress echocardiography as an alternative method to exercise stress testing (EST) and scintigraphic techniques in the detection and localization of coronary artery stenoses relies on the ability of 2-dimensional echocardiography to record left ventricular wall motion and thickening before, during and after

C.A. Nienaber and U. Sechtem (eds): Imaging and Intervention in Cardiology, 105–119.
© 1996 Kluwer Academic Publishers.

Table 1. Stress tests used with echocardiography.

	Transthoracic echocardiography	Transesophageal echocardiography
Dynamic stress:	Treadmill exercise	–
	Supine bicycle ergometry	–
	Upright bicycle ergometry	–
Pharmacologic stress:	*Beta-agonists*: (Dopamine, dobutamine, arbutamine, isoproterenol)	Beta-agonists
	Vasodilators: (Dipyridamole, adenosine)	Vasodilators
Pacing:	Transvenous atrial	
	Transesophageal atrial	Transesophageal atrial
Other:	Cold pressor	–
	Mental stress	

stress application. The identification of stenoses is based on the hypothesis that stress induced ischemia in the perfusion territory of the respective vessel elicits regional wall motion abnormalities which can be evaluated qualitatively or semi-quantitatively by wall motion analysis. Different forms of stress have been used in conjunction with echocardiographic imaging (Table 1). Each of these stress tests has distinct advantages and disadvantages and is based on different mechanisms to create an imbalance between myocardial oxygen demand and supply in the perfusion territory of the stenosed vessel.

Exercise stress

Exercise stress is performed as supine or upright bicycle ergometry or treadmill stress and produces the highest increase in myocardial oxygen demand resulting from an increase in heart rate, systolic blood pressure and contractility [2]. However, this advantage has the price of a more difficult image acquisition due to deep respiratory movements and excessive motion of the chest. In a recent large series of patients approximately 30% of exercise-echocardiography studies were technically suboptimal [7]. Moreover, exercise-echocardiographic information has to be recorded within a critical time window of 90–120 seconds after cessation of exercise stress to ensure optimal accuracy [2]. Ryan et al. [8] previously reported their experience with echocardiography during peak upright bicycle exercise and immediately after exercise in 309 patients. The sensitivity for postexercise images was still 83% as compared with 91% for peak exercise imaging. This contrasts with findings of Presti et al. [9] who has shown that in nearly one third of patients with abnormal wall motion at peak bicycle exercise there was rapid recovery of the wall motion in the postexercise study. Thus it seems prudent to acquire images at the end of the exercise phase and regard negative postexercise images as potentially false negative studies.

Pharmacological stress

Various forms of pharmacological stress have been evaluated for their diagnostic value, clinical safety, side effects and patient tolerance [10]. In general, these agents encompass 2 groups: 1) beta agonists like dobutamine and arbutamine [11, 12] and 2) coronary vasodilators like dipyridamole and adenosine [13, 14]. Beta-agonists increase myocardial oxygen demand through a combined inotropic and chronotropic action. In the presence of a coronary artery stenosis a classic supply-demand mismatch occurs and wall motion abnormalities develop. In contrast, dipyridamole and adenosine induced ischemia is mainly due to a blood flow maldistribution, with a reduction in subendocardial flow in the regions of myocardium supplied by a stenotic coronary artery [15]. The small increase in myocardial oxygen demand which is much smaller than that induced by beta-agonists is not considered relevant for the induction of ischemia. In the presence of a significant coronary artery stenosis dipyridamole and adenosine reduce myocardial oxygen supply, and therefore predominantly affect the supply part of the supply-demand ratio.

Atrial pacing

Pacing stress has also been used in conjunction with echocardiography. Atrial pacing can be performed via the transvenous route, but to preserve the non-invasive nature of the examination transesophageal pacing is more commonly used [16, 17]. With this technique ischemia is induced by an increased heart rate leading to a rise in myocardial oxygen demand.

Stress and transesophageal echocardiography (TEE)

Pharmacological stress using dipyridamole [18] or dobutamine [19–21] and atrial pacing [17, 22] have been used in conjunction with TEE. The transesophageal approach circumvents the problems associated with a poor acoustic window. TEE in conjunction with pharmacological stress has proved to be a feasible, safe and accurate method to assess coronary artery disease. The superior image quality allows a better delineation of endo- and epicardial borders, which facilitates the detection of even slight wall motion abnormalities (Figures 1 and 2) and may even be suitable for quantitative assessment of wall thickening. Moreover, overall sensitivity and specificity for the detection of individual coronary artery stenoses by TEE are encouraging. Panza et al. [21] examined 62 patients with dobutamine-TEE and reported a sensitivity of 83% for detecting stenoses of the left anterior descending coronary artery, 82% for the left circumflex coronary artery and 78% for the right coronary artery. In another TEE-study using atrial pacing stress, Lambertz et al. [17] found sensitivities of 91%, 58% and 83% for the left anterior descending coronary artery, the left circumflex coronary artery and for the right coronary artery, respectively. The main disadvantage of transeso-

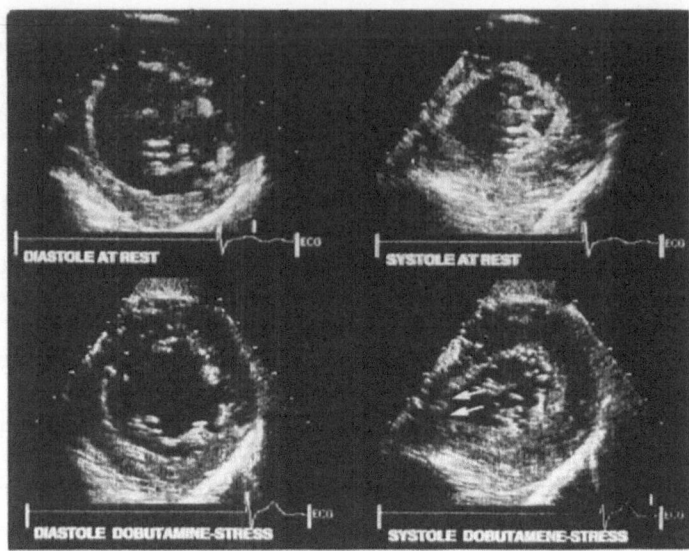

Figure 1. Transesophageal dobutamine-stress echocardiogram of a 56-year-old patient with 90% stenosis of the left anterior descending coronary artery. End-diastolic (left) and end-systolic (right) still frames of a transgastric short axis tomogram are presented in the upper row. The end-systolic still frame shows homogeneous left ventricular wall thickening at baseline conditions. During dobutamine infusion (40 μg/kg/min) inward motion of the endocardial contour and systolic wall thickening (lower right) of the anteroseptal wall (arrows) is reduced.

phageal stress echocardiography is that it requires passage of a probe into the esophagus. Therefore, this technique should be reserved for the examination of patients in whom a transthoracic study is either not feasible or yields ambiguous results.

Selection of the optimal stress for the detection of coronary artery stenoses

Comparison of stress tests in different patient populations

Numerous studies have examined the sensitivity and specificity of exercise and pharmacological stress tests in conjunction with echocardiography. These studies differ with respect to numbers of patients with single and multivessel disease, disease severity and the proportion of patients with infarction so that the comparison between these results is difficult. Table 2 demonstrates the upper and lower range of sensitivities for the detection of significant coronary artery stenoses (% diameter stenosis ≥50%) by either transthoracic or transesophageal echocardiography in conjunction with different stress

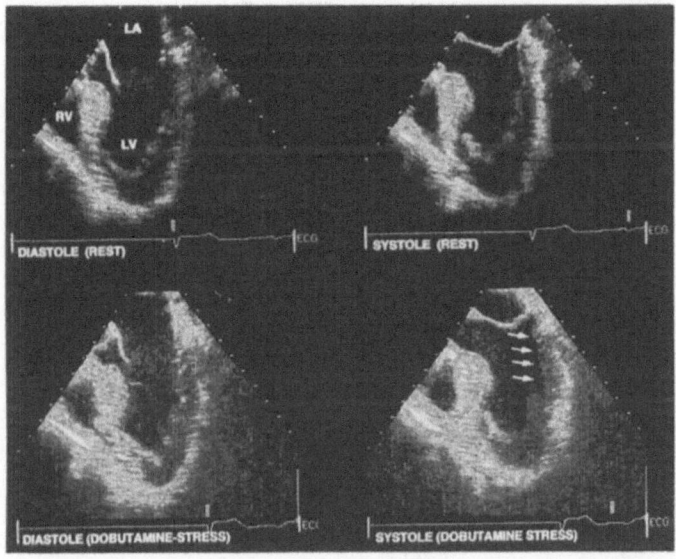

Figure 2. Transesophageal dobutamine-stress echocardiogram of a 47-year-old patient with 95% stenosis of the left circumflex coronary artery. End-diastolic (left) and end-systolic (right) still frames of a transesophageal 4-chamber view are shown. The end-systolic still frame shows homogeneous left ventricular wall thickening at baseline conditions. During dobutamine infusion (30 μg/kg/min) hypokinesis of the lateral wall (lower left, arrows) with significantly reduced inward motion of the endocardial contour developed.

modalities. Sensitivities for multivessel disease are better than for single vessel disease and the transesophageal approach yields better results than transthoracic echocardiography. If only the best values for the various echo-cardiography stress modalities are considered, dynamic- and dobutamine stress achieve the highest sensitivities for the detection of significant coronary artery disease. However, the wide range of reported sensitivities for each of these stress tests reflects the heterogeneity of patient populations and stress protocols and does therefore not allow an accurate comparison.

Comparison of different stress tests in the same patient population

A better approach to compare different stress techniques is to perform these stress tests in the same patients using coronary angiography as the standard of reference. To date, few studies have been performed comparing different echocardiographic stress tests in the same patient population. Table 3 lists all major studies which compared two or more echocardiography stress tests in the same patient population using coronary arteriography as the standard of reference. Picano et al. [33] were the first to compare dynamic stress

Table 2. Sensitivity of different stress tests in conjunction with echocardiography for the detection of functionally relevant coronary artery stenoses (≥ 50% diameter stenosis).

Stress Modality	Transthoracic echocardiography (TTE)		Transesophageal echocardiography (TEE)	
	Single-vessel disease (Sensitivity %)	Multi-vessel disease (Sensitivity %)	Single-vessel disease (Sensitivity %)	Multi-vessel disease (Sensitivity %)
Exercise	58% [23]–92% [24]	75% [8]–100% [25]	–	–
Dobutamine	50% [12]–95% [11]	77% [26]–100% [3]	–	–
Dipyridamole	0% [12]–72% [27]	52% [28]–91% [27]	67% [18]	100% [18]
Adenosine	40% [29]–52% [3]	50% [29]–64% [3]	–	–
Atrial pacing	67% [30]–75% [31]	95% [30]–100% [31]	69% [32]–85% [17]	90% [32]–100% [17]

Table 3. Comparison of different echocardiography stress tests in the same patient population with respect to the extent of CAD.

Study (patients)	Exercise (Sensitivity %)			Dobutamine (Sensitivity %)			Dipyridamole (Sensitivity %)			Adenosine (Sensitivity %)		
	CAD	1-VD	M-VD	CAD	1-VD	M-VD	CAD	1-VD	M-VD	CAD	1-VD	M-VD
Picano et al. [33] (n = 40)	76%	–	–	–	–	–	72%	–	–	–	–	–
Beleslin et al. [27] (n = 136)	88%	88%	91%	82%	82%	82%	74%	72%	91%	–	–	–
Marangelli et al. [31] (n = 60)	89%	81%	95%	–	–	–	43%	25%	58%	–	–	–
Marwick et al. [3] (n = 97)	–	–	–	85%	84%	86%	–	–	–	58%	52%	64%
Bocanelli et al. [34] (n = 68)	–	–	–	–	75%	93%	–	60%	82%	–	–	–
Previtali et al. [35] (n = 35)	–	–	–	68%	59%	92%	57%	31%	92%	–	–	–
Martin et al. [14] (n = 40)	–	–	–	76%	–	–	56%	–	–	40%	–	–
Salustri et al. [38] (n = 46)	–	–	–	79%	40%	67%	82%	50%	72%	–	–	–

CAD = coronary artery disease; 1-VD = single vessel disease; M-VD = multi vessel disease; – = not available.

and high-dose dipyridamole (0.84 mg/kg) in 40 patients and found similar sensitivities and specificities for the detection of coronary artery stenoses (≥70% diameter reduction) with both stress tests. Further evaluation with respect to the localization and extent of coronary artery disease was not provided in this early study. Another study comparing dynamic and pharmacological stress was recently published by Beleslin et al. [27]. This study addressed the overall sensitivity of dynamic, dobutamine and dipyridamole echocardiography and the sensitivity for single and multivessel disease for coronary artery stenoses of ≥50% diameter reduction. In this study, the sensitivity (88%) of exercise echocardiography for detection of single vessel disease was slightly higher than the sensitivity of dobutamine echocardiography (82%) and significantly higher than the sensitivity of dipyridamole echocardiography (72%). The wall motion abnormalities seen in these patients corresponded always to the perfusion territory of the affected vessel. The sensitivity for the detection of multivessel disease was similar for all 3 stress tests (Table 3).

Marangelli et al. [31] compared exercise and dipyridamole echocardiography and atrial pacing using transesophageal echocardiography in the same patient population. This study also demonstrated a significantly higher sensitivity of exercise stress (89%) compared to dipyridamole stress (43%). The sensitivity of transesophageal atrial pacing echocardiography (83%) was comparable to that of dynamic stress echocardiography (89%). Marwick et al. [3] compared dobutamine and adenosine stress and reported a significantly higher overall sensitivity (85%) for dobutamine stress than for adenosine (58%). Sensitivity for single vessel disease using dobutamine stress (84%) was almost the same as the overall sensitivity for coronary artery disease (85%). In contrast, with adenosine stress detection of single vessel disease could be achieved in only 52% of patients. Specificity for dobutamine (82%) and adenosine stress (87%) was in the same range.

Studies by Bocanelli et al. [34], Previtali et al. [35], Martin et al. [14] and Beleslin et al. [27] which also compared dobutamine and dipyridamole stress confirmed the superiority of dobutamine stress for both the detection of single and multivessel disease (Table 3). This is in agreement with magnetic resonance imaging studies in patients with coronary artery disease which also reported higher sensitivities of dobutamine stress in comparison to dipyridamole stress in patients with coronary artery disease [36, 37]. There is only one stress echocardiography study performed by Salustri et al. [38] which demonstrated slightly better results of high dose-dipyridamole than of dobutamine stress.

The lower sensitivity of adenosine and dipyridamole in comparison to exercise and dobutamine is likely due to the fact that flow maldistribution provoked by dipyridamole may not occur or may not be severe enough to induce subendocardial ischemia in patients with only moderately reduced coronary reserve [35]. Even using TEE with its superior image quality in conjunction with dipyridamole stress, wall motion abnormalities were only found in 67% of patients with single vessel disease [18] which is further evidence for the hypothesis that dipyridamole is not the ideal pharmacological stress agent. Dobutamine stress is also more sensitive than dipyridamole in patients taking beta-blockers [27].

Based on the studies mentioned in Table 3 exercise stress is probably the most effective stress test to provoke myocardial ischemia and subsequent wall motion abnormalities. This is in agreement with an animal study reporting that exercise is capable of inducing a slightly greater degree of dissynergy than high-dose dipyridamole and dobutamine [39]. However, in the clinical setting performance of exercise is strongly dependent on patient motivation and the ability to reach adequate exercise levels. Unfortunately, many patients are physically incapable of sufficiently vigorous exercise to provide diagnostically useful data. Stratman et al. [40] reported that as many as 35% of patients with coronary artery disease are unable to complete an exercise treadmill test. This emphasizes the necessity of having a stress mode available that is independent of dynamic exercise. Despite the shortcomings of dipyridamole mentioned above and the higher sensitivity of dobutamine no study has yet demonstrated a significant difference between the diagnostic accuracies of the two agents. Therefore, until we have more precise information the choice of the echocardiographic stress test to detect functionally significant stenoses may be governed by the clinical situation and the preference and experience of the physician.

Comparison of stress echocardiography and myocardial scintigraphy in the same patient population

Exercise-echocardiography versus myocardial scintigraphy

The few studies based on a head to head comparison between exercise-echocardiography and myocardial scintigraphy in the same patient population are listed in Table 4 and discussed briefly below. In a study by Maurer and Nanda [41] 23 patients underwent exercise-echocardiography and thallium-201 planar imaging after a treadmill exercise test. The sensitivity was 74% for thallium-201 scintigraphy and 70% for exercise echocardiography. The specificity was 92% for both techniques. In a similar study using exercise echocardiography and planar thallium-201 imaging with supine bicycle exercise stress Galanti et al. [42] found similar overall sensitivities (93% vs 100%) and specificities (96% vs 92%), but thallium-201 imaging had a significantly higher sensitivity than exercise echocardiography for detecting individual stenoses (85% vs 63%). Pozzoli et al. [43] examined 75 patients by both exercise echocardiography and Tc-99m-methoxy-isobutyl-isonitrile single photon emission computed tomography (MIBI-SPECT) during the same exercise test performed on a bicycle ergometer. Sensitivity was 71% for exercise echocardiography and 84% for MIBI-SPECT. The respective speci-

Table 4. Exercise echocardiography vesus myocardial scintigraphy in the same patient population.

Study	Patients included	Sensitivity		Specificity	
		Echo	MS	Echo	MS
Maurer and Nanda [41]	(n = 23)	70%	74%	92%	92%
Galanti et al. [42]	(n = 53)	93%	100%	96%	92%
Pozzoli et al. [43]	(n = 75)	71%	84%	96%	88%
Quinones et al. [23]	(n = 112)	74%	74%	88%	81%
Amanullah et al. [44]	(n = 27)	82%	95%	80%	100%
Hecht et al. [4]	(n = 71)	90%	92%	80%	65%

Echo = exercise echocardiography; MS = myocardial scintigraphy.

ficities for 26 patients without coronary artery disease were 96% for exercise echocardiography and 88% for MIBI-SPECT. The results of the 2 tests were concordant in 65 of 75 patients (88%). Interestingly, MIBI-SPECT had a higher sensitivity than echocardiography for detection of patients with single vessel disease (82% vs 61%) and detected 64% of all coronary artery stenoses versus 60% by exercise-echocardiography. Quinones et al. [23] studied 289 patients by both echocardiography and thallium-201 SPECT after treadmill exercise. In the 112 patients of this cohort who underwent coronary arteriography, the sensitivity was 74% for both techniques and the specificity was 81% for thallium-201 SPECT and 88% for exercise echocardiography. Amanullah et al. [44] compared exercise echocardiography and thallium-201 SPECT in 27 patients with unstable angina who were referred for coronary arteriography. In the 22 patients with coronary artery disease, exercise echocardiography was positive in 18 (82%) and thallium-201 SPECT in 21 patients (95%). Hecht et al. [4] examined 71 patients with exercise echocardiography during supine bicycle exercise and thallium-201 SPECT during treadmill exercise. The sensitivities in the 51 patients with significant coronary artery disease were 90% and 92%, respectively. Exercise echocardiography detected 88% of all coronary artery stenoses versus 80% for thallium-201 SPECT. Interestingly, exercise echocardiography had a significantly higher sensitivity than thallium-201 SPECT for the detection of left anterior descending coronary artery stenoses (97% vs 82%), although at the expense of diminished specificity (81% vs 94%). The corresponding specificities were 80% and 65%, respectively. The sensitivity, however, of thallium-201 SPECT was higher than that of exercise echocardiography in patients with single vessel disease (95% vs 77%), whereas exercise echocardiography was more sensitive for 1. the prediction of the number of coronary arteries affected (70% vs 46%) and 2. for the detection of patients with three vessel disease (80% vs 47%).

Thus, with the exception of one study, the sensitivity for the detection of coronary artery disease was slightly higher for scintigraphic techniques and similar in the remaining study. However, exercise echocardiography was more sensitive for the identification of the number of affected coronary arteries and the detection of patients with three vessel disease. The specificity was similar with these two methods.

Pharmacological-stress echocardiography versus myocardial scintigraphy

Extensive experience has been accumulated with myocardial scintigraphy and echocardiography during pharmacological stress. However, the number of well conducted comparative studies is still small (Table 5). Some of these studies have already been mentioned in the discussion of different pharmacological stress tests in the same patient population. Marwick et al. [3] compared pharmacological stress with dobutamine and adenosine in combination with both echocardiography and MIBI-SPECT. The sensitivities for echocardiography using dobutamine and adenosine are given in Table 3; the sensitivities for adenosine and dobutamine MIBI-SPECT were 86% and 80%, respectively. The respective specificities were 71% and 74%. Nguyen et al. [29] assessed the use of adenosine echocardiography in comparison to adenosine thallium-201 SPECT. In this study the sensitivity of adenosine echocardiography was only 40%, compared with a sensitivity of 90% by adenosine thallium-201 SPECT. These discrepant findings may be explained by the ability of thallium-201 to detect adenosine induced flow differences whereas the detection of coronary artery disease by echocardiography requires the induction of myocardial ischemia and wall motion abnormalities. In a study by Heinle et al. [45] adenosine echocardiography and adenosine thallium-201 scintigraphy were abnormal in 71% and 86% of patients with multivessel disease; however the corresponding figures for patients with single vessel disease were only 28% and 43%. Amanullah et al. [46] compared

Table 5. Pharmacological stress echocardiography vesus myocardial scintigraphy in the same patient population.

Study	Patients included	Sensitivity		Specificity		Stress agent
		Echo	MS	Echo	MS	
Marwick et al. [3]	(n = 97)	85%	80%*	82%	74%	Dobutamine
Marwick et al. [3]	(n = 97)	58%	86%*	87%	71%	Adenosine
Marwick et al. [47]	(n = 217)	72%	76%*	83%	67%	Dobutamine
Amanullah et al. [46]	(n = 40)	74%	94%*	100%	100%	Adenosine
Foster et al. [48]	(n = 105)	75%	83%*	89%	89%	Dobutamine
Gunalp et al. [49]	(n = 27)	84%	94%*	88%	88%	Dobutamine
Nguyen et al. [29]	(n = 25)	10%	90%	100%	100%	Adenosine

Echo = exercise echocardiography; MS = myocardial' scintigraphy; *studies were based on Tc-99m-methoxy-isobutyl-isonitrile single photon emissin tomography (MIBI-SPECT); the other study was based on thallium-201 SPECT.

MIBI-SPECT and echocardiography during adenosine administration. The sensitivity and specificity in 40 patients were 94% and 100% by MIBI-SPECT and 74% and 100% by echocardiography. In a large study by Marwick et al. [47] comprising 217 patients without prior myocardial infarction who prospectively underwent dobutamine echocardiography and dobutamine MIBI-SPECT, significant coronary artery disease (>50% diameter stenosis) was present in 142 patients. The sensitivities of dobutamine echocardiography and dobutamine MIBI-SPECT were 72% and 76%, respectively. The specificity was significantly higher for dobutamine echocardiography (83%) than for dobutamine MIBI-SPECT (67%). Both techniques had similar sensitivities for the detection of patients with multi vessel disease (77% vs 78%), whereas dobutamine MIBI-SPECT had a slightly higher sensitivity in patients with single vessel disease (74% vs 66%). Foster et al. [48] have also compared the diagnostic value of dobutamine echocardiography with that of dobutamine MIBI-SPECT performed simultaneously during bicycle exercise in 105 patients. In this study the sensitivities were 75% by echocardiography and 83% by MIBI-SPECT, with identical specificities (both 89%). Similar results were reported by Gunalp et al. [49] who found sensitivities of 84% for echocardiography and 94% for MIBI-SPECT, with similar specificities for both imaging techniques (both 89%).

Although few comparative studies are available myocardial scintigraphy appears to be preferable to echocardiography if adenosine or dipyridamole is used. During dobutamine stress sensitivity and specificity of both techniques are similar [3]. In summary, myocardial scintigraphy using the SPECT technique may be superior for the detection of single vessel disease [3], whereas stress-echocardiography may be advantageous in patients with multivessel disease [4].

Conclusions

Stress-echocardiography has become a well-established non-invasive diagnostic approach to patients with known or suspected coronary artery disease. Particularly pharmacological stress echocardiography is increasingly used and has demonstrated a diagnostic accuracy similar to that achieved with exercise-stress and comparable to that of scintigraphic techniques. It is only natural that a certain degree of competition should exist between stress echocardiography and myocardial scintigraphy for the detection of coronary artery disease. The ability to accurately identify individual coronary artery stenoses is shared by both, stress echocardiography and myocardial scintigraphy. In patients with multivessel disease there is a tendency for stress echocardiography to obtain better results. This may be an important point for future research, since the functional relevance and location of ischemia are of paramount importance for clinical decision making in patients with known multivessel coronary artery disease. The common problem in the catheterization laboratory of whether to approach a particular stenosis in a patient with multivessel disease could be addressed by accurate preintervention functional data. Thus, an important goal for non-invasive imaging must be the accurate identification of the physiologic significance of a stenosis in individual coronary arteries with determination of the ischemic burden of myocardium supplied by each separate coronary artery or major branch. With respect to stress echocardiography, an important strength is that a new wall motion abnormality provoked during stress and not present at baseline indicates that true myocardial ischemia, sufficient to impair regional myocardial function, occurred during stress. In contrast, myocardial scintigraphy may only reflect imbalances of flow (vasodilators like dipyridamole and adenosine) and does not allow real time imaging from onset to resolution of myocardial ischemia. One may hypothesize that the region with the earliest onset of a wall motion abnormality in a patient with multivessel disease would be perfused through the culprit lesion. However, there are no echocardiographic data available addressing this important clinical question.

Although cost, radiation exposure and on-line functional information would favour stress echocardiography for the assessment of coronary artery disease, to date the choice of the imaging modality should depend on the quality of the available facilities and the experience of the physician which is particularly important for the adequate evaluation of stress echocardiography studies.

References

1. Wann LS, Faris JV, Childress RH et al. Exercise cross-sectional echocardiography in ischemic heart disease. Circulation 1979; 60: 1300–8.
2. Armstrong WF. Stress echocardiography for detection of coronary artery disease. Circulation 1991; 84 (Suppl I): 43–9.
3. Marwick TH, Willemart B, D'Hondt AM et al. Selection of the optimal nonexercise stress for the evaluation of ischemic regional myocardial dysfunction and malperfusion. Circulation 1993; 87: 345–54.
4. Hecht HS, DeBord L, Shaw R et al. Supine bicycle echocardiography versus tomographic thallium-201 exercise imaging for the detection of coronary artery disease. J Am Soc Echocardiogr 1993; 6: 177–85.
5. Gould KL. Percent coronary stenosis: Battered gold standard; pernicious relic or clinical practility. J Am Coll Cardiol 1988; 11: 886–7.
6. Wilson RF, Johnson MR, Marcus ML et al. The effect of coronary angioplasty on coronary flow reserve. Circulation 1988; 4: 873–85.
7. Marwick TH, Nemec JJ, Pashkow FJ et al. Accuracy and limitations of exercise echocardiography in a routine clinical practice. J Am Coll Cardiol 1992; 19: 74–81.
8. Ryan T, Segar TS, Sawada SG et al. Detection of coronary artery disease with upright bicycle exercise echocardiography. J Am Soc Echocardiogr 1993; 6: 186–97.
9. Presti CF, Armstrong WF, Feigenbaum H. Comparison of echocardiography at peak exercise and after bicycle exercise in evaluation of patients with known or suspected coronary artery disease. J Am Soc Echocardiogr 1988; 1: 119–26.

10. Pennell DJ. Pharmacological cardiac stress: When and how? Nucl Med Commun 1994; 15: 578–85.
11. Marcowitz PA, Armstrong WF. Accuracy of dobutamine stress echocardiography in detecting coronary artery disease. Am J Cardiol 1992; 69: 1269–73.
12. Mazeika PK, Nadizin A, Oakley CM. Dobutamine stress echocardiography for detection and assessemnt of coronary artery disease. J Am Coll Cardiol 1992; 19: 1203–11.
13. Picano E, Masini M, Lattanzi F et al. High dose dipyridamole-echocardiography test in effort angina pectoris. J Am Coll Cardiol 1986; 8: 848–54.
14. Martin TW, Seaworth JF, Johns JP et al. Comparison of adenosine, dipyridamole and dobutamine in stress echocardiography. Ann Intern Med 1992; 116: 190–6.
15. Fung AY, Gallagher KP, Buda AJ. The physiologic basis of dobutamine as compared with dipyridamole stress interventions in the assessment of critical coronary stenosis. Circulation 1987; 76: 943–51.
16. Chapman PD, Doyle TP, Troup PJ et al. Stress echocardiography with transesophageal pacing: Preliminary report of a new method for detection of ischemic wall motion abnormalities. Circulation 1984; 70: 445–50.
17. Lambertz H, Kreis A, Trümper H, Hanrath P. Simultaneous transesophageal atrial pacing and transesophageal two-dimensional echocardiography. A new method of stress echocardiography. J Am Coll Cardiol 1990; 16: 1143–53.
18. Agati L, Renzi M, Sciomer S et al. Transesophageal dipyridamole echocardiography for diagnosis of coronary artery disease. J Am Coll Cardiol 1992; 19: 765–70.
19. Baer FM, Voth E, Deutsch H et al. Assessment of viable myocardium by dobutamine-transesophageal-echocardiography (TEE) and comparison with FDG-PET. J Am Coll Cardiol 1994; 24: 343–53.
20. Prince CR, Stoddard MF, Morris GT et al. Dobutamine two-dimensional transesophageal echocardiographic stress testing for detection of coronary artery disease. Am Heart J 1994; 1: 36–41.
21. Panza JA, Laurienzo JM, Curiel RV et al. Transesophageal dobutamine stress echocardiography for evaluation of patients with coronar artery disease. J Am Coll Cardiol 1994; 24: 1260–7.
22. Hoffmann R, Kleinhans E, Lambertz H et al. Transesophageal pacing echocardiography for detection of restenosis after percutaneous transluminal coronary angioplasty. Eur Heart J 1994; 15: 823–31.
23. Quinones MA, Verani MS, Haichin RM et al. Exercise echocardiography versus thallium-201 single photon computed emission tomography in evaluation of coronary artery disease: Analysis of 292 patients. Circulation 1992; 85: 1026–31.
24. Crouse LH, Harbrecht JJ, Vacek JL et al. Exercise echocardiography as a screening test for coronary artery disease and correlation with coronary arteriography. Am J Cardiol 1991; 67: 1213–8.
25. Limacher MC, Quinones MA, Poliner R et al. Detection of coronary artery disease with exercise two dimensional echocardiography. Circulation 1983; 67: 1211–8.
26. Sawada SG, Segar DS, Ryan T et al. Echocardiographic detection of coronary artery disease during dobutamine infusion. Circulation 1991; 83: 1601–14.
27. Beleslin BD, Ostojic M, Stepanovic J et al. Stress echocardiography in the detection of myocardial ischemia. Circulation 1994; 90: 1168–76.
28. Margonato A, Chierchia S, Cianflone D et al. Limitations of dipyridamole echoardiography in effort angina pectoris. Am J Cardiol 1987; 59: 225–30.
29. Nguyen T, Heo J, Ogilby JD et al. Single photon emission computed tomography with thallium-201 during adenosine induced coronary hyperemia: Correlation with coronary arteriography, exercise thallium imaging and two-dimensional echocardiography. J Am Coll Cardiol 1990; 16: 1375–83.
30. Iliceto S, Sorino M, D'Ambrosio G et al. Detection of coronary artery disease by two-dimensional echocardiography and transesophageal atrial pacing. J Am Coll Cardiol 1985; 5: 118–97.

31. Marangelli V, Iliceto S, Piccini G et al. Detection of coronary artery disease by digital stress echocardiography: Comparison of exercise, transesophageal atrial pacing and dipyridamole echocardiography. J Am Coll Cardiol 1994; 24: 117–24.
32. Kamp O, DeCock CC, Funke AJ et al. Simultaneous transesophageal two-dimensional echocardiography and atrial pacing for detecting coronary artery disease. Am J Cardiol 1992; 69: 1412–6.
33. Picano E, Lattanzi F, Masini M et al. Comparison of the high-dose dipyridamole-echocardiography test and exercise two-dimensional echocardiography for diagnosis of coronary artery disease. Am J Cardiol 1987; 59: 539–42.
34. Boccanelli A, Piazza V, Greco C et al. Comparison of diagnostic value of dipyridamole and dobutamine stress echocardiography in the diagnosis of coronary artery disease. J Am Coll Cardiol 1993 (Abstr); 21: 393A.
35. Previtali M, Lanzarini L, Ferrario M et al. Dobutamine versus dipyridamole echocardiography in coronary artery disease. Circulation 1991; 83 (Suppl III): 27–31.
36. Pennell DJ, Underwood RS, Manzara CC et al. Magnetic resonance imaging during dobutamine stress in patients with coronary artery disease. Am J Cardiol 1992; 70: 34–40.
37. Baer FM, Voth E, Theissen P et al. Comparison of dobutamine-magnetic resonance imaging and dobutamine-99mTc-methoxy-isobutyl-isonitrile SPECT in the diagnosis of coronary artery disease. Radiology 1994; 193: 203–9.
38. Salustri A, Fioretti PM, McNeill AJ et al. Pharmacological stress echocardiography in the diagnosis of coronary artery disease and myocardial ischemia: A comparison between dobutamine and dipyridamole. Eur Heart J 1992; 13: 1356–62.
39. Paulsen PR, Pavek T, Crampton M et al. Which stress is best? Exercise, dobutamine, dipyridamole and pacing in an animal model. J Am Coll Cardiol 1993; (Abstr) 21: 90a.
40. Stratman HG, Kennedy HL. Evaluation of coronary artery disease in the patient unable to exercise. Alternatives to exercise stress testing. Am Heart J 1989; 117: 1344–65.
41. Maurer G, Nanda NC. Two-dimensional echocardiographic evaluation of exercise induced left and right ventricular asynergy: Correlation with thallium scanning. Am J Cardiol 1981; 48: 720–7.
42. Galanti G, Sciagra R, Comeglio M et al. Diagnostic accuracy of peak exercise echocardiography in coronary artery disease: Comparison with thallium-201 myocardial scintigraphy. Am Heart J 1991; 122: 1609–22.
43. Pozzoli MMA, Fioretti PM, Salustri A et al. Exercise echocardiography and technetium-99m MIBI single photon emission computed tomography in the detection of coronary artery disease. Am J Cardiol 1991; 67: 350–5.
44. Amanullah AM, Lindvall K, Bevegard S. Exercise echocardiography after stabilization of unstable angina: Correlation with exercise thallium-201 single photon computed emission tomography. Clin Cardiol 1992; 15: 585–9.
45. Heinle S, Hanson M, Gracey L et al. Correlation of adenosine-echocardiography and thallium scintigraphy. Am Heart J 1993; 125: 1606–13
46. Amanullah AM, Bevegard S, Lindvall K, Aasa M. Assessment of left ventricular wall motion in angina pectoris by two-dimensional echocardiography and myocardial perfusion by technetium-99m sestamibi tomography during adenosine induced coronary vasodilation and comparison with coronary angiography. Am J Cardiol 1993; 72: 983–9.
47. Marwick T, D'Hondt AM, Baudhvin et al. Optimal use of dobutamine stress for the detection and evaluation of coronary artery disease: Combination with echocardiography or scintigraphy or both? J Am Coll Cardiol 1993; 22: 159–67.
48. Foster T, McNeill AJ, Salustri A et al. Simultaneous dobutamine stress echocardiography and technetium-99m isonitrile single-photon emission computed tomography in patients with suspected coronary artery disease. J Am Coll Cardiol 1993; 21: 1591–6.
49. Gunalp B, Dokumaci B, Uyan C et al. Value of dobutamine technetium-99m sestamibi SPECT and echocardiography in the detection of coronary artery disease compared with coronary angiography. J Nucl Med 1993; 34: 889–94.

Corresponding Author: Dr Frank M. Baer, Klinik III für Innere Medizin, University of Cologne, Joseph-Stelzmannstrasse 9, D-50924, Cologne, Germany

9. Perfusion imaging with thallium-201 to assess stenosis significance

EDNA H.G. VENNEKER, BERTHE L.F. VAN ECK-SMIT and ERNST E. VAN DER WALL

Introduction

Since the introduction of coronary angiography in the 1960's, this invasive technique has become the foremost important diagnostic method in the assessment of patients with coronary artery disease. Despite a relatively high interobserver and intraobserver variability, coronary angiography is still considered the gold standard for the assessment of physiological effects of coronary stenosis. In general practice the assumption exists that there is a close correlation between the angiographic diameter of a coronary artery stenosis and the perfusion of the myocardium. This assumption implies that the decision as to whether to revascularize in order to alleviate ischemia is predominantly based on the percent diameter stenosis found during coronary angiography. However, several studies comparing angiographic findings with postmortem findings have shown that coronary angiography underestimates the severity of the lesion [1]. Overestimation of diameter stenosis may also occur due to for instance spasm of the coronary artery or insufficient filling with contrast medium.

A major drawback of using morphological changes as shown by coronary angiography is the poor relation between stenosis severity and the functional significance of a stenosis. Also the length of the stenosis, the absolute cross-sectional luminal area of the segment, and the presence or absence of collateral vessels are of major importance for the hemodynamic significance of the arterial lesion.

In clinical practice it is often necessary to define whether a lesion detected at coronary angiography is indeed the cause of the patient's symptoms. This is especially difficult in a patient with atypical chest pain. Such patients undergo coronary angiography with increasing frequency because it is well known that high grade stenoses can be present despite the absence of ischemic signs in the exercise electrocardiogram at high exercise levels. If an eccentric stenosis of intermediate severity is then found, ischemia in the corresponding myocardial region should be demonstrated by perfusion imaging to avoid cosmetic angioplasty. Perfusion imaging may also be helpful for

C.A. Nienaber and U. Sechtem (eds): Imaging and Intervention in Cardiology, 121–134.
© 1996 *Kluwer Academic Publishers.*

decision making in a patient with multivessel disease, in whom identification of the culprit lesion would allow to angioplasty only this lesion to gain immediate relief of chest pain. The amount of ischemia in specific vascular beds can be evaluated [2] and those vessels with the greatest ischemia can be dilated first. Later on, the other vessels can be revascularized in a staged procedure.

Because of the abovementioned issues it is obvious that assessment of functional significance of a certain coronary stenosis plays an important role in the management of coronary artery disease even after coronary angiography has been performed. Several methods are available for assessing the impairment of coronary flow caused by a coronary stenosis or the functional consequences of such impaired blood flow to regional myocardial contraction. These techniques include myocardial scintigraphy using thallium-201 or technetium-99 labeled isonitriles, positron emission tomography (PET) using F-18-fluorodeoxyglucose (FDG) (see Chapter 10), echocardiographic (see Chapter 8) and magnetic resonance imaging techniques (see Chapters 11–13).

This chapter will review the diagnostic accuracy of scintigraphic techniques for the detection of coronary artery disease. In addition, the role of perfusion imaging following coronary angiography to direct decisions regarding therapeutic intervention will be discussed.

Myocardial perfusion

In normal coronary arteries myocardial blood flow is primarily regulated by the resistance of the arteriolar vessels. Epicardial arteries provide little resistance under physiological circumstances. However, in case of vessel stenosis a transstenotic pressure gradient develops which leads to arteriolar vasodilatation and subsequently results in normal flow to the myocardium distal from the stenosis. In animals, it has been reported that resting coronary blood flow can be maintained at normal levels if less than 90% of the cross-sectional area is obstructed. In case of increasing myocardial oxygen demand the distal arteriolar bed is unable to dilate further if there is an arterial cross-sectional obstructed area of more than 90% [3]. Coronary stenoses that are unable to maintain myocardial blood by arteriolar vasodilatation are considered to be physiologically significant. Under conditions of increased workload, coronary plaques obstructing more than 65% of the luminal cross-sectional area have been shown to be of physiological significance [3].

As myocardial blood flow at rest is normal even in the presence of a significant coronary stenosis, patients with stable coronary artery disease are usually asymptomatic at rest. However, the insufficient coronary flow reserve will result in myocardial ischemia during periods of increased myocardial oxygen demand e.g. during exercise or during positive inotropic stimulation. Assessment of myocardial perfusion abnormalities by perfusion scintigraphy is based on the principle of depicting transient flow inhomogeneities caused

Table 1. Characteristics of available myocardial perfusion imaging agents

	Thallium-201	Tc-99 m-sestamibi	Tc-99 m-teboroxime
Half-life within the heart	3–4 hours	5–6 hours	<10 minutes
Dose	2.0–3.5 mCi	30 mCi	30 mCi
Injections/exercise study	1 (2)	2	2
Myocardial extraction fraction	85%	65%	90%
Start imaging after	5–10 minutes	1–2 hours	2 minutes
Planar imaging time	30 minutes	10–15 minutes	3–6 minutes
SPECT imaging time	30 minutes	15–20 minutes	
Ventricular function	No	Yes	Yes
ECG gating	No	Yes	No

by increased workload or pharmacologically induced vasodilation. Several radiopharmaceuticals are currently used for perfusion imaging (Table 1).

Thallium characteristics and kinetics

Thallium-201 has been used extensively for noninvasive assessment of myocardial perfusion in cardiovascular disease. The long physical half-life of thallium-201 (73 hours) restricts the maximal dose which can be administered to 4 mCi. This low dose results in a low count rate which in turn is detrimental for image quality. Distribution of thallium is closely related to regional blood flow [4, 5]. The myocardium extracts 85% of the thallium after an intravenous bolus injection. The uptake of thallium into the myocardium is mainly mediated by an active process involving the sodium-potassium ATP-ase pump [6]. Peak activity of thallium in the myocardium is reached within a few minutes after injection of thallium at maximum exercise followed by a gradual decrease of myocardial thallium activity. The washout rate of thallium is again related to myocardial blood flow. The higher the flow, the faster the washout from the myocardium, and the lower the flow, the slower the washout. This means that nonischemic regions have a more rapid washout than ischemic regions which is one process leading to equalization or near equalization of counts in redistribution images. The other process contributing to the equalization of counts in late images is the continued uptake of thallium in areas with low flow due to the gradient between the higher thallium blood levels and the lower thallium concentration in the ischemic cell.

New technetium-99m perfusion agents

Due to the imperfect imaging characteristics of thallium-201, new perfusion agents labeled with Tc-99m have been developed. Currently, only Tc-99m sestamibi and Tc-99m-teboroxime have been approved for clinical use.

Tc-99m-sestamibi

Tc-99m-sestamibi is a lipophilic cationic complex that is regionally distributed to the myocardium in proportion to blood flow. In contrast to thallium-201, it is bound within the cytoplasm and has minimal redistribution over time. The mechanism of uptake into the myocardium involves passive diffusion and extraction of sestamibi from the blood is lower (65%) than for thallium. However, because of the intracellular retention and additional subsequent myocardial uptake during recirculation, the absolute retention of Tc-99m-sestamibi several minutes after administration is comparable with that of thallium-201. The absence of redistribution means that 1) imaging can be performed even several hours after injection of the tracer without alteration of the initial blood flow related distribution and 2) two separate injections are required to differentiate between ischemia (lower uptake during exercise but normal uptake at rest) and infarction (lower uptake during exercise which remains unchanged after rest injection). Image quality of Tc-99m-sestamibi images is better than of thallium-201 images because higher doses of Tc-99m-sestamibi can be injected. This higher dose of Tc-99m-sestamibi is possible because the estimated absorbed radiation dose to the whole body is one order of magnitude lower per mCi than for thallium-201 (0.02 rad/mCi instead of 0.21 rad/mCi).

TC-99 m-teboroxime

Tc-99 m-teboroxime is also highly lipophilic but neutral and is taken up by the myocardium in proportion to blood flow with a 90% extraction fraction. Clearance from the circulation is very rapid, which means that images must be acquired *within* the first 10 minutes after injection. Therefore, planar imaging is the preferred method of acquisition although single photon emission computed tomography (SPECT) imaging using two- and three-headed gamma cameras is possible. Because experience with this agent has been limited, its use will be no further discussed in this chapter.

Simultaneous assessment of ventricular function and perfusion

One of the advantages of technetium labeled perfusion agents is that they can be administered as an intravenous bolus and first-pass assessment of right and left ventricular function can be performed. If perfusion images are acquired in a gated mode after injection of Tc-99m-sestamibi, myocardial thickening between end-diastole and end-systole can be measured, which may be helpful to differentiate attenuation artifact from myocardial scar.

Performance of myocardial perfusion studies

Various protocols have been evaluated in order to achieve the best protocol for the assessment of myocardial perfusion but no consensus about the optimal method has been reached. One of the most widely used methods for assessing myocardial perfusion is scintigraphy after injection of thallium-201 at maximum physical exercise followed by a redistribution scintigram after 4 hours. Since thallium-201 is distributed proportional to flow, the differences between regional coronary flow can be visualized as regional differences in thallium-201 accumulation. As a result of slower wash-out an ischemic defect initially seen on the exercise scintigram will completely fill in or even turn into a region with higher count rate on the delayed rest scintigram.

When patients are unable to perform physical exercise, pharmacological stress with intravenous dipyridamole or adenosine can be applied. Both drugs cause vasodilation, leading to an increase in myocardial blood flow of three to four times the normal blood flow in normal coronary arteries. In contrast, myocardial blood flow fails to increase to the same extent in coronary arteries with significant stenoses. This leads to heterogeneity in thallium accumulation, without necessarily producing myocardial ischemia. Recently, alternative forms of pharmacological stress with dobutamine and other inotropic agents have been introduced. These drugs produce an increase of myocardial oxygen demand resulting in heterogeneity of blood flow in normal and narrowed coronary arteries, leading to true regional ischemia.

Several imaging protocols have been proposed for sestamibi imaging. Separate injections at peak exercise and at rest can be performed on the same day or on separate days. Whereas the separate day protocol offers the advantage of better images due to two full 30 mCi doses for both injections, and also may obviate the need for a rest study in patients with normal exercise studies, it is associated with an unwanted delay in getting the results. Therefore, a one-day protocol with a rest study followed by a stress study is often preferred. The stress-rest protocol is less often employed [7]. Pharmacologic stress testing using sestamibi yields similar diagnostic accuracy as exercise stress imaging.

Detection of coronary artery disease by scintigraphic perfusion imaging

Scintigraphic assessment of myocardial perfusion may be performed by planar or SPECT imaging. In planar scintigraphy images are acquired from three views (i.e. anterior, left anterior oblique, left lateral view). However, superposition of myocardial segments limits accurate discrimination of vascular regions. Moreover, attenuation of thallium activity and scatter caused by variable amounts of overlying soft tissue may cause artifacts limiting the accuracy for detection of perfusion defects.

Visual interpretation of planar thallium images has been extensively employed to detect coronary artery disease and the largest clinical experience and largest number of published results has accumulated with this technique. The sensitivity of visually interpreted planar thallium imaging for detecting coronary artery disease in published studies with arteriographic confirmation is in the order of 80–90% [8]. Specificity has initially been in the order of 90% [8] but disappointingly low rates of specificity have recently been published, which may relate to some form of referral bias because patients with normal perfusion scans are not any longer selected for catheterization.

Since there is a significant intraobserver and interobserver variability for visual analysis of perfusion images, quantitative methods have been developed, which have a slightly higher sensitivity for the detection of coronary artery disease. One of the major advantages of quantitative scintigraphy is an enhanced rate of detecting stenoses in individual coronary vessels [9]. The use of quantitative scintigraphic techniques significantly enhances the detection rate in patients with single vessel disease. Wackers et al. [10] compared visual and quantitative techniques in patients with chest pain and found a sensitivity of 55% for detection of single vessel disease by visual analysis compared to 84% sensitivity by quantitative scintigraphy. Nevertheless, quantitative analysis of planar thallium images does not abolish the inherent limitations of planar imaging.

In SPECT, imaging data are acquired from multiple views (20–30). From these data tomographic slices are reconstructed in three orientations, i.e. the short axis, the vertical long axis, and the horizontal long axis. The main advantage of this technique is that individual coronary territories can be better separated. Several studies comparing SPECT with planar imaging have indicated that in this respect SPECT is superior to planar imaging [11, 12]. This aspect is of course especially important in patients undergoing scintigraphy after cardiac catheterization to assess the functional relevance of an angiographically detected stenosis. The detection of disease in individual coronary arteries with greater than 50% stenosis can be accomplished by thallium-SPECT with sensitivities ranging from 78% to 81% for the left anterior descending artery [12–16], 75% to 89% for the right coronary artery, and 65% to 79% for the left circumflex coronary artery (Table 2). Specificities

Table 2. SPECT thallium-201 exercise imaging: Evaluation of coronary artery disease in specific coronary arteries. (Reprinted from Hecht et al. Cardiology Clinics 1994; 12: 373–83 with permission from the author and publisher.)

Study	Technique	Sensitivity (%)			
		All vessels	LAD	RCA	LCX
DePasquale et al. [13]	Exercise	79	78	89	65
Maddahi et al. [14]	Exercise	80	78	82	79
Mahmarian et al. [15]	Exercise	77	81	75	77
Van Train et al. [16]	Exercise	77	78	84	68

of 83% to 92% for the left anterior descending coronary artery, 71% to 95% for the left circumflex coronary artery, and 60% to 99% for the right coronary artery have been reported.

The detection of mild coronary artery disease as well as the identification of multivessel disease are two other important advantages of SPECT over planar imaging. However, the higher sensitivity of thallium SPECT imaging as compared to planar thallium imaging is accompanied by a lower specificity, which is related to the higher number of artifacts (mainly by patient motion) in tomographic imaging. Only if quality of SPECT imaging is rigorously controlled is it possible to minimize the number of false positive studies and achieve similar specificities as for planar thallium imaging.

Similar to planar imaging quantitative analysis of SPECT data reduces interobserver and intraobserver variability and can be considered as a valuable complentary tool to visual analysis. For SPECT several quantitative methods for analyzing data have been developed. In order to quantify and analyze the data in one single functional image, the so-called bull's eye image is usually constructed, which provides easy detection and localization of flow abnormalities. In a study performed by Mahmarian et al. [16], the sensitivity and specificity for detection of coronary artery disease with thallium-SPECT by quantitative analysis were 87% and 83%, respectively.

The use of sestamibi does not result in higher sensitivity or specificity than that of thallium in the detection of coronary artery disease [17, 18]. However, sestamibi imaging may have advantages over thallium imaging in identifying individual stenoses. In a study by Kahn et al. [19], sestamibi identified 59/75 (79%) significantly stenosed arteries compared with only 45/75 (60%) by thallium-201 (p < 0.05). The increased detection of individual coronary artery stenoses was most marked in the vessels with mild stenoses (50–75% diameter stenosis); 65% of these lesions caused perfusion defects on sestamibi images as compared to only 35% on thallium images. Assuming that the detection of perfusion defects in patients with chest pain and moderate stenoses represents a true positive finding, the use of sestamibi seems advantageous to assess the significance of such a stenosis observed at coronary arteriography. However, in the intermediate range of stenosis severity, it is also possible that the more frequent observation of perfusion defects by sestamibi represents false positive findings leading to unnecessary revascularizations whereas the more conservative thallium approach could represent a more realistic estimate of stenosis significance. Ultimately, this question can only be resolved by measuring flow reserve either by PET or by invasive Doppler wire techniques.

A new issue has arisen with the more frequent use of ad hoc coronary angioplasty [27]. This development may result in detecting stenoses of intermediate severity and performing angioplasty without the proof of ischemia in the related myocardial region. Therefore, in patients with atypical chest pain and borderline stress electrocardiograms it may be advisable to perform imaging studies before angiography.

Coronary angiography: Correlation of anatomical with functional measurements of stenosis severity

The poor correlation between angiographically estimated or measured diameter stenosis and the functional significance of the observed coronary narrowing was confirmed in a study by Folland et al. [20] in 227 patients who had a >70% diameter stenosis in a single vessel by visual estimation. There was no consistent relationship between the angiographically defined severity of the stenosis and the exercise capacity of the patient irrespective whether the severity of the stenosis was assessed by visual or quantitative methods.

Basic considerations of fluid mechanics indicate that the obstruction to blood flow caused by a coronary artery stenosis varies directly with the length of the stenosis and inversely with the fourth power of the radius (Bernoulli's theorem). Therefore, despite its limitations the minimal diameter of a stenosis is undoubtedly the best single parameter to describe the functional significance of the lesion. However, as shown in Chapter 19, angiographic measurement even of this simple parameter is not entirely straightforward, especially in eccentric stenoses, and perfusion imaging may be helpful to demonstrate or exclude ischemia in the myocardium perfused by a vessel with a geometrically complex stenosis.

Abnormalities of the coronary microcirculation, which cannot be assessed by coronary angiography, may also influence myocardial perfusion and cause myocardial ischemia [21, 22]. In contrast to coronary angiography, perfusion imaging is able to detect abnormalities at the level of these very small arteries and may thus explain anginal symptoms in patients with normal coronary angiograms. Consequently, perfusion imaging has been advocated in patients with normal angiograms suffering from angina.

In recent years the assessment of coronary flow reserve has been introduced as a reliable measure to determine the functional status of a coronary artery stenosis. White et al. [23] studied 39 patients with isolated, discrete coronary lesions in whom the reactive hyperemic responses were measured using a Doppler catheter and who were subsequently compared to the cineangiogram. In these patients with lesions varying in severity from 10–95% stenosis, the percentage stenosis observed on the angiogram did not significantly correlate with the reactive hyperemic response (Figure 1). Underestimation of the severity of the lesion occurred in 95% of the vessels with >60% diameter stenosis on coronary angiography. Both overestimation and underestimation occurred in lesions with less than 60% stenosis. The authors concluded that the physiological effects of the majority of coronary stenoses cannot accurately be determined by means of coronary angiography, indicating the need for better analytical methods to assess coronary stenosis such as coronary videodensitometry and improved radionuclide perfusion techniques.

Wilson et al. [24] performed a study on the prediction of the physiologic

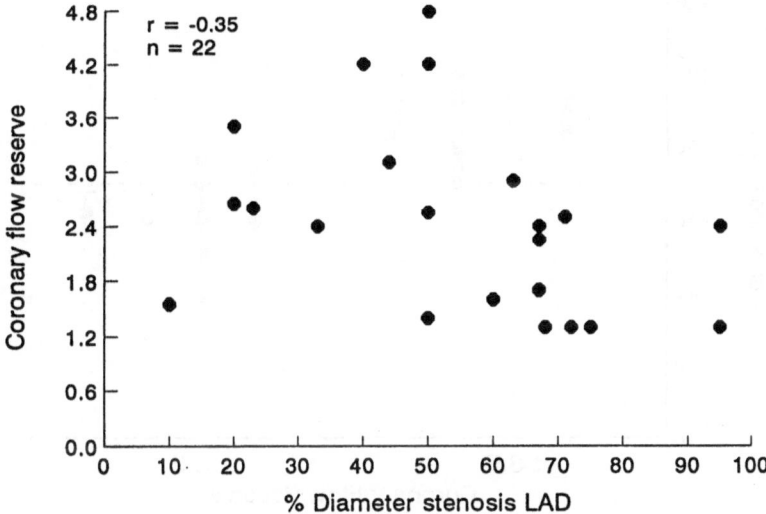

Figure 1. Relation between the coronary artery diameter stenosis and the coronary flow reserve in 22 patients with one discrete lesion in the left anterior descending coronary artery (LAD). (Modified from White et al. N Engl J Med 1984; 310: 819–24 [23].)

significance of coronary arterial lesions by quantitative lesion geometry in patients with limited coronary artery disease. They studied 50 patients with a single discrete coronary artery stenosis in only one (84%) or two vessels (16%) and determined coronary flow reserve by the Doppler technique using papaverine as the vasodilating substance. In contrast to previous studies from their institution demonstrating a poor relationship between quantitative estimates of coronary luminal stenosis and intra-operative measurements of coronary flow reserve obtained in patients with multi-vessel coronary artery disease, the coronary flow reserve measured in patients with discrete limited coronary artery disease correlated closely with luminal stenosis determined precisely with quantitative coronary angiography. Coronaries arteries with <70% area stenosis uniformly had normal coronary flow reserve (lower limit of normal 3.5) (Figure 2). Coronary arteries with >90% area stenosis were associated with a wide range of coronary flow reserves (1.0 to 2.8). They concluded that the evaluation of coronary flow reserve should facilitate the assessment of the physiological significance of coronary arterial lesions in the catheterization laboratory.

Zijlstra et al. [25] compared quantitative arteriographic analysis with measured coronary flow reserve and thallium-201 exercise perfusion scintigraphy. They studied 38 patients with single vessel disease and the myocardial perfusion defects on thallium scintigram were analyzed quantitatively and by visual interpretation. They showed that both percent diameter stenosis and obstruction area generally correlated well with functional measurements of

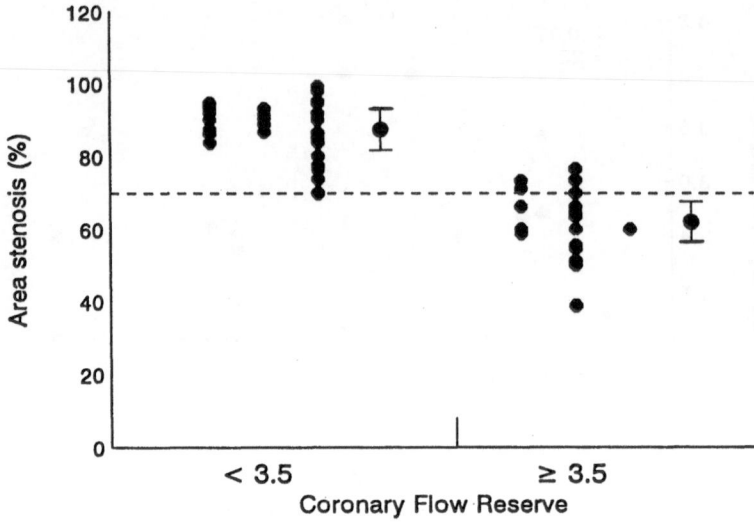

Figure 2. The percent area stenosis of lesions associated with normal (>3.5) and abnormal (≤3.5) coronary flow reserve. Coronaries arteries with <70% area stenosis uniformly had normal coronary flow reserve. (Modified from Wilson et al. Circulation 1987; 75: 723–32 [24].)

stenoses severity such as radiographically measured coronary flow reserve and thallium-201 scintigraphy. However, for individual patients the relation between pressure drop and coronary flow reserve was better than between obstruction area or percent diameter stenosis and coronary flow reserve. This indicated that the calculated pressure drop over the stenoses was more accurate than any anatomic description in assessing the functional consequences of a coronary artery lesion. The pressure drop also served as a better variable to distinguish patients with normal and abnormally coronary flow reserve and predicted the results of thallium-201 scintigraphy more accurately. They further showed that thallium-201 scintigraphy was only partly useful to predict the measured coronary flow reserve in individual patients. Thallium perfusion was usually normal when coronary flow reserve was moderately reduced (between 2.5 and 3.4). However, almost all patients with a severe reduction in flow reserve (<2.5) had a positive thallium-201 scintigram (Figure 3). The authors concluded that thallium-201 scintigraphy can be useful in selected patients, for instance to assess the occurrence of restenosis after angioplasty for single vessel coronary artery disease. The assessment of coronary flow reserve is an indispensible addition to quantitative angiography especially to determine the functional importance of moderately severe coronary artery lesions.

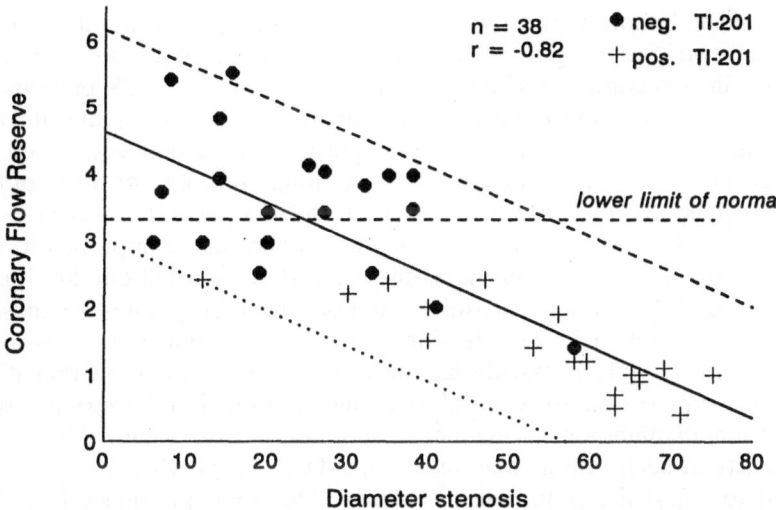

Figure 3. Relation between coronary flow reserve (CFR), thallium-201 scintigraphy and percent diameter stenosis (DS) in 38 patients. The dashed horizontal line is the lower limit of normal coronary flow reserve. The closed circles represent 18 patients with a positive thallium scintigram. The open circles represent 20 patients with a negative thallium scintigram. (Modified from Zijlstra et al. J Am Coll Cardiol 1988; 12: 686–91 [25].)

Perfusion imaging as a tool to select patients for PTCA

The small risk to the patient and the substantial cost of cardiac catheterization make it desirable to restrict this examination to patients in whom the procedure is most likely to have therapeutic consequences. The selection of these high risk patients who need catheter intervention or bypass surgery is an important strength of perfusion imaging techniques. Numerous studies could demonstrate that perfusion imaging and coronary angiography yield similar prognostic power in mildly symptomatic patients with coronary artery disease. However, the issue has not yet been settled whether coronary angiography should not be performed and PTCA thus be avoided in patients with symptoms suggestive of coronary artery disease but a perfectly normal perfusion scintigram.

The evaluation of patients with multivessel coronary disease for percutaneous transluminal coronary angioplasty raises the question: Is incomplete revascularization an acceptable procedure in these patients, or does complete revascularization need to be performed, as in coronary artery bypass grafting? To provide an answer Breisblatt et al. [2] utilized exercise thallium imaging as a guide to the performance of angioplasty in 85 patients with multivessel coronary disease. Preangioplasty exercise thallium imaging helped to identify the primary stenosis ("culprit lesion") in 93% of patients.

Two weeks to 1 month after dilation of this lesion, repeated thallium imaging identified two patient groups: Group 1, 47 patients with no evidence of ischemia in a second vascular distribution and Group 2, 38 patients who needed further angioplasty because of ischemia in another vascular territory. In Group 2, 47% of patients had angioplasty of a second vessel and 79% required multivessel angioplasty at 1 year follow-up. In contrast, only six Group 1 patients (13%) required angioplasty of a second vessel at 1 year. Thus, incomplete revascularization may be an acceptable approach in many patients with multivessel coronary disease and stress thallium-201 imaging may be a useful technique in the evaluation and management of these patients. In this context it is interesting that a recent publication assessing the effects of incomplete revascularization came to the conclusion that it does not improve prognosis to revascularize mild stenoses in coronary arteries > or =1.5 mm in diameter serving modest amounts of myocardium [26]. Hence, angioplasty in such lesions may not be justified except when they are documented to cause life-style-limiting angina. The good prognosis in patients with normal scintigrams after coronary angioplasty is entirely compatible with these findings and strengthens the prognostic role of scintigraphy in patients with multivessel disease.

Another potential role for scintigraphy is in the selection of the optimal revascularization strategy in patients with multivessel disease and vessels which cannot be treated by angioplasty. Demonstration of the presence or absence of significant amounts of ischemia in such vessels would either favour bypass grafting or angioplasty of the other vessel(s).

Conclusions

Coronary angiography continues to be the main tool in the diagnosis and management of patients with coronary artery disease. After all, the decision on whether or not to revascularize depends a great deal on the suitability of the coronary arteries for bypass grafting or PTCA. Also, collateral vessels may be detected by coronary angiography, although there may be a discrepancy between collateral function and angiographic appearance. The clinical decision making is still mainly guided by the presence of an anatomical stenosis as assessed by coronary angiography. In this chapter we emphasized that myocardial perfusion imaging can assist in clinical decision making before and after coronary angiography. We see the main role of perfusion imaging in determining the clinical relevance of an anatomical stenosis of intermediate severity to avoid cosmetic angioplasty in asymptomatic patients or those with atypical chest pain.

As scintigraphy using thallium-201 or sestamibi is a widely available, relatively easy, and noninvasive method for the assessment of myocardial perfusion it should play an important role in the diagnosis of myocardial ischemia and in the management of these patients. At present, several protocols are available for the assessment of myocardial perfusion which seem to be similar with respect to sensitivity and specificity. Since no large comparative multicenter trials have been performed yet, it is difficult to say which protocol should be used in the current setting. In terms of patient convenience, one should preferably head for a simple time-saving imaging protocol.

References

1. Arnett EN, Isner JM, Redwood DR et al. Coronary artery narrowing in coronary heart disease: Comparison of cineangiographic and necropsy findings. Ann Intern Med 1979; 91: 350–6.
2. Breisblatt WM, Barnes JV, Weiland F, Spaccavento LJ. Incomplete revascularization in multivessel percutaneous transluminal coronary angioplasty: The role for stress thallium-201 imaging. J Am Coll Cardiol 1988; 11: 1183–90.
3. Gould KL. Noninvasive assessment of coronary stenoses by myocardial perfusion imaging during pharmacologic coronary vasodilation. I. Physiologic basis and experimental validation. Am J Cardiol 1978; 41: 267–72.
4. Belgrave E, Lebowitz E. Development of thallium-201 for medical use (Abstr). J Nucl Med 1992; 13: 781.
5. Strauss HW, Harrison K, Langan JK et al. Thallium-201 for myocardial imaging. Relation of thallium-201 to regional myocardial perfusion. Circulation 1975; 51: 641–5.
6. Weich HF, Strauss HW, Pitt B. The extraction of thallium-201 by the myocardium. Circulation 1977; 56: 188–91.
7. Taillefer R. Technetium-99m sestamibi myocardial imaging: Same-day stress-rest studies and dipyridamole. Am J Cardiol 1990; 66: 80E–4.
8. Kaul S. Cardiac imaging in conjunction with exercise stress testing in patients with suspected coronary artery disease: A comparison of the techniques. Cardiovasc Imaging 1989; 1: 20–8.
9. Berger BC, Watson DD, Taylor GJ et al. Quantitative thallium-201 exercise scintigraphy for detection of coronary artery disease. J Nucl Med 1981; 22: 585–93.
10. Wackers FJT, Fetterman, RC, Mattera JA et al. Quantitative planar thallium-201 stress scintigraphy: A critical evaluation of the method. Semin Nucl Med 1985; 15: 46–59.
11. Fintel DJ, Links JM, Brinker JA et al. Improved diagnostic performance of exercise thallium-201 single photon emission computed tomography over planar imaging in the diagnosis of coronary artery disease: A receiver operating characteristic analysis. J Am Coll Cardiol 1989; 13: 600–12.
12. Kiat H, Berman DS, Maddahi J. Comparison of planar and tomographic exercise thallium-201 imaging methods for the evaluation of coronary artery disease. J Am Coll Cardiol 1989; 13: 613–6.
13. DePasquale EE, Nody AC, DePuey EG et al. Quantitative rotational thallium-201 tomography for identifying and localizing coronary artery disease. Circulation 1988; 77: 316–27.
14. Maddahi J, Van Train K, Prigent F et al. Quantitative single photon emission computed thallium-201 tomography for detection and localization of coronary artery disease: Optimization and prospective validation of a new technique. J Am Coll Cardiol 1989; 14: 1689–99.
15. Van Train KF, Maddahi J, Berman DS et al. Quantitative analysis of tomographic stress thallium-201 myocardial scintigrams: A multicenter trial. J Nucl Med 1990; 31: 1168–79.
16. Mahmarian JJ, Boyce TM, Goldberg RK et al. Quantitative exercise thallium-201 single photon emission computed tomography for the enhanced diagnosis of ischemic heart disease. J Am Coll Cardiol 1990; 15: 318–29.
17. Wackers FJ, Berman DS, Maddahi J et al. Technetium-99m hexakis 2-methoxyisobutyl

isonitrile: Human biodistribution, dosimetry, safety, and preliminary comparison to thallium-201 for myocardial perfusion imaging. J Nucl Med 1989; 30: 301–11.

18. Kiat H, Maddahi J, Roy LT et al. Comparison of technetium-99m methoxy isobutyl isonitrile and thallium 201 for evaluation of coronary artery disease by planar and tomographic methods. Am Heart J 1989; 117: 1–11.

19. Kahn JK, McGhie I, Akers MS et al. Quantitative rotational tomography with 201Tl and 99 mTc 2-methoxy-isobutyl-isonitrile. A direct comparison in normal individuals and patients with coronary artery disease. Circulation 1989; 79: 1282–93.

20. Folland ED, Vogel RA, Hartigan P et al. Relation between coronary artery stenosis assessed by visual, caliper and computer methods and exercise capacity in patients with single-vessel coronary artery disease. Circulation 1994; 89: 2005–14.

21. James TN. The spectrum of diseases of small coronary arteries and their physiologic consequences. J Am Coll Cardiol 1990; 15: 763–74.

22. James TN, Bruschke AVG. Seminar on small coronary artery disease. Introduction. Structure and function of small coronary arteries in health and disease. J Am Coll Cardiol 1990; 15: 511–2.

23. White CW, Wright CB, Doty DB et al. Does visual interpretation of the coronary arteriogram predict the physiological importance of a coronary stenosis. N Engl J Med 1984; 310: 819–24.

24. Wilson RF, Marcus ML, White CW. Prediction of the physiologic significance of coronary arterial lesions by quantitative lesion geometry in patients with limited coronary artery disease. Circulation 1987; 75: 723–32.

25. Zijlstra F, Fioretti P, Reiber JHC, Serruys PW. Which cineangiographically assessed anatomic variable correlates best with functional measurements of stenosis severity? A comparison of quantitative analysis of the coronary cineangiogram with measured coronary flow reserve and exercise/redistribution thallium-201 scintigraphy. J Am Coll Cardiol 1988; 12: 686–91.

26. Cowley MJ, Vandermael M, Topol EJ et al. Is traditionally defined complete revascularization needed for patients with multivessel disease treated by elective coronary angioplasty? Multivessel Angioplasty Prognosis Study (MAPS) Group. J Am Coll Cardiol 1993; 22: 1289–97.

27. Lund GK, Nienaber CA, Hamm CW et al. One-session cardiac catherization and balloon dilation ('prima vista'-PTCA): Results and risks. Dtsch Med Wschr 1994; 119: 169–74.

Corresponding Author: Prof. Ernst E. van der Wall, Department of Cardiology C1–P25, University Hospital Leiden, Rijnsburgerweg 10, 2333 AA Leiden, The Netherlands

10. Perfusion imaging by PET to assess stenosis significance

GUNNAR K. LUND and CHRISTOPH A. NIENABER

Introduction

Quantification of coronary flow and coronary flow reserve is an attractive concept to assess stenosis significance, because the ultimate severity of a coronary stenosis depends on the reduced ability to increase myocardial blood flow by reserve vasodilation at the arteriolar level [1]. By arteriolar autoregulation coronary flow reserve follows the myocardial demand, in other words, coronary circulation remains at a constant level with either decreased coronary pressure or increased stenosis severity to meet the actual metabolic demand (Figure 1). Nevertheless, the quantitative magnitude of vasodilator flow reserve is inversely related to the increasing severity of a stenosis. The complexity of this concept of coronary flow reserve is outlined in Figure 2. The autoregulatory capacity allows resting coronary blood flow to stay constant over a wide range of diameter stenoses but decreases gradually with a stenotic diameter reduction of 85% to 90%, and is reduced under resting conditions with diameter stenoses >90%. This relationship is the basic concept of coronary flow reserve measurements for defining stenosis severity (Figure 2). In normal arteries coronary flow can be increased 3 to 5 times by vasodilation of the periphereal coronary bed, thus absolute coronary flow reserve, defined as maximal flow in the stenosed artery devided by resting blood flow in the same region, ranges from 3 to 5 in humans. With increasing stenosis severity coronary flow reserve decreases almost linearly and in severely stenosed arteries with exhausted coronary reserve, maximal vasodilation does not even result in any flow increase; hence, absolute coronary flow reserve has the minimal value of one.

There are two fundamentally different concepts of assessing coronary flow reserve: one is based on anatomic information, the other on a physiologic approach [2]. Both concepts are related and provide independent and complementary information for the quantification of stenosis significance and subsequent clinical decision making.

The anatomic-geometric approach to assess coronary stenosis severity uses morphologic dimensions of a given stenosis derived from an amplified

C.A. Nienaber and U. Sechtem (eds.) Imaging and Intervention in Cardiology. 135–147.
© 1996 *Kluwer Academic Publishers.*

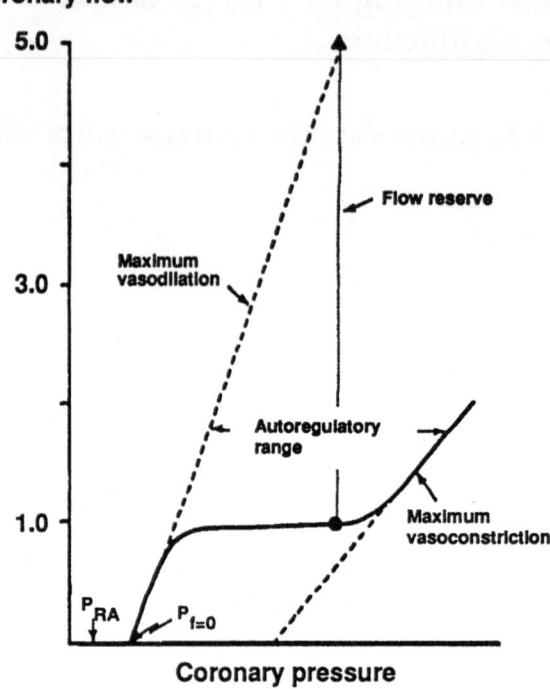

Figure 1. Steady-state relationship between coronary flow and coronary arterial pressure. The solid line depicts the normal relationship. At a constant level of myocardial metabolic demand, coronary flow is maintained constant over a wide range of intracoronary pressures, between the bounds of maximum coronary vasodilation and constriction (dashed lines). The solid circle represents the normal operating point under basal conditions; the solid triangle is the flow observed at the same pressure during maximum vasodilation. Flow reserve, the ratio of flow during vasodilation to that measured before vasodilation, is in this case 5.0. PRA = right arterial pressure; Pf = 0 = "back pressure" opposing coronary flow. (From Klocke FJ. Measurements of coronary flow reserve: Defining pathophysiology versus making decisions about patient care. Circulation 1987; 76: 1183–9, by permission of the American Heart Journal, Inc.)

coronary angiogram, such as percent diameter stenosis, absolute diameter reduction, shape and length of the stenosis, integrated to calculate stenosis flow reserve. This stenosis flow reserve derived from quantitative coronary arteriography (QCA) is a single integrated functional measure of stenosis severity [3]. However, QCA-determined stenosis flow reserve is designed to assess the severity of a given stenosis under standardized, rather than under real physiological and steadily changing "in vivo" conditions. Conversely, measurements of absolute coronary flow reserve (maximal flow/resting flow) is possible with invasive electromagnetic flowmeters, a parameter highly variable and dependable on aortic pressure and rate-pressure product [4]. Flowmeter measurements of relative coronary flow reserve, defined as maxi-

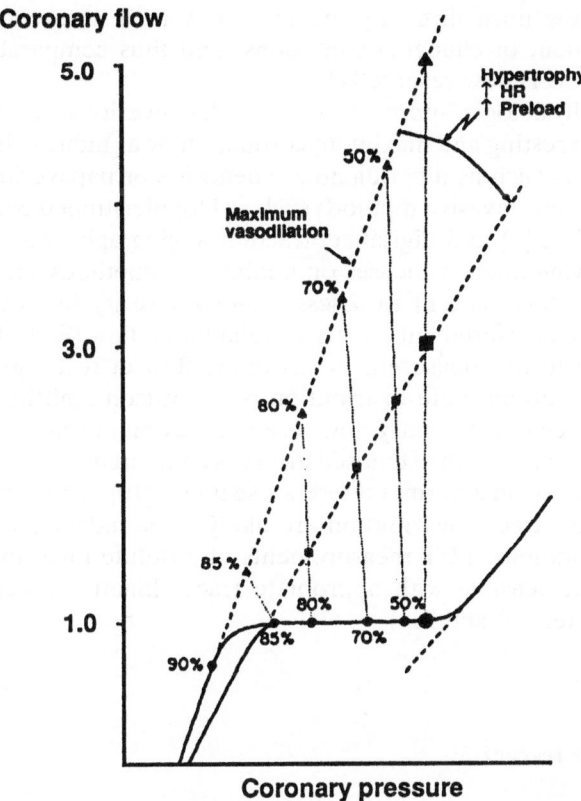

Figure 2. Complexities of the coronary flow reserve concept. Due to autoregulatory reserve the coronary resting flow stays constant over a wide range of 50–85% diameter reduction, becomes exhausted between 85 and 90% diameter stenosis and is dramatically reduced even under basal conditions with a stenosis of more than 90% diameter reduction. The intersections with the pressure-flow relationship for maximum vasodilation define the reciprocal variation of flow reserve with stenosis severity and demonstrate the attractiveness of the concept to utilize measurements of flow reserve for the definition of stenosis severity. Chronic reductions in maximum flow during vasodilation with corresponding reductions in calculated flow reserve have been documented in various forms of hypertrophy. The shift to the right of the pressure-flow relationship corresponds to a reduction in flow reserve from 5.0 (large solid triangle) to 3.0 (large solid square) at a normal coronary artery pressure; that means that flow reserve would be essentially the same for an 80% diameter coronary stenosis subtending normal myocardium and a 50% diameter stenosis subtending hypertrophied myocardium operating on the shifted pressure-flow relationship. (From: Klocke FJ. Measurements of coronary flow reserve: Defining pathophysiology versus making decisions about patient care. Circulation 1987; 76: 1183–9, by permission of the American Heart Journal, Inc.)

mal stenotic flow normalized by maximal flow to a nonstenotic segment, are less dependent of changing conditions, and thus comparable to QCA-determined stenosis flow reserve [4].

Thus, the physiologic approach assesses the severity of a given stenosis by its impact on resting and maximum coronary flow as induced by pharmaco-logic vasodilators such as dipyridamole, adenosine or papaverine. Following this concept various invasive methods such as Doppler-tipped coronary artery catheters or wires [5] and digital subtraction angiography were used [6, 7]. However, growing interest focuses on noninvasive methods such as positron emission tomography (PET) to assess stenosis severity by both qualitative and quantitative measurements of myocardial blood flow [8, 9]. PET imaging may be employed for measurements of blood flow at rest and stress based on the relative and absolute distribution of a positron emitting flow tracer. For analysis of relative coronary flow reserve, maximum tracer concentration in a segment supplied by the stenosed artery is compared to or normalized for maximum perfusion in a normal reference segment [10]. Thus, measurements based on relative tracer distribution are likely to be independent of varying physiologic conditions. PET measurements of absolute myocardial flow and flow reserve are feasible with appropiate tracer kinetic modeling [11–14]. (See also Chapters 19 and 21.)

PET blood flow tracers

Nitrogen-13 ammonia, oxygen-15 water, rubidium-82 and copper-62 PTSM (Cu II pyruvaldehyde bis N^4-methylthiose micarbazone) are tracers for PET perfusion imaging (Table 1). Their physical and biochemical properties allow rapid exchange and diffusion at the myocyte surface, thus reflecting true tissue perfusion. However, none of these tracers combines all characteristics for optimal quantification, such as ultra-short physical half-life, minimal radiation dose, uptake directly related to flow and thus, independent of metabolic conditions, and last but not least generator-produced rather than cyclotron dependent. At present, quantification requires sophisticated mathe-matical modeling and analysis [11–14], including rapid data acquisition free of detector saturation, and concomitant use of a blood pool tracer to correct

Table 1. Characteristics of blood flow tracers used with positron emission tomography.

Tracer	Physical half-time	Dose
N-13 ammonia	10.0 min	10–20 mCi
0–15 water	2.1 min	30–40 mCi (0.5 mCi/kg)
Rb-82	1.25 min	20–50 mCi
Cu-62 PTSM	9.7 min	20 mCi

for blood pool spillover of activity. These procedures, however, will soon be automated.

Nitrogen-13 ammonia

Because N-13 labeled ammonia is rapidly cleared from blood, avidly retained in myocardial tissue and provides high image contrast. Both, extraction and clearance have been described in terms of compartmental analysis [15]. Nitrogen-13 ammonia has a 10-minute physical half-time, allowing sequential studies. The radiation dose for the patient is approximately 6 to 7 mrad/mCi [16]. Because it is lipid soluble, $^{13}NH_3$ diffuses readily into myocardial cells and is trapped as glutamine. At a physiologic pH ammonia exists primarily in the form of NH^{4+} and its myocardial concentration is not only depending on blood flow, but on the total amount of nitrogen-13 ammonia administered as a function of time, on its extraction and retention fraction at an instantaneous flow, and only marginally on the metabolic state of the myocardium [17, 18]. Tracer kinetic modeling is required for absolute quantitative flow measurements, since myocardial uptake of N-13 ammonia correlates nonlinearly with blood flow [19–21].

Oxygen-15 water

Oxygen-15 water is a tracer probably best suited for quantification of myocardial perfusion due to the essentially free diffusion into myocardial tissue and an almost complete extraction rate of this tracer [20]. However, oxygen-15 remains in the blood pool, and contaminates the image with spillover of activity from the blood pool and from surrounding structures. To overcome this problem, oxygen-15 carbon monoxide is administered by inhalation after each perfusion scan to label the blood pool. The myocardial activity is then identified by digital subtraction of the blood pool oxygen-15 carbon monoxide activity from the oxygen-15 activity. With current techniques, the signal-to-noise ratio is not as high as with nitrogen-13 ammonia or with rubidium-82. However, with faster data acquisition rates larger tracer doses may be used to overcome this limitation. As a rule and because of their ultra-short physical half-lives, oxygen-15 and nitrogen-13–labeled tracers are used only at major centers with on-site cyclotrons.

Rubidium-82 and copper-62 PTSM (generator-produced)

In contrast to $^{13}NH_3$ and $H_2^{15}O$, rubidium-82, a potassium analog, can be eluted from a strontium-82 generator system using normal saline, which eliminates the need for an on-site cyclotron [22–24]. Over 30 years ago Rubidium isotopes were first used to assess myocardial blood flow, since the external detection of myocardial rubidium uptake has been demonstrated. Due to its short, 74 second half-life, rubidium-82 is particularly convenient for frequent sequential examinations under rapidly changing conditions, such as ischemia or acute myocardial infarction [25]. In 10 to 20 ml saline solution 30 to 50 mCi are intravenously given as a bolus. The radiation dose to the patient is approximately 1.6 to 2 mrad/mCi [26]. The predicted flow, derived from rubidium-82 uptake after correction for the extraction fraction, is linearly related to microsphere flow, and minimally influenced by acidosis, alkalosis, digoxin, propranolol, and glucose-insulin levels [27]. The rubidium-82 solution is pumped over a calibrated dosimeter and is passed through a Millipore filter prior to intravenous infusion. Since the parent strontium has a half-life of 25 days, one generator provides sufficient concentration of rubidium-82 for 4 to 6 weeks. Copper-62 PTSM has more recently been introduced as a generator produced tracer of myocardial perfusion. Its uptake characteristics, however, are not ideal with a relatively low extraction fraction.

PET perfusion imaging

There are basically two different approaches in the use of PET perfusion imaging to assess stenosis severity. The first is a qualitative approach based on the relative distribution of myocardial tracer activity; the qualitative use of PET for the evaluation of myocardial blood flow enables detection of coronary artery disease with similar or greater accuracy than any other conventional noninvasive radionuclide method [28–30]. The second represents a quantitative approach utilizing the unique ability of PET for the entirely noninvasive measurement of absolute myocardial blood flow based on appropiate tracer kinetic modeling [11–14]. The quantitative approach provides measurements of net blood flow in absolute terms.

Detection of coronary artery disease by qualitative PET perfusion imaging

The practical limits of emission tomography perfusion imaging for the detection of impaired flow reserve was first observed in animals experiments using labeled microspheres and direct gamma-camera imaging of cross-sectional myocardial slices after sacrifice. The minimal coronary narrowing detected by this method was 40 to 50% diameter stenosis [31]; a similar detection threshold is achieved with pharmacologic vasodilation using dipyridamole. Dogs instrumented with adjustable stenoses of the left circumflex artery were imaged with PET after injection of nitrogen-13 ammonia. By visual analysis defects were identified with tracer administration at vasodilation and coronary narrowings of as little as 47% diameter stenosis by quantitative coronary angiography could be detected. Human coronary flow reserve begins to diminish progressively if diameter stenoses exceeded 40% [9]. In 193 patients Demer et al. [8] found a correlation between results of visual PET analysis

Stenosis flow reserve

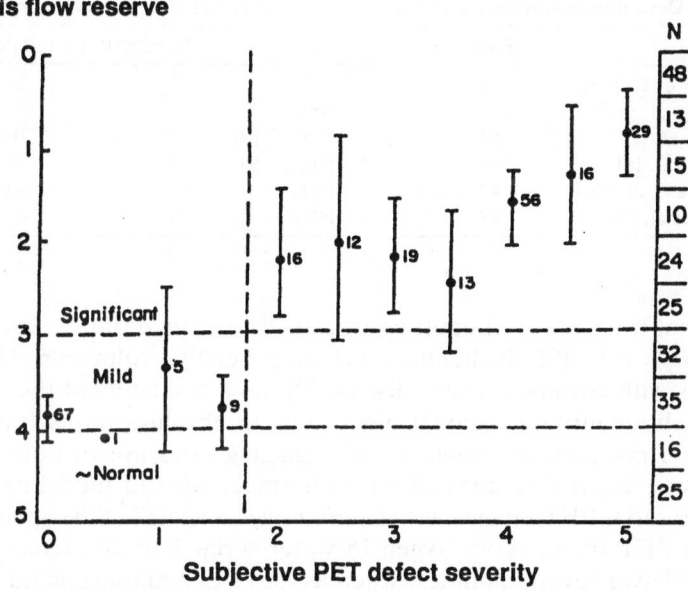

Subjective PET defect severity

Figure 3. Relation between angiographic stenosis flow reserve and subjective PET defect severity in corresponding anatomic regions for 243 coronary stenoses. The mean value of stenosis flow reserve is plotted as a funtion of PET defect severity. The horizontal dashed lines identify the ranges of normal, mildly reduced, and significantly reduced stenosis flow reserve. The vertical dashed line indicates that a PET defect score of 2 or more predicts the presence of either a mild or a significant stenosis. The error bars represent the 90% confidence intervals. The number of patients represented is shown adjacent to each point. (From: Demer LL, Gould KL, Goldstein RA et al. Assessment of coronary artery disease severity by positron emission tomography: Comparison with quantitative arteriography in 193 patients. Circulation 1989; 79: 825, by permission of the American Heart Association,. Inc.)

of defect severity and the stenosis flow reserve as derived from quantitative coronary angiography (Figure 3).

Both rubidium-82 and N-13 ammonia have comparable diagnostic accuracies and the reported sensitivities for detection of coronary artery disease range from 87 to 97% with specificities from 78 to 100% (Table 2). Appropriate correction for photon attenuation together with both high contrast and spatial resolution account for the diagnostic performance of PET.

Quantitative assessment of myocardial blood flow and stenosis flow reserve

The main asset of positron emission tomography that distinguishes this technique from other myocardial perfusion imaging methods, is the capability to provide accurate quantitative information. The dual photon release allows emission images to be corrected for the specific photon attenuation, thus,

Table 2. Detection of coronary artery disease by PET: correlation with coronary arteriography.

Study	Patients	Tracer	Sensitivity (%)	Specificity (%)
Schelbert et al. [33]	32	$^{13}NH_3$	97	100
Tamaki et al. [29]	25	$^{13}NH_3$	95	100
Gould et al. [2]	50	$^{13}NH_3$, ^{82}Rb	95	100
Demer et al. [8]	193	$^{13}NH_3$, ^{82}Rb	94	95
Yonekura et al. [34]	49	$^{13}NH_3$	97	100
Tamaki et al. [35]	48	$^{13}NH_3$	98	–

the signal from positron emitting tracers can be quantitated. Several studies in animals [11, 12], in humans including healthy volunteers [13, 14] and patients with coronary artery disease [9] have documented the feasiblity to accurately quantitate regional blood flow in absolute terms (i.e. milliliters per gram per min) by dynamic PET imaging (and use of both blood pool and tissue input functions along with tracer kinetic modeling). For that purpose serial PET images are acquired over a specific time span tailored to a given PET tracer. For oxygen-15 water serial 1 to 20 second images are recorded over several minutes, whereas for N-13 ammonia an aditional static image is recorded for 10 to 15 minutes to obtain high count density images. Tracer activity concentrations in arterial blood and in myocardial tissue is derived from regions of interest in both left ventricular cavity and myocardium and time activity curves are generated that represent the arterial input function and the myocardial response to it. The kinetics of a tracer in blood and tissue is described by a model of two or more functional compartments that reflect the volume of tracer distribution and tracer exchange between compartments is described by linear rate constants [32].

A recent study by Uren [9] demonstrated the relationship between stenosis severity and degree of myocardial blood flow impairment, as determined by quantitative PET imaging. They found that in a range from 17 to 87% diameter stenosis resting coronary flow remains constant. Hyperemia or vasodilation induced maximal coronary flow diminishes progressively if a diameter stenosis is 40% or greater. Both findings are consistent with the concept of stenosis flow reserve first proposed by Gould [4, 31], whereas resting myocardial blood flow remains constant up to 80–90% diameter reduction. During vasodilation, however, flow progressively decreases beginning at a stenosis severity of 40%. Uren showed a significant inverse relation between myocardial blood flow during adenosine or dipyridamole induced hyperemia and percent diameter stenosis (Figure 4A), as well as a significant positive correlation between maximal myocardial blood flow and minimal lumen diameter (Figure 4B). These findings are consistant with previous experimental results [4]. Thus, noninvasive quantification of blood flow as measured with PET allows to assess stenosis flow reserve and carries important functional information on the physiological severity of a given morphological lesion as assessed from angiography.

Myocardial blood flow (ml/min/g)

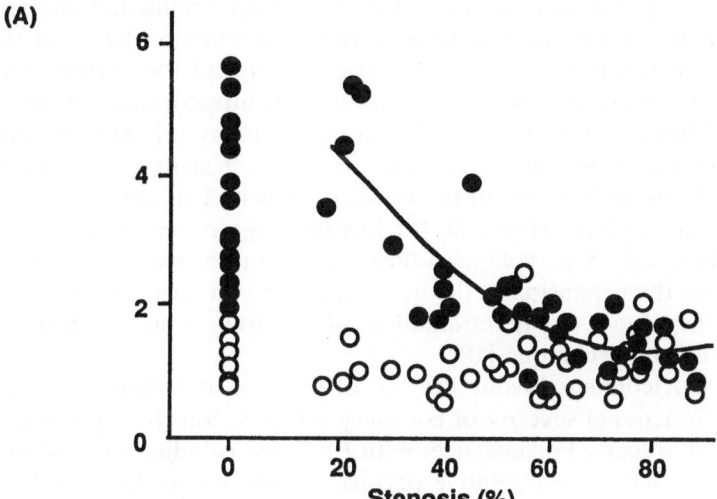

Myocardial blood flow (ml/min/g)

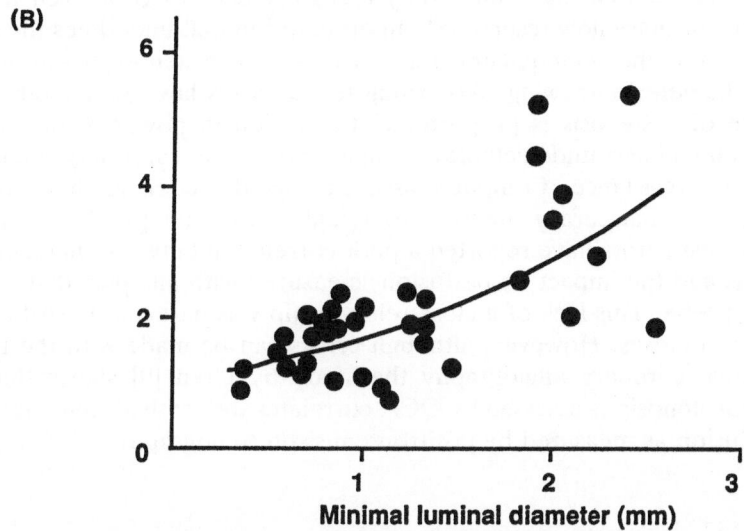

Figure 4. Myocardial blood flow versus stenosis severity as percent diameter stenosis (A) and as minimal lumen diameter (B). There was no significant correlation between blood flow in the 35 patients at base line (open circles) and the degree of their stenosis; flow during hyperemia (solid circles) however, was significantly impaired as stenosis severity increased. The values in the 21 controls are shown at 0% stenosis; some circles represent more than one control (A). There was a significant correlation between blood flow during hyperemia and the stenosis severity (B). (From: Uren NG, Melin JA, De Bruyne B et al. Relation between myocardial blood flow and the severity of coronary artery stenosis. N Engl J Med 1994; 330: 1782, by permission of the New England Jounal of Medicine.)

Previous investigators tried to integrate all geometric characteristics of a coronary artery stenosis, including diameter or area reduction and length of the lesion. Kirkeeide demonstrated a strong correlation between the flow reserve predicted from angiographic assessment and the coronary flow reserve measured with flowmeters [3]. In humans, intracoronary Doppler catheters have been used to measure blood flow velocity [5]. The measurement of absolute blood flow however from the Doppler signal is only possible if the cross-sectional diameter of the vessel is known. This approach, however, has several limitations: above all, the fact that measurements with a Doppler catheter do neither take collateral flow and flow to branches proximal to the stenosis, nor the expansion of the distal vascular bed during vasodilation into account; therefore, the determination of nutritive tissue perfusion is not feasible with this technique [18].

These shortcomings favour the use of positron emission tomography to assess the functional severity of coronary artery lesions by the tissue uptake of PET flow tracers. For instance, with PET and rubidium-82 and nitrogen-13 labeled ammonia, the relative perfusion reserve correlated with stenosis severity expressed as percent vessel diameter or area reduction in a curvilinear fashion [32]. Stenosis flow reserve, however, varies widely in patients with stenosis of 50–60% diameter. For instance, 38% of patients with stenoses greater than 50% have only a slightly decreased or even normal estimated coronary flow reserve [8], an observation that underlines the problem of defining the hemodynamic relevance of a given stenosis based only on percent diameter narrowing. According to Laplace's law the hemodynamic relevance of a stenosis is proportional to the fourth power of the radius, thus, small changes undetectable by angiography may cause larger changes in coronary resistance. Computer assisted edge-detection methods reduce the error and inaccuracy inherent to visual assessment [3]. Nevertheless, several investigators have reported a poor correlation between the degree of a stenosis and the impact on perfusion, measured with an epicardial suction Doppler probe. This lack of a close relationship was particularly striking for moderate stenoses. However, although errors can be made with the use of quantitative coronary angiography the study by Uren [9] shows that the severity of stenosis as assessed by QCA correlates well with absolute myocardial perfusion as measured by positron emission tomography.

QCA, positron emission tomography and stenosis severity

Quantitative coronary arteriography accounting for parameters of stenosis dimension such as percent narrowing, absolute lumen area, and length is thought to provide a single integrated measure of anatomic geometry with sufficient accuracy, both for an investigative purpose and for clinical decision making. This concept has been theoretically and experimentally both validated and challenged, but has been demonstrated to be somewhat clinically useful. Conversely, positron emission tomography provides a physiological and truely quantitative approach to myocardial perfusion and for the evaluation of specific therapeutic interventions in the management of coronary heart disease. PET technology for quantifying myocardial blood flow in humans has reached a point at which it can be applied routinely and reliably for the study of coronary stenosis significance and objectively assesses the result of interventional revascularization. Both, the accurate noninvasive physiological and the angiographic anatomic definition of stenosis severity are complementary. Together, they provide a complete morphological and functional description of a given coronary artery narrowing. (See also Chapters 8, 9, 11, 22 and 19.)

References

1. Klocke FJ. Measurements of coronary flow reserve: Defining pathophysiology versus making decisions about patient care. Circulation 1987; 76: 1183–9.
2. Gould KL. Identifying and measuring severity of coronary artery stenosis. Quantitative coronary arteriogragrphy and positron emission tomograpy. Circulation 1988; 78: 237–45.
3. Kirkeeide RL, Gould KL, Parsel L. Assessment of coronary stenoses by myocardial perfusion imaging during pharmacologic coronary vasodilation. VII. Validation of coronary flow reserve as a single integrated functional measure of stenosis severity reflecting all its geometric dimensions. JACC 1986; 7: 103–13.
4. Gould KL, Kirkeeide RL, Buchi M. Coronary flow reserve as a physiologic measure of stenosis severity. JACC 1990; 15: 459–74.
5. Wilson RF, Marcus ML, White CW. Prediction of the physiologic significance of coronary arterial lesions by quantitative lesion geometry in patients with limited coronary artery disease. Circulation 1987; 75: 723–32.
6. Nissen SE, Elion JL, Booth DC et al. Value and limitations of computer analysis of digital subtraction angiography in the assessment of coronary flow reserve. Circulation 1986; 73, 562–71.
7. Vogel RA, LeFree M, Bates E et al. Application of digital techniques to selective coronary arteriography: Use of myocardial contrast appearence time to measure coronary flow reserve. Am Heart J 1984; 107: 153–64.
8. Demer LL, Gould KL, Goldstein RA et al. Assessment of coronary artery disease severity by positron emission tomography: Comparison with quantitative arteriography in 193 patients. Circulation 1989; 79: 825–35.
9. Uren NG, Melin JA, De Bruyne B et al. Relation between myocardial blood flow and the severity of coronary artery stenosis. N Engl J Med 1994; 330: 1782–8.
10. Gould KL, Goldstein RA, Mullani NA et al. Noninvasive assessment of coronary stenoses by myocardial perfusion imaging during pharmacologic coronary vasodilation. VIII. Clinical feasibility of positron cardiac imaging without a cyclotron using generator-produced rubidium-82. JACC 1986; 7: 775–89.
11. Bol A, Melin JA, Vanoverschelde JL et al. Direct comparison of ^{13}N ammonia and ^{15}O water estimates of perfusion with quantification of regional myocardial blood flow by mircopheres. Circulation 1993; 87: 512–25.
12. Bergmann SR, Herrero P, Markham J et al. Noninvasive quantification of myocardial blood flow in human subjects with oxygen-15-labeled water and positron emission tomography. JACC 1989; 14: 639–52.
13. Hutchins GD, Schwaiger M, Rosenspire KC et al. Noninvasive quantification of regional

blood flow in the human heart using N-13 Ammonia and dynamic positron emission tomographic imaging. JACC 1990; 15: 1032–42.

14. Krivokapich J, Smith GT, Huang SC et al. ^{13}N ammonia myocardial imaging at rest and with exercice in normal volunteers: Quantification of absolute myocardial perfusion with dynamic positron emission tomography. Circulation 1989; 80: 1328–37.

15. Krivokapich J, Huang SC, Phelps ME et al. Dependence of 13-NH1$_3$ myocardial extraction and clearance on flow and metabolism. Am J Physiol 1982; 242: H536.

16. Lockwood AH. Absorbed doses of radiation after an intravenous injection of N-13 ammonia in man: Concise communication. J Nucl Med 1980; 21: 276.

17. Gould KL, Lipscomb K, Hamilton GW. Physiologic basis for assessing critical coronary stenosis. Am J Cardiol 1974; 33: 87–94.

18. Sibley DH, Millar HD, Hartley CJ et al. Subselective measurement of coronary blood flow velocity using a steerable Doppler catheter. J Am Coll Cardiol 1986; 8: 1332–40.

19. Nienaber C, Ratib O, Gambhir S et al. A quantitative index of regional blood flow in canine myocardium derived noninvasively with N-13 ammonia and dynamic positron emission tomography. J Am Coll Cardiol 1991; 17: 260–9.

20. Bergmann SR, Fox KAA, Rand AL et al. Quantification of regional myocardial blood flow in vivo with H$_2$^{15}O. Circulation 1984; 70: 724.

21. Rosenspire KC, Schwaiger M, Mangner TJ et al. Metabolic fate of N-13 ammonia in human and canine blood. J Nucl Med 1990; 31(3): 163–7.

22. Goldstein RA, Kirkeeide RL, Demer LL et al. Relation between geometric dimensions of coronary artery stenoses and myocardial perfusion reserve in man. J Clin Invest 1987; 79: 1473–8.

23. Brown BG, Bolson E, Frimer M et al. Quantitative coronary arteriography: Estimation of dimensions, hemodynamic resistance, and atheroma mass of coronary artery lesions using the arteriogram and digital computation. Circulation 1977, 55: 329–37.

24. Gould KL. Assessment of coronary stenoses with myocardial perfusion imaging during pharmacologic vasodilation. IV. Limits of detection of stenosis with idealized experimental cross-sectional myocardial imaging. Am J Cardiol 1978, 42: 761–8.

25. Gould KL, Schelbert HR, Phelps ME et al. Noninvasive assessment of coronary stenosis with myocardial perfusion imaging during pharmacologic coronary vasodilation. V. Detection of 47% diameter coronary stenosis with intravenous 13-N ammonia and emission-computed tomography in intact dogs. Am J Cardiol 1979, 43: 200–8.

26. Kearfot KJ. Radiation absorbed dose estimates for positron emission tomography (PET): K-38, Rb-81, Rb-82 and Dx-130. J Nucl Med 1982; 23: 1128.

27. Goldstein RA, Mullani NA, Marsani SK et al. Myocardial perfusion with rubidium-82. II. Effects of metabolic and pharmacologic interventions. J Nucl Med 1983; 24: 907.

28. Budinger TF, Derenzo SE, Gullbert GT et al. Emission computer-assisted tomography with single-photon and positron annihilation photons. J Comput Assist Tomogr 1977; 1: 131–45.

29. Tamaki N, Yonekura Y, Senda M et al. Value and limitation of stress thallium-201 single photon emission computed tomography: Comparison with nitrogen-13 ammonia positron tomography. J Nucl Med 1988; 29: 1181–8.

30. Stewart R, Schwaiger M, Molina E et al. Comparison of rubidium-82 positron emission tomography and thallium-201 SPECT imaging for detection of coronary artery disease. Am J Cardiol 1991; 67: 1303–8.

31. Gould KL. Assessment of coronary stenoses with myocardial perfusion imaging during pharmacologic vasodilatation. IV. Limits of detection of stenosis with idealized experimental cross-sectional myocardial imaging. Am J Cardiol 1978; 42: 761.

32. Schelbert HR. Consideration of measurements of myocardial blood flow with positron-emission tomography. Investigative Radiology 1993; 28 (Suppl 4): S47–55.

33. Schelbert HR, Phelps ME, Hoffmann E et al. Regional myocardial perfusion assessed with N-13 labelled ammonia and positron emission computerized axial tomography. Am J Cardiol 1979; 43: 209.

34. Yonekura Y, Tamaki N, Senda M et al. Detection of coronary artery disease with 13-N-ammonia and high resolution positron emission computed tomography. Am Heart J 1987; 113: 645.
35. Tamaki N, Yonekurea Y, Senda M et al. Value and limitation of stress TI-201 tomography. Comparison with perfusion and metabolic imaging with positron tomography. Circulation 1987; 76 (Suppl. IV): IV-4.

Corresponding Author: Dr Gunnar K. Lund, Department of Cardiology, University Hospital Eppendorf, Martinistrasse 52, D-20246, Hamburg, Germany

11. Contrast enhanced magnetic resonance imaging for assessing myocardial perfusion and reperfusion injury

LEONARD M. NUMEROW, MICHAEL F. WENDLAND,
MAYTHEM SAEED and CHARLES B. HIGGINS

Introduction

Noninvasive cardiac imaging techniques are being used with increasing frequency to guide interventional procedures as they are being applied to ischemic heart disease and to assess their effects. These interventions relieve coronary artery stenoses that produce myocardial ischemia, and improve myocardial perfusion after thrombolytic therapy. New fast and ultra-fast magnetic resonance imaging (MRI) techniques have ameliorated previous limitations of slow temporal resolution. With these methods, high resolution images of the heart are obtained in seconds or fractions of a second. Thus, MRI may now image the first pass of a contrast agent bolus through the heart. Recent experimental, and some limited clinical experience indicate that dynamic contrast enhanced cardiac MRI is a valuable imaging technique for myocardial perfusion imaging. Contrast enhanced MRI might be used to 1) define zones of myocardial ischemia (perfusion defects) based upon rapid imaging during the first pass of a contrast agent; 2) differentiate occlusive from reperfused infarctions; and 3) determine myocardial viability.

MR contrast media in cardiac imaging

In general, MRI contrast media [1] consist of paramagnetic ions such as gadolinium (Gd), manganese (Mn), or dysprosium (Dy) complexed to chelates, such as DTPA. The distribution space of a MR contrast agent depends on the nature of the ligand forming the complex. These MR contrast media may be primarily intravascular or extravascular, and extravascular agents may be located in the intracellular or extracellular spaces.

An important imaging characteristic of a MR contrast medium is its basic influence on myocardial signal intensity: T1 relaxation enhancement or magnetic susceptibility effect (Figure 1A). T1 enhancing agents such as Gd-DTPA shorten the T1 relaxation time of perfused myocardial tissue, increasing signal intensity on T1-weighted images (Figure 1B). This contrast-produc-

C.A. Nienaber and U. Sechtem (eds): Imaging and Intervention in Cardiology, 149–165.
© 1996 Kluwer Academic Publishers.

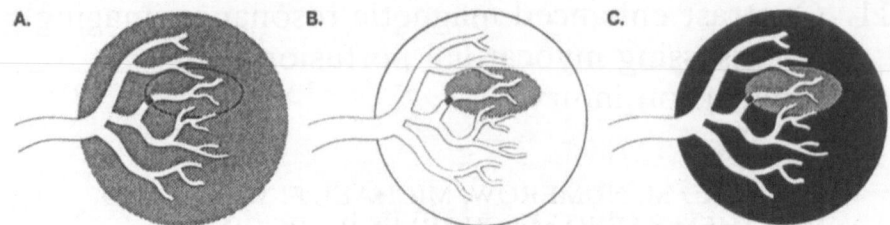

Figure 1. MR imaging scheme to demonstrate myocardial ischemia using T1 enhancing and magnetic susceptibility contrast media. (Reprinted, with permission, from MR Imaging of the Body. Higgins CB, Hricak H, Helms C. New York, Raven Press, 1992: 1291.) (A) Without MR contrast media there is no contrast between normal and ischemic myocardium, in the early hours after occlusion. (B) Following administration of a T1 enhancing contrast agent, signal intensity in normal myocardium is increased and the ischemic zone is demarcated as a region of low signal intensity ("cold spot"). (C) After administration of a magnetic susceptibility contrast agent, signal intensity of normal myocardium is reduced (negative enhancement) and the ischemic zone is demarcated as a zone of high signal intensity ("hot spot").

ing effect of the agent depends upon delivery by myocardial perfusion and tissue water content, for it is upon the abundant water proton that the contrast medium exerts its T1 enhancing effect. Following contrast agent administration, normally perfused myocardium experiences the T1 shortening effect of the delivered contrast molecules, and signal intensity is increased. In hypoperfused myocardium, delivery of contrast medium is reduced, so these zones initially encounter less of the T1 shortening effect and appear hypointense compared to greatly enhanced normal myocardium. T1 enhancing media also cause a decrease in the T2 relaxation time, causing signal intensity to be reduced at higher doses.

Magnetic susceptibility agents shorten the T2 relaxation time, which causes signal intensity to decrease in areas to which they are distributed (Figure 1C). With these contrast media, visualized image signal intensity depends on delivery by perfusion as well as compartmentalization of the agent. Contrast molecules restricted to (compartmentalized in) the extracellular space surrounding viable cardiac myocytes cause local signal to be depleted (negative enhancement). However, if these contrast molecules are distributed in both the intracellular and extracellular spaces due to loss of myocardial cell membrane integrity, then the tissue signal intensity persists since the agent does not exert its effect. Therefore, when imaged with magnetic susceptibility contrast media, normally perfused myocardial regions (which compartmentalize the contrast molecules) are depleted of MR signal. Regions having reduced perfusion appear hyperintense. As well, zones with intact delivery but no contrast molecule compartmentalization (reperfused infarctions) are relatively hyperintense.

Thus, both families of MR contrast media produce differential signal (contrast) between normal and abnormal myocardium by preferentially influencing the signal of tissue that is normally perfused. With T1 enhancing agents, perfusion defects are "cold spots" and with magnetic susceptibility agents they are "hot spots".

Evaluation of myocardial perfusion and identification of perfusion defects

MRI techniques for assessing perfusion

For cardiac MRI studies, traditional electrocardiogram-gated spin echo and cine-gradient recalled echo (GRE) MRI sequences have been used extensively. These high spatial resolution techniques depict cardiac and extracardiac anatomy, wall motion, and regional wall thickening [2]. However, with spin echo methods, first pass perfusion studies of a contrast agent bolus cannot be performed because of inherent slow temporal resolution.

Recently developed fast and ultra-fast MRI sequences have overcome the limitations of spin echo and cine-GRE techniques, and allow noninvasive assessment of myocardial perfusion [3]. Among the most popular of these methods are fast gradient recalled echo (GRE) strategies [3, 4] and echo planar imaging (EPI) [5]. Fast GRE methods provide tomographic cardiac perfusion images at 1 to 3 second intervals. With slight variations in MR pulse sequences, these imaging techniques can either be T1-weighted (inversion recovery prepared fast GRE) [3] or T2-weighted (driven equilibrium prepared fast GRE) [4]. The MR contrast media used for these studies are T1 enhancing agents and magnetic susceptibility agents, respectively. Another technique for monitoring the transit of a contrast agent through the heart is EPI [5]. Tomographic images are typically obtained with a short exposure time, in the range of 30–50 milliseconds. Because of these ultra-fast imaging times, motion artifacts are reduced and there is no need for electrocardiogram-gated acquisitions. Similar to the fast GRE techniques, EPI pulse sequences can be modified to emphasize T1 or T2 (T2*) effects. In these studies a single contrast agent may produce T1 enhancing effects or magnetic susceptibility effects depending on the echo-planar sequence used and the concentration of the contrast agent. However, at the present time, availability of EPI is limited because of special hardware requirements. In the near future, this capability may be available on standard MR imagers.

Coronary artery occlusion: Animal studies

Contrast enhanced fast and ultra-fast MRI techniques have been applied in animal models to examine differences in myocardial tissue signal intensity caused by coronary artery occlusions. Ligating the left coronary artery in an isolated perfused rat heart model, Atkinson et al. [3] performed T1–weighted fast GRE MR imaging after infusion of a T1 enhancing contrast agent. Compared to pre contrast images, signal intensity increased four-fold in nonischemic myocardium and was essentially unaltered in zones of ischemia. Perfusion defects were observed almost immediately and for several hours following coronary artery occlusion. In vivo studies of rat hearts have also been conducted with ultra-fast MR techniques within 2 hours of left coronary artery occlusion [6]. After the bolus administration of T1 enhancing or magnetic susceptibility contrast agents, T1 or T2*-weighted EPI was performed. On the T1–weighted images, normal myocardial tissue enhanced (brightened) following contrast agent infusion and nonenhanced ("cold spot") perfusion defects were observed. For T2*-weighted experiments, contrast medium influence on normal myocardium was seen as signal depletion (negative enhancement), and ischemic myocardium maintained signal, so perfusion defects were "hot spots". Myocardial perfusion defects have also been observed in other rat experiments using T1 and T2*-weighted EPI sequences and other contrast agents, Gd-BOPTA/Dimeg [7] or Gd-DTPA-BMA [5] (Figure 2).

In a similar model of LAD occlusion in dogs, Saeed et al. [8] used fast GRE sequences to demonstrate perfusion defects in zones of myocardial ischemia with both T1 relaxation enhancing and magnetic susceptibility effect agents. A positive correlation [9] has been found between the alteration of myocardial MR signal induced by the T1 enhancing agent, Gd-DTPA, and myocardial blood flow assessed by microsphere distribution. Of interest, quantification of the peak signal change as a function of injected dose of a magnetic susceptibility agent has been performed [10]. Results suggest a linear relationship between injected dose and relaxation rate $(1/T2^*)$. The quantification of myocardial perfusion will be discussed in a subsequent section.

Clinical studies in myocardial infarction

Clinical experience with contrast enhanced fast and ultra-fast MRI in patients with myocardial infarction is limited. A recent study [11] examined dynamic signal intensity changes on contrast enhanced fast MR images in 14 patients

---

→

Figure 2. Myocardial perfusion defects demonstrated by inversion recovery (T1-weighted) and gradient echo (T2*-weighted) echo-planar MRI, two hours after left coronary artery occlusion in a rat. Selected transaxial images before as well as 6, 12, and 28 seconds after Gd-DTPA-BMA injection at low dose (T1 enhancing effects) and high dose (magnetic susceptibility effects) are shown. (RV = right ventricular cavity; LV = left ventricular cavity.) (A) Inversion recovery EPI initially demonstrates increased signal (enhancement) of the LV at 6 seconds followed by enhancement of normal myocardium. Note the hypointense perfusion defect (arrows) in the anterolateral wall of the left ventricle. (B) Gradient echo EPI demonstrates signal depletion (negative enhancement) in RV and LV at 6 seconds, and subsequent signal loss from normal myocardium at 12 seconds. The perfusion defect in the anterolateral wall of the left ventricle (arrows) is hyperintense.

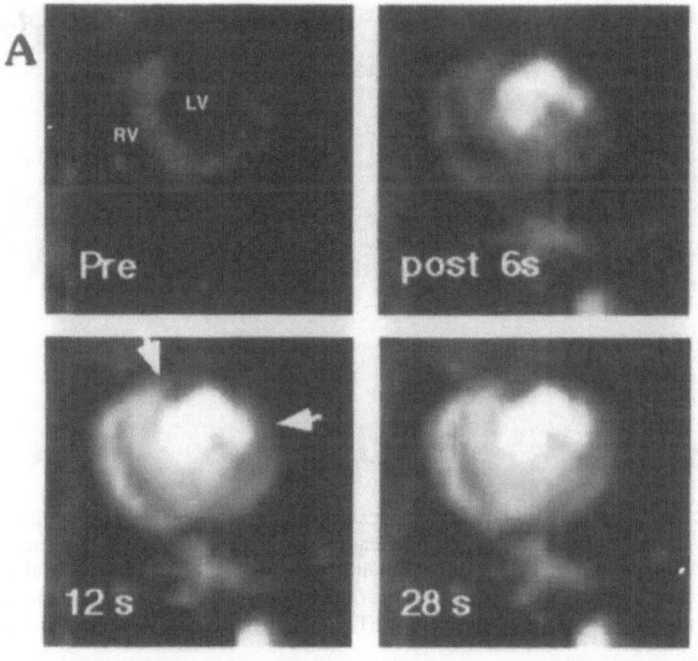

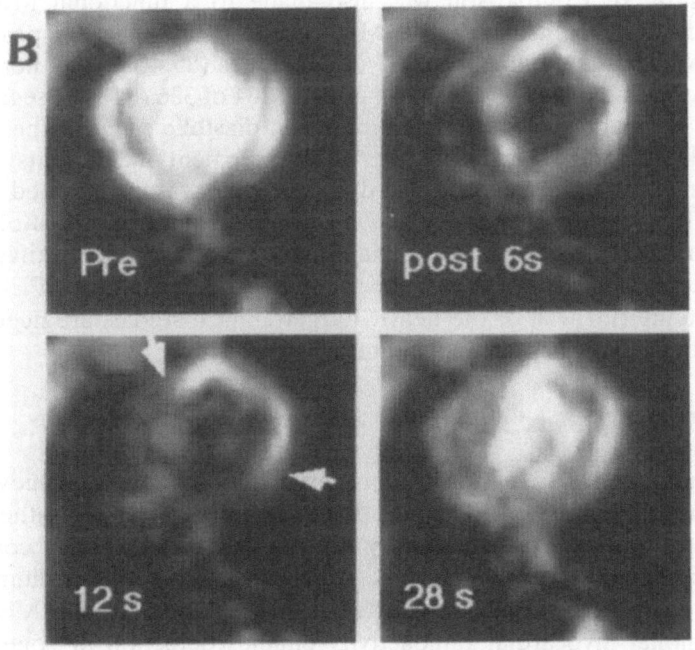

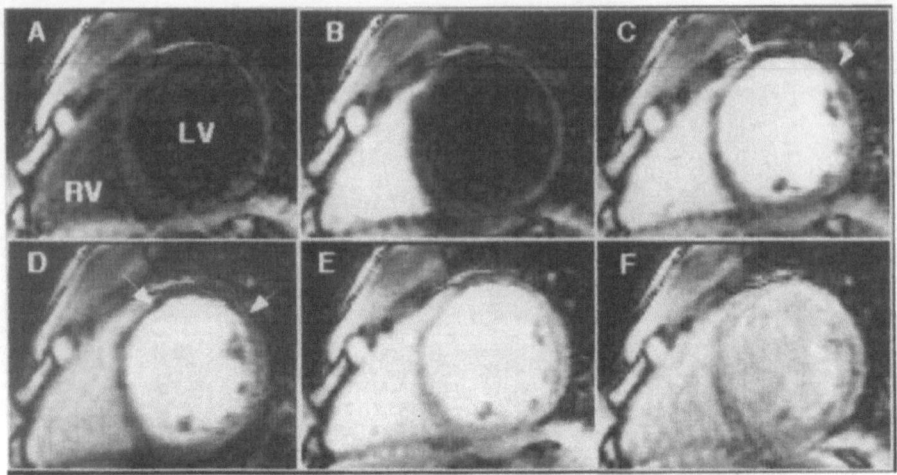

Figure 3. Selected transaxial ultra-fast MR images at the mid-ventricular level demonstrate the pattern of dynamic contrast enhancement in a patient with previous anterior wall myocardial infarction. After pre-contrast image A, note sequential brightening (enhancement) of RV (image B) and LV (image C), followed by normal myocardium (images C, D). A hypointense anterior wall perfusion defect is demarcated by arrows. (RV = right ventricular cavity, LV = left ventricular cavity.)

with fixed myocardial perfusion defects (infarctions) on SPECT thallium studies (Figure 3). Comparison was also made to a functional MR wall motion study in each instance. The MR perfusion images were positively correlated with thallium images in 287 of 336 zones (85.4%). MR perfusion results also correlated well with MR function in 284 of 336 (84.5%) segments. Of interest, normal myocardial signal intensity, diastolic wall thickness, and systolic thickening were seen in the inferior wall segment of 2 patients, where thallium tomograms portrayed a fixed defect that was interpreted as an infarction. This observation raises the possibility that these zones of fixed thallium perfusion defect represent diaphragmatic attenuation artifact and that contrast enhanced MRI may be more specific than thallium SPECT for assessing the inferior wall of the heart. Larger clinical studies are needed to provide further evidence to substantiate this possibility.

Coronary artery stenosis: Animal studies

Presently, noninvasive detection of coronary artery stenosis is achieved by observing myocardial tissue alterations due to reduced perfusion, rather than by direct visualization of the coronary arteries. One of the most common techniques is radionuclide scintigraphy, which images the myocardium after delivery of a radiotracer that is extracted from the blood stream. Measurement of regional myocardial radioactivity enables detection of zones with reduced relative perfusion. In an analogous fashion, contrast enhanced dynamic MRI studies can provide evidence of coronary artery disease (CAD) by depicting myocardial perfusion defects during the first pass of a bolus of contrast agent. Image contrast is predominantly due to decreased delivery of the contrast agent in ischemic myocardium versus normal tissue (see also Chapters 9–12).

MR perfusion studies ideally are performed in both the basal resting state and during stress, which evokes disparate flow at higher flow rates. However, because of physical space restrictions and MRI motion artifacts during exercise, dynamic forms of stress such as treadmill or bicycle exercise are impractical when inside an MR imager. As a result, pharmacologic forms of stress such as intravenous dipyridamole, adenosine or dobutamine infusion are more widely used.

Perfusion defects have been successfully depicted using intravenous dipyridamole in a canine model of myocardial ischemia, produced by surgical creation of coronary artery stenosis. In one experiment, Wilke et al. [9] used contrast enhanced T1-weighted fast MRI to examine 24 dogs at rest and following dipyridamole (0.8 mg/kg) infusion. Radioactive microspheres confirmed regional myocardial blood flow levels. During vasodilation, hypoperfused myocardium appeared as a hypointense perfusion defect on MR images. In another 5 dogs [12], contrast enhanced fast MRI was used with an intravascular T1 enhancing agent and the vasodilator adenosine to successfully differentiate myocardium affected by a subtotal LAD occlusion (intracoronary pressure 40–50 mm Hg) from normal myocardium. Most recently, T1-weighted fast MRI after dipyridamole administration has demonstrated perfusion defects with the T1 enhancing contrast agent Gd-BOPTA/Dimeg, in a canine model of coronary artery stenosis (Figure 4). In the basal state, hypoperfused could not be distinguished from normal myocardium. However, following dipyridamole hyperemia, perfusion defects were identified as zones of delayed and reduced peak enhancement.

Coronary artery stenosis: *Clinical studies*

Contrast enhanced dynamic MR imaging of patients with non occlusive CAD has been performed in the basal state alone and also in basal followed by vasodilated states. Manning et al. [14] studied 12 patients with severe (>80% luminal diameter reduction) coronary artery stenoses at rest. Because stenoses were severe, it was expected that perfusion might be reduced in the basal state [15]. Examining the first pass signal intensity versus time curve, myocardium supplied by severely stenotic vessels had a lower peak signal intensity and a lower rate of signal increase compared to myocardium perfused by coronary arteries without stenoses (p = 0.001 for both measurements). Following revascularization, peak signal intensity in these ischemic myocardial zones became virtually normal, although the rate of signal intensity increase remained unchanged.

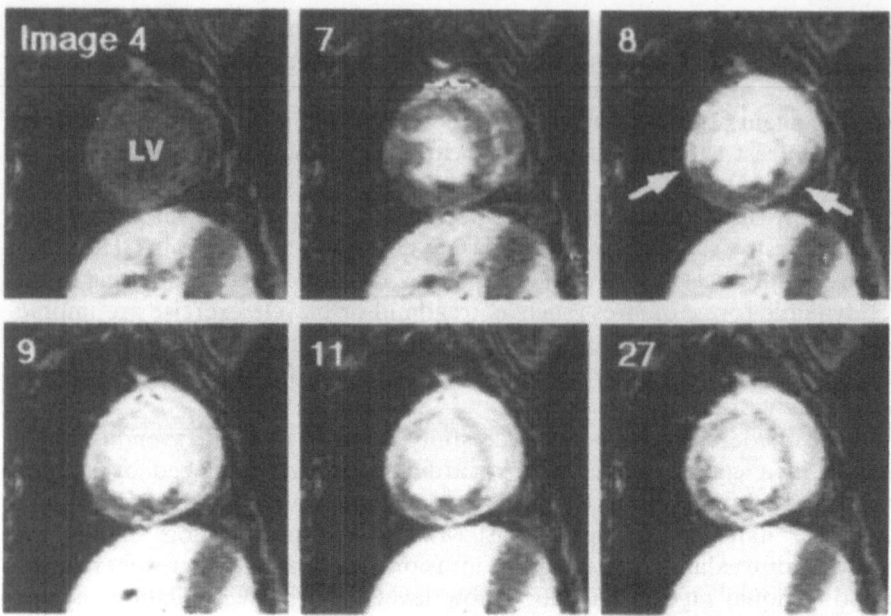

Figure 4. Selected transaxial inversion recovery (T1-weighted) fast GRE MR images obtained during the first pass of a gadolinium chelate (Gd-BOPTA/Dimeg, 0.05 mmol/kg) following infusion of dipyridamole (0.5 mg/kg) in a canine model of left circumflex coronary artery stenosis. Baseline image 4 is obtained before injection of the contrast agent. After contrast administration, signal intensity of the left ventricular cavity (LV) increases (image 7). Image 8 depicts enhancement of normal myocardium and a perfusion defect in the diaphragmatic segment of the left ventricle is defined by arrows. Subsequently, the hypoperfused myocardial zone enhances in a delayed manner.

Other studies have included pharmacologic vasodilation aiming to increase sensitivity for detecting CAD. Schaefer et al. [16] examined 6 patients with CAD using contrast enhanced T1-weighted fast MRI before and after dipyridamole administration, demonstrating reduced peak MRI signal in 9 myocardial zones. Thallium-201 scintigraphy perfusion defects were seen at 8 of 9 of these MRI perfusion defects, and angiography confirmed CAD involving the supplying vessels. Another study of 19 patients with angiographically defined CAD (>75% stenosis) [17] compared MRI to 99 m-Technetium Sestamibi (MIBI) SPECT perfusion imaging before and after dipyridamole. Compared to MIBI, contrast enhanced fast MRI detected hypoperfused myocardium in 15/19 patients at rest, and in 18/19 patients during hyperemia. In addition, certain flow parameters derived from sequential MR images (inverse mean transit time and time to peak signal intensity) provided an estimation of reduced coronary flow reserve in hypoperfused myocardium. However, these studies did not address the sensitivity of MRI for detecting CAD. Klein et al. [18] used contrast enhanced fast MRI before and after dipyridamole to study 5 patients, comparing results to contrast angiography and MIBI scintigraphy. With coronary arteriography as a gold standard, pre- and post-dipyridamole MRI depicted 13 true-positive segments, 9 true-negative segments, 3 false-negative segments, and no false-positive segments, yielding 81% sensitivity and 100% specificity for detecting chronically ischemic myocardium. Agreement with MIBI in these patients was somewhat less, with sensitivity 77–92% and specificity 75%. Thus, fast MRI methods show potential for the noninvasive detection of CAD.

MR quantification of regional myocardial blood flow

Recent applications of ultra-fast MRI techniques for detection of myocardial ischemia and infarction have raised interest in using MR for the measurement of tissue perfusion. However, to quantitate perfusion, a number of conditions must be fulfilled: 1) true first pass conditions must be present so that recirculation does not contribute to MR signal intensity; 2) the contrast medium must be administered as a rapid bolus (<2 seconds); 3) temporal MR resolution must be adequate; and (4) an accurate kinetic model is required to describe the arterial bolus input function. This model should integrate kinetics of the contrast agent, taking into account intercompartmental water exchange as well as other complex factors such as water kinetics and tissue compartmentalization.

The simplest model for measuring myocardial perfusion was described almost a century ago by Stewart [19] and is described more recently by Rosen et al. [20]. The Central Volume Theorem states that tissue blood flow (F) can be determined from the ratio

$$F = V/Tm$$

where V is the volume of distribution of the contrast agent in tissue, and Tm is the mean transit time, the time it takes for any given particle of the contrast agent to traverse the tissue. Wilke et al. [21] selected this model in an early attempt to quantify myocardial perfusion with contrast enhanced MRI in a canine model of myocardial ischemia. A preliminary experiment had shown that with fast MRI, measurement of inverse T1 ($1/T1 = \Delta R1$) values due to varying the concentration of Gd-DTPA in an isotonic saline solution was linearly related to the concentration of contrast agent. Fast MR imaging monitored the first pass of a T1 enhancing agent through the heart, before and after dipyridamole stress. By generating MR image signal intensity versus time curves, the parameter $1/Tm$ correlated closely with absolute myocardial blood flow, determined by simultaneous radiolabeled micros-

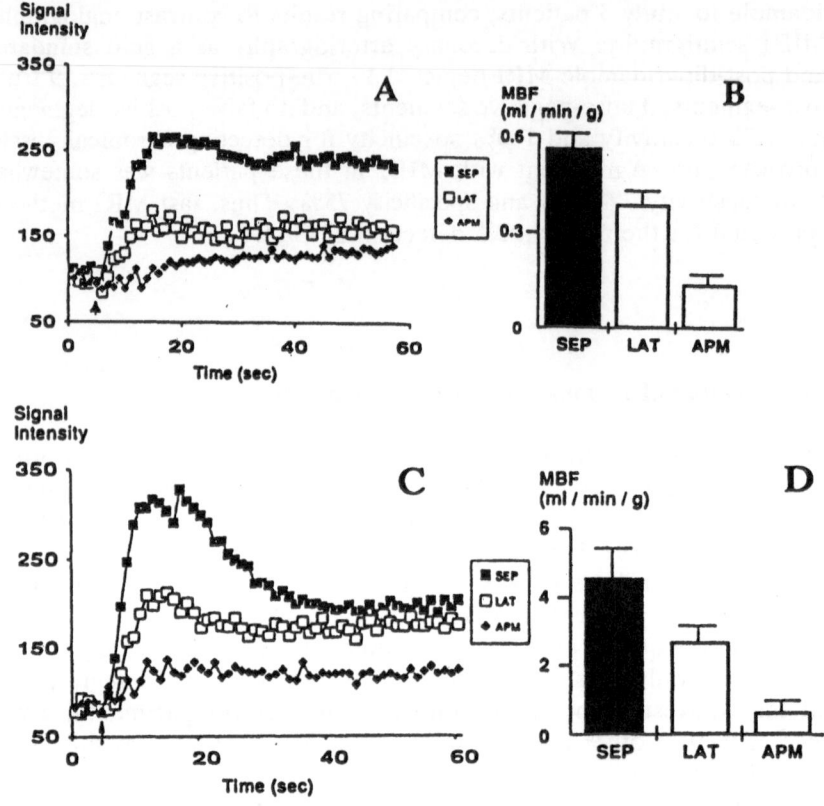

Figure 5. MR quantitation of myocardial perfusion following severe subtotal left coronary artery occlusion: signal intensity-time curves during myocardial first pass of a Gd-DTPA bolus and myocardial blood flow determined from microsphere measurements in three different myocardial segments (SEP = septum, LAT = lateral wall of the left ventricle, APM = anterior papillary muscle). (A) and (B) illustrate MRI and microsphere data, respectively, under resting (basal) conditions; and (C) and (D) show the data from the same animal after dipyridamole induced stress. Under resting conditions, perfusion differences among hypoperfused (APM), intermediate (LAT), and well perfused myocardium (SEP) are well differentiated, and agree qualitatively with the measured blood flow. During hyperemia, shortening of the rise time to peak signal intensity and a higher peak signal are observed in the normally perfused septal region. These changes are less marked in the intermediately perfused LAT, and absent in severely hypoperfused APM. (Reprinted, with permission, from [21], p. 493.)

phere injections (Figure 5). Thus, estimation of myocardial blood flow with MRI seems feasible.

On the other hand, Wendland et al. [22] used EPI to monitor the passage of incremental doses of intravascular and extracellular T1 enhancing contrast agents through normal rat myocardium and described current limitations of MR perfusion quantitation. They concluded that $\Delta R1$ of myocardium was not monoexponential and that models that are used to calculate myocardial blood flow from signal intensity changes require consideration of complex water kinetics in myocardial compartments. Also, extravascular contrast had a significantly altered first pass signal intensity-time profile compared to intravascular contrast, presumably due to extraction into the extracellular space. Such low molecular weight compounds may not be ideal for quantifying myocardial perfusion.

Perhaps the approach of Diesbourg et al. [23] will overcome some of the quantification limitations outlined above. A mathematical model, the modified Kety equation [24], was selected to pattern the myocardial tissue distribution and clearance of an extravascular contrast agent under first pass conditions. Use of this formula required MR measurement of myocardial contrast agent concentration following bolus injection. In an excised dog heart model, MR-calculated myocardial blood flow correlated positively with radioactive microsphere-determined flow. Relative myocardial blood flow in canine myocardium has also been predicted by the Kety equation using fast MR techniques [25]. In this study, results compared favorably with calculations from positron emission tomography ($p < 0.05$).

Differentiation of occlusive from reperfused infarctions

After thrombolytic therapy, it is crucial to determine that reperfusion has occurred at the tissue level and whether irreversibly injured myocardial tissue is present in the jeopardized region. Ito et al. [26] studied patients with acute myocardial infarctions who had angiographic evidence of reflow, using myocardial contrast echocardiography (MCE). Compared to patients with residual MCE perfusion defects (n = 9), those without defects (n = 30) had significant improvement in global and regional LV function when examined four weeks later. Thus, the demonstration of residual perfusion defects at the tissue level can be useful for predicting poor recovery of function in reperfused myocardium.

In animal experiments, contrast enhanced MRI with a T1 enhancing agent has been shown to be effective in differentiating occlusive infarction from reperfused myocardial infarction. Saeed et al. [27] showed in rats that reperfused, irreversibly injured myocardium enhanced significantly greater than either reperfused reversibly injured or normal myocardium (Figure 6A). In a separate study, the same group [28] also demonstrated that following T1 enhancing contrast medium administration, occlusive infarctions had a complicated enhancement pattern consisting of multiple zones (Figure 6B). Epicardial and endocardial margins of the infarctions enhanced immediately and homogeneously, while central zones, which were initially hypointense, gradually increased in intensity over 60 minutes following contrast administration. Enhancing occlusive infarction margins were observed and have since been referred to as the "peri-infarction zone" [29]. Occlusive and reperfused infarctions have also been studied with a magnetic susceptibility agent and

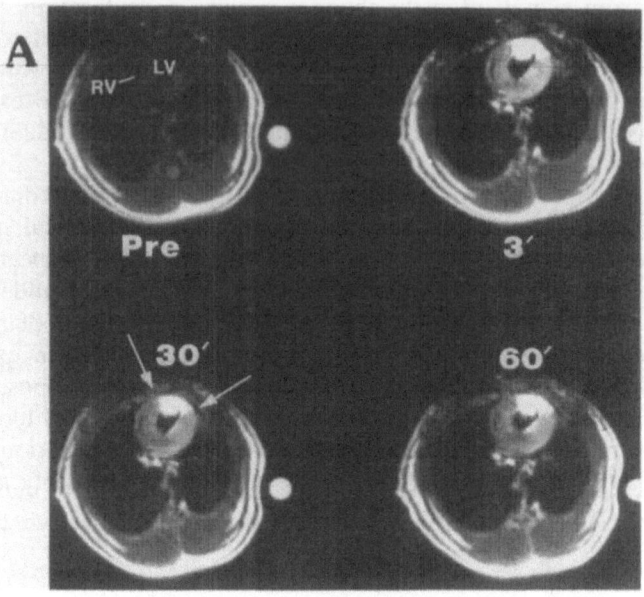

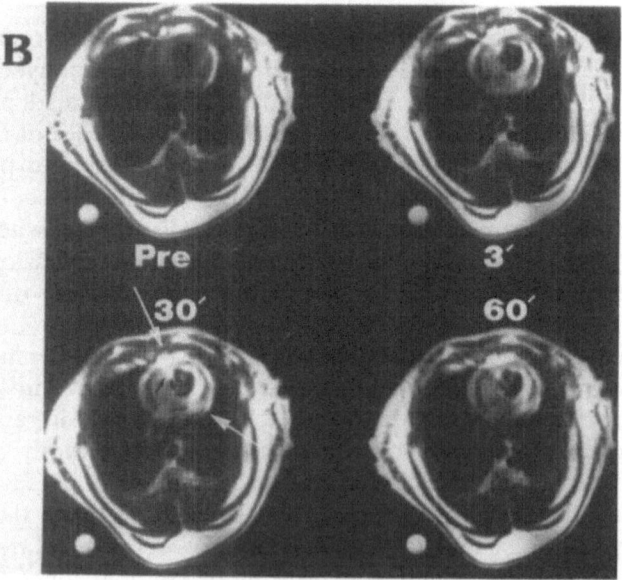

Figure 6. Sequential transaxial contrast enhanced T1-weighted MR images of a rat model of reperfused and occlusive myocardial infarction. (RV = right ventricular cavity, LV = left ventricular cavity.) (A) Prominent homogeneous enhancement of the injured anterolateral wall of the left ventricle (demarcated by arrows) is demonstrated after 2 hours of left coronary artery occlusion and 1.5 hours of reperfusion. (B) Complex pattern of contrast enhancement in a 3.5-hour-old occlusive infarction. Images demonstrate hypointense infarcted myocardium in the anterior and lateral walls of the left ventricle (larger white arrows), high signal intracavitary rim along the infarcted wall, and the peri-infarction zone (small black arrows), at the margins of the myocardial infarction.

T2-weighted MR imaging [30]. Following contrast administration, normal myocardium was almost completely depleted of signal, occlusive infarctions maintained most of their signal (74 ± 5% of baseline), and reperfused infarctions had intermediate signal (35 ± 3% of baseline).

To date, only one experiment has employed ultra-fast MR techniques to differentiate occlusive from reperfused myocardial infarctions. Saeed et al. [31] showed that occlusive infarctions had delayed or no enhancement during the first pass of a T1 enhancing agent. In reperfused infarctions, signal intensity rose continually during the first few minutes to a level of intensity exceeding normal myocardium.

Unfortunately, clinical circumstances in patients frequently do not involve pure circumstances of occlusive or reperfused myocardial infarctions, but rather a heterogeneous myocardial injury with components of both. Consequently, it has been difficult to determine the effectiveness of contrast enhanced MRI to reliably differentiate these two conditions. In patients with recent myocardial infarctions, de Roos et al. [32, 33] performed an electrocardiogram-gated spin-echo MRI sequence with a T1 enhancing agent, finding significant enhancement of occlusive and reperfused infarctions relative to normal myocardium. Enhancement patterns were complicated, and there was extensive overlap, precluding discrimination between the two. Van Rossum et al. [34] were able to distinguish occlusive from reperfused infarctions by the relative reduced enhancement of the occlusive infarction. This was seen only on their earliest images, at 6 to 8 minutes following contrast administration, suggesting that the difference was due to decreased initial delivery of Gd-DTPA. Increased and persistent MR signal has been found in reperfused myocardial infarctions [35]. Perhaps the temporal resolution of fast and ultra-fast MR methods will be useful in assessing for tissue reperfusion.

Contrast enhanced MRI for determining myocardial viability in reperfused infarction

An exciting new possibility has been suggested for determining myocardial necrosis in reperfused infarctions based upon examining the effects of MR contrast media on the myocardium [36, 37]. This approach utilizes both T1 enhancing and magnetic susceptibility agents (Figure 7). A T1 enhancing contrast agent is first used to define myocardial regions that are effectively perfused, either normal myocardium or reperfused infarctions. Subsequent administration of a magnetic susceptibility contrast agent causes signal depletion in myocardium that compartmentalizes contrast molecules, either normal myocardium or viable cells within the reperfused infarction. Nonviable zones, on the other hand, are not affected by the susceptibility agent because cellular compartments have collapsed. In other words, regions with reperfused necrotic myocardium show enhancement (signal increase) with a T1 relaxation

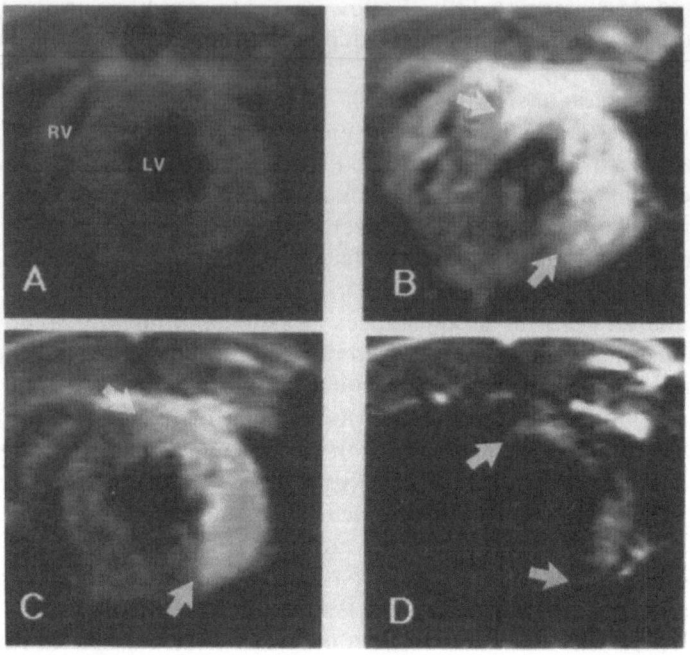

Figure 7. Selected transaxial MR images of a rat subjected to 2 hours of left coronary artery occlusion and 2 hours of reperfusion. T1-weighted images pre-contrast (A) and post-administration of Gd-DTPA-BMA (B) demonstrate increased signal intensity (enhancement) in the anterolateral wall of the LV (arrows), confirming reperfusion at the tissue level. A T2-weighted image before (C) the administration of magnetic susceptibility agent depicts increased signal anterolaterally (arrows) consistent with myocardial edema. Following Dy-DTPA-BMA (D), signal depletion (negative enhancement) involves all myocardium except the anterolateral wall of the LV (arrows), where nonviability (infarction) was confirmed by histopathologic staining. (RV = right ventricle, LV = left ventricle.)

enhancing agent but reduced or no enhancement (signal does not decrease) with a magnetic susceptibility contrast medium.

This strategy has been recently tested in experimental in vivo and in vitro rat models of reperfused myocardial infarction [36, 37]. The T1 enhancing and magnetic susceptibility contrast agents were injected following 1–2 hours of LAD occlusion and then 1–3 hours of reperfusion. The concentrations of both contrast agents measured by biochemical assay were higher in reperfused infarction than in normal myocardium. On MR images in vivo and following extirpation of the heart, reperfused infarctions appeared as bright zones on T1-weighted images, confirming delivery of T1 enhancing agents. On T2-weighted images, these reperfused zones had less signal depletion than normal myocardium and therefore appeared bright, despite having a higher concentration of the magnetic susceptibility agent (Figure 7). This combination of findings is consistent with cellular nonviability. Thus, reperfused infarcted tissue can be characterized by showing delivery of the T1 enhancing agent to the jeopardized tissue and lack of enhancement with a magnetic susceptibility contrast medium.

Conclusion

Because of exciting recent improvements in temporal resolution, development of new contrast media, and novel imaging strategies, MRI has considerable potential for the evaluation of ischemic heart disease. Future clinical uses will include detection of myocardial ischemia and infarction, quantification of regional myocardial perfusion, differentiation of reperfused from occlusive infarction, and determination of myocardial viability.

Acknowledgements

Special thanks to Drs Scott Flamm and Luc Jutras for their helpful suggestions during the preparation of this manuscript. Dr Numerow is supported by a grant from the Alberta Heritage Foundation for Medical Research.

References

1. Higgins CB, Saeed M, Wendland MF et al. Contrast media for cardiothoracic MR imaging. JMRI 1993; 3: 265–76.
2. Higgins CB. Essentials of cardiac radiology and imaging. Philadelphia: J.B. Lippincott Company, 1992: 253–82.
3. Atkinson JA, Burstein D, Edelman RR et al. First pass cardiac perfusion: Evaluation with ultrafast MR imaging. Radiology 1990; 174: 757–62.
4. Sakuma H, O'Sullivan M, Lucas J et al. Effect of magnetic susceptibility contrast medium on myocardial signal intensity with fast gradient-recalled echo and spin-echo MR imaging: Initial experience in humans. Radiology 1994; 190: 161–6.
5. Wendland MF, Saeed M, Masui T et al. Echo-planar MR imaging of normal and ischemic myocardium with gadodiamide injection. Radiology 1993; 186: 535–42.
6. Wendland MF, Saeed M, Higgins CB. Strategies for differential enhancement of myocardial ischemia using echoplanar imaging. Invest Radiol 1991; 26: S236–8.
7. Yu KK, Saeed M, Wendland MF et al. Real-time dynamics of an extravascular magnetic resonance contrast medium in acutely infarcted myocardium using inversion recovery and gradient-recalled echo-planar imaging (EPI). Invest Radiol 1992; 27: 927–34.
8. Saeed M, Wendland MF, Sakuma H et al. Detection of myocardial ischemia using first pass contrast-enhanced inversion recovery and driven equilibrium fast GRE imaging. Book of Abstracts of the Twelfth Annual Scientific Meeting of the Society of Magnetic Resonance in Medicine, August 14–20, 1993, New York. Berkeley: Society of Magnetic Resonance in Medicine, 1993: 536.
9. Wilke N, Simm C, Machnig T et al. First pass myocardial perfusion imaging with gadolinium: correlation with myocardial flow in dogs. Book of Abstracts of the Tenth Annual Scientific

Meeting and Exhibition of the Society of Magnetic Resonance in Medicine, August 10–16, 1991, San Francisco. Berkeley: Society of Magnetic Resonance in Medicine, 1991: 244.

10. Wendland MF, Saeed M, Masui T et al. First Pass of an MR susceptibility contrast agent through normal and ischemic heart: Gradient-recalled echo-planar imaging. JMRI 1993; 3: 755–60.

11. Bourne MW, Numerow L, Amidon L et al. The assessment of the extent of myocardial functional and perfusion abnormality with fast gradient echo (FGRE) magnetic resonance imaging in patients with chronic myocardial infarction: Comparison with Thallium 201 SPECT. Book of Abstracts of the Second Meeting and Exhibition of the Society of Magnetic Resonance, August 6–12, 1994, San Francisco. Berkeley: Society of Magnetic Resonance, 1994.

12. Wilke N, Xu Y, Zhang Y et al. MR First Pass Imaging in the Assessment of Myocardial Perfusion using a Blood Pool Contrast Agent. Book of Abstracts of the Twelfth Annual Scientific Meeting of the Society of Magnetic Resonance in Medicine, August 14–20, 1993, New York. Berkeley: Society of Magnetic Resonance in Medicine, 1993: 537.

13. Saeed M, Wendland MF, Sakuma H et al. MR-enhanced myocardial perfusion imaging: Identification of hemodynamically significant coronary artery stenosis in dogs. Book of Abstracts of the Second Meeting and Exhibition of the Society of Magnetic Resonance, August 6–12, 1994, San Francisco. Berkeley: Society of Magnetic Resonance, 1994.

14. Manning WJ, Atkinson DJ, Grossman W et al. First-pass nuclear magnetic resonance imaging studies using gadolinium-DTPA in patients with coronary artery disease. J Am Coll Cardiol 1991; 18: 959–65.

15. Gould KL, Kelley KO. Physiological significance of coronary flow velocity and changing stenosis during coronary vasodilation in awake dogs. Circ Res 1982; 50: 695–704.

16. Schaefer S, van Tyen R, Saloner D. Evaluation of myocardial perfusion abnormalities with gadolinium-enhanced snapshot MR imaging in humans. Radiology 1992; 185: 795–801.

17. Wilke N, Koronaeos A, Engels G et al. First pass contrast-enhanced myocardial perfusion magnetic resonance imaging at rest and during dipyridamole in humans with coronary artery disease. Book of Abstracts of the Eleventh Annual Meeting of the Society of Magnetic Resonance in Medicine, August 8–14, 1992, Berlin, Germany. Berkeley: Society of Magnetic Resonance in Medicine, 1992: 605.

18. Klein MA, Collier BD, Hellman RS, Bamrah VS. Detection of chronic coronary artery disease: Value of pharmacologically stressed, dynamically enhanced turbo-fast low-angle shot MR images. AJR 1993; 161: 257–63.

19. Stewart GN. Researches on the circulation time in organs and on the influences which affect it. J Physiol (London) 1894; 15: 1–89.

20. Rosen BR, Belliveau JW, Vevea JM, Brady TJ. Perfusion imaging with NMR contrast agents. Magn Reson Med 1990; 14: 249–65.

21. Wilke N, Simm C, Zhang J et al. Contrast-enhanced first pass myocardial perfusion imaging: Correlation between myocardial blood flow in dogs at rest and during hyperemia. Magn Reson Med 1993; 29: 485–97.

22. Wendland MF, Saeed M, Yu K et al. Inversion recovery EPI of bolus transit in rat myocardium using intravascular and extravascular gadolinium-based MR contrast media: Dose effects on peak signal enhancement. Magn Reson Med 1994 (accepted).

23. Diesbourg LD, Prato FS, Wisenberg G et al. Quantification of myocardial blood flow and extracellular volumes using a bolus injection of Gd-DTPA: Kinetic modeling in canine ischemic disease. Magn Reson Med 1992; 23: 239–53.

24. Kety, SS. The theory and applications of the exchange of inert gas at the lungs and tissues. Pharmacol Rev 1951; 3: 1–41.

25. Watson MT, Lorenz CH, Delbeke D et al. Quantification of regional myocardial perfusion: A comparison of contrast-enhanced magnetic resonance imaging and positron emission tomography. Book of abstracts of the Twelfth Annual Scientific Meeting of the Society of Magnetic Resonance in Medicine, August 14–20, 1993, New York. Berkeley: Society of Magnetic Resonance in Medicine, 1993: 636.

26. Ito H, Tomooka T, Sakai N et al. Lack of myocardial perfusion after successful thrombolysis: A predictor of poor recovery of left ventricular function in anterior myocardial infarction. Circulation 1992; 85: 1699–1705.

27. Saeed M, Wendland MF, Takehara Y, Higgins CB. Reversible and irreversible injury in the reperfused myocardium: Differentiation with contrast material-enhanced MR imaging. Radiology 1990; 175: 633–7.

28. Saeed M, Wagner S, Wendland MF et al. Occlusive and reperfused myocardial infarcts: Differentiation with Mn-DPDP-enhanced MR imaging. Radiology 1989; 172: 59–64.

29. Masui T, Saeed M, Wendland MF, Higgins CB. Occlusive and reperfused myocardial infarcts: MR imaging differentiation with nonionic Gd-DTPA-BMA. Radiology 1991; 181: 77–83.

30. Saeed M, Wendland MF, Higgins CB. Characterization of reperfused myocardial infarctions with T1-enhancing and magnetic susceptibility-enhancing contrast media. Invest Radiol 1991; 26: S239–41.

31. Saeed M, Wendland MF, Yu KK et al. Identification of myocardial reperfusion using echoplanar MR imaging: Discrimination between occlusive and reperfused infarctions. Circulation 1994 (accepted).

32. de Roos A, van Rossum AC, van der Wall E et al. Reperfused and nonreperfused myocardial infarction: Diagnostic potential of Gd-DTPA-enhanced MR imaging. Radiology 1989; 172: 717–20.

33. de Roos A, Matheijssen NAA, Doornboos J et al. Myocardial infarct size after reperfusion therapy: Assessment with Gd-DTPA-enhanced MR imaging. Radiology 1990; 176: 517–21.

34. van Rossum AC, Visser FC, van Eenige MJ et al. Value of gadolinium-diethylene-triamine pentaacetic acid dynamics in magnetic resonance imaging of acute myocardial infarction with occluded and reperfused coronary arteries after thrombolysis. Am J Cardiol 1990; 65: 845–51.

35. Bazille A, Lima JAC, Judd RM et al. Persistent MR contrast enhancement of reperfused myocardial infarction in humans. Book of Abstracts of the Twelfth Annual Scientific Meeting of the Society of Magnetic Resonance in Medicine, August 14–20, 1993, New York. Berkeley: Society of Magnetic Resonance in Medicine, 1993: 559.

36. Saeed M, Wendland MF, Masui T, Higgins CB. Myocardial infarctions on T1– and susceptibility-enhanced MRI: Evidence for loss of compartmentalization of contrast media. Magn Reson Med 1994; 31: 31–9.

37. Geschwind JF, Saeed M, Wendland MF et al. Identification of myocardial cell death in reperfused myocardial injury using dual mechanisms of contrast enhanced magnetic resonance imaging. In: Proceedings of the 42nd Annual Meeting of the Association of University Radiologists, May 3–8, 1994, Boston. Reston, Virginia: Association of University Radiologists, 1994.

Corresponding Author: Dr Charles B. Higgins, Department of Radiology, University of California, 505 Parnassus Avenue, San Francisco, CA 94143-0628, USA

12. Non-invasive visualization of the coronary arteries using magnetic resonance imaging – is it good enough to guide interventions?

WARREN J. MANNING and ROBERT R. EDELMAN

Introduction

Despite advances in both prevention and treatment, cardiovascular disease remains a leading cause of morbidity and mortality in developed nations. The current "gold standard" for the evaluation of the coronary arteries is contrast coronary angiography. The data acquired from such diagnostic procedures (i.e. presence, location and severity of stenoses) is utilized both for diagnostic and prognostic purposes. For those with significant disease, information gained from contrast angiography is currently the standard by which mechanical interventions (coronary artery bypass graft (CABG) surgery or percutaneous revascularization techniques (balloon angioplasty, intracoronary stents, intracoronary atherectomy) as well as pharmacologic therapies are planned.

Need for non-invasive coronary angiography

In addition to their high cost ($3–5K/procedure), contrast coronary angiography carries a low complication rate, including local vascular/infectious complications, myocardial infarction, stroke or peripheral emboli, and death [1]. Furthermore, while there are semi-quantitative techniques for estimating the flow restriction caused by a focal coronary artery stenosis based on the conventional contrast angiogram, they do not provide a *quantitative* assessment of coronary artery blood flow.

The ability to perform non-invasive coronary angiography and thereby identify patients with and without stenoses within the major epicardial vessels would represent a major advance in patient care. Patients free of significant coronary stenoses on non-invasive coronary angiography would avoid the cost, inconvenience, and potential risks of conventional contrast coronary angiography. Non-invasive coronary angiography would serve to identify those patients at particularly high risk for complications during conventional angiography (e.g. left main coronary artery stenosis), or eliminate the need

C.A. Nienaber and U. Sechtem (eds): Imaging and Intervention in Cardiology. 167–190.
© 1996 *Kluwer Academic Publishers.*

for contrast coronary angiography among patients requiring cardiac surgery for primary valvular heart disease. In addition, non-invasive coronary angiography could be used to facilitate scheduling of a mechanical intervention (i.e. angioplasty, atherectomy, stents, etc.), thereby obviating the need for separate diagnostic and therapeutic procedures. Non-invasive coronary angiography would also assist in the scheduling of invasive procedures (e.g. the patient with single vessel disease on non-invasive coronary angiography would be scheduled to undergo directed angioplasty at a time when an operating room is available to treat potential complications of angioplasty, while a patient with left main and/or three vessel disease on non-invasive coronary angiography might undergo confirmatory diagnostic catheterization without such "back-up" available, or even proceed directly to surgery). Finally, follow-up angiographic information in patients undergoing revascularization procedures would also be more readily obtained (see also Chapters 7, 8, 9 and 20).

Current options for non-invasive visualization of the coronary arteries

Current options for non-invasive coronary angiography include cardiac ultrasound (echocardiography), ultrafast or cine CT, and magnetic resonance coronary angiography (MRCA). Conventional two-dimensional (2D) transthoracic echocardiography imaging has been successful at identification of the ostia of left main and right coronary artery in 60–90% of adult patients [2] but imaging of the left anterior descending and circumflex coronary arteries has proven more difficult despite advances in transducer and imaging technology. Few data are available on the accuracy of this technique for the identification of coronary stenoses.

Transesophageal echocardiography (TEE) is often able to identify the ostia of the left main coronary artery, (Figure 1) with images of the full length of the left main coronary artery and its bifurcation reported in 90% of subjects [3]. Two-dimensional imaging may be combined with Doppler techniques to identify patients with left main coronary artery stenoses [3]. TEE visualization and evaluation of the proximal left anterior descending and left circumflex have also been described [4]. While clinically relevant, left main coronary artery disease is found in only a small minority of patients referred for angiography and data on the ability of TEE to reliably image the right coronary artery or identify significant disease of that vessel is as yet unknown. Finally, utilizing pharmacologic stress, recently published data suggest transesophageal echocardiography may be useful for the identification of stenoses in the proximal left anterior descending coronary artery [5]. Though transesophageal echocardiography does not require contrast injection or arterial access, it is minimally invasive and has associated risks of esophageal perforation, laceration, aspiration, and dysrhythmias [6].

Coronary artery calcification is both a sensitive and a specific marker

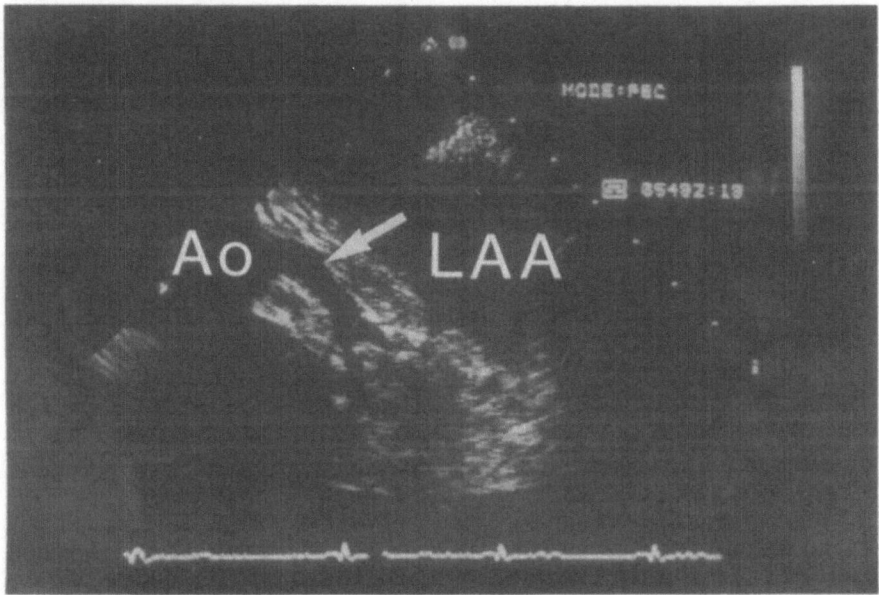

Figure 1. Transesophageal echocardiographic image of left main coronary artery (white arrow) extending to bifurcation Ao = ascending aorta. LAA = left atrial appendage. (Reprinted with permission [20].)

for the presence of coronary artery atherosclerosis [7]. While not directly visualizing the coronary arteries, cine or ultrafast CT is very sensitive for identifying and quantifying coronary artery calcium. Unfortunately, not all obstructive lesions have detectable calcium within the atherosclerotic plaque and *non-obstructive* calcified atherosclerotic plaques are common in apparently healthy men over 50 years and women over 60 years [7]. While non-invasive, cine CT does expose the patient to considerable amounts of potentially harmful ionizing radiation (making it less desirable for screening or repetitive studies) and the presence of epicardial calcium serves only as an indirect method to identify significant coronary artery stenoses. Its role as a screening test for coronary artery disease remains unproved.

Visualization of the native coronary arteries by magnetic resonance imaging

Magnetic resonance (MR) imaging is ideally suited for evaluating the heart, with excellent soft tissue discrimination and the ability to image the heart in double-oblique, tomographic sections. Using electrocardiographic (ECG) gated techniques, MR imaging has already established itself as the non-invasive "gold standard" for the assessment of cardiac anatomy and biven-

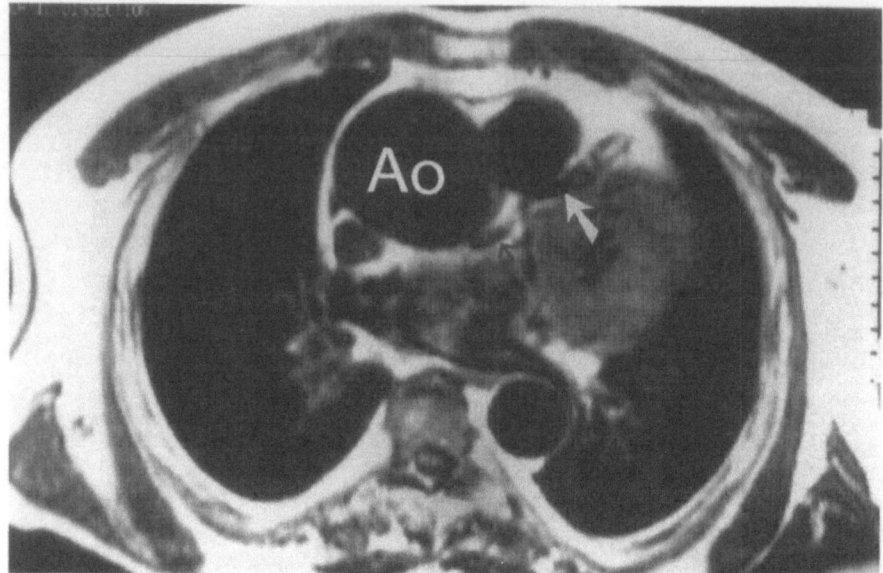

Figure 2. Conventional ECG-gated multi-phase spin-echo axial section at the proximal aorta in a patient referred for evaluation of a dilated ascending aorta. Note the left main coronary artery (black arrow) and extension into the left anterior descending (LAD) coronary artery (solid white arrow). (Reprinted with permission [20].)

tricular systolic function [8–10]. Conventional MR imaging is now widely accepted as the technique of choice for the evaluation of the thoracic aorta in the hemodynamically stable patient with suspected aortic dissection [11]. MR imaging also offers the opportunity to non-invasively characterize blood flow within the aorta and great vessels [12]. The coronary arteries, however, have a diameter 10 times *smaller* than the ascending thoracic aorta. In addition, the coronary vessels are tortuous and there is extensive motion during both the cardiac cycle and with normal respiration.

Using conventional multi-phase ECG-gated spin-echo techniques, in which data for each image is acquired over 2–8 minutes, images of the proximal aorta will occasionally include the origin of the major epicardial coronary arteries (Figure 2). Despite data acquisition over several minutes and lack of respiratory gating, the presence and location of both coronary artery ostia may be successfully obtained in selected patients [13]. Unfortunately, using this technique, visualization of even the proximal portion of the major coronary arteries and identification of stenoses have not been reported.

Greater success at visualization of the coronary arteries has been achieved utilizing MR subtraction methods [14], 3D techniques [15], spiral scanning [16] and segmentation gradient echo sequences [17]. Echo planar MRCA has also been recently described [18, 19] and offers great promise. A common theme of the majority of these magnetic resonance coronary angiographic (MRCA) techniques includes the use of multiple 10 to 20 second breath holds to minimize respiratory motion artifacts (blurring) and imaging during mid-diastole, a period of relative diastasis, so as to minimize the artifacts related to cardiac motion. Specific merits and detractions of each technique is explained elsewhere [20].

At the time of this writing, the greatest amount of clinical investigation has been performed using 2D segmented k-space gradient echo approaches. With this method, multiple phase encoding steps are acquired during a brief period of diastole during each of a series of heart beats [17]. Typically, 160 phase encoding steps (matrix 160×256) are acquired (8/heart beat for 20 beats) with a field-of-view of 240×240 mm, resulting in a spatial resolution of 1.5×0.9 mm. Each 2D image may be acquired with a 2–4 mm slice thickness. Thirty to forty breath-hold images are generally needed to define the major coronary anatomy. As with other gradient echo sequences, rapidly moving, laminar blood flow results in a "bright" signal due to the inflow of unsaturated protons, while stagnant blood (or tissue) appear "dark" because of saturation effects due to repeated proton stimulation. Focal areas of turbulence within blood vessels also appear "dark" due to proton dephasing.

Typically the coronary ostia are identified in the transverse plane (Figure 3). An example of a transverse MR image at the level of the right coronary artery is shown in Figure 3a, with a more inferior section depicted in Figure 3b. Taking advantage of the unique ability of MR to directly acquire images in any orientation, these initial images may be followed by obliquely oriented images acquired along the major or minor axis of the vessels. Oblique images along the major axis of the right coronary artery are shown in Figure 3c, with adjacent sections delineating portions of the vessel which deviated into adjoining imaging sections (Figure 3d–f). The left main coronary artery may also be visualized in transverse (Figure 4) section, with superior and inferior sections delineating the left anterior descending and left circumflex coronary arteries. The left main and left circumflex coronary arteries are also frequently seen with oblique images. Double-oblique images may also be obtained along the axis of the left main and left anterior descending coronary arteries, resulting in large portions of the left coronary artery being identified within a single section (Figure 5).

Using this approach in a series of young adult volunteers [17], it is possible to identify the left main coronary artery in 96% of subjects, the left anterior descending and right coronary arteries in all subjects, and the left circumflex coronary artery in 76% of subjects. In addition to these major vessels, diagonal branches of the left anterior descending coronary artery were identified in 80% of subjects and the great cardiac vein in 88% of subjects. The obtuse marginal branches of the left circumflex coronary artery are more difficult to visualize using this technique [21], a problem likely related to the choice of imaging planes, and potentially overcome by 3D approaches. The

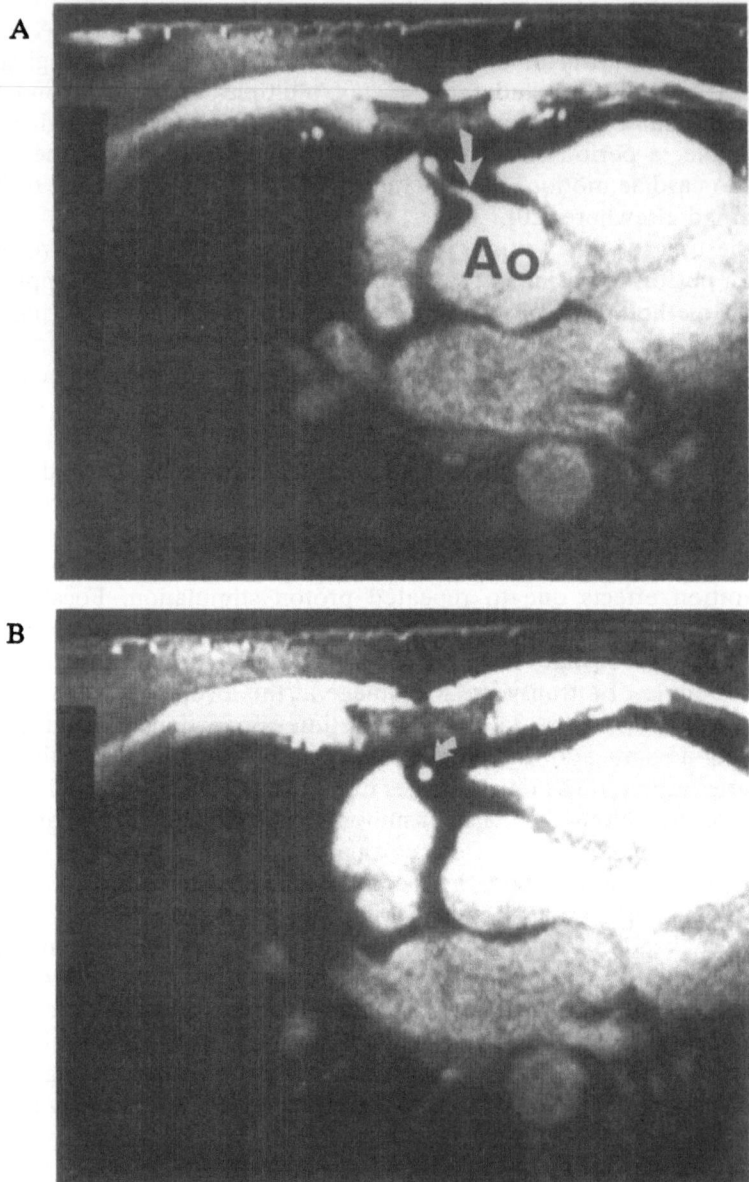

Figure 3. Two mm thick breath-hold axial MR sections in a healthy volunteer at: a) the level of the proximal right coronary artery (RCA; solid white arrow); b) subsequent transverse section of RCA at a more inferior level (white arrow) identifying the vessel in cross-section. c) Oblique MR section taken along the major axis of the vessel as defined by (a); d–e) adjacent sections depicting the mid-RCA (arrows); f) bifurcation of the distal RCA (solid white arrow). LV = left ventricular cavity. RV = right ventricular cavity. Ao = aortic root. (Reprinted with permission of the American Heart Association [17].)

C

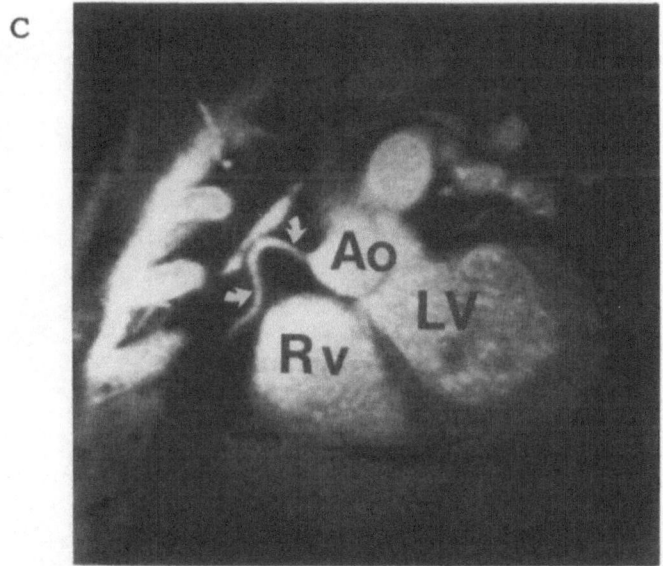

D

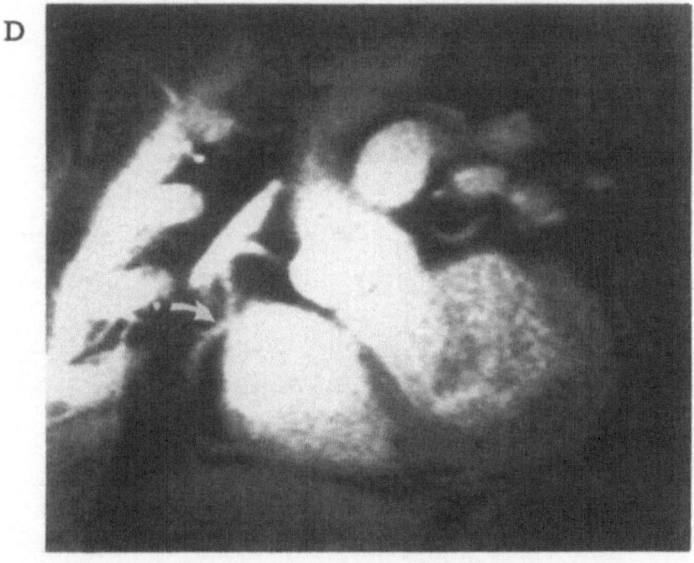

Figure 3 Continued.

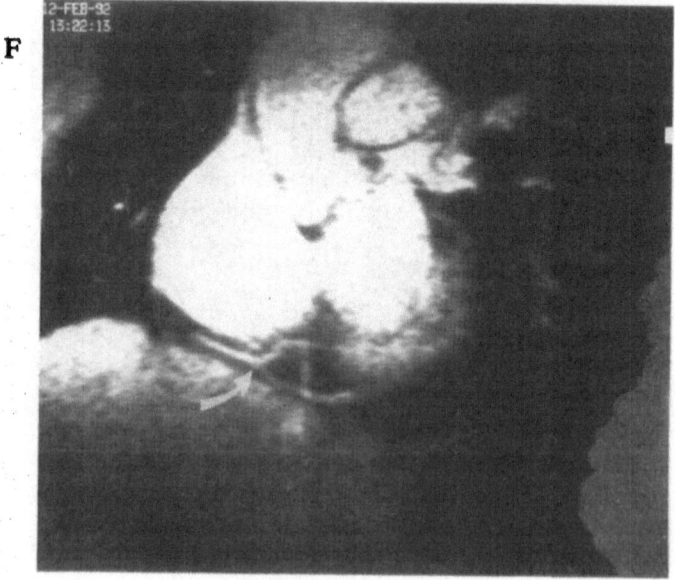

Figure 3 Continued.

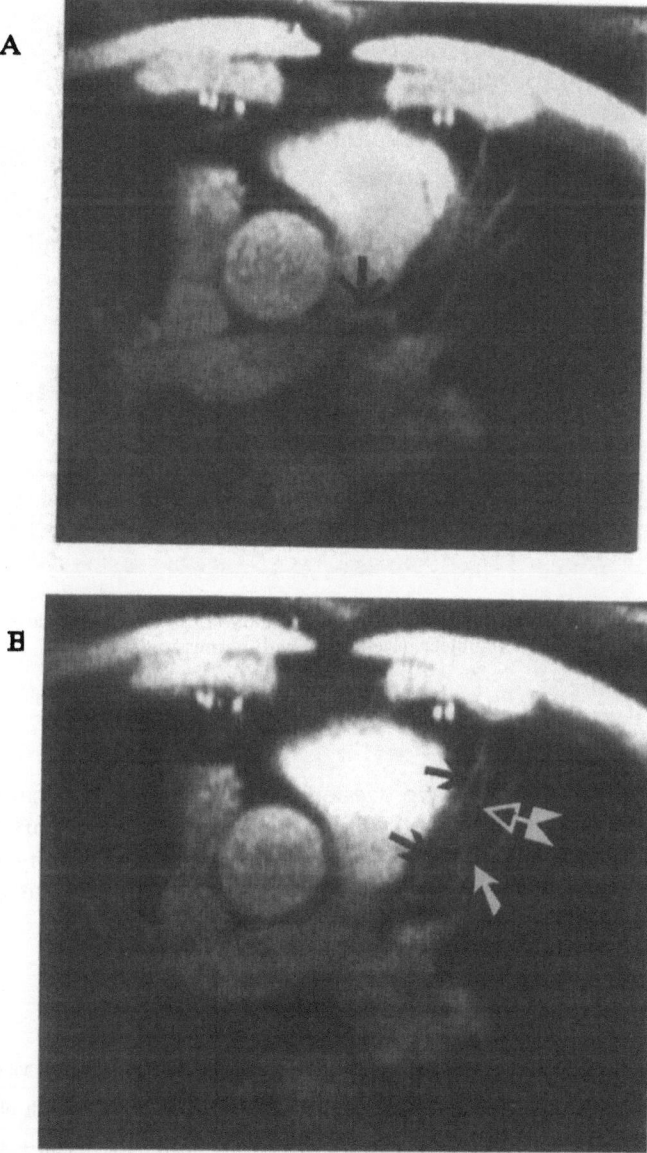

Figure 4. a) Axial MR section of the left main coronary artery (solid white arrow) continuing on into the b) LAD (black arrows) coronary artery. Note the diagonal branches off the LAD (solid white arrows) and the great cardiac vein (open white arrow). (Reprinted with permission of the American Heart Association [17].)

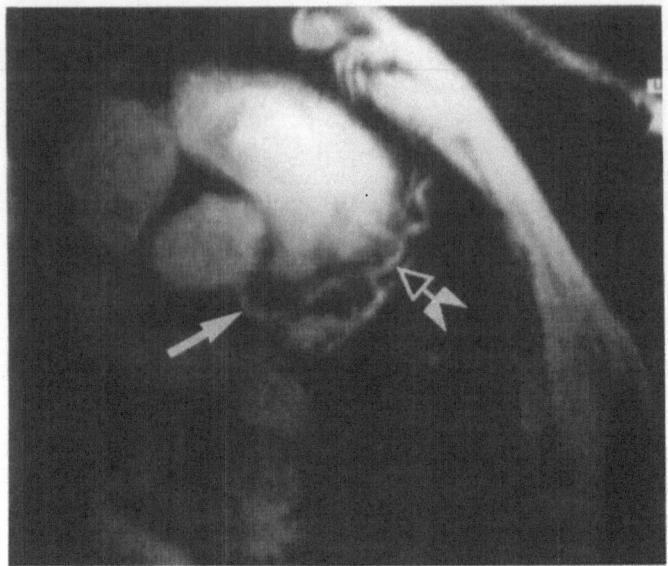

Figure 5. Oblique section depicting the left main coronary artery (solid white arrow) and LAD (open white arrow) in another subject. (Reprinted with permission [20].)

average vessel diameter and average length of contiguously observed coronary artery are shown in Table 1. Similar results have been reported utilizing 3D MRCA techniques [22]. Quantitative contrast angiography of *normal* proximal vessel lumen are in good correlation with quantitative MRCA diameter data [23] (Figure 6). (See also Chapters 8, 9 and 10.)

Table 1. MRA assessment of proximal coronary diameter and length of vessel visualized.

Vessel	Proximal diameter		Length observed[a]		Length observed[b]
	Mean (mm)	(range)	Mean (mm)	(range)	Mean ± SD (mm)
RCA	3.7	(2.7–5.1)	58	(24 – 122)	60 ± 14
LM	4.8	(3.4–6)	10	(8–14)	10 ± 3
LAD	3.6	(3–4)	44	(28–93)	61 ± 31
LCX	3.5	(3–4)	25	(9–42)	40 ± 15

[a]Reprinted with permission of the American Heart Association [17].
[b]Adapted from [22].
RCA = right coronary artery; LM = left main coronary artery; LAD = left anterior descending coronary artery; LCX = left circumflex coronary artery.

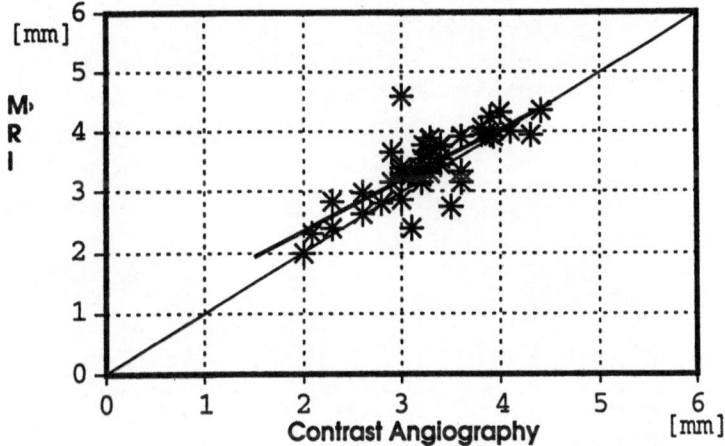

Figure 6. Comparison of coronary artery diameter. (Reprinted with permission [23].)

Identification of native coronary artery disease by magnetic resonance coronary angiography

The small caliber of the native coronary arteries (diameter 3–4 mm) and relatively limited spatial resolution of current MRCA techniques (1.5×0.9 mm), makes quantitative MRCA improbable using current technology, though such quantitation is possible for larger arteries such as the aorta and carotid arteries. The development of stronger gradient systems and specialized surface coils [24] may permit quantitative MRCA in the future. Though quantitative MRCA is not currently possible, as previously mentioned, gradient-echo MRCA techniques are sensitive to laminar and absent or turbulent blood flow, with laminar blood flow depicted as a "bright" signal, whereas regions of turbulent, markedly diminished, or absent blood flow are displayed as signal "voids". A total occlusion or severe stenosis with poor distal blood flow might be expected to appear as an abrupt loss of signal (Figure 7), while arteries with severe stenoses but significant antegrade blood flow might be expected to demonstrate a focal loss of signal, corresponding to an area of turbulence at the stenotic site, followed by bright signal depicting laminar flow in the more distal lumen (Figure 8). This MRCA technique, however, is also insensitive to *direction* of blood flow. Thus a situation in which a vessel with a total occlusion but extensive collaterals to the distal vessel could result in visualization of the distal vessel (after a region of signal void corresponding to the occlusion) while vessels with subtotal occlusions may have very slowly moving blood in the post-stenotic lumen, resulting in absence of signal in the distal lumen due to saturation effects. MRCA techniques in which blood in the aortic root is "tagged" followed by a delay of several hundred msec during which the "tagged blood" is allowed to flow

A

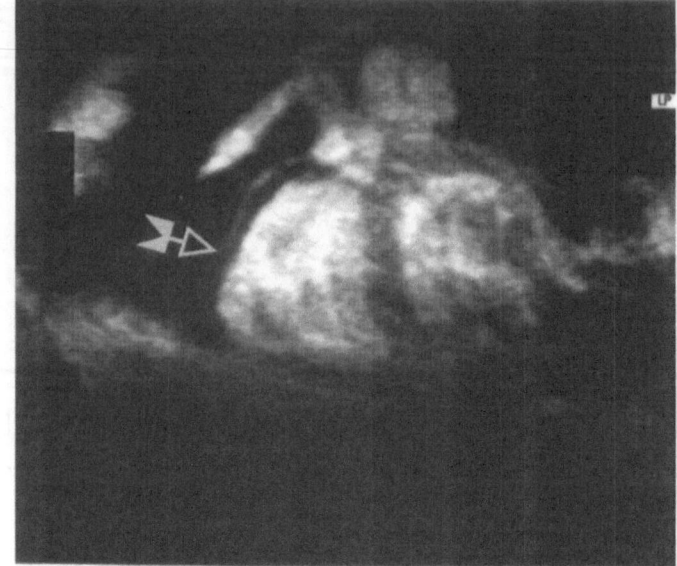

B

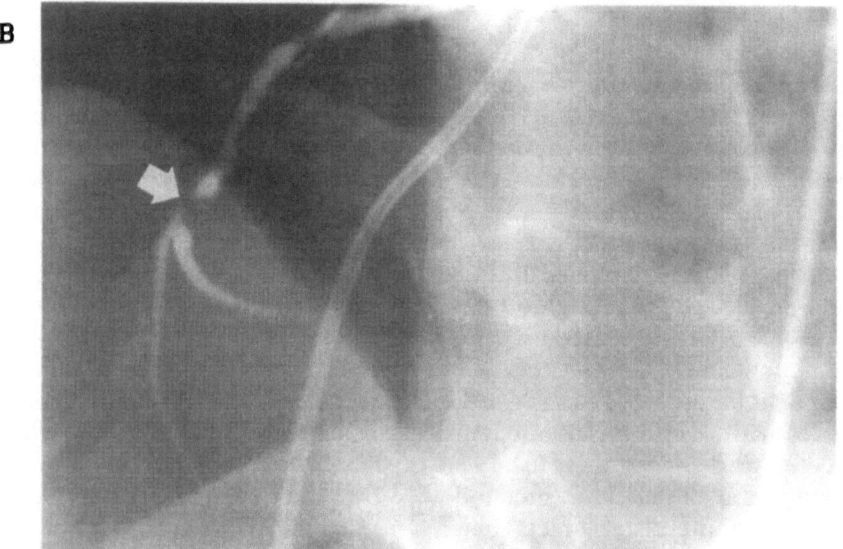

Figure 7. a) Oblique sections of the proximal RCA. Note the abrupt loss of signal in the proximal artery (open white arrow). The more distal artery was not visualized in adjacent sections. b) corresponding conventional angiogram demonstrating the sub-total occlusion of the proximal RCA (white arrow). (Reprinted with permission of the New England Journal of Medicine [25].)

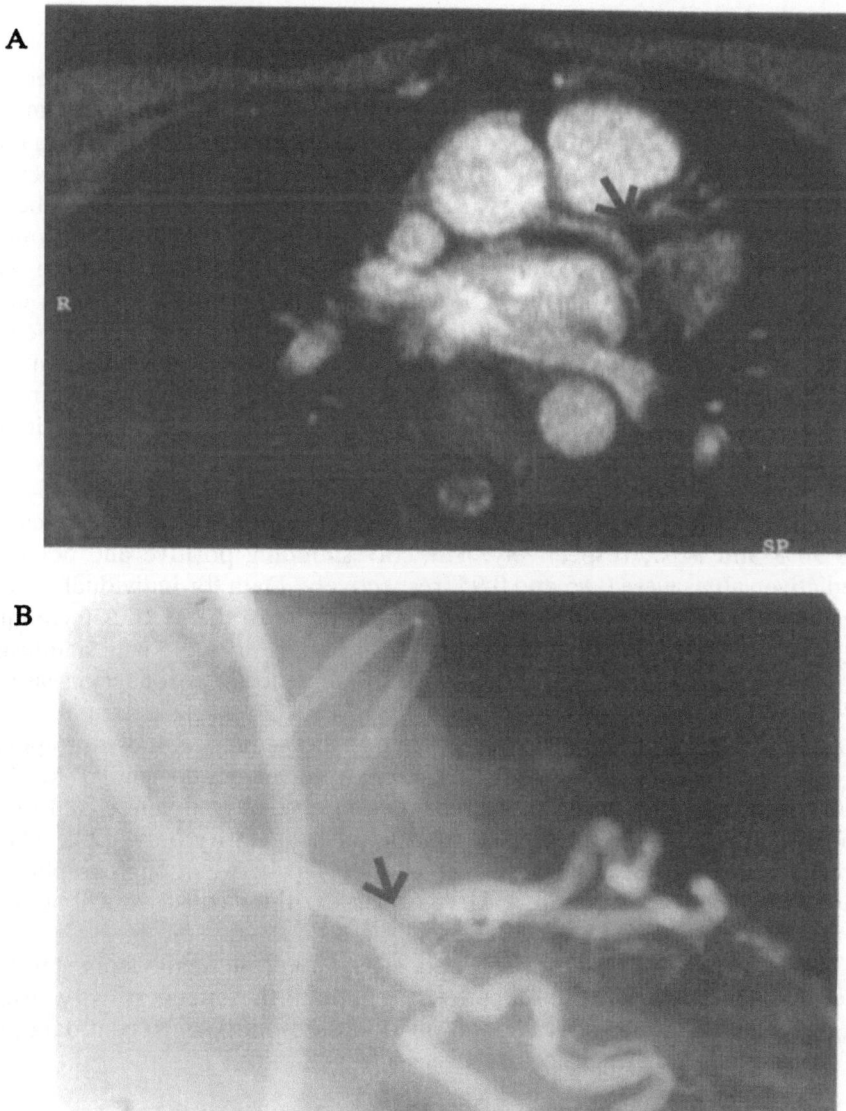

Figure 8. a) Axial section demonstrating the left main and LCX with a signal void (black arrow) in the proximal LAD. Also note the more distal LAD and diagonal (white arrow) are seen. b) corresponding RAO caudal conventional angiogram confirming the tight proximal LAD stenosis (black arrow). (Reprinted with permission [20].)

antegrade into the coronary arteries [14, 19a] would not suffer from this limitation and may be useful for distinguishing these two situations.

A recent study correlated findings on 39 patients referred for elective coronary angiography who also underwent MRCA examination either immediately before or after conventional contrast angiography [25]. Since quantitative MRCA was not possible, the sensitivity of the MRCA sequence to abnormalities of blood flow was used to grade individual vessels as being "normal or having minimal disease" if there were minimal or no luminal irregularities on MRCA, or as having "substantial disease" if there was marked attenuation of the luminal diameter or a signal void. MRCA data and conventional contrast angiographic data were analyzed independently by blinded observers, with a 50% or greater diameter stenosis by contrast angiography as the standard for disease; MRCA images of 98% of the major arteries were adequate for evaluation. Overall sensitivity and specificity of the 2D MRCA technique for correctly classifying individual vessels as with (50% or greater diameter stenosis on conventional contrast angiography) or without disease, for a population with a 36% likelihood of diseased vessels was 90% and 92%, respectively. The corresponding positive and negative predictive values were 0.85 and 0.95, respectively. Data for individual vessels are shown in Table 2. The sensitivity and specificity of the MRCA technique for correctly classifying individual patients as having or not having significant coronary disease, in this population with an incidence of coronary disease of 0.74, was 97% and 70%, respectively.

Absolute signal intensity in 2D gradient echo sequence does not appear to correlate with focal stenoses [26]. Others have graded similar MRCA studies according to arterial signal changes as severe (complete signal loss), moderate (partial signal loss) and mild (wall irregularity only) [27]. These investigators have found a significant relationship between angiographic diameter stenoses based on these MRCA classifications (see also Chapters 8, 9, 13 and 19).

The widespread use of intracoronary stents, typically made from stainless steel or tantalum, has raised a concern regarding the effects of very strong magnetic fields on these devices and possible stent motion. Recent data [28]

Table 2. Sensitivity, specificity, positive/negative predictive value of MR coronary angiography.

	Numbers with disease (%)	Sensitivity (%)	Specificity (%)	PV (+)	PV (−)
LM	2 (5%)	100	100	1.00	1.00
LAD	23 (64%)	87	92	0.95	0.80
LCX	7 (20%)	71	90	0.63	0.93
RCA	20 (53%)	100	78	0.83	1.00
Patient	29 (74%)	97	70	0.90	0.88

PV (+) = predictive value positive; PV (−) = predictive value negative.
Modified from [25] and printed with permission of the New England Journal of Medicine.

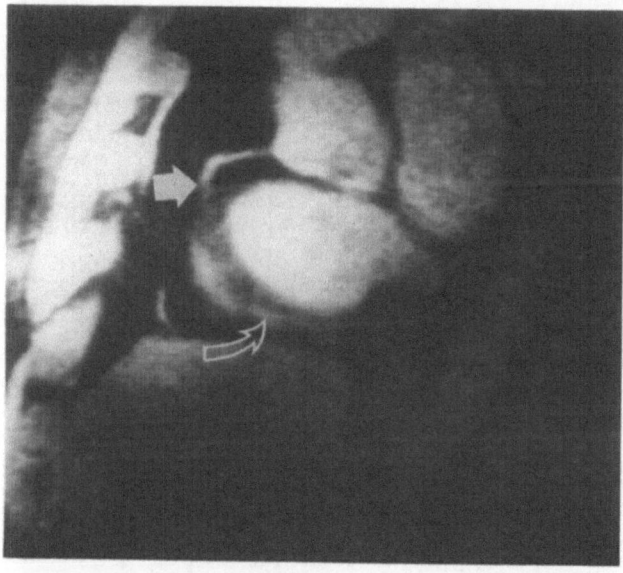

Figure 9. Oblique image taken along the long axis of the RCA. Note the abrupt signal void in the proximal portion of the vessel (white arrow) with the more distal vessel well seen (open white arrow). The signal void corresponded to an intracoronary stent with widely patent lumen.

suggest, however, that these stents are not significantly influenced by the magnetic fields currently used (< 1.5 Tesla) for clinical imaging. Imaging of the vessel lumen along the length of the stent, however, does result in a local image artifact, precluding evaluation of this portion of the vessel (Figure 9).

MR assessment of coronary artery flow velocity

In addition to imaging of the coronary arteries, MR imaging techniques also hold the potential for assessment of coronary artery blood flow. Currently, such assessment is limited to invasive techniques such as intracoronary Doppler flow probes [29] and transesophageal echocardiography [30]. Recently, phase contrast MR techniques, in which signal intensity is proportional to blood flow velocity have been validated for the assessment of ventricular stroke volume and cardiac output as well as for quantification of intracardiac shunts by assessing blood flow within the great arteries [31]. Sequences analogous to the segmented 2D turbo-FLASH approach for MRCA have been developed for phase contrast assessment of coronary artery blood flow [32, 33]. This method has presently only been described in volunteers with in-vivo quantification of blood flow velocity at sites of

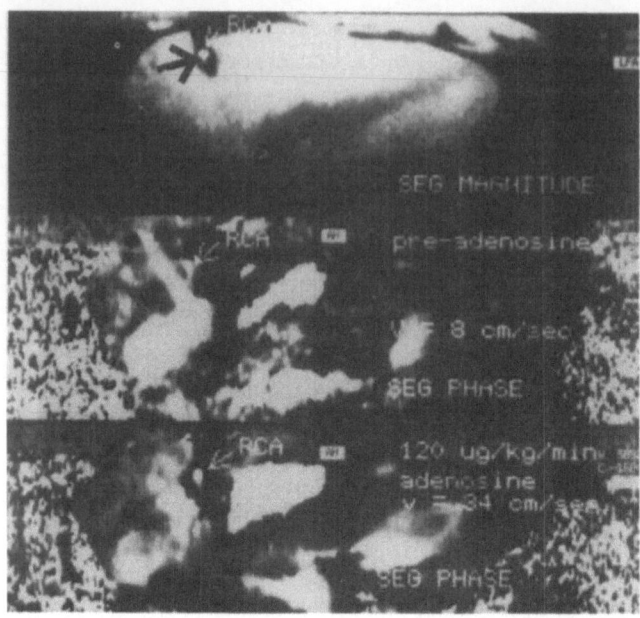

Figure 10. Top: Axial magnitude (anatomic) identifying the right coronary artery (black arrow), Bottom 2 panels: phase difference (flow) images obtained using velocity quantification method during a single breath-hold. Phase difference image gives flow velocity of 8 cm/sec at rest (middle panel) and 34 cm/sec after administration of adenosine, 120 μg/kg/min (bottom panel). (Reprinted with permission [32].)

coronary stenoses yet to be described. While in theory cross sectional area of the coronary artery could also be assessed so as to measure coronary flow (e.g cc/min of blood flow), the previously mentioned relative spatial resolution of current MRCA precludes accurate measurement of native coronary artery cross sectional area at the present time. Following administration of intravenous adenosine a four-fold increase in diastolic right coronary artery velocity has been found (Figure 10). A recent study using time-of-flight echo planar imaging to measure coronary artery flow reserve documented a 52% increase in left anterior descending artery flow velocity among volunteers during isometric exercise [34]. While few data in patients with coronary disease either at rest or following pharmacologic stress has been published, this technique holds particular promise for assessing the physiological significance of a coronary artery stenosis and assessing coronary artery flow reserve. Should this technique be successful at identifying a particular *resting* flow profile which is characteristic for those with significant coronary stenosis, then it would be a particularly valuable adjunct to non-invasive MRCA, as both techniques could be performed in the absence of intravenous access or medication (see also Chapters 8, 9 and 18–20).

MRCA of anomalous coronary arteries

The ability of MRCA to acquire data in double-oblique orientations is un-iquely suited for the evaluation of anomalous coronary arteries. While rare, occurring in only 0.6–1.2% of adults referred for coronary angiography [35] and generally not associated with impaired myocardial perfusion, hemodyn-amically significant anomalies, with abnormalities of myocardial perfusion are seen and frequently associated with sudden death [36]. These hemodyn-amically significant lesions include the origin of the left coronary artery from the pulmonary artery, coronary artery fistulae and the origin of the left coronary artery from the right sinus of Valsalva with subsequent passage of the vessel between the aorta and right ventricular infundibulum. While the diagnosis of anomalous coronary arteries is easily made by contrast angio-graphy, definition of the subsequent course of these vessels (anterior or posterior to the right ventricular outflow tract) is often difficult. Such infor-mation is important, since it is the posteriorly (to the pulmonary artery) directed course that is associated with a poor prognosis. Both conventional gradient echo [37] and the 2D segmented approaches [38] have been de-scribed as techniques to visualize the course of these vessels (Figure 11). While data from blinded studies have not been reported, MRCA is probably the best non-invasive technique for delineation of the anatomic relationship of these anomalous vessels with the great arteries.

MRCA of coronary artery bypass grafts

Venous bypass grafts and internal mammary coronary arteries have been found to be easier to image using conventional MR imaging techniques due to their larger size (typically 5–10 mm in diameter) and more limited mobility associated with cardiac and respiration motion. Conventional spin-echo [39–41] and gradient echo [42, 43] techniques have both been studied for their ability to assess bypass graft patency. For most of these investigations, trans-verse images are obtained at a level corresponding to that expected for the bypass graft. A graft is then characterized as "patent" if the normal signal void (spin echo) or bright signal (gradient echo) (Figure 12) of laminar blood flow is seen in at least two anatomic levels in the expected region of the bypass graft. If a signal void was seen at only one level, a graft was considered "indeterminate", and if no signal voids were identified, the graft was con-sidered to be occluded. Data from several studies comparing MR imaging data with contrast angiography are summarized in Table 3.

Major obstacles to imaging of bypass grafts are the local signal loss/artifacts associated with hemostatic clips or sternal wires. Avoidance of these clips is likely to improve MRCA results, but it may be premature to advocate their exclusion in all patients based on the future potential of MRCA. Such a recommendation does appear reasonable for younger patients who are likely

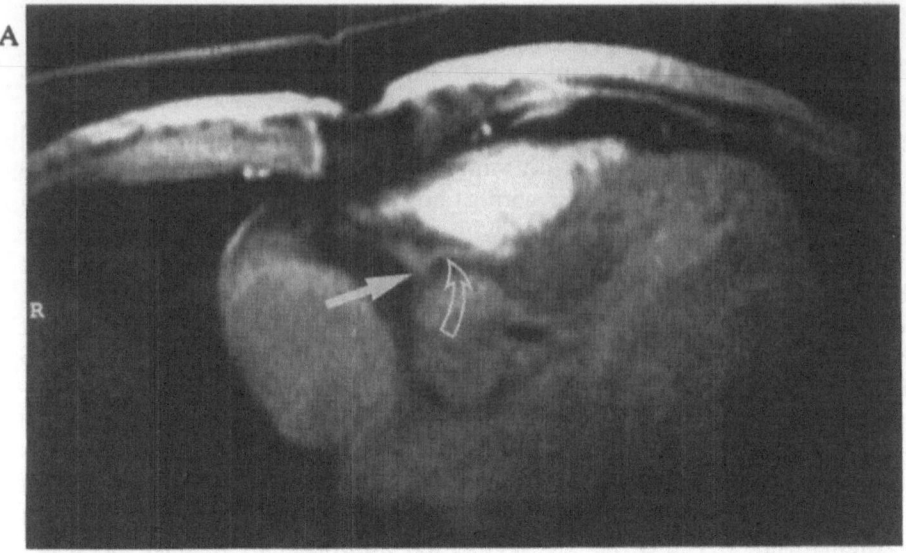

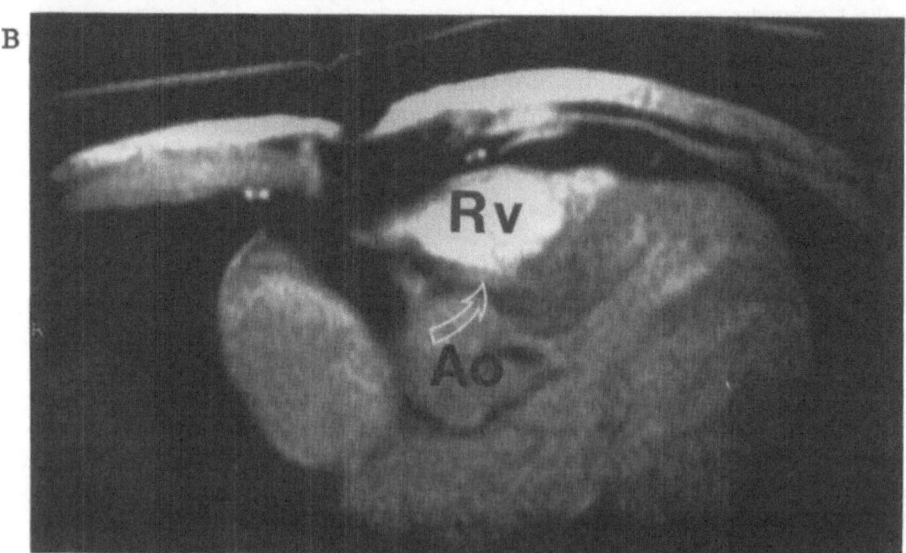

Figure 11. a) Transverse MRCA at the level of the right coronary artery ostia (solid white arrow) and origin of the anomalous left coronary artery (open white arrow); b–c) successive transverse images depicting the course (open white arrows) of the left coronary artery into the interventricular groove; d) Contrast angiogram demonstrating the right coronary artery with anomalous origin (open white arrow) of the left coronary artery. AO = ascending aorta. LA = left atrium. PA = pulmonary artery. RV = right ventricular outflow tract. (Reprinted with permission [38].)

C

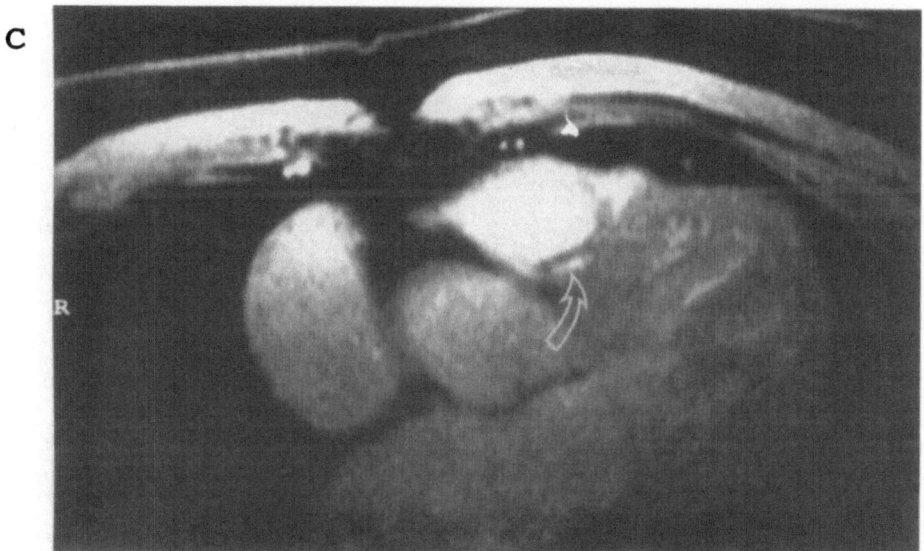

D

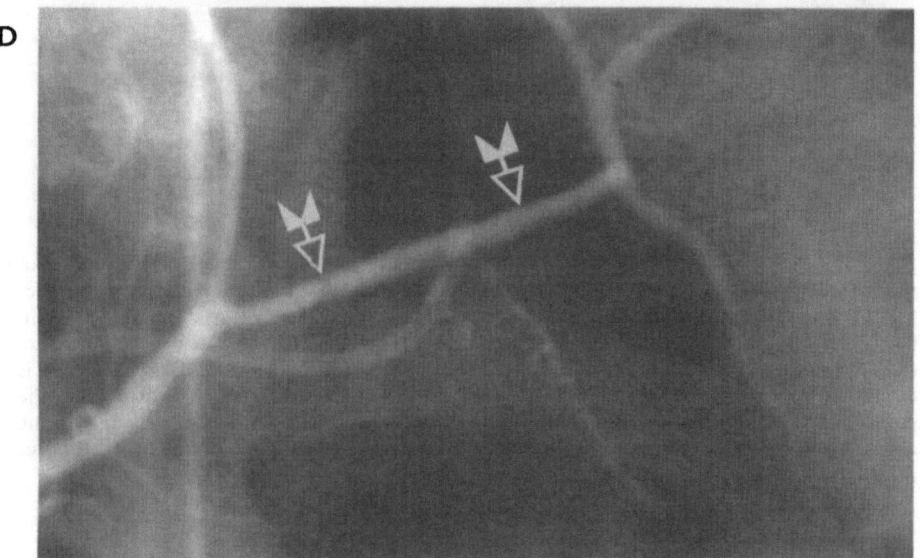

Figure 11. Continued.

to need repeated angiographic data as their bypass grafts age and develop focal stenoses. Signal voids induced by these prostheses were sometimes difficult to distinguish from those related to blood flowing rapidly through the bypass graft. In addition, grafts with very tight stenoses, in which blood

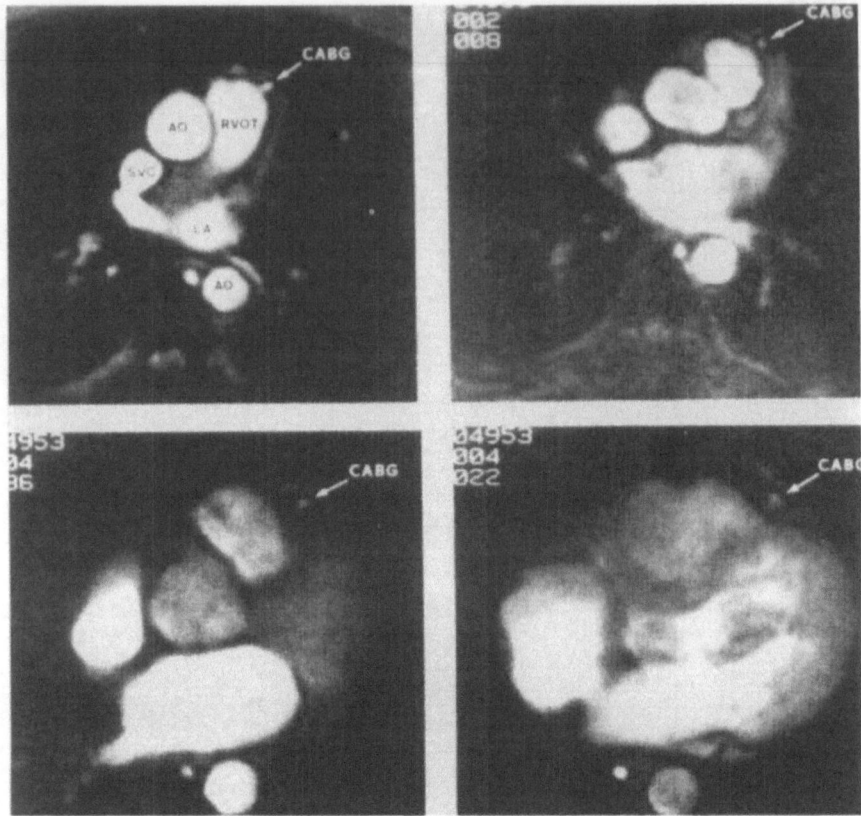

Figure 12. Cine gradient refocused scan with retrospective ECG synchronization at the level of the ascending aorta and moving inferiorly. Flip angle 30°, TR = R-R interval, TE = 20 msec, 128 × 256 image matrix (reconstructed to 256 × 256). Top left panel: Reverse saphenous vein bypass graft (CABG) to the LAD is shown draped over the right ventricular outflow tract (RVOT) in an axial diastolic image. Top right panel: 2 cm lower, the LAD bypass graft is displayed over the RVOT. Bottom left panel: 2 cm lower, the LAD bypass graft overlies the proximal RVOT. Bottom right panel: the LAD bypass graft and native LAD connect in the anteroseptal region. AO = aorta; SVC = superior vena cava. (Reprinted with permission of the American Heart Association [40].)

flow would be expected to be low, often result in insufficient contrast to identify a graft as patent [40].

While both the spin-echo and standard gradient-echo techniques appear promising as a non-invasive method to assess bypass graft patency, patency of an individual graft with this technique is inferred by visualization of a patent portion of the graft somewhere along its length. Certainly identification of occluded grafts is an important first step, but it would be far more valuable to identify bypass vessels which are patent but have significant diameter stenoses. Such stenoses may certainly be the cause of ongoing

Table 3. Sensitivity/specificity of MR for characterizing CABGs as patent or occluded.

Author	Technique	# patients	# grafts	% SVG	% patent	Sensitivity	Specificity
White [39]	Spin-echo	25	72	88	69	0.86	0.72
Rubinstein [40]	Spin-echo	20	47	100	62[a]	0.90	0.72
Jenkins [41]	Spin-echo	16[b]	41	100	63	0.89	0.73
White [42]	Cine gradient-echo	10	28	96	52	0.93	0.86
Aurigemma [43]	Cine gradient-echo	20	45	91	73	0.88	1.00

[a]Graft with 99% diameter stenosis was considered occluded.
[b]Number of patients who had comparison angiograms.
SVG = reverse saphenous vein bypass graft.

myocardial ischemia, yet for the studies as yet reported, a bypass graft with a significant stenosis would be "correctly" classified as patent using conventional spin-echo or gradient-echo imaging. Recently, very preliminary data has been reported on the use of segmented gradient echo techniques (similar to that utilized for imaging of the native vessels) for imaging of vein grafts [44], but stenoses have not been visualized.

Phase velocity mapping has also been utilized to measure blood flow in native and grafted internal mammary arteries [45] as well as reverse saphenous vein grafts [46]. Graft flow is characterized by a biphasic pattern with an average flow of almost 100 ml/min.

Conclusion

In conclusion, MRCA of both native coronary arteries and bypass grafts and the identification of diseased vessels is now possible, though insufficient data has been published at the time of this submission to advocate the use of MRCA to guide interventions. Clinical indications for MRCA would include evaluation of the course of anomalous coronary arteries, though MRCA is not advocated as an imaging tool to screen patients for this rare disorder. Rapid progress is being made in both MR software and hardware which may allow the acquisition of coronary artery anatomic and functional data, including blood flow in the near future.

Supported in part by the Edward Mallinckrodt Jr. Foundation, St. Louis, MO, and grants from the National Institutes of Health (ROI HL45180, ROI HL48538) Bethesda, MD, USA.

References

1. Johnson LW, Lozner EC, Johnson S et al. Coronary arteriography 1984–1987: A report of

the Registry of the Society for Cardiac Angiography and Interventions. I. Results and complications. Cathet Cardiovasc Diagn 1989; 17: 5–10.

2. Douglas PS, Fiolkoski J, Berko B, Reichek N. Echocardiographic visualization of coronary artery anatomy in the adult. J Am Coll Cardiol 1988; 11: 565–71.

3. Yoshida K, Yoshikawa J, Hozumi T et al. Detection of left main coronary artery stenosis by transesophageal color Doppler and two-dimensional echocardiography. Circulation 1990; 81: 1271–6.

4. Memmola C, Iliceto S, Rizzon P. Detection of proximal stenosis of left coronary artery by digital transesophageal echocardiography: Feasibility, sensitivity, and specificity. J Am Soc Echocardiogr 1993; 6: 149–57.

5. Samdarshi TE, Nanda NC, Gatewood RP et al. Usefulness and limitations of transesophageal echocardiography in the assessment of proximal coronary artery stenosis. J Am Coll Cardiol 1992; 19: #N572–80.

6. Daniel WB, Erbel R, Kasper W et al. Safety of transesophageal echocardiography: A multicenter survey of 10,419 examinations. Circulation 1991; 83: 817–21.

7. Moore EH, Greenberg RW, Merick SH et al. Coronary artery calcifications: Significance of incidental detection on CT scans. Radiology 1989; 172: 711–6.

8. Shapiro EP, Rogers WJ, Beyar R et al. Determination of left ventricular mass by magnetic resonance imaging in hearts deformed by acute infarction. Circulation 1989; 79: 706–11.

9. NE, Fujita N, Caputo GR, Higgins CB. Measurement of right ventricular mass in normal and dilated cardiomyopathic ventricles using cine magnetic resonance imaging. Am J Cardiol 1992; 69: 1223–8.

10. Cranney GB, Lotan CS, Dean L et al. Left ventricular volume measurement using cardiac axis nuclear magnetic resonance imaging: Validation by calibrated ventricular angiography. Circulation 1990; 82: 154–63.

11. Nienaber CA, von Kodolitsch Y, Nicolas V et al. The diagnosis of thoracic aortic dissection by noninvasive imaging procedures. N Engl J Med 1993; 328: 1–9.

12. Mostbeck GH, Caputo GR, Higgins CB. MR measurement of blood flow in the cardiovascular system. Am J Roent 1992; 159: 453–61.

13. Paulin S, von Schulthess GK, Fossel E, Krayenbuehl HP. MR imaging of the aortic root and proximal coronary arteries. Am J Roent 1987; 148: 665–70.

14. Wang SJ, Hu BS, Macovski A, Nishimura DG. Coronary angiography using fast selective inversion recovery. Magn Reson Med 1991; 18: 417–23.

15. Debiao L, Paschal CB, Haacke EM, Adler LP. Coronary arteries: Three-dimensional MR imaging with fat saturation and magnetization transfer contrast. Radiology 1993; 187: 401–6.

16. Meyer CH, Hu BS, Nishimura DG, Macovski A. Fast spiral coronary artery imaging. Magn Reson Med 1992; 28: 202–13.

17. Manning WJ, Li W, Boyle NG, Edelman RR. Fat-suppressed breath-hold magnetic resonance coronary angiography. Circulation 1993; 87: 94–104.

18. Börnert P, Jensen D. Coronary artery imaging at 0.5T using echo planar imaging (Abstr). Soc Magn Reson 1994; 372.

19. Wielopolski PA, Manning WJ, Edelman RR. Breath-hold volumetric imaging of the heart using magnetization prepared 3D segmented echo planar imaging. J Magn Reson Imag 1995; 4: 403–9

19a. Hundley WG, Clarke GD, Landau C et al. Noninvasive determination of infarct artery patency by cine magnetic resonance angiography. Circulation 1995; 91: 1347–53.

20. Manning WJ, Edelman RR. MR coronary angiography. Magn Reson Q 1993; 9: 131–51.

21. Post JC, van Rossum AC, Hofman MBM et al. Current limitations of two-dimensional breath-hold MR angiography in coronary artery disease (Abstr). Soc Magn Reson 1994; 508.

22. Post JC, van Rossum AC, Hofman MBM, Valk J, Visser CA. Respiratory-gated three-dimensional MR angiography of coronary arteries and comparison with X-ray contrast angiography (Abstr). Soc Magn Reson 1994; 509.

23. Scheidegger MB, Vassalli G, Hess OM, Boesiger P. Validation of coronary artery MR angiography: Comparison of measured vessel diameters with quantitative contrast angiography (Abstr). Soc Magn Reson 1994; 497.
24. Chien D, Anderson C. Breathhold magnetic resonance angiography of coronary arteries using a circularly polarized phased array system (Abstr). Soc Magn Reson 1994; 502.
25. Manning WJ, Li W, Edelman RR. A preliminary report comparing magnetic resonance coronary angiography with conventional angiography. N Engl J Med 1993; 328: 828–32.
26. Rogers WJ, Kramer CM, Simonetti OP, Reichek N. Quantification of human coronary stenoses by magnetic resonance angiography (Abstr). Soc Magn Reson 1994; 370.
27. Pennell DJ, Bogren HG, Keegan J et al. Detection, localisation and assessment of coronary artery stenosis by magnetic resonance imaging (Abstr). Soc Magn Reson 1994; 369.
28. Scott NA, Pettigrew RI. Absence of movement of coronary stents after placement in a magnetic resonance imaging field. Am J Cardiol 1994; 73: 900–1.
29. Yamagishi M, Hotta D, Tamai J et al. Validity of catheter-tip Doppler technique in assessment of coronary flow velocity and application of spectrum analysis method. Am J Cardiol 1991; 67: 758–62.
30. Iliceto S, Marangelli V, Memmola C, Rizzon P. Transesophageal Doppler echocardiography evaluation of coronary blood flow velocity in baseline conditions and during dipyridamole-induced coronary vasocilation. Circulation 1991; 83: 61–9.
31. Brenner LD, Caputo GR, Mostbeck G et al. Quantification of left to right atrial shunts with velocity-encoded cine nuclear magnetic resonance imaging. J Am Coll Cardiol 1992; 20: 1246–50.
32. Edelman RR, Manning WJ, Gervino E, Li W. Flow velocity quantification in human coronary arteries using fast, breath-hold MR angiography. J Magn Reson Imag 1993; 3: 699–703.
33. Keegan J, Firmin D, Gatehouse P, Longmore D. The application of breath hold phase velocity mapping techniques to the measurement of coronary artery blood flow velocity: Phantom data and initial in vivo results. Magn Reson Medicine 1994; 31: 526–36.
34. Poncelet BP, Weisskoff RM, Wedeen VJ et al. Time of flight quantification of coronary flow with echo-planar MRI. Magn Reson Med 1993; 30: 447–57.
35. Kimbiris D, Iskandrian AS, Segal BL, Bemis CE. Anomalous aortic origin of coronary arteries. Circulation 1978; 58: 606–15.
36. Cheitlin MD, Decastro CM, McAllister HA. Sudden death as a complication of anomalous left coronary origin from the anterior sinus of Valsalva: A not-so-minor congenital anomaly. Circulation 1974; 50: 780–7.
37. Doorey AJ, Wills JS, Blasetto J, Goldenbert EM. Usefulness of magnetic resonance imaging for diagnosing an anomalous coronary artery coursing between aorta and pulmonary trunk. Am J Cardiol 1994; 74: 198–9.
38. Manning WJ, Li W, Cohen SI et al. Anomalous left coronary artery: Improved definition with magnetic resonance coronary angiography. Am Heart J 1995; 130 (in press).
39. White RD, Caputo GR, Mark AS et al. Coronary artery bypass graft patency: Non-invasive evaluation with MR imaging. Radiology 1987; 164: 681–6.
40. Rubinstein RI, Askenase AD, Thickman D et al. Magnetic resonance imaging to evaluate patency of aortocoronary bypass grafts. Circulation 1987; 76: 786–91.
41. Jenkins JPR, Love HG, Foster CJ et al. Detection of coronary artery bypass graft patency as assessed by magnetic resonance imaging. Br J Radiol 1988; 61: 2–4.
42. White RD, Pflugfelder PW, Lipton MJ, Higgins CB. Coronary artery bypass grafts: Evaluation of patency with cine MR imaging. Am J Roent 1988; 150: 1271–4.
43. Aurigemma GP, Reichek N, Axel L et al. Noninvasive determination of coronary artery bypass graft patency by cine magnetic resonance imaging. Circulation 1989; 80: 1595–602.
44. Pennell DJ, Keegan J, Firmin DN et al. Magnetic resonance coronary angiography: early experience in coronary artery disease and visualisation of vein grafts (Abstr). Soc Magn Reson Med 1993; 219.

45. Debatin JF, Strong JA, Sostman HD et al. MR characterization of blood flow in native and grafted internal mammary arteries. J Magn Reson Imag 1993; 3: 443–50.
46. Galjee MA, van Rossum AC, Doesburg T et al. Value of cine gradient-echo phase velocity imaging in assessment of coronary artery bypass graft patency and function: An angiographically controlled study (Abstr). Soc Magn Reson 1994; 499.

Corresponding Author: Dr Warren J. Manning, Departments of Medicine (Cardiovascular Division) and Radiology, Charles A. Dana Research Institute and Harvard-Thorndike Laboratory of the Beth Israel Hospital and Harvard Medical School, Boston, MA 02215, USA

13. MRI as a substitute for scintigraphic techniques in the assessment of inducible ischaemia

DUDLEY J. PENNELL

Introduction

The response of the electrocardiogram to exercise has been the mainstay of the non-invasive cardiological assessment of chest pain since ST-depression in association with angina was first described early this century, despite the poorly understood physiological cause. The overall results for the detection of coronary artery disease by exercise electrocardiography are mediocre with an 81% sensitivity and 66% specificity [1], and the site of ST segment changes is poorly correlated with the underlying site of arterial disease [2]. This results because electrocardiographic changes occur late in the cascade of physiological changes associated with ischemia [3], numerous conditions exist where exercise ST segment depression occurs for other reasons, and exercise tolerance is often limited by physical or psychological problems. For these reasons exercise electrocardiography has important limitations and other imaging techniques to assess myocardial ischemia have been developed. Magnetic resonance imaging (MRI) is the latest to be evaluated and has particular strengths with tomographic imaging in any plane, good tissue contrast, high resolution and the lack of ionising radiation.

Dynamic exercise in the magnet

There are no published reports of the diagnostic use of dynamic exercise with MRI, though exercise devices for fitting to the rear of the magnet have been made from non-ferromagnetic materials [4, 5]. Low level prone exercise during magnetic resonance spectroscopy has been reported [6]. Significant supine exercise in the magnet is awkward, particularly as the workload increases, and this leads to movement artefact exacerbated by hyperventilation. The sensation of exercising in a confined environment is unpleasant and sustaining peak exercise for the duration of scanning is difficult. These problems may be ameliorated by the use of ultrafast imaging techniques

C.A. Nienaber and U. Sechtem (eds): Imaging and Intervention in Cardiology. 191–209.
© 1996 *Kluwer Academic Publishers.*

however, such as spiral flow velocity mapping [7]. Results in normals have been reported, with collection of flow data throughout systole from a single heartbeat [5]. Significant increases were documented in mean and peak aortic flow, whilst the time to peak flow fell. These results are encouraging, and suggest that there may be a happy marriage between exercise and ultrafast imaging, but improvements in image resolution are necessary and direct comparisons need to be made with the pharmacological techniques in the induction of ischaemia.

Alternatives to dynamic exercise

A number of stress techniques other than exercise have been used for the diagnosis of coronary artery disease and these might be considered for stress in the magnet (Figure 1). Isometric exercise using the hand dynamometer is

Isometric exercise	Handgrip	
Pacing	Atrial	
Thermal	Cold pressor	
Neural	Mental stress	
Pharmacological	Vasodilator	Dipyridamole
		Adenosine
	Vasoconstrictor	Ergonovine
		Vasopressin
		Angiotensin
	Beta agonists	Adrenaline
		Isoprenaline
		Dopamine
		Dobutamine

Figure 1. The alternatives to dynamic exercise for cardiac stress. Only the pharmacological techniques are presently suitable for use in the magnet.

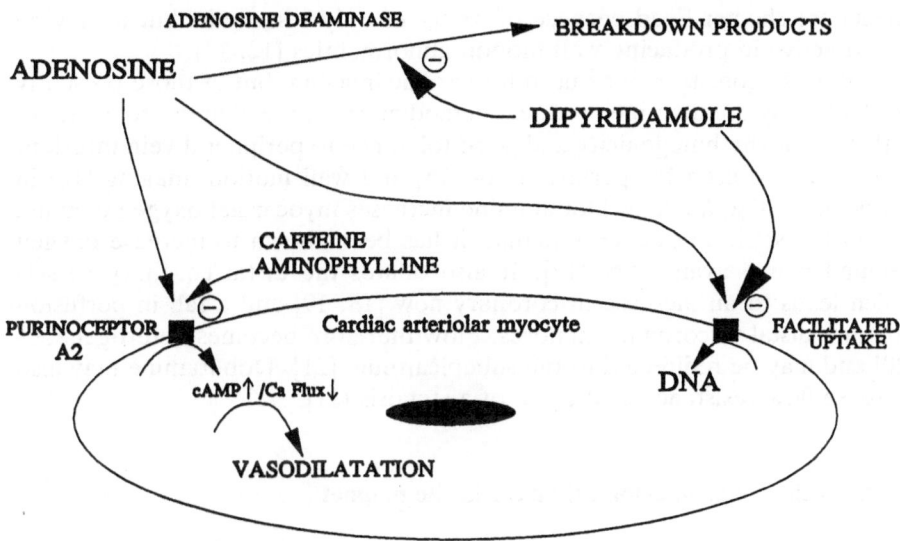

Figure 2. The action of dipyridamole is to raise interstitial adenosine by blocking its breakdown and facilitated cellular uptake. The adenosine acts on the A2 receptor to cause vasodilatation. This binding is competitively antagonised by caffeine and methylxanthines such as aminophylline. Infused adenosine acts directly on the A2 receptor and is greatly potentiated by oral dipyridamole treatment. The electrophysiological effects of adenosine are mediated by the A1 receptor and include slowed atrioventricular conduction and hyperpolarisation of atrial cells.

possible, however the results of its use are unimpressive and muscle fatigue rapidly occurs. Atrial pacing is useful for invasive stress studies, but intracardiac electrodes are unsuitable for MRI. Cold pressor stress is impractical because of the difficulties of using iced water in the scanner and the capricious results with its use. Mental stress requires considerable patient cooperation and, together with the small changes observed, it too does not appear suitable. Therefore the most suitable alternative to exercise is the use of pharmacological stress.

The vasodilator dipyridamole has been widely studied. Its mechanism of action in raising interstitial levels of adenosine is shown in Figure 2. It is simple to administer in a 4 minute infusion of 0.56 mg/kg and causes an increase in human coronary flow of up to 6 times baseline [8], with a $t_{1/2}$ of up to 30 minutes [9]. In the presence of significant coronary stenoses, myocardial flow heterogeneity occurs which can be detected by perfusion techniques. Reduction in perfusion pressure distal to a stenosis, reduction in collateral pressure and flow, and redistribution of flow from subendocardium to subepicardium can cause ischemia and wall motion abnormalities [10], which can be detected by MRI. Adenosine at 140 μg/kg/min may also be given for a direct effect and it causes similar changes in coronary flow [11]. Its side effects are shorter lived because of its $t_{1/2}$ of only 4 seconds, but it may be less effective in producing wall motion abnormalities [12, 13].

The beta agonists may be used for cardiac imaging, but of those presently available only dobutamine produces hemodynamic effects similar to exercise, with a low arrhythmogenicity and good tolerance to peripheral vein infusion. It too may be used for perfusion [14, 15] and wall motion imaging [16] in doses up to 40 µg/kg/min. Dobutamine increases myocardial oxygen demand and in the setting of acute ischemia, it has been shown to increase oxygen demand above availability [17]. It also dilates the distal coronary vessels which leads to an increase in coronary flow [18, 19] and a fall in perfusion pressure distal to coronary stenoses. Flow therefore becomes heterogeneous [20] and may be redirected to the subepicardium [21]. Dobutamine may also increase flow resistance at the site of a stenosis [21].

Studies using pharmacological stress in the magnet

Dipyridamole magnetic resonance wall motion imaging

Pennell et al. first reported the detection by MRI of reversible wall motion abnormality in coronary artery disease using dipyridamole at a dose of 0.56 mg/kg with a 10 mg bolus after 10 minutes [22]. Gradient echo cine imaging with velocity compensation at 0.5 T was used, with TE 14 ms, flip angle 45° 16 frames/cardiac cycle and 2 repetitions. Cines were acquired in the vertical and horizontal long axes and 2 short axis planes. A subsequent study of this technique was performed in 40 patients, 23 of whom had previous infarction. This showed a sensitivity of 67% by induction of new wall motion abnormality different to any found at rest, when compared with areas of reversible ischemia assessed by thallium tomography (Figure 3) [23]. The sensitivity for detection of significant coronary artery disease was 62%. The poor sensitivity of detection of disease occurred because of the inability to detect smaller areas of ischemia (Figure 4). The procedure was well tolerated, but side effects from the dipyridamole, both cardiac and non-cardiac were common. Imaging time before and after dipyridamole was 30 and 15–20 minutes.

An unexpected finding was the small but significant (4% $p < 0.05$) fall in signal from areas of ischemic myocardium. Signal changes were seen in 38% of ischemic segments. This was not explicable by changes in relaxation times with ischemia because such changes occur over a longer time frame, nor was it related to hypokinesis which would be expected to increase the myocardial signal. The likeliest explanation was thought to be a reduction in myocardial blood content, and this was supported by the finding of signal loss predominantly in the subendocardium where the most severe ischemia would be expected from the action of dipyridamole.

Two further studies using dipyridamole during gradient echo imaging have

A

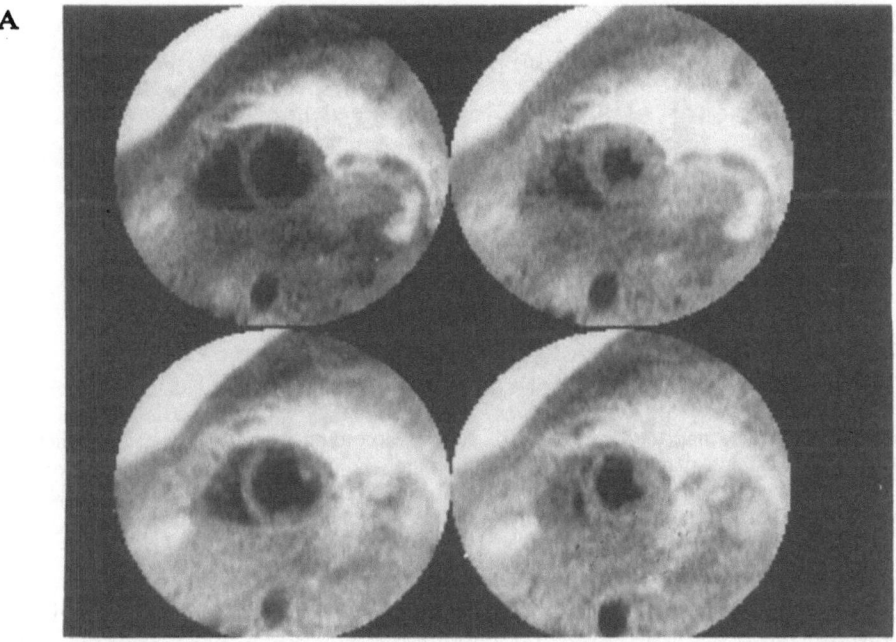

B

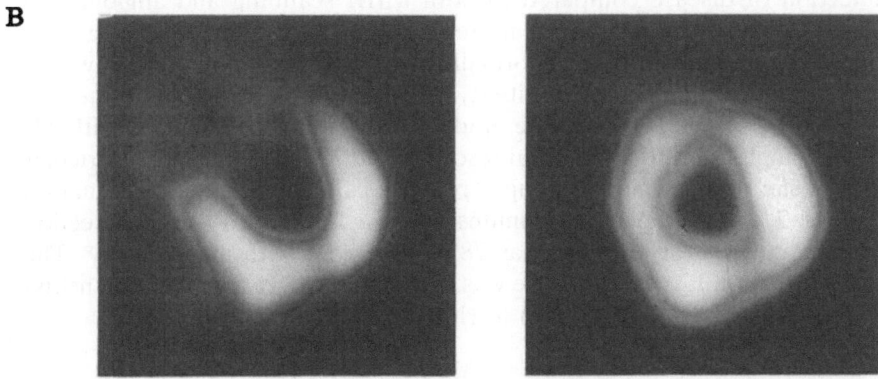

Figure 3. Dipyridamole MRI in a patient with left anterior descending artery disease. Pre-dipyridamole images are in the top row with post-dipyridamole images below. On the left is end-diastole, with end-systole on the right. The pattern of left ventricular contraction is normal prior to vasodilatation, but reduced contraction is seen in the anteroseptal region after dipyridamole. b) The MRI abnormality is closely matched by the perfusion defect (left) seen during dipyridamole thallium myocardial perfusion tomography which shows (right) full reversibility. (Reproduced from Pennell et al. with permission [31].) (For colour plate of Figure 3b see page 533.)

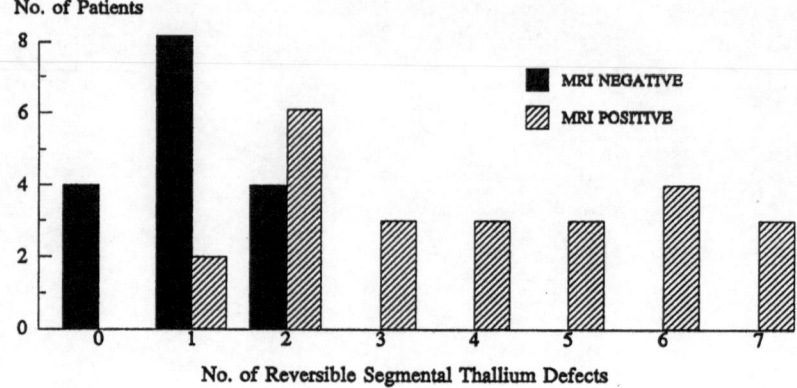

Figure 4. Chart showing the distribution of patients according to size of reversible ischemia found by dipyridamole thallium myocardial perfusion tomography (maximum number of myocardial segments was 9). The solid columns show those patients in whom the MR study failed to show a reversible wall motion abnormality. This was in patients with small defects.

confirmed these findings. Casolo et al. studied 10 patients (7 with previous infarction) at 0.5 T, and infused 0.7 mg/kg dipyridamole over 5 minutes with comparison of wall motion changes with $Tc^{99\,m}$-MIBI perfusion tomography and angiography [24]. Cine gradient echo imaging with a temporal resolution of 50 ms was used, with a single midventricular short axis slice. The sensitivity of detection of disease compared to both MIBI scanning and angiography was 100%. Baer et al. studied a more homogeneous group of 23 patients with no resting wall motion abnormality at 1.5 T [25] and this allowed a more confident estimation of sensitivity of detection of ischaemia in individual arterial territories. Again, cine gradient echo imaging was used with TE 12 ms, flip angle 30° and a temporal resolution of 28 ms. Two mid-ventricular short axis slices were imaged using 4 repetitions to improve image quality. A dose of 0.75 mg/kg over 10 minutes was used and the overall detection rate of coronary artery disease was 78% compared with angiography. The sensitivity for 1 and 2 vessel disease was 69% and 90%, respectively. Sensitivity and specificity for each arterial territory are shown in Figure 5.

Dobutamine magnetic resonance wall motion imaging

Dobutamine has also been used for stress wall motion imaging by MRI. It has a number of advantages in the magnet including operator controlled level of stress, a short half life of 120 seconds, physiological effects mimicking exercise more closely than dipyridamole, and stress induced tachycardia which considerably shortens the stress imaging period when conventional MRI techniques are used.

Pennell et al. reported the use of dobutamine for MRI and showed a

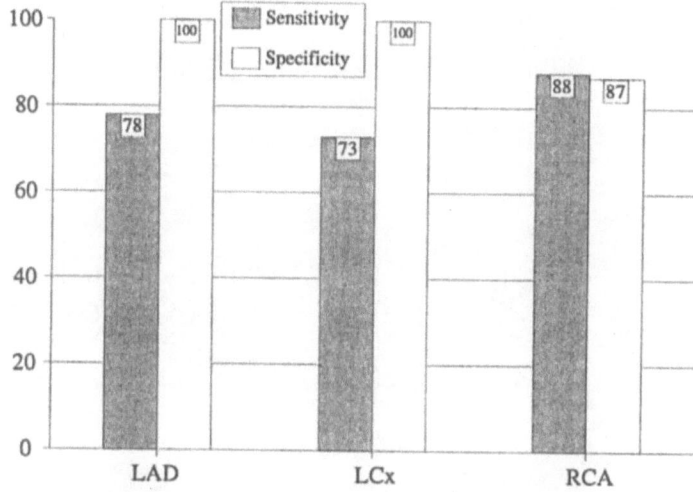

Figure 5. The sensitivity and specificity using dipyridamole MRI of wall motion for the detection of coronary artery disease in each coronary artery in 23 patients without resting wall motion abnormality (data from Baer et al. [25]). LAD-left anterior descending artery, LCx-left circumflex artery, RCA-right coronary artery.

considerable improvement in diagnostic performance [26], when compared with the results with dipyridamole in similar patients [23]. In 25 patients with coronary artery disease, gradient echo cine imaging with velocity compensation was used at 0.5 T, with an echo time of 14 ms, flip angle 45° at rest, 35° during stress, and 12 frames per cardiac cycle. Cines were once again acquired in the vertical and horizontal long axes and 2 short axis planes. Dobutamine was infused up to 20 µg/kg/min increasing the heart rate, systolic blood pressure and double product substantially. This shortened the imaging time during stress to 10–15 minutes. Of the patients with reversible ischemia identified by dobutamine thallium tomography, 95% had reversible myocardial wall motion abnormalities (Figure 6). This represented a sensitivity for detection of significant coronary artery disease of 91%. There was a close concordance in site and extent of the perfusion and wall motion abnormalities, with 96% agreement at rest, 90% during stress and a 91% agreement for the assessment of reversible ischemia. There were no significant differences between MRI and thallium in the detection or location of coronary stenoses (Figure 7), but determination of specificity was hampered by small patient numbers. A 9.2% reduction in signal was found in the ischemic segments, and areas of signal reduction were seen in half of the patients with a new wall motion abnormality, but occasional areas of reduced signal were seen in non-ischemic segments and therefore the specificity of signal reduction for

A

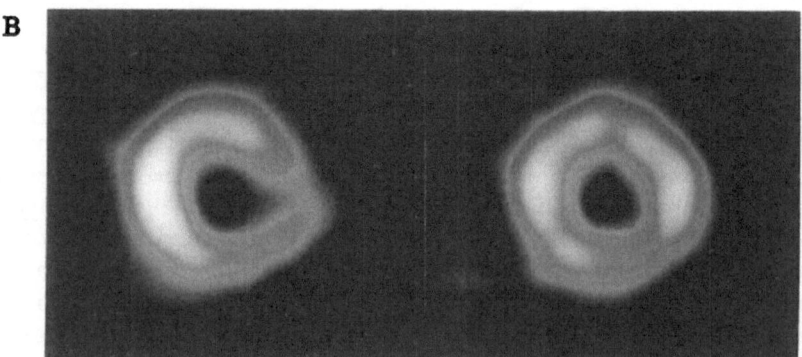

B

Figure 6. a) Dobutamine MRI of a patient with left circumflex artery disease. The format is the same as Figure 3. The contraction pattern at rest is normal but during dobutamine an abnormality of contraction is seen in the lateral wall which matches b) the reversible perfusion defect seen during dobutamine thallium myocardial perfusion tomography. (Reproduced from Pennell et al. with permission [26].) (For colour plate of Figure 6b see page 533.)

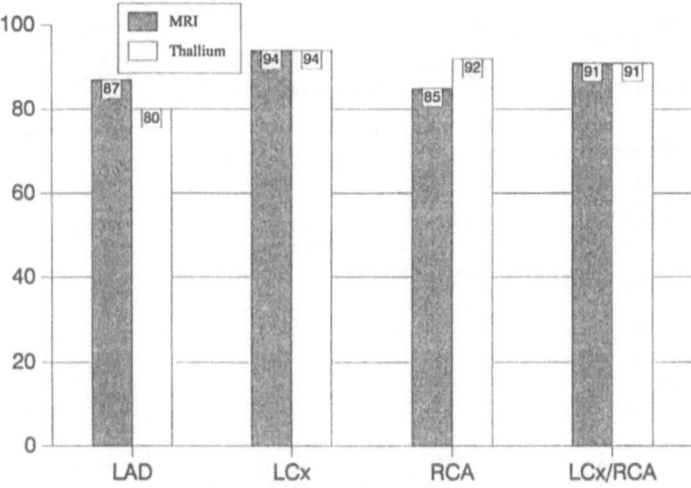

Figure 7. Comparison of sensitivity of detection of coronary artery disease by thallium tomography with MRI of wall motion during dobutamine stress (data from Pennell et al. [26]). Abbreviations as in Figure 5 and LCx/RCA-combined left circumflex and right coronary artery territories.

ischemia was reduced. The dobutamine was well tolerated in the magnet but cardiac and non-cardiac side effects were common.

Results with dobutamine MRI have also been reported by 2 other European groups. Van Rugge et al. studied normals and subsequently patients with coronary artery disease. In the first study, 23 normal subjects were given dobutamine to a maximum dose of 15 µg/kg/min [27]. Imaging was performed at 1.5 T using the cine gradient echo technique with TE 13 ms, flip angle 30° repetition time 30 ms and 8 short axis slices covering the left ventricle from base to apex. Normal ranges were established using a quantitative analysis for global ventricular function and regional wall thickening during rest and stress in the true short axis plane. Heterogeneous values for resting wall thickening were found, as has been described using echocardiography, and significant increases in thickening occurred during stress. At rest, greatest thickening occurred at the apex with a decline in wall thickening in slices towards the base. However, the change in wall thickening from baseline with dobutamine stress was greatest at the base with non-significant changes occurring in the apical portion of the left ventricle and the apex. By recording wall thickening in 20 segments around each short axis slice, the thickening could be displayed graphically to show regional variation, with comparison of rest and dobutamine stress (Figure 8). Van Rugge et al. then proceeded to report their experience with dobutamine stress wall motion imaging in patients with coronary artery disease, with qualitative [28] and quantitative [29] analyses. In the qualitative study, the authors examined short axis cines only, using 6 slices to cover from base to apex. Otherwise the imaging

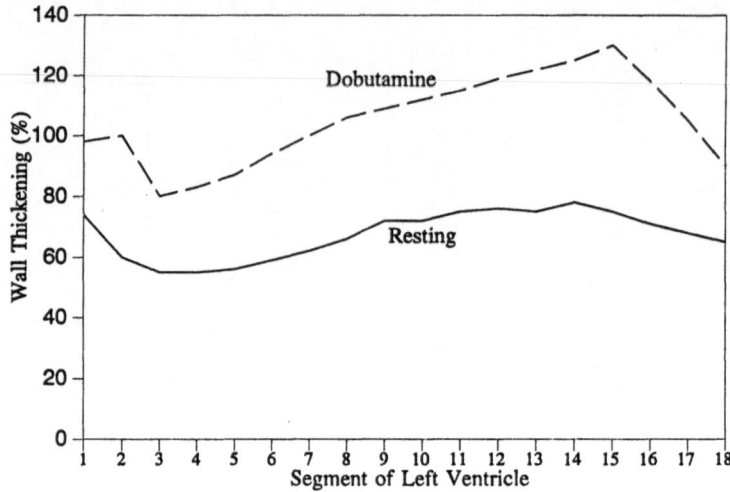

Figure 8. Variation in wall thickening of 18 segments from around the left ventricle at mid-papillary muscle level, at rest and during dobutamine infusion as measured by MRI. Such graphs may potentially be used to define limits of normality for quantitative analysis of stress wall contraction. Wall thickening was defined as (end-systolic – end-diastolic thickness)/end-diastolic thickness. (Adapted from van Rugge et al. [27].)

parameters were the same as above. Of 45 patients studied, 37 had coronary artery disease and 30 (81%) showed wall motion abnormality with dobutamine stress. The specificity in this series was 100%. The results were better than exercise electrocardiography (70/63%) or dobutamine electrocardiography (51/63%). Single, double and triple vessel disease was detected with 75%, 80% and 100% sensitivity respectively. In the quantitative study, 39 patients without rest wall motion abnormality and 10 normal volunteers were stressed with dobutamine concentrations up to 20 µg/kg/min. A short axis stress cine which was judged to show wall motion abnormality was analysed with a modified centerline method. In these preselected cuts, stress wall motion was considered abnormal if 4 or more adjacent chords (100 encompassed the ventricle) showed systolic wall thickening below 2SD of that obtained from the normals. This resulted in a 91% sensitivity and a 80% specificity for detection of disease. Single, double and triple vessel disease were detected with 88%, 91% and 100% sensitivity respectively, whilst the sensitivity of detection of individual coronary artery stenosis was 75%, 87% and 63% for the left anterior descending, right coronary and left circumflex arteries respectively. Unfortunately no direct comparison of the quantitative and qualitative methods was given in this paper to determine in the same patients if the time consuming task of endo- and epicardial tracing yielded a significant diagnostic improvement. Further questions to be answered include whether the quantification is significantly disturbed by the presence of resting wall motion abnormalities.

Baer et al. have also studied the role of dobutamine MRI of wall motion in 28 patients with coronary artery disease but without previous infarction [30]. Imaging was performed at 1.5 T, with a gradient echo sequence with a TE of 12 ms and a flip angle of 30°. The peak dobutamine dose was 20 μg/kg/min. Although the peak rate pressure product was lower during dobutamine MRI than exercise electrocardiography, the relative sensitivities were 85% and 77%. Single and multivessel disease was detected with 73% and 100% sensitivity, respectively. The sensitivity and specificity for detection of disease in the individual arteries was 87/100% in the left anterior descending, 78/88% for the right coronary and 62/93% for the left circumflex arteries.

All three groups who have now studied wall motion during dobutamine stress report good results and excellent patient tolerance. However, the studies presently last too long and the need to perform these studies with breath-hold fast MRI would immediately assist the determination of any likely clinical role. Comparison with thallium imaging and stress electrocardiography shows excellent correlation with the former, and significant improvement over the latter.

Dobutamine magnetic resonance myocardial velocity imaging

The steady state haemodynamics generated by infusion of dobutamine allows imaging of other aspects of cardiac function during stress using conventional imaging techniques with longer image acquisition times. Karwatowski et al. have studied ventricular long axis motion before and after dobutamine stress in normal subjects [31] and in patients with coronary artery disease [32]. Long axis motion of the left ventricle is thought to be a particularly sensitive indicator of contractile dysfunction because the myocardial fibres in the subendocardium are aligned longitudinally and the subendocardium is the first portion of the myocardium to be affected by reduced perfusion [33]. The technique uses velocity mapping of the myocardium in the short axis plane just below the mitral annulus, with through plane velocity sensitisation (0.3–0.5 m/s) to measure the long axis velocities (Figure 9). Karwatowski et al. defined normal long axis dynamics in 31 normal subjects [31]. The peak velocity of long axis motion always occurred in early diastole and significant heterogeneity occurred around the ventricular wall with greatest velocities in the lateral wall. A mean figure for long axis velocity was generated by considering the myocardial slice as a whole, or regional velocities were calculated by dividing the slice into 16 segments. These can be graphically displayed as shown in Figure 10.

Following this study of normals, Karwatowski et al. have also studied 9 normal subjects and 25 patients with coronary artery disease before and during dobutamine stress [32]. The study concentrated on diastolic function, because highest long axis velocities occur at this time, and abnormalities of

Early Systole   Early Diastole

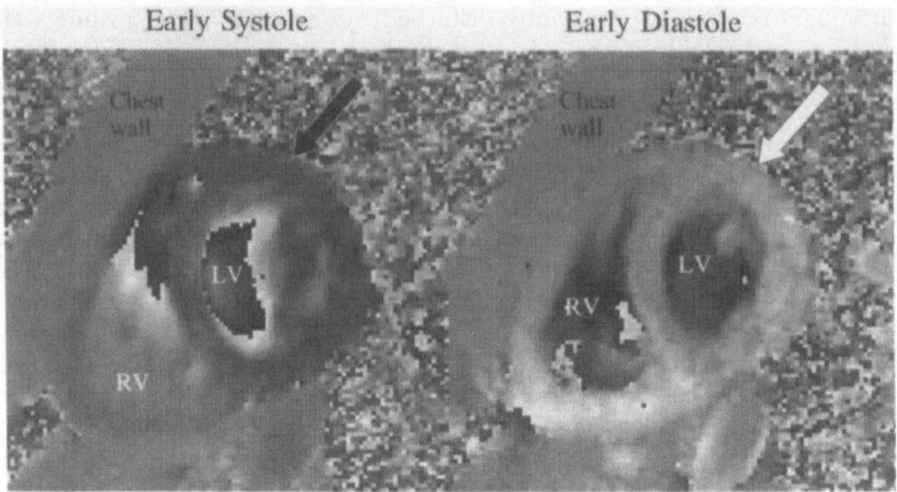

Figure 9. Velocity maps of the myocardium in the short axis plane in early systole (left) and early diastole (right). Mid-grey represents stationary velocity. In early systole the myocardium is relatively thin and in a dark shade (black arrow) representing increased velocities towards the apex. In early diastole the myocardium is thicker and the shading of the myocardium is light (white arrow), showing recoil towards the base. There is considerable aliasing of the velocities in the blood within the ventricular cavities because the velocity window is set very low. Regional variations in velocity may be determined from segments around the myocardial circumference. RV = right ventricle, LV = left ventricle. (Reproduced with permission from Karwatowski et al. [31].)

left ventricular function during ischaemia may occur first in diastole [34]. Diastolic function was assessed by measuring the time to peak early diastolic velocity, and at this time point the mean velocity of the myocardium, and the maximum and minimum regional segmental velocity. The time to peak diastolic velocity decreased in both normals and patients from baseline to low dose dobutamine (5–7.5 μg/kg/min), and from low to high dose dobutamine (10–15 μg/kg/min). The mean long axis velocity increased in the normals with low dose dobutamine and remained elevated with the high dose. In the patients with reversible ischaemia however, 62% developed a reduced mean long axis velocity. Patients with previous infarction but no reversible ischaemia behaved similarly to normals. Regional changes in long axis velocity were also examined. In the normals, regional long axis velocity increased with low dose dobutamine, but with high dose some reduction was seen particularly in the inferoseptal wall. In patients with reversible ischaemia, 62% developed abnormal regional velocities with dobutamine. Overall, 67% of patients with reversible ischaemia had an abnormal global or regional response to stress. The patients with anterior ischaemia were more likely to develop abnormal velocity values during stress, because of the greater

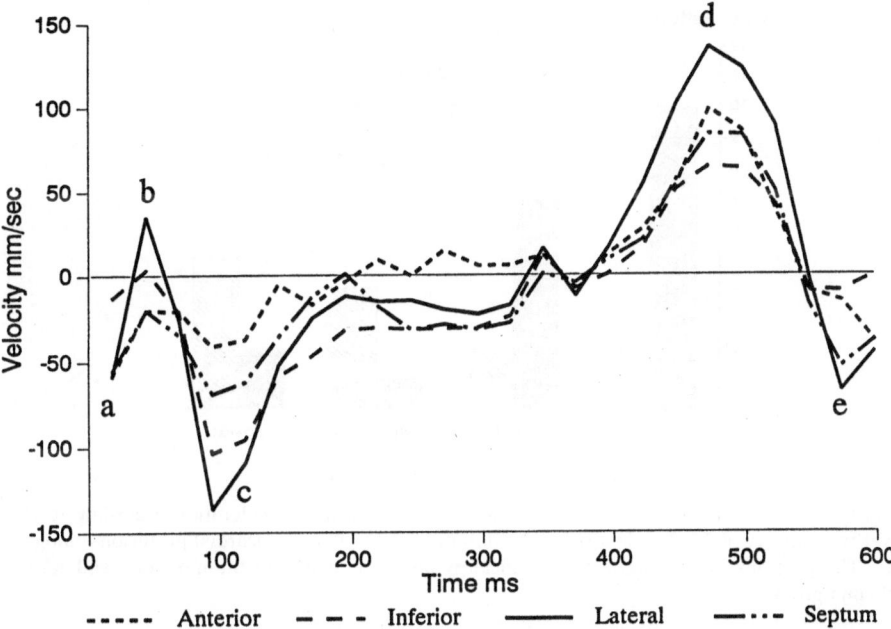

Figure 10. Graphical representation of regional myocardial velocity. Point a) represents displacement of the heart with shape change, b) isovolumic contraction prior to the descent of the base towards the apex in systole, c) peak systolic long axis velocity followed by rapid motion of the base away from the apex, d) peak early diastolic velocity and e) brief period of movement back towards the base. Measurements of peak diastolic timing of velocity are made at point d). (Reproduced with permission from Karwatowski et al. [31].)

contribution to mean myocardial long axis velocity from these segments. Therefore there was a lower sensitivity for uncovering inferior ischaemia.

Dobutamine magnetic resonance aortic flow imaging

The steady state hemodynamics created by dobutamine infusion also allow the measurement of aortic flow during stress by MRI velocity mapping. Simultaneous area and velocity measurements of the ascending aorta yield accurate measurements of absolute flow, and by also measuring the heart rate and blood pressure during stress, the stroke volume, cardiac output, aortic acceleration, cardiac power output and flow wave velocity may be calculated. Pennell et al. have reported studies in normal subjects and patients with coronary artery disease [35]. The data were examined to determine which parameters were predictive of the extent of reversible myocardial ischemia determined from dobutamine thallium tomography.

In the normal subjects, an increase in all parameters was seen with dobutamine stress, except for the stroke volume which rose and then fell, and the

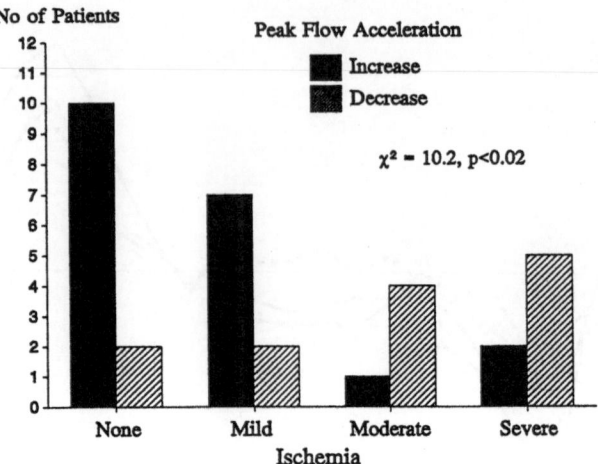

Figure 11. Chart showing the occurrence of a fall in peak flow acceleration according to the severity of myocardial ischemia assessed by dobutamine thallium myocardial perfusion tomography. The peak flow acceleration fell significantly more frequently in the moderate and severe ischemia groups.

diastolic blood pressure which remained unchanged. In patients with coronary artery disease, the qualitative pattern of change in parameters was similar, except that a fall in peak flow acceleration at peak stress was found to occur significantly more frequently in patients with moderate and severe ischemia than in patients with mild or no ischemia (Figure 11). The quantitative change from baseline to peak stress in 5 parameters was significantly related to the extent of myocardial ischemia (peak flow acceleration, peak flow, cardiac power output, maximum dobutamine dose tolerated and systolic blood pressure). Using multivariate analysis, the peak flow acceleration was found to be the most predictive variable ($p < 0.00001$), and alone explained 58.4% of the variation in the observed myocardial ischemia (Figure 12). Only the cardiac power output retained predictive significance after allowing for the peak flow acceleration but its contribution to the predictive accuracy of the model was small (4.2%).

This study showed that an assessment of global ventricular function by MRI could be performed during dobutamine stress. Peak acceleration has been measured with echocardiography in coronary artery disease during exercise and has been found to be a useful parameter of global left ventricular contractility [36, 37], whereas results of acceleration measurements during dipyridamole infusion are contradictory [38, 39]. Controversy exists over its clinical diagnostic use because of the dependence on preload and afterload [40, 41]. This failing is shared by other global function parameters such as

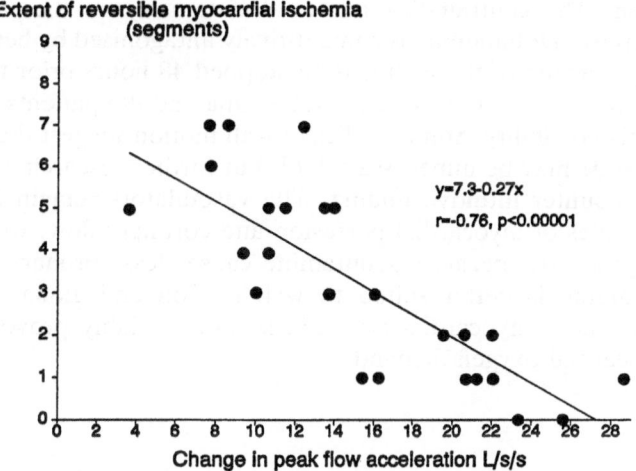

Figure 12. Graph of the regression of the change in peak flow acceleration against the extent of reversible myocardial ischemia (maximum number of segments was 9).

the ejection fraction and might confound the comparison of results obtained on different occasions rather than with a single assessment.

Magnetic resonance perfusion imaging

The passage of an intravenous bolus of magnetic resonance contrast may be used in the evaluation of cardiac perfusion in combination with ultrafast techniques such as FLASH or echo-planar imaging. It is highly likely that a clinical test would employ vasodilators to accentuate the difference in flow between normal and stenosed arteries. This has been reported for both FLASH [42–44] and echo planar imaging [45, 46], and comparison of thallium and dipyridamole MRI has showed good agreement using FLASH imaging [43] (see also Chapters 13, 14 and 23).

Choice of pharmacological agent

It is likely that the role of pharmacological vasodilatation and stress in the magnet will grow for the functional assessment of heart disease. This will require familiarity of the strengths of each technique and the important contraindications [47]. The vasodilators should not be administered to asthmatics because of the risk of provocation of severe bronchospasm [48, 49]. Adenosine infusion in sinoatrial disease may lead to sinus arrest, and should also be avoided [50]. Caffeine is a competitive antagonist of adenosine and should be avoided for at least 12 hours prior to scanning to avoid attenuated vasodilatation. The contraindications to dobutamine are the same as for dynamic exercise. Dobutamine is competitively antagonised by beta-blockers and the longer acting of these should be stopped 48 hours prior to imaging. This may occasionally lead to withdrawal angina and the patients need to be warned of this possibility. Some studies of wall motion suggest that cessation of beta blockade may be unnecessary [16], but further research is needed to confirm this counter intuitive finding. The vasodilators remain first choice agents for studies of myocardial perfusion and coronary flow, which should be feasible presently, because dobutamine causes less coronary hyperemia [10]. Dobutamine is better suited to wall motion and global ventricular studies [10], where myocardial ischemia is more reliably provoked by increased myocardial oxygen demand.

Conclusions

There are a number of MRI stress techniques being developed which will be direct competitors with scintigraphic techniques for the evaluation of reversible myocardial ischaemia. The most well developed is wall motion imaging which has been performed in a number of centres using both dipyridamole and dobutamine. This technique is analogous to stress echocardiography, but MRI has the inherent advantages of better resolution, and true long and short axis imaging with contiguous parallel slices. The results in comparison with myocardial perfusion imaging are reasonable, especially with dobutamine, but all the studies reported to date have been conducted in patients with a very high pre-test likelihood of disease and much more intense scrutiny in patient populations with intermediate and low pre-test risk are necessary before a confident and clinically robust investigation can be envisaged. A simple and rapid technique for quantification of wall motion would greatly help clinical use. The other techniques described above are more experimental at present. Long axis velocity imaging and aortic flow imaging during dobutamine stress have only been performed in one centre and their overall sensitivity needs further evaluation. They therefore remain speculative. Myocardial perfusion imaging by MRI is very attractive because of the lack of ionising radiation, despite the need for intravenous cannulae (probably in a central vein or right atrium for quantitative work) and a contrast agent injection. Although FLASH imaging has been used by most investigators to date, coverage of the entire ventricle is difficult with this technique and multislice echo-planar imaging may be necessary in the clinical arena [51]. Exercise stress in the magnet remains difficult despite some modest success and many patients fail to exercise fully because of physical of psychological reasons, and therefore there is every likelihood that pharmacological stress will continue to be the technique of choice for stress MRI in the long term.

References

1. Detrano R, Gianrossi R, Mulvihill D et al. Exercise induced ST segment depression in the diagnosis of multivessel coronary disease: A meta analysis. J Am Coll Cardiol 1989; 14: 1501–8.
2. Abouantoun A, Ahnve S, Savvides M et al. Can areas of myocardial ischemia be localised by the exercise electrocardiogram? A correlative study with thallium-201 scintigraphy. Am Heart J 1984; 108: 933–41.
3. Nesto RW, Kowalchuk GJ. The ischemic cascade: Temporal sequence of hemodynamic, electrocardiographic and symptomatic expressions of ischemia. Am J Cardiol 1987; 57: 23C–30C.
4. Schaefer S, Peshock RM, Parkey RW, Willerson JT. A new device for exercise MR imaging. Am J Roentgenol 1986; 147: 1289–90.
5. Mohiaddin RH, Gatehouse PD, Firmin DN. Exercise related changes in aortic flow measured by magnetic resonance spiral echo-planar phase-shift velocity mapping. J Magn Reson Imag 1995; 5: 159–63.
6. Conway MA, Bristow JD, Blackledge MJ et al. Cardiac metabolism during exercise in healthy volunteers measured by ^{31}P magnetic resonance spectroscopy. Br Heart J 1991; 65: 25–30.
7. Gatehouse PD, Firmin DN, Collins S, Longmore DB. Real time blood flow imaging by spiral scan phase velocity mapping. Magn Reson Med 1994; 31: 504–12.
8. Wilson RF, Laughlin DE, Ackell PH et al. Transluminal, subselective measurement of coronary artery blood flow velocity and vasodilator reserve in man. Circulation 1985; 72: 82–92.
9. Brown G, Josephson MA, Petersen RD et al. Intravenous dipyridamole combined with isometric handgrip for near maximal coronary flow in patients with coronary artery disease. Am J Cardiol 1981; 48: 1077–85.
10. Fung AY, Gallagher KP, Buda AJ. The physiological basis of dobutamine as compared with dipyridamole stress interventions in the assessment of critical coronary stenosis. Circulation 1987; 76: 943–51.
11. Wilson RF, Wyche K, Christensen BV et al. Effects of adenosine on human coronary arterial circulation. Circulation 1990; 82: 1595–606.
12. Zoghbi WA, Cheirif J, Kleiman NS et al. Diagnosis of ischemic heart disease with adenosine echocardiography. J Am Coll Cardiol 1991; 18: 1271–9.
13. Nguyen T, Heo J, Ogilby D, Iskandrian AS. Single photon emission computed tomography with thallium-201 during adenosine induced coronary hyperaemia: Correlation with coronary arteriography, exercise thallium imaging and two-dimensional echocardiography. J Am Coll Cardiol 1990; 16: 1375–83.
14. Pennell DJ, Underwood SR, Swanton RH et al. Dobutamine thallium myocardial perfusion tomography. J Am Coll Cardiol 1991; 18: 1471–9.
15. Pennell DJ, Underwood SR, Ell PJ. Safety of dobutamine stress for thallium myocardial perfusion tomography in patients with asthma. Am J Cardiol 1993; 71: 1346–50.
16. Sawada SG, Segar DS, Ryan T et al. Echocardiographic detection of coronary artery disease during dobutamine infusion. Circulation 1991; 83: 1605–14.
17. Willerson JT, Hutton I, Watson JT et al. Influence of dobutamine on regional myocardial blood flow and ventricular performance during acute and chronic myocardial ischemia in dogs. Circulation 1976; 53: 828–33.
18. Vasu MA, O'Keefe DD, Kapellakis GZ et al. Myocardial oxygen consumption: Effects of epinephrine, isoproterenol, dopamine, norepinephrine and dobutamine. Am J Physiol 1978; 235: 237–41.
19. Fowler MB, Alderman EL, Oesterle SN et al. Dobutamine and dopamine after cardiac surgery: Greater augmentation of myocardial blood flow with dobutamine. Circulation 1984; 70 (Suppl I): 103–11.

20. Meyer SL, Curry GC, Donsky MS et al. Influence of dobutamine on hemodynamics and coronary blood flow in patients with and without coronary artery disease. Am J Cardiol 1976; 38: 103–8.

21. Warltier DC, Zyvlowski M, Gross GJ et al. Redistribution of myocardial blood flow distal to a dynamic coronary arterial stenosis by sympathomimetic amines. Comparison of dopamine, dobutamine and isoproterenol. Am J Cardiol 1981; 48: 269–79.

22. Pennell DJ, Underwood SR, Longmore DB. The detection of coronary artery disease by magnetic resonance imaging using intravenous dipyridamole. J Comput Assist Tomogr 1990; 14: 167–70.

23. Pennell DJ, Underwood SR, Ell PJ et al. Dipyridamole magnetic resonance imaging: A comparison with thallium-201 emission tomography. Br Heart J 1990; 64: 362–9.

24. Casolo GC, Bonechi F, Taddei T et al. Alterations in dipyridamole induced LV wall motion during myocardial ischaemia studied by NMR imaging. Comparison with Tc-99m-MIBI myocardial scintigraphy. G Ital Cardiol 1991; 21: 609–17.

25. Baer FM, Smolarz K, Jungehulsing M et al. Feasibility of high dose dipyridamole magnetic resonance imaging for detection of coronary artery disease and comparison with coronary angiography. Am J Cardiol 1992; 69: 51–6.

26. Pennell DJ, Underwood SR, Manzara CC et al. Magnetic resonance imaging during dobutamine stress in coronary artery disease. Am J Cardiol 1992; 70: 34–40.

27. Van Rugge FP, Holman ER, van der Wall EE et al. Quantitation of global and regional left ventricular function by cine magnetic resonance imaging during dobutamine stress in normal human subjects. Eur Heart J 1993; 14: 456–63.

28. Van Rugge FP, van der Wall EE, de Roos A, Bruschke AVG. Dobutamine stress magnetic resonance imaging for detection of coronary artery disease. J Am Coll Cardiol 1993; 22: 431–9.

29. Van Rugge FP, van der Wall EE, Spanjersberg SJ et al. Magnetic resonance imaging during dobutamine stress for detection and localisation of coronary artery disease. Quantitative wall motion analysis using a modification of the centerline method. Circulation 1994; 90: 127–38.

30. Baer FM, Voth E, Theissen P et al. Gradient echo magnetic resonance imaging during incremental dobutamine infusion for the localisation of coronary artery stenosis. Eur Heart J 1994; 15: 218–25.

31. Karwatowski SP, Mohiaddin RH, Yang GZ et al. Noninvasive assessment of regional left ventricular long axis motion using magnetic resonance velocity mapping in normal subjects. J Magn Reson Imag 1994; 4: 151–5.

32. Karwatowski SP, Forbat SM, Mohiaddin RH et al. Regional left ventricular long axis function in controls and patients with ischaemic heart disease pre and post angioplasty (Abstr). Circulation 1993; 88 (Suppl): I–83.

33. Jones CHJ, Raposo L, Gibson DG. Functional importance of the long axis dynamics of the left ventricle. Br Heart J 1990; 63: 1228–37.

34. Reduto LA, Wickermeyer WJ, Young JB et al. Left ventricular diastolic performance at rest and during exercise in patients with coronary artery disease. Assessment with first pass radionuclide ventriculography. Circulation 1981; 63: 1228–37.

35. Pennell DJ, Firmin DN, Burger P et al. Assessment of **magnetic** resonance velocity mapping of global ventricular function during dobutamine infusion in coronary artery disease. Br Heart J 1995; 74: 163–70.

36. Harrison MR, Smith MD, Friedman BJ, DeMaria AN. Uses and limitations of exercise Doppler echocardiography in the diagnosis of ischeamic heart disease. J Am Coll Cardiol 1987; 10: 809–17.

37. Fisman EZ, Ben-Ari E, Pines A et al. Pronounced reduction of aortic flow velocity and acceleration during heavy isometric exercise in coronary artery disease. Am J Cardiol 1991; 68: 485–91.

38. Labowitz AJ, Pearson AC, Chaitman BR. Doppler and two-dimensional echocardiographic

assessment of left ventricular function before and after intravenous dipyridamole stress testing for detection of coronary artery disease. Am J Cardiol 1988; 62: 1180–5.

39. Grayburn PA, Popma JJ, Pryor SL et al. Comparison of dipyridamole-Doppler echocardiography to thallium-201 imaging and quantitative coronary arteriography in the assessment of coronary artery disease. Am J Cardiol 1989; 63: 1315–20.

40. Harrison MR, Clifton D, Berk MR, DeMaria AN. Effect of heart rate on Doppler indexes of systolic function in humans. J Am Coll Cardiol 1989; 14: 929–35.

41. Wilke N, Engels G, Koronaeos A et al. First pass myocardial perfusion imaging with ultrafast Gadolium enhanced MR imaging at rest and during dipyridamole administration (Abstr). Radiology 1992; 185(P): 133.

42. Schaefer S, van Tyen R, Saloner D. Evaluation of myocardial perfusion abnormalities with gadolinium enhanced snapshot MR imaging in humans. Radiology 1992; 185: 795–801.

43. Eichenberger AC, Schuiki E, Kochli VD et al. Ischemic heart disease: Assessment with gadolinium enhanced ultrafast MR imaging and dipyridamole stress. J Magn Reson Imag 1994; 4: 425–31.

44. Kantor HL, Rzedzian RR, Pykett IL et al. Transient effects of Gadolinium-DTPA and Dysprosium-DTPA intravenous infusion on myocardial NMR image intensity using high speed NMR imaging (Abstr). Proc Soc Magn Reson Med 1988; 246.

45. Hunter GJ, Kantor HL, Weisskopf RM et al. Assessment of myocardial perfusion by MRI: Correlation with radiolabelled microspheres (Abstr). Proc Soc Magn Reson Med 1991; 119.

46. Pennell DJ. Cardiac stress in nuclear medicine. In: Murray IPC, Ell PJ, editors. Nuclear medicine in clinical diagnosis and management. London, UK: Churchill Livingstone, 1994.

47. Homma S, Gilliland Y, Guiney TE et al. Safety of intravenous dipyridamole for stress testing with thallium imaging. Am J Cardiol 1987; 59: 152–4.

48. Taviot B, Pavheco Y, Coppere B et al. Bronchospasm induced in an asthmatic by the injection of adenosine. Press Med 1986; 15: 1103.

49. Pennell DJ, Mahmood S, Ell PJ, Underwood SR. Bradycardia progressing to cardiac arrest during adenosine thallium myocardial perfusion imaging in covert sino-atrial disease. Eur J Nucl Med 1994; 21: 170–2.

50. Edelman RR, Li W. Contrast enhanced echo planar MR imaging of myocardial perfusion: Preliminary study in humans. Radiology 1994; 190: 771–7.

Corresponding Author: Dr Dudley Pennell, Magnetic Resonance Unit, Royal Brompton Hospital, Sydney Street, London SW3 6NP, UK

14. Assessment of viability by MR-techniques

UDO SECHTEM, FRANK M. BAER, EBERHARD VOTH,
PETER THEISSEN, CHRISTIAN SCHNEIDER and HARALD
SCHICHA

Introduction

Magnetic resonance techniques are in an early phase of their application to detect viable myocardium after myocardial infarction. However, magnetic resonance imaging (MRI) seems ideally suited to detect the regional wall thinning associated chronic myocardial scar [1–5]. In contrast to akinetic and thinned transmural *chronic* infarcts [6–9], *acutely* infarcted myocardium may be transmurally necrotic and akinetic but may not yet exhibit myocardial thinning [9]. Therefore, assessment of wall thickness by MRI is not sufficient to determine viability. Stimulation of residual contractility by catecholamines, which is well known from viability studies using left ventricular angiography [10], radionuclide ventriculography [11], or echocardiography [12], can also be used in conjuction with MRI to demonstrate residual viability in these patients [13]. It is also possible to employ magnetic resonance spectroscopy, especially in the setting of acute myocardial infarction, where substantial myocardial wall thinning has not yet occurred to document the presence or absence of high-energy phosphates as indicators of viable myocardium [14].

This chapter will review features of viable and scarred myocardium as characterized by MRI and compare MRI to scintigraphic techniques currently used for the identification of viable myocardium. In addition, the potential of magnetic resonance spectroscopy (MRS) for diagnosis of viability will be discussed.

Acute and chronic contractile dysfunction of viable myocardium

In contrast to acutely necrotic or chronically scarred myocardium, the contractile dysfunction of viable myocardium is potentially reversible. The failure of viable myocardium to contract may be due to two different mechanisms: stunning or hibernation. Stunning describes the dysfunctional state of the myocardium caused by a brief occlusion of a coronary artery with subsequent restoration of blood flow [15]. Clinically, stunning can be observed after acute myocardial infarction with early reperfusion, after mechanical interven-

C.A. Nienaber and U. Sechtem (eds): Imaging and Intervention in Cardiology. 211–236.
© 1996 *Kluwer Academic Publishers.*

tions such as balloon angioplasty, and after ischemic episodes due to intense exercise [16]. The time course of recovery after myocardial stunning depends on the extent of the perfusion abnormality during the preceding phase of ischemia and dysfunction may be present for several weeks although coronary blood flow is normal [17].

In contrast to stunning, hibernation refers to a condition characterized by a prolonged dysfunction of the myocardium due to prolonged periods of ischemia or chronically reduced perfusion in severe coronary artery disease [18]. Clinically, this condition may be seen in patients with occluded coronary arteries with or without a history of myocardial infarction. In these patients, some residual perfusion, for instance through collaterals, may completely or partially prevent irreversible structural damage of the myocardial region perfused by the occluded artery. Identification of hibernating myocardium is clinically important because revascularization of these regions may result in restitution of contractile function [19]. The pathophysiology of hibernation is, however, not entirely clear due to the inability to develop an animal model of hibernation in which a state of low perfusion and absent contraction could be preserved for a prolonged period of time. The results of a recent study [20] have initiated a discussion whether hibernation is a truly independent entity or whether it is merely the result of repetitive ischemia with delayed recovery of the myocardium, i.e. a form of repetitive stunning.

MR-techniques and viability in acute myocardial infarcts

Infarct healing leads to structural changes within the infarct zone [9]. Therefore, it is necessary to distinguish between the application of MR-techniques in acute or recent infarcts and chronic infarcts, i.e. infarcts that are more than 16 weeks old. After this time, practically all infarcts have transformed into a contracted, firm, white scar [9]. In contrast, both acutely stunned myocardium and acutely necrotic myocardium may have normal wall thickness.

Signal intensity changes on spin-echo images

An increase in signal intensity of freshly infarcted myocardium, which appears on T2 weighted spin-echo MR images only a few hours after occlusion of a coronary artery [21], can be used to determine the extent of irreversible myocardial damage [22]. It is not clear, however, whether this area of increased myocardial signal intensity that is seen within the first week after the event (Figure 1) represents necrotic myocardium or incorporates some edematous viable myocardium (Figure 2) [23, 24]. After 3 weeks, true infarct size may be more closely approximated by the area of increased signal intensity because the edema surrounding the infarct has presumably regressed

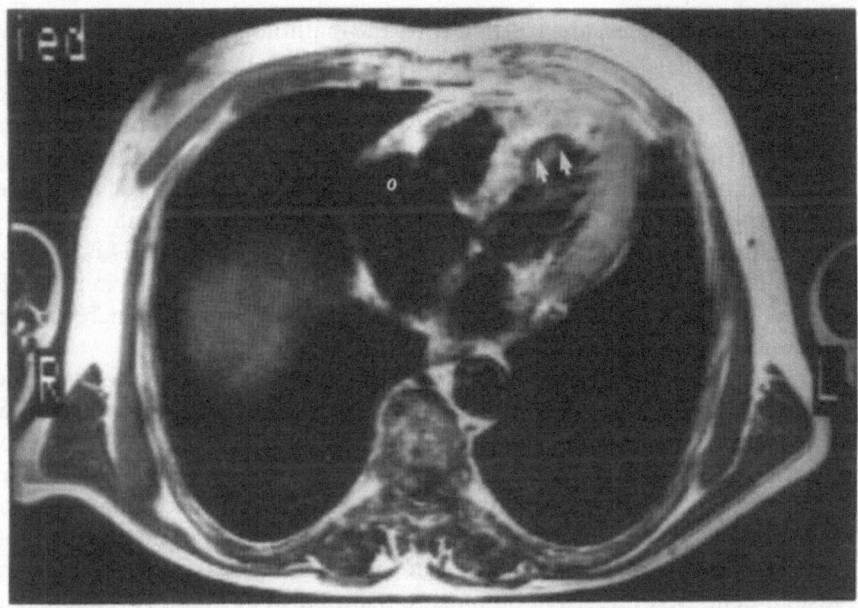

Figure 1. Transverse spin-echo-image (TE = 30 ms) in a patient with seven day old reperfused anteroseptal myocardial infarction. Signal intensity is increased in the anterior wall and the interventricular septum (arrows) as compared to the lateral wall of the left ventricle. (Reproduced from: Baer FM et al. Herz 1994; 19: 51–64 with permission from the publisher.)

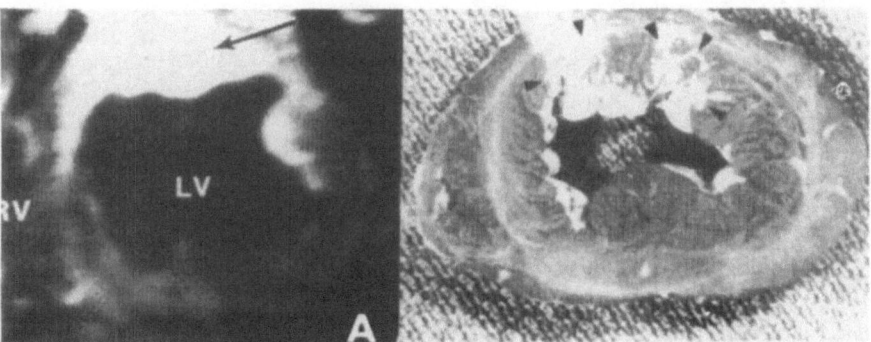

Figure 2. Short-axis spin-echo image (echo time 60 ms) of ex vivo dog heart (A) and corresponding triphenyltetrazolium chloride-stained specimen (B). The heart was subjected to 3 hours of coronary artery occlusion. The infarct is small, patchy, and predominantly subendocardial (black arrowheads). The region of increased signal intensity on the MR image (large arrow) is more transmural and clearly overestimates true infarct size. LV = left ventricle; RV = right ventricle. (Reprinted with permission from the American College of Cardiology. Source: Ryan T et al. J Am Coll Cardiol 1990; 15: 1355–1364.)

and signal abnormalities are restricted to the pathologically determined infarct area [25].

When measuring the area of increased "myocardial" signal intensity, one
has to consider that slow blood flow adjacent to an area of severe hypokinesia
also results in high signal intensity of the blood. This signal from blood may
blend with the myocardium and may give the false impression of increased
signal intensity *within* the myocardium [26]. The use of signal intensity
changes for making a diagnosis of complete myocardial necrosis is further
complicated by the fact that in vivo MR imaging sometimes results in artifacts
caused by breathing and cardiac arrhythmias. Thus spurious increases in
signal intensity may also be found in normal persons [27].

Only one paper directly addresses the question, whether reversibly and
irreversibly injured myocardium can be distinguished on the basis of signal
intensity measurements [28]. Transient occlusion of a coronary artery of
various durations was used in dogs to produce stunned and infarcted myocardium. In contrast to infarcted myocardium, stunned myocardium did not
show increases in a signal intensity despite regional systolic dysfunction
(Figure 3). There are no reports about signal intensity measurements on
native spin-echo MR images in humans to distinguish between reversible and
irreversible damage to the myocardium.

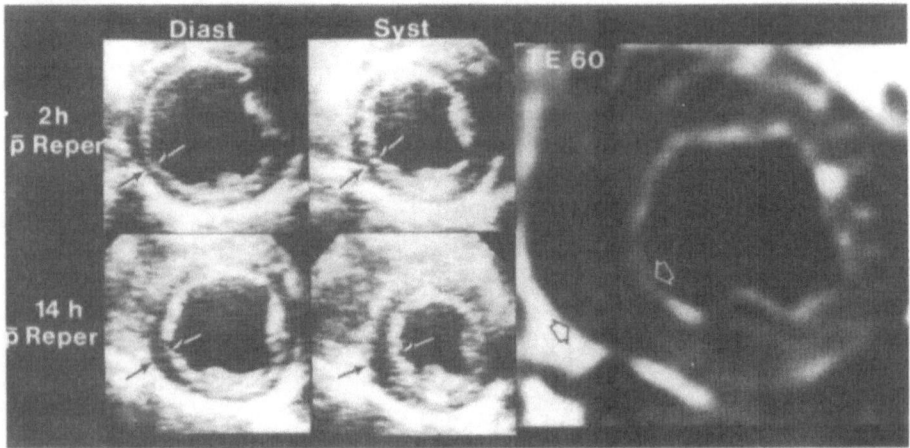

Figure 3. Short-axis echocardiograms at end-diastole (Diast) and end-systole (Syst) and the
corresponding MR image (echo time = 60 ms) in a dog undergoing 1 hour of coronary occlusion
before reperfusion (p Reper). At 2 hours of reperfusion (just before MR imaging), diastolic
thinning and reduced systolic thickening are apparent in the ischemic but viable zone (arrows).
After 14 hours of reperfusion (bottom two images) wall thickening has improved. There is no
visually apparent change in signal intensity in the corresponding anterior region on the MR
image on the right consistent with the absence of acute necrosis. (Reprinted with permission
from the American College of Cardiology. Source: Ryan T et al. J Am Coll Cardiol 1990; 15:
1355–1364.)

Contrast agents

Gadolinium and manganese chelates have been employed in animal models to differentiate between reversible and irreversible injury (stunning and necrosis) on the basis of signal enhancement [29, 30]. Reperfused, reversibly injured myocardium enhances in a similar way as normal myocardium. In contrast, irreversibly injured myocardium shows more signal enhancement than either normal or reversibly injured myocardium [29, 30].

In contrast to the above mentioned T1-enhancing contrast agents, T2* enhancing agents cause a decrease of signal intensity in normal myocardium by dephasing water molecules, which diffuse through local magnetic field gradients induced by a heterogeneous distribution of the contrast agent. The heterogeneous distribution in normal myocardium occurs because cell membranes act as a barrier and limit access of the contrast agent to the intracellular space. If cell death has occurred cell membranes are destroyed and the contrast agent is distributed more homogeneously throughout the cells and the interstitium. Therefore, spin dephasing will be less affected and less signal loss will occur. This was recently confirmed in an animal model of reperfused myocardial infarcts, which showed less signal loss after administration of dysprosium-DTPA-bis(methylamide) than normal myocardium on T2-weighted spin-echo images [31]. However, these interesting findings have yet to be confirmed in humans.

MR-spectroscopy

Localized ^{31}P-MR spectroscopy is able to directly observe the metabolism of myocardial cells from ischemia to infarction [14]. High energy phosphates such as phosphocreatine and ATP decrease early after the onset of ischemia whereas the inorganic phosphate peak increases (Figure 4).

It has been shown in vivo in animal models using coils directly applied to the surface of the heart that phosphocreatine recovers after brief coronary occlusion and reperfusion [32, 33]. Based on these spectroscopic measurements during acute myocardial ischemia, phosphocreatine was proposed as an indicator for the balance of myocardial perfusion and actual energy requirements [32]. After the onset of ischemia, the concentration of phosphocreatine decreases much faster than that of ATP, which results in a rapid increase of the ratio of ATP/creatinephosphate [32, 33]. In contrast to these changes in acutely ischemic myocardium, chronically hypoperfused hibernating myocardium should be characterized by a balanced reduction of both, ATP and phosphocreatine, because it has been shown that phosphocreatine levels can recover under these circumstances after a longer waiting period [34–36]. However, no spectroscopy data have been reported from the only clinically relevant model of hibernation, the patient with decreased myocardial function which recovers after revascularization.

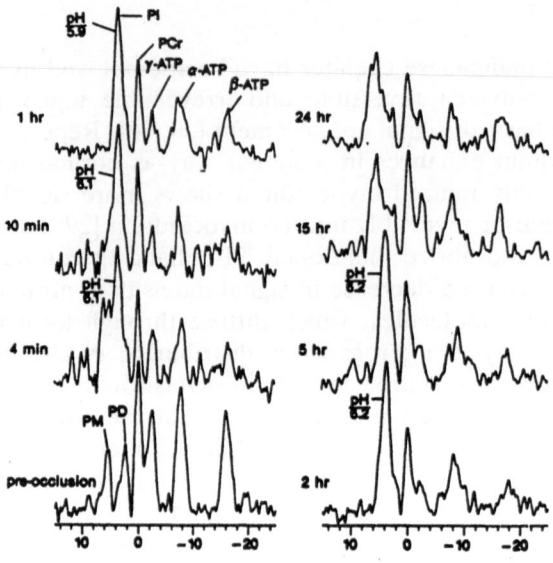

Figure 4. Metabolism of ischemic myocardium over 24 hours after coronary occlusion as observed by magnetic resonance spectroscopy. The signal of high-energy phosphates is received by a coil located outside the dog's chest. Localization of spectra was achieved by using depth-resolved surface coil spectroscopy (DRESS). Scan times per spectrum were 10 minutes. Times coincide with commencement of spectral acquisition relative to coronary occlusion. The ratio of phosphocreatine to inorganic phosphate (PCr/Pi) decreased from 8 preocclusion to 0.5 postocclusion. It is also possible to monitor the course of the pH-value over time. Phosphate peaks are labelled in the one hour spectrum. Pi = inorganic phosphate; PCr = phosphocreatine; PM = phosphomonoesters; PD = phosphodiesters; α-ATP, β-ATP, γ-ATP denote the three peaks of ATP. (Reproduced from: Bottomley PA et al. Magn Reson Med 1987; 5: 129–42 with permission from the publisher.)

More recently, new pulse sequences and high field magnets have permitted separate observation of the endocardial and epicardial portion of left ventricular wall in animal models [37, 38]. This ability may further improve the detection of residual tissue viability, which is preferentially located near the epicardium [39].

In contrast to the spectra of viable myocardium, which exhibit various amounts of phosphocreatine, completely infarcted myocardium should not contain any measurable amount of phosphocreatine and ATP and could thus be distinguished from myocardium which harbours surviving myocardial cells. Unfortunately, the quantification of metabolism by MR-spectroscopy in humans is not without problems because volumes of interest are relatively large as compared to myocardial wall thickness. Further technical progress is necessary in order to correctly quantify the amount of viable myocardium contained within a small volume of interest [37], and only then will MR spectroscopy be able to provide clinically meaningful information for the diagnosis of myocardial viability [40].

Wall motion abnormalities

Severe wall motion abnormalities, which are typical of myocardial necrosis, can be easily depicted using MRI [41]. However, severe disturbances of left ventricular wall motion may also be observed in stunned myocardium and are therefore not helpful to differentiate both entities. Consequently, quantification of a severely hypokinetic region from MR-images is not sufficient to determine the volume of *infarcted* myocardium even though these measurements correlate well with the size of wall motion abnormalities on left ventriculography [42].

Inotropic stimulation by various pharmacological agents, which results in improved contractile function of viable but not of necrotic myocardium, can be employed with MR imaging to assess residual viability in patients with recent infarcts after thrombolysis [43]. An increase of systolic myocardial wall thickening after intravenous administration of dobutamine of more than 20% as compared to the resting value has been proposed as an index of myocardial viability [43] and was found to be more sensitive in the detection of viability than thallium imaging at rest with rest-redistribution. Up to now, only preliminary results in a few patients have been reported [43] and further experience using recently developed fast imaging sequences [44] is necessary before the clinical value of dobutamine MRI in the detection of viability in patients with acute infarcts can be assessed.

Viability in chronic myocardial infarcts

Wall thinning takes place in transmural infarcts approximately 12 to 16 weeks after the event and can be detected in systole and diastole during spin-echo or gradient-echo MRI [1–5] (Figure 5). The consistent finding of wall thinning in large chronic Q-wave infarcts on MR images [45] and data from experimental and pathology studies led to the hypothesis that scarred myocardium could be distinguished from viable myocardium on the basis of diastolic wall thickness.

Pathology findings in chronic myocardial infarcts

When transmural infarcts are produced in rats [46], which have little collateral circulation, wall thickness in the region of healed transmural infarcts is only $35 \pm 1\%$ of normal whereas the wall thickness of non-transmural infarcts remains almost normal. In contrast, infarcts in dogs are usually non-transmural due to abundant collaterals and result only in minor reductions of enddiastolic wall thickness [47].

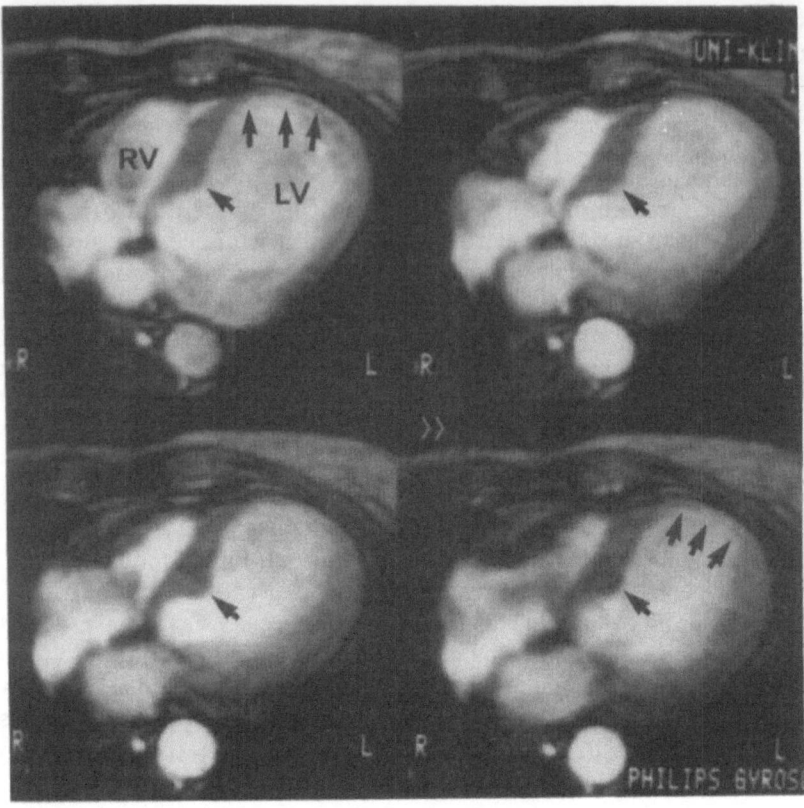

Figure 5. Four phases of the cardiac cycle in a patient with a remote Q-wave anterior myocardial infarct. Transverse gradient-echo MR images of the heart (upper left: end-diastole; upper right: early systole; lower left: mid-systole; lower right: end-systole). Severe thinning of the anterior wall (three arrows, upper left) is evident at end-diastole. There is no thickening of the area with severely reduced enddiastolic wall thickness, whereas the posterior septum and the lateral wall thicken normally during systole. (Reproduced from: Baer FM et al. Herz 1994; 19: 51–64 with permission from the publisher.)

In humans, there is confusion of terms as to what should be regarded as transmural or non-transmural infarcts [48]. Pathologists define transmural scars as infarcts which span the full wall from the endocardium to the epicardium at least at one point of the left ventricular circumference [49]. The infarct may extend through the full thickness of the myocardium over most of the left ventricular region supplied by the infarct artery or it may be transmural only at one point of this territory [49] which translates into a large variation of the percentage of infarcted myocardium within the perfusion territory of the infarct related vessel. Similarly, non-transmural infarcts may be subendocardial, which means restricted to the inner third of the left ventricular wall, or may extend far into the outer third of the wall without reaching the epicardium. Therefore, both transmural and non-transmural infarcts may result in variable amounts of myocardial necrosis and hence in very different amounts of wall thinning after healing of the infarct. This was confirmed in a histopathologic study, which examined thickness of viable myocardium in more than 200 autopsies after a single fatal myocardial infarct [50]. Measurements were made at the point of greatest gross thinning and revealed that only 37 of 204 infarcts were truly transmural and failed to show any viable myocardium. In the majority of the infarcts, the thickness of the surviving myocardium formed a continuum ranging from less than 10% to 83% of neighbouring normal wall thickness. The relationship between enddiastolic wall thickness as measured from MR images and viability was addressed by a study by Dubnow and coworkers which demonstrated that the total wall thickness of chronic transmural myocardial infarcts was usually less than 6 mm [51].

Thus, there is evidence that most infarcts are incomplete with respect to the perfusion territory of the occluded vessel and that some viable cells survive even in the core of the infarct. Importantly, viable myocardium can be found in most infarct border zones. Wall thinning occurs in large chronic transmural infarcts and a wall thickness of < 6 mm is typically found in these infarcts which do not harbour relevant amounts of viable myocardium in the perfusion bed of the infarct related artery.

Wall thickness by MRI and viability

Despite the difficulties of deriving the amount of viable myocardium from a measurement of wall thickness alone, some basic facts permit conclusions from MRI measured left ventricular wall thickness on myocardial viability. First, we know from the calculation of wall thickness from FDG-PET images that even FDG-avid hibernating myocardium must measure at least 4 mm plus some scar tissue to reach the 50% threshold for viability set for FDG-PET [52–56]. Second, pathology data show, as discussed above, that chronic transmural scar measures <6 mm in thickness [51]. Third, intraoperative biopsies from asynergic left ventricular regions showed <10% muscle loss if regional function was improved postoperatively (viable myocardium) whereas muscle loss was more than 50% in regions without recovery (scar) [19]. Thus, non-contractile myocardium thinner than 6 mm is very likely to be completely scarred or so severely damaged that recovery of regional function after revascularization is highly unlikely.

Comparison of wall thickness and wall thickening at rest by MRI with FDG-uptake by PET

The hypothesis that thinned and akinetic myocardium represents chronic scar has been tested by comparing MR-findings to PET and SPECT findings in identical myocardial regions [13, 57]. Comparison of MRI with scintigraphic techniques, especially the matching of identical regions, is facilitated by the fact that MRI provides a three-dimensional set of sections through the left ventricle which is very similar to reconstructed PET or SPECT sections.

A recent study used wall thickness measurements from short axis MR tomograms in 35 patients with chronic infarcts (infarct age at least four months) and regional akinesia on left ventricular angiograms to compare with PET criteria of viability [13]. An initially akinetic segment was considered viable if enddiastolic wall thickness was ⩾5.5 mm, which was the mean regional left ventricular wall thickness on gradient-echo MR images minus 2.5 standard deviations obtained from a group of normal volunteers [58]. Segments were graded viable by PET if FDG-uptake was ⩾50% of the maximum FDG-uptake in a region perfused by a coronary artery without significant stenosis (⩽50% diameter stenosis) and normal wall motion by left ventriculography. Preserved end-diastolic wall thickness in akinetic regions was found in 17/35 (48%) patients at rest, whereas 18/35 showed severe wall thinning indicating scar (Figure 6). Viability of the infarct region was diagnosed by FDG-PET in 23/35 (66%) patients and gradings based on FDG-uptake and myocardial morphology were identical in 29/35 (83%) patients. There was a total of 2200 segments, 482 of which (23%) were akinetic at rest (Figure 7). Of these akinetic segments, 234 (48%) had preserved end-diastolic wall thickness and 299 (62%) were viable by FDG-PET yielding a sensitivity of 72%. Specificity was 89% and the positive predictive accuracy was 91%. The correlation of endiastolic wall thickness and FDG-uptake is shown in Figure 8. There was a significant difference in FDG-uptake between segments with preserved diastolic wall thickness and those with substantial myocardial thinning (Figure 9). Importantly, relative FDG-uptake did not differ between segments with systolic wall thickening at rest or akinesia at rest, as long wall thickness was preserved (Figure 9). Thus, enddiastolic left ventricular wall thickness as measured from MR images predicts myocardial viability accurately and gives results similar to FDG-PET.

Other authors [59] who compared PET and MRI in patients with coronary artery disease and global left ventricular dysfunction came to different conclusions. They showed that FDG-uptake was largely *independent* of regional end-diastolic wall thickness. Although FDG-uptake was significantly lower in regions which were akinetic or dyskinetic as compared to hypokinetic and normokinetic regions on MRI, there was a large overlap between groups making wall thickness measurements not helpful for the prediction of FDG-uptake and viability. There are two possible explanations for their finding of a lack of metabolic activity in regions with normal enddiastolic wall thickness (almost 20% of segments without metabolic activity had wall thickness of 10 mm). First, both patients with recent and with chronic infarcts could have been included in the study and the regions with acute necrosis were the ones without metabolism but with normal wall thickness. The second explanation could be overestimation of myocardial thickness by MRI which could have

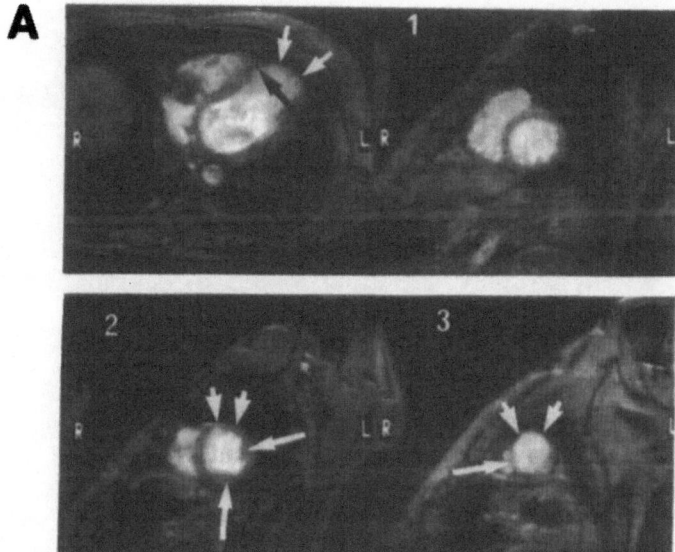

Figure 6. (A) Diastolic gradient-echo MR images of a patient who had a large transmural myocardial infarct 2 years previously. Upper left: Severe thinning of the anterior wall (small white arrows) and the anterior portion of the interventricular septum (small black arrow) is evident on this transverse section through the left ventricle slightly below the inferior portion of the mitral valve ring. Upper right: The most posterior short axis section (1), close to the mitral valve plane, demonstrates homogeneous and normal wall thickness throughout the entire cicumference of the left ventricle. Lower left: The midventricular short axis section (2), at the level of the papillary muscles (large white arrows), shows some thinning of the anterior wall (small white arrows) with preserved septal thickness. Lower right: Anterior wall (small white arrows) and interventricular septum (long white arrow) are maximally thinned on this apical short axis section (3).

occurred because a spin-echo technique with short echo-times (20 ms) was used. There is often slow blood flow adjacent to regions with wall motion abnormalities, which may get confused with myocardium on first spin-echo images [60], especially if shorter echo times are employed. In view of the arguments presented above, it is quite difficult to understand that some regions had a normal regional FDG-uptake despite the presence of severe wall thinning to values of 4 mm and less [59].

Viability in regions with wall thickening by MRI

Perrone-Filardi and coworkers also reported comparative findings in 25 patients with chronic myocardial infarcts from PET, [201]thallium (^{201}Tl) tomographic imaging and magnetic resonance imaging [61]. Regional systolic wall thickening as determined from spin-echo MR images was regarded as the

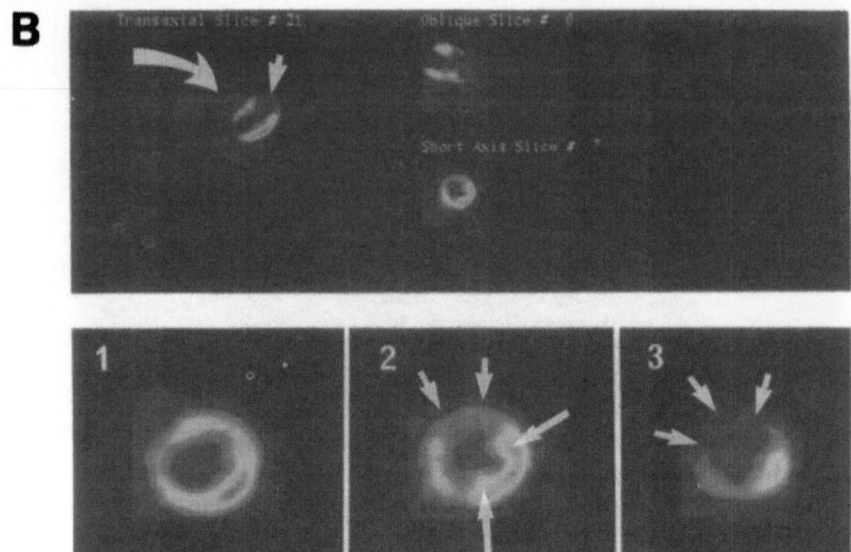

Figure 6. (B) FDG-PET images of the same patient. The corresponding transverse image is seen in the upper left of the figure (curved arrow). The region without FDG-uptake (small white arrow) matches exactly the region with severe wall thinning on the diastolic gradient-echo MR image. The basal short axis section is seen in the lower left of the figure (1) and shows normal tracer uptake throughout the myocardium. The somewhat lower uptake of the interventricular septum is due to partial volume effects with the neighbouring aortic root. There is reduced FDG-uptake in the anterior wall (small arrows) of the midventricular section (2) which corresponds exactly to the regional wall thinning in the MR image. Both papillary muscles are visible (longer arrows). In the apical section (3), there is severely reduced FDG-uptake in the anterior wall and the septum (arrows), which fits nicely with the MR image. (Reproduced from: Sechtem U et al. Int J Card Imaging (Suppl 1) 1993; 9: 31–40.) (For colour plate of Figure 6B see page 534.)

standard of reference for viability. FDG-uptake was classified as normal (>80% uptake relative to a normal reference region), moderately reduced (50% to 79% uptake) or severely reduced (<50% uptake). As compared to regions with severely reduced FDG-activity, regions with only moderately reduced activity showed a slightly but significantly greater enddiastolic wall thickness (9.4 ± 2.6 vs 8.0 ± 3.7 mm) and wall thickening (1.7 ± 2.7 vs −0.7 ± 2.1 mm). Irreversible ^{201}Tl-defects after 3–4-hour redistribution on SPECT imaging were also classified as slight (>65% to <85% of maximal ^{201}Tl-activity), moderate (50%–65% of maximal activity) and severe (<50% of maximal activity). Regions with mild or moderate irreversible ^{201}Tl-defects showed systolic wall thickening which was similar to that observed in regions with reversible ^{201}Tl-defects. In contrast, regions with severe irreversible ^{201}Tl-defects showed no wall thickening. The authors concluded that preserved wall thickness and systolic wall thickening on MRI was another piece of

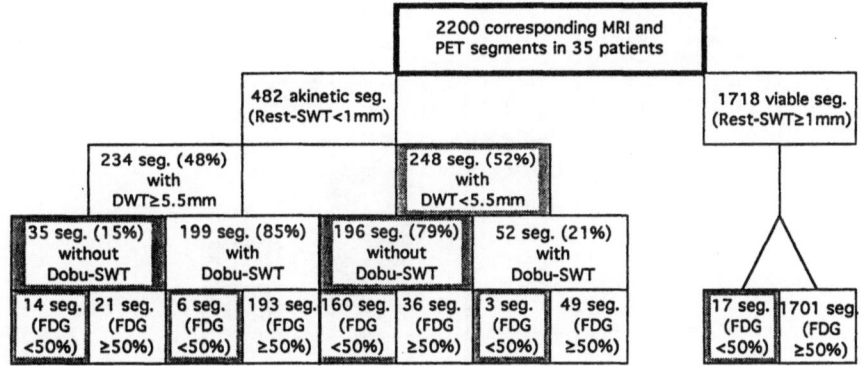

Figure 7. Distribution of segmental gradings based on wall thickening at rest (Rest-SWT) in the second row, diastolic wall thickness (DWT) in the third row, systolic wall thickening of ≥1 mm during dobutamine infusion (Dobu-SWT), and relative FDG uptake on PET images (last row). Shaded boxes indicate scarred segments based on the definition of scar in that particular row. FDG = ^{18}F-fluorodeoxyglucose; MRI = gradient-echo magnetic resonance imaging; PET = positron emission tomography; Seg = segment.

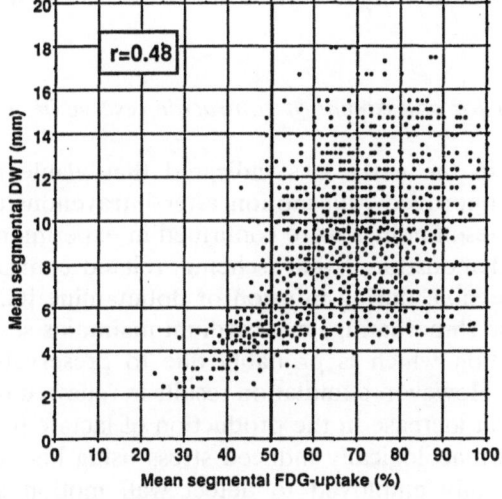

Figure 8. Correlation between enddiastolic wall thickness measured from gradient-echo MR images and relative FDG-uptake in PET images.

evidence that regions with moderate reductions in blood flow and FDG-activity or regions with only slight to moderate irreversible ^{201}Tl-defects represent viable myocardium. On the other hand, these data also support the notion that MRI is useful to establish the presence of viable myocardium

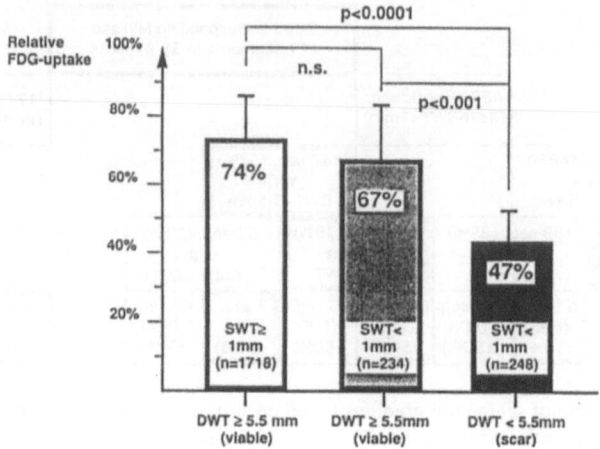

Figure 9. Mean segmental FDG-uptake related to diastolic wall thickness and systolic wall thickening at rest as assessed by MRI. DWT = enddiastolic wall thickness; FDG = ^{18}F-fluorodeoxyglucose; SWT = systolic wall thickening at rest.

in patients with chronic myocardial infarcts based on wall thickness and thickening.

Dobutamine-MRI for assessment of contractile reserve in chronic infarcts

Invasive studies in the early 70's indicated that viable myocardium was characterized by improved wall motion after intravenous administration of adrenalin [10]. These findings were confirmed in experiments with anesthetized pigs which demonstrated that ischemia-related contractile dysfunction may become reversible during infusion of dobutamine [62, 63]. Underperfused and akinetic (hibernating) myocardium maintains sensitive to positive inotropic stimulation which is probably due to preservation of anaerobic energy resources. However, stimulation results in renewed reduction of phosphocreatine and an increase in the production of lactate [62].

MRI with pharmacologically induced stress using high-dose dobutamine has been successfully employed to detect wall motion abnormalities secondary to high grade coronary stenoses [64, 65]. Low-dose dobutamine can be employed in patients with chronic myocardial infarcts to induce improved wall motion in viable but initially akinetic myocardial regions. Such a response would be another indicator of viability in a region with preserved wall thickness. In patients with chronic myocardial infarcts and regions of akinesia in the left ventricular angiogram diagnostic agreement between FDG-uptake and dobutamine induced contraction reserve as seen by MRI was found in 31 of 35 (89%) patients [13] (Figure 10). Of 251 initally akinetic myocardial regions, which showed wall thickening of ≥1 mm after

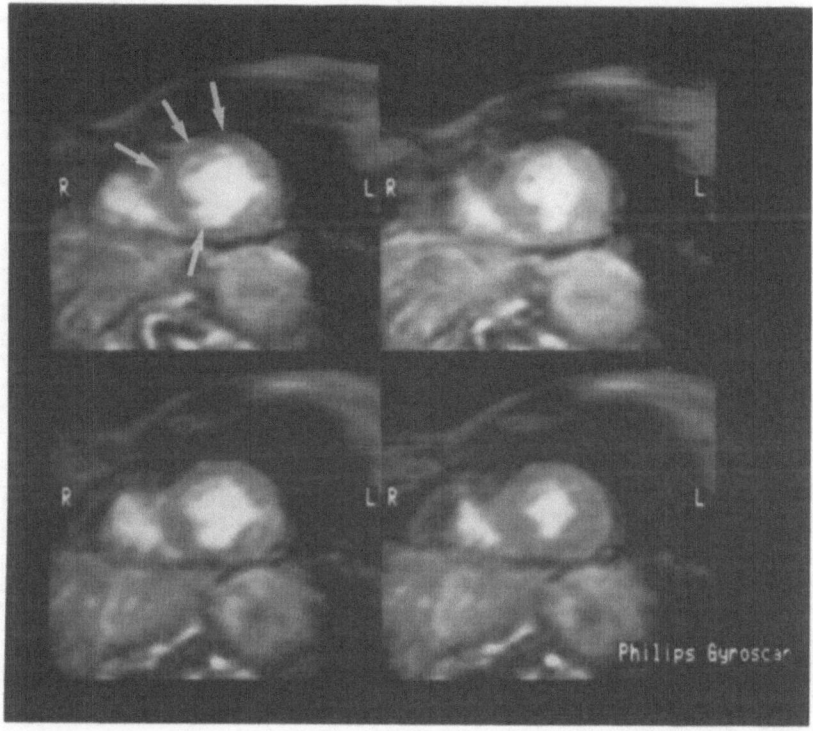

Figure 10. A: Short axis gradient-echo MR images (TR = 28 ms, TE = 12 ms) during dobutam-ine infusion (10 mg/kg/min) in a patient with chronic anteroseptal myocardial infarction. Upper left: Enddiastolic image. There is some wall thinning in the anteroseptal region (3 white arrows) and less pronounced in the inferior wall (single white arrow). Upper right: The endsystolic image demonstrates akinesia of the anteroseptal region, the inferior region shows minimal wall thickening. Lower left: Enddiastolic image during dobutamine: Lower right: At endsystole, there is perfectly normal wall thickening of the inferior wall and obvious dobutamine-induced wall thickening of the anteroseptal region.

dobutamine stimulation, 242 (96%) had FDG-uptake of >50% on PET-images (Figure 11). The combination of the morphologic MR-parameter "enddiastolic wall thickness" and the functional MR-parameter "dobutamine induced systolic wall thickening" gave the best result for sensitivity (88%) and positive predictive accuracy (92%). The detailed segmental comparison between MRI and PET parameters is shown in Figure 7. Interestingly, mean FDG-uptake did not differ between regions which were normokinetic or hypokinetic and regions which were akinetic but showed contractile reserve after application of dobutamine (Table 1). However, there was a significant difference in FDG-uptake between segments thought to be viable by MRI and those found to be scarred by MRI (Table 1).

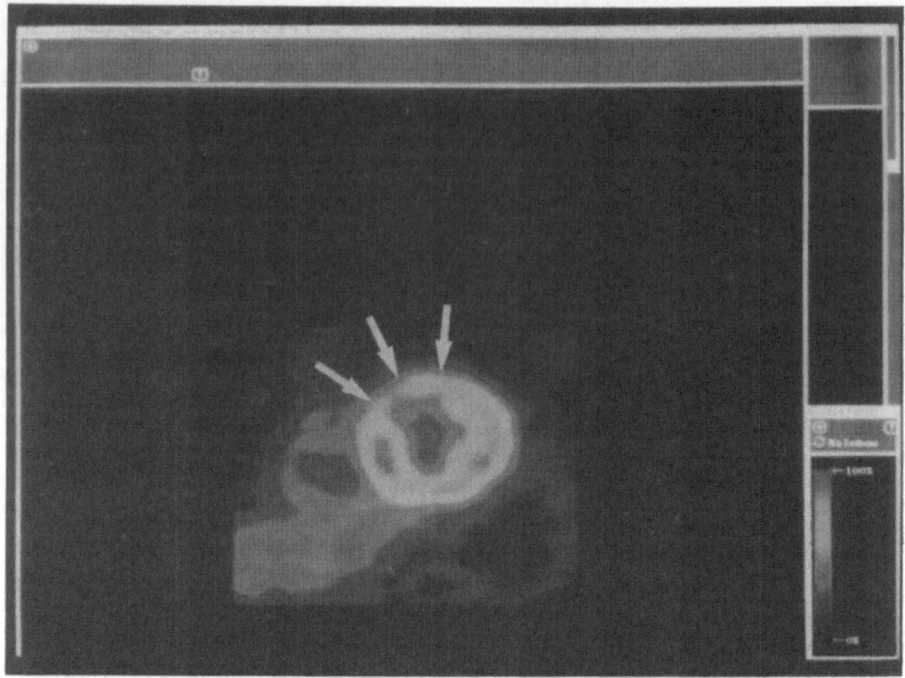

Figure 10. B: The corresponding FDG-PET image shows reduced uptake in the anteroseptal region (arrows), but relative uptake is larger than 50%. Therefore, this region is also viable by PET-criteria. The inferior wall shows normal FDG-uptake. (For colour plate of Figure 10B see **page 535.**)

Comparison of MRI with ^{99}Tc-MIBI-SPECT

We could recently demonstrate [45, 57] that regions with significantly reduced MIBI uptake at rest also had significantly reduced enddiastolic wall thickness and systolic wall thickening (Figure 12). In patients with large areas of akinesis after remote myocardial infarction, infarct size determined from MIBI-SPECT images and MR images correlated well for anterior infarcts but less good for inferior infarcts. For the latter, infarct size tended to be larger on SPECT-images [58] (Figure 13).

MRI is also useful to identify morphologic differences in patients with chronic Q-wave and non-Q-wave infarcts (Figure 14). In patients with angiographically documented coronary artery disease and chronic non-Q-wave infarcts, enddiastolic wall thickness is usually normal and systolic wall thickening is present in most regions. In a study comparing left ventricular morphology of patients with non-Q-wave and Q-wave infarcts, 93% of segments in the non-Q-wave patients were viable by MR criteria and only 7%

FDG-PET	**Rest-MRI** MRI-DWT				**Dobutamine-MRI (10 µg/kg/min)** MRI-SWT				**Rest or Dobutamine-MRI** MRI-DWT or SWT		
	viable	scar			viable	scar			viable	scar	
viable	214	85	299	viable	242	57	299	viable	263	36	299
scar	20	163	183	scar	9	174	183	scar	24	159	183
	234	248	482		251	231	482		287	195	482

Figure 11. Comparison of MRI viability gradings in 35 patients with 482 left ventricular myocardial segments, which were akinetic at rest MRI, based on enddiastolic wall thickness (left), dobutamine induced systolic wall thickening (middle), and combination of both parameters (right) with viability gradings based on relative FDG-uptake on PET images. DWT = enddiastolic wall thickness; FDG-PET = ^{18}F-fluorodeoxyglucose positron emission tomography; MRI = gradient-echo magnetic resonance imaging; SWT = systolic wall thickening during dobutamine infusion.

Table 1. Quantitation of FDG-uptake, enddiastolic wall thickness and wall thickening during dobutamine infusion in relation to functional MRI viability criteria.

	Normokinesia or hypokinesia at rest (n = 1718)	Akinesia at rest and dobu-SWT (n = 251)	Akinesia at rest and no dobu-SWT (n = 188)	Dyskinesia at rest and no dobu-SWT (n = 43)
FDG [%]	74 ± 12*·**	68 ± 16*·**	46 ± 13**	39 ± 7**
DWT [mm]	11.5 ± 2.9	8.8 ± 3.3	4.8 ± 1.7	3.5 ± 0.9
Dobu-SWT [mm]	5.3 ± 2.3	2.5 ± 1.7	0.2 ± 0.3	−0.5 ± 0.3
(% of DWT)	(46%)	(28%)	(4%)	(−14%)

Dobu-SWT = systolic wall thickening (≥ 1 mm) during dobutamine infusion; DWT = enddiastolic wall thickness; FDG = relative uptake of ^{18}F-fluorodeoxyglucose; MRI = gradient-echo magnetic resonance imaging; *no significant difference in FDG-uptake between column 2 and 3 of the table; **$p < 0.01$ for (column 2 and column 3) versus (column 4 and column 5).

were scarred [45]. This was significantly different in the group with large Q-wave-infarcts, in which 27% of segments were scarred and only 63% were viable (Figure 15). Concordance of MRI and MIBI-SPECT classifications was also high in the patients with non-Q-wave infarcts although MIBI slightly overestimated the size of the infarct.

MR spectroscopy in chronic infarcts

The wall thinning normally found in chronic transmural infarcts makes the acquisition of interpretable MR spectra difficult because the smallest volumes

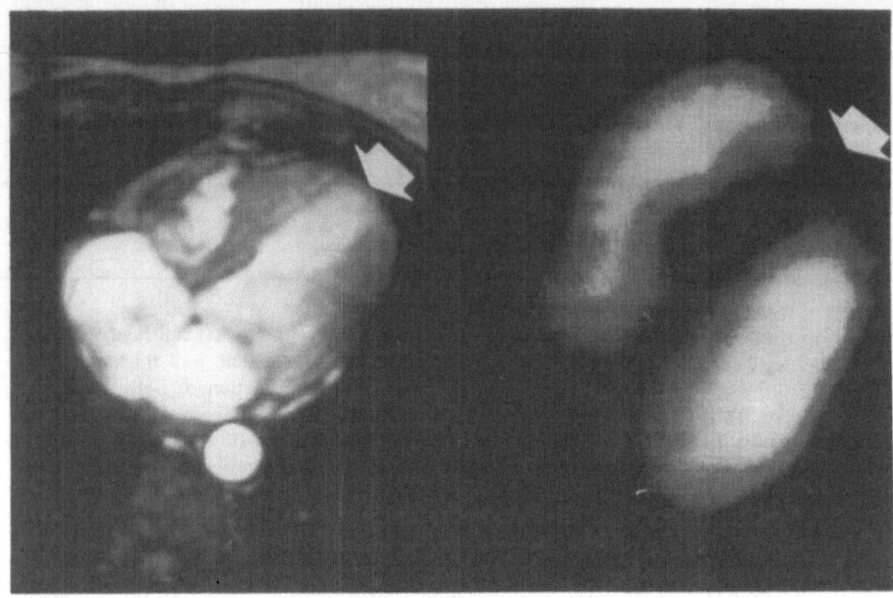

Figure 12. Corresponding gradient-echo MR and MIBI-SPECT images. The zone of severe wall thinning seen on the MR image (arrow) corresponds exactly to the region with severely reduced MIBI-uptake (arrow). (Reproduced from: Sechtem U et al. Int J Card Imaging (Suppl 1) 1993; 9: 31–40.) (For colour plate of this figure see **page 536.**)

of interest achievable with any spatial localization technique are much larger than the amount of thinned myocardium within the measurement volume. This may be one reason why data on the application of MR-spectroscopy to identify viable myocardium in patients with chronic infarcts are not available.

Conclusions

MRI relies on indirect signs of viability such as signal characteristics, wall thickening at rest or after stimulation by dobutamine, and wall thickness, but the technique is not able to directly demonstrate preserved myocardial metabolism in the region of interest. Nevertheless, comparative studies with FDG-PET and MIBI-SPECT indicate the potential of MRI to correctly identify regions with residual viability and clearly distinguish them from regions with predominant chronic scar, which could be used to decide whether revascularization of a particular region is indicated or not. Results about the reliability of enddiastolic wall thickness measurements alone to

a

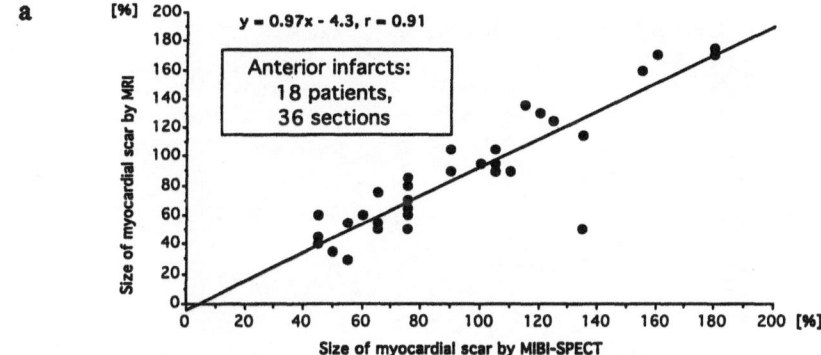

b

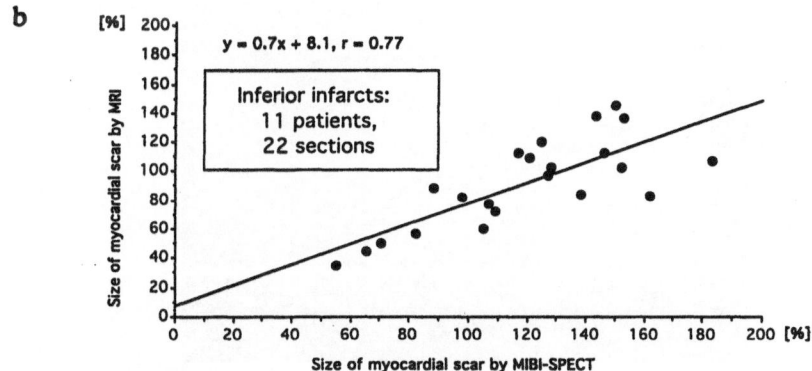

Figure 13. Comparison of scintigraphic and morphologic infarct extension as assessed by MIBI-SPECT and MRI in patients with anterior (a) and inferior myocardial infarction (b). Infarct size was measured in degrees [°] of the circumference in the section with the largest defect and varied between 40° and 180° for anterior infarcts and 55° and 185° for inferior myocardial infarcts. Correlation of infarct size measured from MRI and MIBI-SPECT tomograms was better for anterior than for inferior infarcts. (Reproduced from: Baer FM et al. Herz 1994; 19: 51–64 with permission from the publisher.)

diagnose viability are conflicting and more data are needed to clarify this matter. However, if a region shows dobutamine induced wall thickening by MRI it is very likely to also show FDG-uptake on PET images. No data have been published on the ability of MRI to predict functional recovery of akinetic areas after revascularization which is the ultimate verification of viability tests. These data are needed to make a final judgment about the precision of MR diagnoses of viability.

MR scanning of the entire ventricle using standard gradient-echo sequences is still very time consuming and examination times are in the order of 45 to 75 minutes. However, fast MR-imaging techniques are now available,

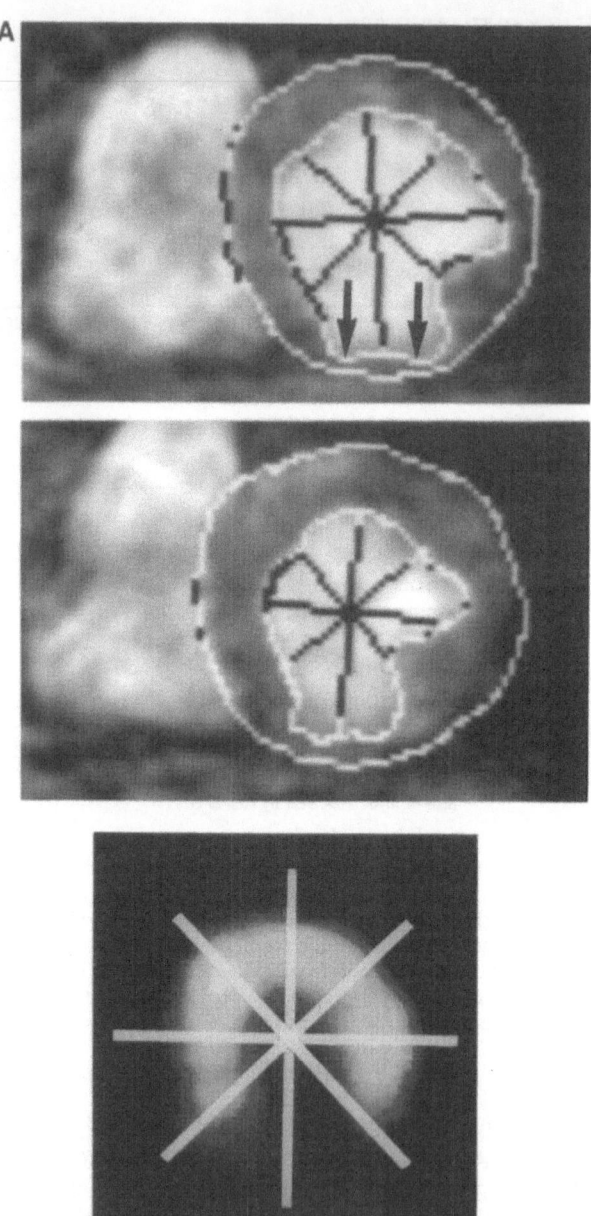

Figure 14. Mid-ventricular MRI and MIBI-SPECT short axis tomograms of patients with previously documented inferior myocardial infarction. Note the corresponding standardized segmental evaluation pattern for both imaging techniques. A: Upper panel: The inferior segments
of the patient with the Q-wave infarct contain myocardium with markedly reduced diastolic wall
thickness (black arrows). Middle panel: There is only minimal systolic wall thickening in the
thinned area. Lower panel: The SPECT tomogram shows a severe MIBI-uptake defect in the
corresponding region.

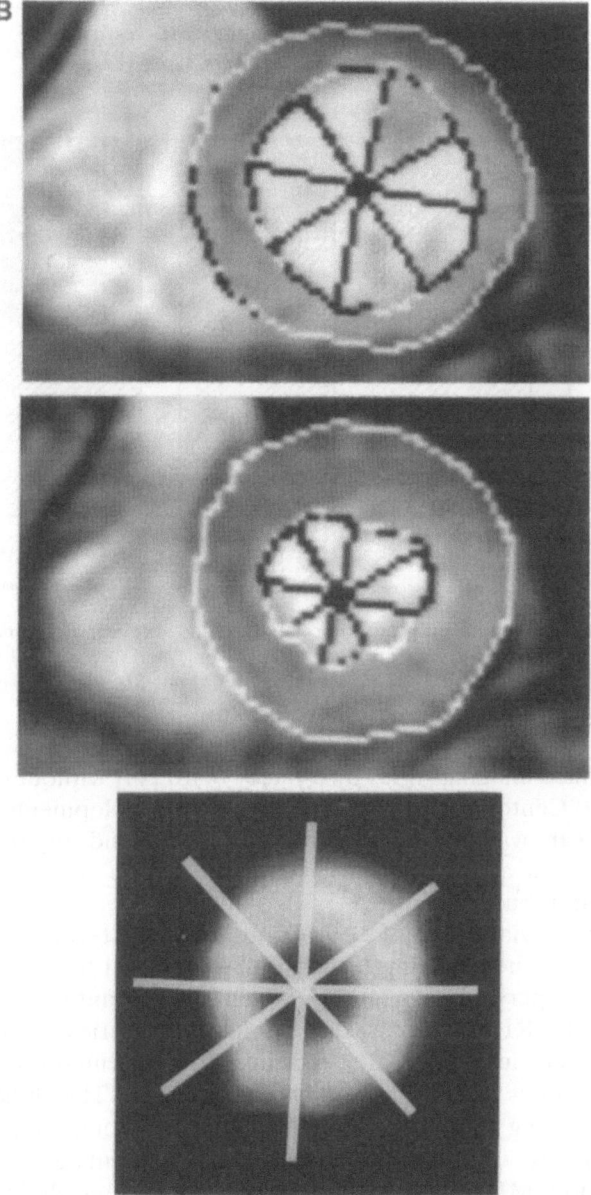

Figure 14. B: Upper panel: The inferior segments of the patient with non-Q-wave infarct show normal diastolic wall thickness and systolic wall thickening is almost normal (middle panel). Lower panel: There is no significant reduction of MIBI-uptake. (Reproduced from: Baer et al. Eur Heart J 1994; 15: 97–107 with permission from the publisher.)

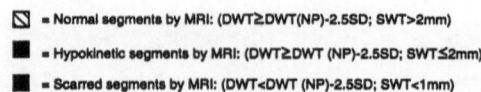

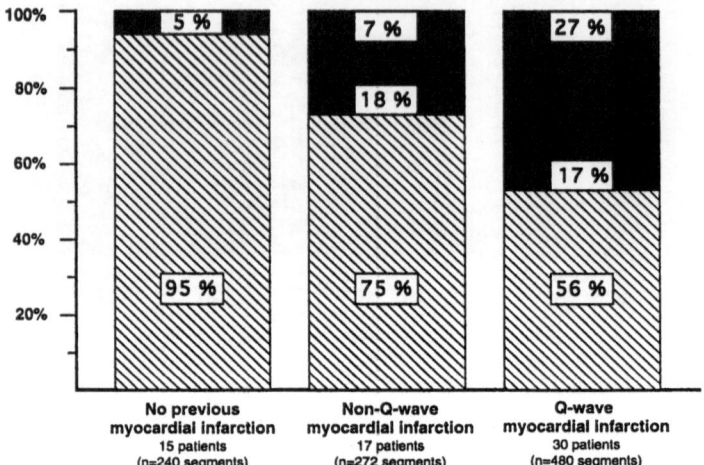

Figure 15. Percentage of segments graded normal, hypokinetic or scar according to MRI criteria in patients without previous myocardial infarction, chronic non-Q-wave and Q-wave infarcts. (Reproduced from: Baer et al. Am J Cardiol 1994; 74: 430–4 with permission of the publisher.)

which will reduce imaging times by a factor of 10 [44] without compromising image quality. Centers equipped with the latest developments in MR hardware and software will have a powerful tool at their hands to provide clinically useful information about myocardial viability within short scan times and without radiation burden.

Assessment of viability by fast gradient-echo MR techniques has several advantages over other imaging techniques. Compared to echocardiography, MRI often has superior image quality, which is important for deriving quantitative data, and MRI gives a truly three-dimensional series of images covering the entire left ventricle. Compared to scintigraphic techniques, MRI is faster to perform and does not require radioactive material. The clinical usefulness of MRI for assessing viability can only be defined by comparing fast gradient-echo MRI directly with the other modalities in patients groups undergoing revascularization. MRS is less likely than MRI to become clinically employed for diagnosing myocardial viabiliy. Nevertheless, MRS provides unique physiologic information and may enhance the understanding of metabolic changes occurring in acute ischemia.

Acknowledgements

We would like to thank the staff of the Department of Nuclear Medicine who performed the MR and scintigraphic examinations shown in this chapter.

References

1. Akins EW, Hill JA, Sievers KW, Conti CR. Assessment of left ventricular wall thickness in healed myocardial infarction by magnetic resonance imaging. Am J Cardiol 1987; 59: 24–8.
2. Higgins CB, Lanzer P, Stark D et al. Imaging by nuclear magnetic resonance in patients with chronic ischemic heart disease. Circulation 1984; 69: 523–31.
3. Pflugfelder PW, Sechtem UP, White RD, Higgins CB. Quantification of regional myocardial function by rapid cine MR imaging. Am J Roentgenol 1988; 150: 523–9.
4. White RD, Holt WW, Cheitlin MD et al. Estimation of the functional and anatomic extent of myocardial infarction using magnetic resonance imaging. Am Heart J 1988; 115: 740–8.
5. Sechtem U, Sommerhoff BA, Markiewicz W et al. Regional left ventricular wall thickening by magnetic resonance imaging: Evaluation of normal persons and patients with global and regional dysfunction. Am J Cardiol 1987; 59: 145–51.
6. Roberts CS, Maclean D, Maroko P, Kloner RA. Early and late remodeling of the left ventricle after acute myocardial infarction. Am J Cardiol 1984; 54: 407–10.
7. Schlichter J, Hellerstein HK, Katz LN. Aneurysm of the heart. A correlative study of 102 proven cases. Medicine 1954; 33: 43–86.
8. Fishbein MC, Maclean D, Maroleo PR. The histopathologic evolution of myocardial infarction. Chest 1978; 73: 843–9.
9. Mallory GK, White PD, Salcedo-Galger J. The speed of healing of myocardial infarction: A study of the pathologic anatomy in 72 cases. Am Heart J 1939; 18: 647–71.
10. Horn HR, Teichholz LE, Cohn PF et al. Augmentation of left ventricular contraction pattern in coronary artery disease by an inotropic catecholamine. Circulation 1974; 49: 1063–71.
11. Rozanski A, Berman D, Gray R et al. Preoperative prediction of reversible myocardial asynergy by postexercise radionuclide ventriculography. N Engl J Med 1982; 307: 212–6.
12. Pierard LA, De Landsheere CM, Berthe C et al. Identification of viable myocardium by echocardiography during dobutamine infusion in patients with myocardial infarction after thrombolytic therapy: Comparison with positron emission tomography. J Am Coll Cardiol 1990; 15: 1021–31.
13. Baer FM, Voth E, Theissen P et al. Comparison of low-dose dobutamine-gradient-echo magnetic resonance imaging and position emission tomography with [18F] fluorodeoxyglucose in patients with coronary artery disease. A functional and morphologic approach to the detection of residual myocardial viability. Circulation 1995; 91: 1006–15.
14. Bottomley PA, Smith LS, Brazzamano S et al. The fate of inorganic phosphate and pH in regional myocardial ischemia and infarction: A noninvasive 31P NMR study. Magn Reson Med 1987; 5: 129–42.
15. Braunwald E, Kloner RA. The stunned myocardium: Prolonged, postischemic ventricular dysfunction. Circulation 1982; 66: 1146–9.
16. Kloner RA, Allen J, Cox TA et al. Stunned left ventricular myocardium after exercise treadmill testing in coronary artery disease. Am J Cardiol 1991; 68: 329–34.
17. Bolli R, Zhu WX, Thornby JI et al. Time course and determinants of recovery of function after reversible ischemia in conscious dogs. Am J Physiol 1988; 254: 102–14.
18. Rahimtoola SH. The hibernating myocardium. Am Heart J 1989; 117: 211–21.
19. Bodenheimer MM, Banka VS, Hermann GA et al. Reversible asynergy. Histopathologic

and electrographic correlations in patients with coronary artery disease. Circulation 1976; 53: 792–6.

20. Vanoverschelde JLJ, Wijns W, Depre C et al. Mechanisms of chronic regional postischemic dysfunction in humans. Circulation 1993; 87: 1513–23.

21. Tscholakoff D, Higgins CB, McNamara MT, Derugin N. Early-phase myocardial infarction: Evaluation by MR imaging. Radiology 1986; 159: 667–72.

22. Rokey R, Verani MS, Bolli R et al. Myocardial infarct size quantification by MR imaging early after coronary occlusion in dogs. Radiology 1986; 158: 771–4.

23. Buda AJ, Aisen AM, Juni JE et al. Detection and sizing of myocardial ischemia and infarction by nuclear magnetic resonance imaging in the canine heart. Am Heart J 1985; 110: 1284–90.

24. Bouchard A, Reeves RC, Cranney G et al. Assessment of myocardial infarct size by means of T2–weighted 1H nuclear magnetic resonance imaging. Am Heart J 1989; 117: 281–9.

25. Wisenberg G, Prato FS, Carroll SE et al. Serial nuclear magnetic resonance imaging of acute myocardial infarction with and without reperfusion. Am Heart J 1988; 115: 510–8.

26. McNamara MT, Higgins CB, Schechtmann N et al. Detection and characterization of acute myocardial infarction in man with use of gated magnetic resonance. Circulation 1985; 71: 717–24.

27. Filipchuk NG, Peshock RM, Malloy CR et al. Detection and localization of recent myocardial infarction by magnetic resonance imaging. Am J Cardiol 1986; 58: 214–9.

28. Ryan T, Tarver RD, Duerk JL et al. Distinguishing viable from infarcted myocardium after experimental ischemia and reperfusion by using nuclear magnetic resonance imaging. J Am Coll Cardiol 1990; 15: 1355–64.

29. McNamara MT, Tscholakoff D, Revel D et al. Differentiation of reversible and irreversible myocardial injury by MR imaging with and without gadolinium-DTPA. Radiology 1986; 158: 765–9.

30. Saeed M, Wendland MF, Takehara Y, Higgins CB. Reversible and irreversible injury in the reperfused myocardium: Differentiation with contrast material-enhanced MR imaging. Radiology 1990; 175: 633–7.

31. Saeed M, Wendland MF, Masui T, Higgins CB. Myocardial infarctions on T1- and susceptibility-enhanced MRI: Evidence for loss of compartmentalization of contrast media. Magn Res Med 1994; 31: 31–9.

32. Guth BD, Martin JF, Heusch G, Ross JJ. Regional myocardial blood flow, function and metabolism using phosphorus-31 nuclear magnetic resonance spectroscopy during ischemia and reperfusion in dogs. J Am Coll Cardiol 1987; 10: 673–81.

33. Camacho SA, Lanzer P, Toy BJ et al. In vivo alterations of high-energy phosphates and intracellular pH during reversible ischemia in pigs: A 31P magnetic resonance spectroscopy study. Am Heart J 1988; 116: 701–8.

34. Arai AE, Pantely GA, Anselone CG et al. Active downregulation of myocardial energy requirements during prolonged moderate ischemia in swine. Circ Res 1991; 69: 1458–69.

35. Pantely GA, Malone SA, Rhen WS et al. Regeneration of phosphocreatine in pigs despite continued moderate ischemia. Circ Res 1990; 67: 1481–93.

36. Schulz R, Guth PD, Pieper K et al. Recruitment of inotropic reserve in moderately ischemic myocardium at the expense of metabolic recovery: A model of short-term hibernation. Circ Res 1992; 70: 1282–95.

37. Menon RS, Hendrich K, Hu X, Ugurbil K. 31P NMR spectroscopy of the human heart at 4 T: Detection of substantially uncontaminated cardiac spectra and differentiation of subepicardium and subendocardium. Magn Reson Med 1992; 26: 368–76.

38. Gober JR, Schaefer S, Camacho SA et al. Epicardial and endocardial localized 31P magnetic resonance spectroscopy: Evidence for metabolic heterogeneity during regional ischemia. Magn Reson Med 1990; 13: 204–15.

39. Bottomley PA, Herfkens RJ, Smith LS, Bashore TM. Altered phosphate metabolism in myocardial infarction: P-31 MR spectroscopy. Radiology 1987; 165: 703–7.

40. Rehr RB, Tatum JL, Hirsch JI et al. Reperfused-viable and reperfused-infarcted myocardium: differentiation with in vivo P-31 MR spectroscopy. Radiology 1989; 172: 53–8.
41. Meese RB, Spritzer CE, Negro VR et al. Detection, characterization and functional assessment of reperfused Q-wave acute myocardial infarction by cine magnetic resonance imaging. Am J Cardiol 1990; 66: 1–9.
42. Johns JA, Leavitt MB, Newell JB et al. Quantitation of acute myocardial infarct size by nuclear magnetic resonance imaging. J Am Coll Cardiol 1990; 15: 143–9.
43. Nienaber CA, Rochau T, Chatterjee T, Nicolas V. Dobutamin-Magnet resonanz tomographie und 201–Thallium-SPECT: Nachweis von vitalem Myokard in der Postinfarktphase (Abstr). Z Kardiol 1993; 82 (Suppl 1): 17.
44. Atkinson DJ, Edelman RR. Cineangiography of the heart in a single breath hold with a segmented turboFLASH sequence. Radiology 1991; 178: 357–60.
45. Baer FM, Smolarz K, Theissen P et al. Assessment of myocardial viability by quantification of $^{99\,m}$Tc-methoxyisobutyl-isonitrile uptake at rest: Comparison with parameters of myocardial viability obtained from gradient-echo magnetic resonance imaging. Eur Heart J 1994; 15: 97–107.
46. Roberts CS, Maclean D, Braunwald E et al. Topographic changes in the left ventricle after experimentally induced myocardial infarction in the rat. Am J Cardiol 1983; 51: 872–6.
47. Sasayama S, Gallagher KP, Kemper WS et al. Regional left ventricular wall thickness early and late after coronary occlusion in the conscious dog. Am J Physiol 1981; 240: H293–9.
48. Phibbs B. "Transmural" versus "subendocardial" myocardial infarction: An electrocardiographic myth. J Am Coll Cardiol 1983; 1: 561–4.
49. Freifeld AG, Schuster EH, Bulkley BH. Nontransmural versus transmural myocardial infarction. A morphologic study. Am J Med 1983; 75: 423–32.
50. Pirolo JS, Moore GW, Hutchins GM. Continuum of the thickness of surviving myocardial wall with single myocardial infarcts. Arch Pathol Lab Med 1986; 110: 382–4.
51. Dubnow MH, Burchell HB, Titus JL. Postinfarction left ventricular aneurysm. A clinico-morphologic and electrocardiographic study of 80 cases. Am Heart J 1965; 70: 753–60.
52. Hoffman EJ, Huang SC, Phelps ME. Quantitation in positron emission computed tomography: 1. Effect of object size. J Comput Assist Tomogr 1979; 3: 299–308.
53. Bonow RO, Dilsizian V, Cuocolo A, Bacharach SL. Myocardial viability in patients with chronic coronary artery disease and left ventricular dysfunction: Thallium-201 reinjection versus 18F-fluorodeoxyglucose. Circulation 1991; 83: 26–37.
54. Parodi O, Schelbert H, Schwaiger M et al. Cardiac emission computed tomography: Underestimation of regional tracer concentration due to wall motion abnormalities. J Comput Assist Tomogr 1984; 8: 1083–92.
55. Wienhard K, Eriksson L, Grootoonk S et al. Performance evaluation of the positron scanner ECAT EXACT. J Comput Assist Tomogr 1992; 16: 854–863.
56. Schelbert HR, Phelps ME, Selin C et al. Regional myocardial ischemia assessed by 18–fluoro-2–deoxyglucose and positron emission tomography. In: Heiss HW, editor. Advances in clinical cardiology. Vol. I. Quantification of myocardial ischemia. New York: Gerhard Witzstrock, 1980: 437–49.
57. Baer FM, Smolarz K, Jungehulsing M et al. Chronic myocardial infarction: Assessment of morphology, function, and perfusion by gradient echo magnetic resonance imaging and 99 mTc-methoxyisobutyl-isonitrile SPECT. Am Heart J 1992; 123: 636–45.
58. Baer FM, Smolarz K, Jungehülsing M et al. Magnetresonanztomographische Darstellung transmuraler Myokardinfarkte im Vergleich zur 99Tc-methoxyisobutyl-isonitrile-SPECT. Z Kardiol 1992; 81: 423–31.
59. Perrone-Filardi P, Bacharach SL, Dilsizian V et al. Metabolic evidence of viable myocardium in regions with reduced wall thickness and absent wall thickening in patients with chronic ischemic left ventricular dysfunction. J Am Coll Cardiol 1992; 20: 161–8.
60. von Schulthess GK, Fisher MR, Crooks LE, Higgins CB. Gated MR imaging of the heart: Intracardiac signal in patients and healthy subjects. Radiology 1985; 156: 125–32.
61. Perrone-Filardi P, Bacharach SL, Dilsizian V et al. Regional left ventricular wall thickening.

Relation to regional uptake of 18–fluoro-deoxyglucose and 201Tl in patients with chronic coronary artery disease and left ventricular dysfunction. Circulation 1992; 86: 1125–37.

62. Schulz R, Miyazaki S, Miller M et al. Consequences of regional inotropic stimulation of ischemic myocardium on regional myocardial blood flow and function in anesthetized swine. Circ Res 1989; 64: 1116–26.

63. Vatner SF. Correlation between acute reductions in myocardial blood flow and function in conscious dogs. Circ Res 1980; 47: 201–7.

64. Pennell DJ, Underwood SR, Manzara CC et al. Magnetic resonance imaging during dobutamine stress in coronary artery disease. Am J Cardiol 1992; 70: 34–40.

65. Baer FM, Smolarz K, Theissen P et al. Identification of hemodynamically significant coronary artery stenoses by dipyridamole-magnetic resonance imaging and 99 mTc-methoxyisobutyl-isonitrile-SPECT. Int J Card Imaging 1993; 9: 133–45.

Corresponding Author: Prof. Dr. Udo Sechtem, Klinik für Innere Medizin, University of Cologne, Joseph-Stelzmannstrasse 9, D-50924, Cologne, Germany

15. Assessment of viability in severely hypokinetic myocardium before revascularization and prediction of functional recovery: Contribution of thallium-201 imaging

JACQUES A. MELIN, JEAN-LOUIS VANOVERSCHELDE, BERNHARD GERBER and WILLIAM WIJNS

Introduction

Myocardial imaging with thallium-201 (^{201}Tl) has been proposed and extensively used for the assessment of myocardial viability because tracer uptake and retention require tracer delivery through adequate perfusion, sarcolemmal integrity and intact metabolic function. These three properties have been shown to be important requirements in order to permit recovery of systolic function after restoration of normal perfusion in dysfunctional myocardium. The aim of this chapter is to review the experimental studies providing a rationale for the use of ^{201}Tl for viability studies and the clinical data suggesting that exercise and resting ^{201}Tl imaging provide relevant information for the assessment of dysfunctional myocardium.

Experimental validation

Two phases of ^{201}Tl kinetics have to be distinguished: the myocardial uptake early after intravenous injection of the tracer and the late phase of ^{201}Tl redistribution. The early myocardial uptake is proportional to regional blood flow and extraction fraction [1–3]. Extraction fraction has been found to be unaltered in experimental conditions such as hypoxia [4] and stunned myocardium [5]. Also, in short-term hibernating myocardium [6], myocardial ^{201}Tl uptake is not impaired out of proportion to the flow decrease.

In necrotic myocardium, a good agreement was also observed between ^{201}Tl initial myocardial trapping and microspheres determined flow in the intact animal [7–10]. The correlation between ^{201}Tl uptake and regional myocardial blood flow was less satisfactory in the acute phase of reperfusion after myocardial infarction with an underestimation of flow by ^{201}Tl in reperfused samples [7]. Additionally, early after reperfusion, ^{201}Tl activity in the necrotic samples did not significantly differ from that in the viable samples for a similar amount of myocardial blood flow [11–13].

Thus, the initial trapping of ^{201}Tl by the myocardium appears to be pro-

C.A. Nienaber and U. Sechtem (eds): Imaging and Intervention in Cardiology, 237–248.
© 1996 *Kluwer Academic Publishers.*

portional to flow in different experimental conditions without an independent influence of the viable or necrotic status of the myocardium.

Following the first pass myocardial uptake phase after intravenous tracer injection, there is a constant exchange of ^{201}Tl between the myocardium and the extracellular compartments, with a clearance from normal myocardium and replacement by residual ^{201}Tl blood pool activity. This continuous kinetics exchange forms the basis of ^{201}Tl redistribution [14].

Redistribution or delayed defect resolution is observed when ^{201}Tl is injected during transient myocardial hypoperfusion [15] or with a chronic reduction in myocardial blood flow which is referred to as rest redistribution [16]. The mechanism for rest redistribution during chronic ischemia is both a diminution in the initial ^{201}Tl uptake and a subsequent decrease in the tracer's intrinsic efflux rate [15]. There is a substantially slower ^{201}Tl washout over time from the stenosis region compared with the ^{201}Tl washout from nonischemic regions.

When ^{201}Tl is given during coronary occlusion, ^{201}Tl gradients between normal and ischemic zones after reperfusion are significantly lower than the gradients measured during coronary occlusion and, thus, delayed redistribution of ^{201}Tl injected before reperfusion is an indication of viable myocardium [17–19]. When myocardial necrosis is present, no delayed ^{201}Tl redistribution is observed in the zone of irreversibly injured myocardial tissue [9].

Thus, this experimental work suggests that the early uptake of ^{201}Tl is proportional to blood flow regardless of altered metabolic conditions. The indirect estimate of flow by the initial trapping has already some potential relevance for viability assessment because a minimal level of myocardial blood flow is required to maintain cell membrane integrity and hence viability [20–25]. The redistribution process, on the other hand, could be used as an index of myocardial viability if a sufficient time interval allows to complete the kinetics exchange and if sufficient residual ^{201}Tl activity remains in the blood pool.

Resting ^{201}Tl clinical imaging

When the clinical question pertains to the presence or absence of myocardial viability and not to the detection of inducible ischemia, such as in patients with severe left ventricular dysfunction, rest-redistribution ^{201}Tl imaging may be the procedure of choice. Gewirtz et al. [26] were first to report that ^{201}Tl defects may occur on resting images in patients with severe chronic coronary artery disease, and that a substantial number of defects which redistribute have a normal or hypokinetic wall motion. Berger et al. [27] reported that 80% of patients showing initial resting defects with delayed rest redistribution preoperatively demonstrated an increase in left ventricular ejection fraction postoperatively. In that study, only 22% of patients with persistent defects preoperatively at rest showed comparable improvement. Rest and redistribution were also quantitatively analyzed in terms of postrevascularization functional assessment by Iskandrian et al. [28] in 26 patients with a mean left ventricular ejection fraction of 33%. Normal rest ^{201}Tl images or reversible resting defects correctly identified 12 of 14 patients with improvement in left ventricular function postoperatively, while only 2 of 9 patients with a fixed resting perfusion defects showed a similar improvement.

In a series of 17 patients with a mean left ventricular ejection fraction of 37%, Mori et al. [29] reported that four of six patients with improved global ejection fraction after revascularization showed resting ^{201}Tl redistribution while 8 out of 11 patients who did not improve significantly after revascularization had no resting ^{201}Tl redistribution. In terms of asynergic regions, 11 of 14 regions with resting redistribution had improved wall motion after revascularization. However, 14 of 37 regions without redistribution also improved. It is noteworthy that some of these regions without redistribution and with improved function after revascularization had a higher early ^{201}Tl uptake.

Ragosta et al. [30] performed pre- and postoperative resting quantitative ^{201}Tl scintigraphy and radionuclide angiography in 21 coronary patients with ejection fraction of under 35%. The prospectively defined criteria for viability included normal initial uptake, an initial resting defect with delayed partial or total redistribution, or a mild persistent defect with over 50% reduction in ^{201}Tl activity. Lack of viability was defined as persistent defect showing more than 50% reduction in ^{201}Tl activity. Of the severely asynergic segments showing a normal pattern or mild reduction of thallium uptake preoperatively, 62% and 54%, respectively, improved function after surgery while only 8 of 35 segments (23%) with no evidence of viability by preoperative thallium imaging improved function 2 months after coronary artery bypass surgery. In this study, the improvement in left ventricular function after surgery was related to the number of asynergic segments with ^{201}Tl criteria of viability. In patients with more than 7 viable asynergic segments left ventricular ejection fraction rose by more than 12% after revascularization while it remained unchanged in patients with 7 or less viable asynergic segments.

Alfieri et al. [31] studied 13 patients with a mean ejection fraction of 35%. The segmental analysis showed a high sensitivity (93%) but a low specificity (43%). Two recent studies [32, 33] examined the impact of redistribution or delayed imaging on the recovery of regional dysfunction. Marzullo et al. [32] reported a sensitivity of 86% and a specificity of 92% in a group of 14 patients with 75 dysynergic segments. A recent study of a group of 18 patients with a mean ejection fraction of 35% analyzed quantitatively redistribution ^{201}Tl activity one hour after rest injection with SPECT [33]. Sensitivity for segments with ^{201}Tl activity of more than 60% and improved wall motion after revascularization was 88% and specificity was 83%.

Rest-redistribution planar ^{201}Tl imaging was also used to identify residual myocardial viability after myocardial infarction [34]. Early (2 ± 1 days) after

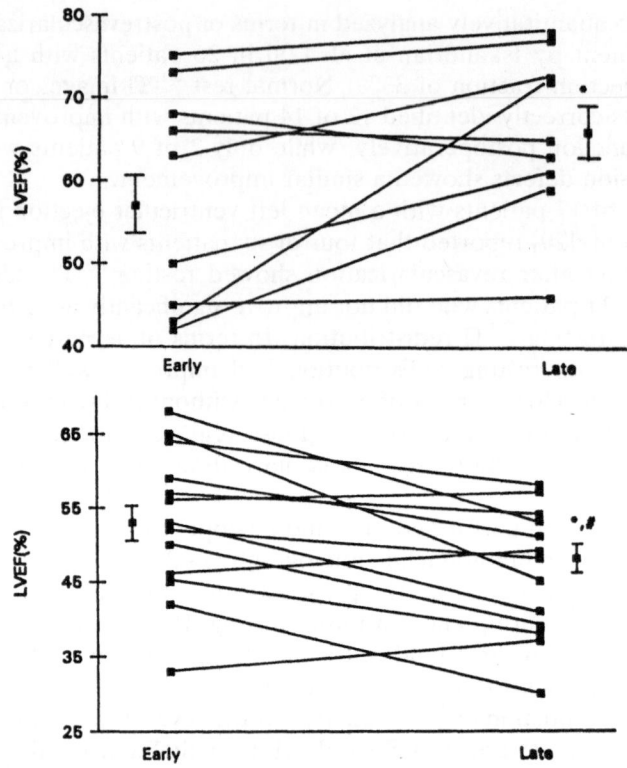

Figure 1. Early and late left ventricular ejection fraction (LVEF) in patients after myocardial infarction with (top panel) and without (lower panel) predicted viable myocardium by ^{201}Tl rest-redistribution imaging (from [34]).

myocardial infarction, viability was defined by the rest ^{201}Tl scan as an initial mild rest defect or any defect with redistribution. Those patients who were predicted to have viable myocardium in the infarct zone (Figure 1, top panel) had a better early and late left ventricular ejection fraction and infarct-related regional wall motion than patients predicted to have non viable myocardium. In the subgroup of patients with revascularization, only those patients predicted to have viable myocardium on the basis of rest ^{201}Tl scintigraphy had improved global and regional ventricular function.

Lastly, a study compared quantitative rest-redistribution ^{201}Tl data with PET patterns of viability [35]; 49 of the 59 myocardial regions (83%) with severely reduced FDG uptake by PET had severe ($\leq$50% of peak activity) irreversible ^{201}Tl defects, and only 2% of the normal and 5% of the mismatch myocardial regions by PET had severe irreversible ^{201}Tl defects.

Taken together, the rest-redistribution studies with postrevascularization functional assessment show sensitivity and specificity values of about 70% in

Table 1. Accuracy of thallium-201 scintigraphy for predicting improvement in left ventricular ejection fraction after revascularization.

	No. patients	EF (%)	Sensitivity	Specificity
Iskandrian, 1983	26	33	12/14 (86%)	8/12 (67%)
Mori, 1991	17	37	4/6 (67%)	8/11 (73%)
Ragosta, 1993	21	27	8/11 (73%)	7/10 (70%)
Vanoverschelde, 1994	34	27	9/15 (60%)	13/19 (68%)

terms of patient analysis (Table 1). Segmental analysis (Table 2) shows good sensitivity values and somewhat lower specificity at least in two recent studies [30, 31]. It is important to emphasize that the two studies which used quantitative analysis and redistribution uptake for viability assessment had the best sensitivity and specificity figures [32, 33]. This is consistent with the experimental data previously discussed (see also Chapters 3–5 and 15–18).

Exercise ^{201}Tl scintigraphy

Clinical assessment and therapeutic management in many coronary patients with left ventricular dysfunction require evaluation of both inducible ischemia and viability. Therefore, stress and redistribution imaging would be used as a first choice test for a comprehensive assessment of the extent and severity of myocardial ischemia. Uptake of ^{201}Tl at redistribution or after reinjection of a small dose of ^{201}Tl would then be indicative of viable myocardium in analogy to the ^{201}Tl rest-redistribution protocol.

Redistribution imaging

After exercise, an initial defect showing complete or partial delayed redistribution implies ischemia and viability. Defects that remain persistent from the initial to the delayed images are suggestive of scar. However, persistent ^{201}Tl defects may represent viable myocardium rather than scar if the redistri-

Table 2. Accuracy of perfusion scintigraphy for recovery of regional left ventricular dysfunction after revascularization.

	No. patients (segments)	Sensitivity	Specificity
Mori, 1991	17 (51)	11/25 (44%)	23/26 (88%)
Marzullo, 1993	14 (75)	42/49 (86%)	24/26 (92%)
Ragosta, 1993	21 (176)	81/89 (93%)	27/87 (31%)
Alfieri, 1993	13 (120)	82/88 (93%)	14/32 (44%)
Udelson, 1994	18 (46)	15/17 (88%)	24/29 (83%)
Dilsizian, 1990	20 (23)	13/13 (100%)	8/10 (80%)
Ohtani, 1990	24 (61)	33/37 (89%)	12/24 (50%)

bution ^{201}Tl defects are mild, i.e. a ^{201}Tl uptake of over 50% as compared to the normal zone [36]. This phenomenon can be assessed by looking at the amount of ^{201}Tl activity on delayed ^{201}Tl imaging [37, 38]. Greater amounts of ^{201}Tl present in these images indicate larger amounts of viable myocardium. The presence or absence of redistribution by itself does not influence the results. Severe persistent defects demonstrating more than 50% reduction in ^{201}Tl counts compared to a normal region should be further assessed for potential viability by late redistribution imaging at 18 to 24 hours [39–41] or preferentially by ^{201}Tl reinjection at rest following acquisition of the 4-hour redistribution images [42]. A proposed mechanism for ^{201}Tl fill-in after 24 hours or after reinjection of ^{201}Tl is that ^{201}Tl may be unavailable for additional uptake at 4 hours due to low blood concentration of ^{201}Tl and continued hypoperfusion. Even late imaging will result in an overestimation of scar since one-third of the segments irreversible at 18–72 hours reveals contractile recovery after revascularization [40]. The underestimation of viability on 24-hour ^{201}Tl imaging was also confirmed by the demonstration that the majority of myocardial regions with fixed ^{201}Tl defects on late images has preserved metabolic activity [43]. An additional limitation of the 24-hour imaging to detect late redistribution is the suboptimal count statistics.

Reinjection imaging

An alternative to 24-hour delayed redistribution imaging for the detection of myocardial viability is the reinjection of a second small dose of ^{201}Tl at rest following the 4-hour redistribution images. In a study of 20 revascularized patients, Dilsizian et al. [42] showed that 87% (13/15) of regions showing enhanced ^{201}Tl uptake on reinjection study showed normal ^{201}Tl uptake and improved regional wall motion after angioplasty in contrast to those regions (n = 8) which were irreversible after reinjection and had all abnormal ^{201}Tl uptake and abnormal regional wall motion after dilation.

Ohtani et al. [44] studied 24 patients before coronary artery bypass surgery with the stress-redistribution-reinjection protocol. Improvement in wall motion after surgery was observed in 23 of 31 segments (74%) exhibiting visual redistribution and 14 of 30 segments (47%) without redistribution on the delayed images. The reinjection identified new redistribution in 10 of the 14 improved segments that were undetected on the delayed images.

Additional evidence for the value of the ^{201}Tl reinjection method was shown when this technique was compared with PET using the presence of metabolic activity as evidence for viability [45, 46]. In the study of Bonow et al. [46], detection of myocardial viability by the two techniques was concordant in 88% of segments with severe persistent defects. Also, most mild persistent defects on serial early and 4-hour imaging showed evidence of viability as assessed by [18]FDG uptake.

When the reinjection protocol is used for the assessment of viability, the 4-hour delayed redistribution imaging should not be omitted because some of

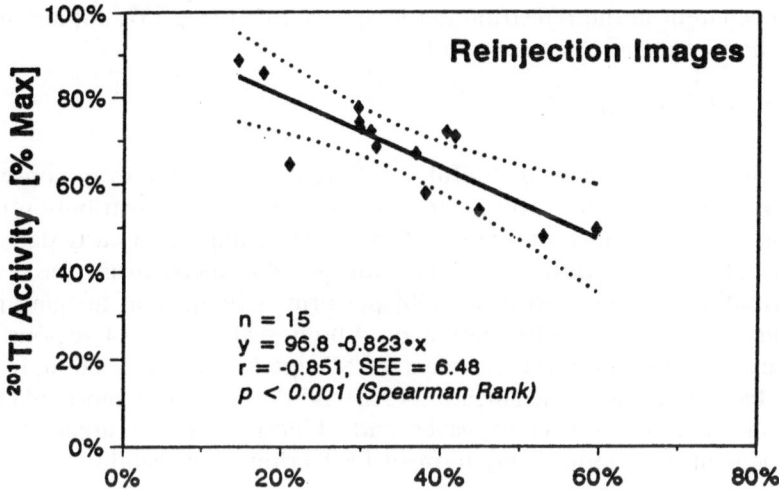

Figure 2. Relation between the amount of interstitial fibrosis and the level of regional ^{201}Tl activity at reinjection in 15 patients with persistent defects in their stress-redistribution images (from [48]).

the defects that demonstrate redistribution at 4 hours will revert to persistent defects after reinjection. Dilsizian and Bonow [47] observed this phenomenon in 25% of regions showing redistribution at 4 hours. Nearly one quarter defects will be misclassified as non reversible if redistribution imaging is not performed before reinjection.

The importance of quantifying residual ^{201}Tl activity after reinjection has been emphasized by a recent study showing that the level of regional ^{201}Tl activity after reinjection was significantly related to the mass of preserved viable myocytes [48]. The authors qualified ^{201}Tl activity on stress-redistribution-reinjection planar ^{201}Tl images in 37 patients who underwent transmural biopsies at the time of bypass surgery. In patients with persistent defects on conventional stress-redistribution images, interstitial fibrosis was significantly lower in patients who had enhanced regional ^{201}Tl activity after tracer reinjection compared with those who did not have enhancement of tracer activity after reinjection. Additionally, there was an inverse relation between the amount of fibrosis and the level of regional ^{201}Tl activity in the reinjection images (Figure 2). This relation obtained on continuous values is important to note because the level of fibrosis is directly related to the absence of improvement of function after revascularization [49].

Thus, the sequence of poststress, 4-hour redistribution and reinjection imaging is the most clinically appropriate protocol for the evaluation of inducible ischemia and detection of viability. The data relevant for predicting recovery of regional dysfunction can be provided by the quantitative analysis of ^{201}Tl content in the redistribution image as a first step [37, 38] and in the reinjection image as a second step [42].

Reverse redistribution

[201]Tl reinjection may also be useful in differentiating viable from non-viable myocardial regions with reverse redistribution. Reverse redistribution is defined as the appearance of a new defect or worsening of an early defect on redistribution scans. In order to elucidate possible mechanisms for reverse redistribution, Marin-Neto et al. [50] performed reinjection imaging in 39 patients with reverse redistribution on 4-hour scans. 82% of regions with reverse redistribution showed enhanced ^{201}Tl uptake with reinjection; in 18% the defects remained unchanged. Persistent defects were more likely to occur in an area showing Q waves and akinesis, whereas areas showing improvement were more likely to meet PET criteria for viability.

Dual-isotope imaging

A possible alternative protocol to later injection ^{201}Tl imaging which combines the potential for optimal viability detection with increased efficiency, is separate dual- isotope imaging with ^{201}Tl and ^{99m}Tc-Sestamibi [51]. This approach uses the resting ^{201}Tl image to assess resting perfusion and viability immediately followed by a stress test with injection of Sestamibi at stress for the diagnosis of myocardial ischemia. Concern about this method is that it may be difficult to compare changes in tracer distribution when different radionuclides are used. Also, resting ^{201}Tl imaging without the redistribution imaging may significantly underestimate perfusion defect reversibility in up to 75% of myocardial segments [27–29]. Additionally, the true extent of the ischemic defect may be underestimated with Sestamibi injection following stress [52, 53].

Alternative methods for viability and conclusions

Other approaches such as Positron Emission Tomography and low-dose dobutamine echocardiography have been proposed to predict the reversibility of left ventricular dysfunction after coronary revascularization. Only two studies have directly compared dobutamine echocardiography and ^{201}Tl scintigraphy in the same patient population. Mazullo et al. [32] studied 14 patients with resting-redistribution planar ^{201}Tl scintigraphy and dobutamine echocardiography. Delayed ^{201}Tl scintigraphy and dobutamine echocardiography showed similar predictive accuracy for viable myocardium (sensitivity of 80% for ^{201}Tl and 82% for dobutamine echocardiography; specificity of 92% for both techniques). Vanoverschelde et al. [54] studied 52 patients with left ventricular ejection fraction of 36% prior to coronary revascularization. The patients underwent dobutamine echocardiography and exercise-redistribution-reinjection ^{201}Tl SPECT imaging. Dobutamine echocardiography correctly identified 88% of the patients with and 75% of the patients without viable myocardium. Overall accuracy was 83%. With ^{201}Tl, the presence of more than 50% tracer uptake at reinjection on left ventricular short-axis cross sections of the dysfunctional area had a sensitivity of 75%, specificity of 70% and an overall accuracy of 73%. In this study, low dose dobutamine echocardiography and quantitative exercise-redistribution-reinjection ^{201}Tl SPECT had comparable accuracy for identification of viability and reversible dysfunction.

Only one study using ^{201}Tl and PET metabolic imaging was performed in the same patients with reduced ejection fraction and with a post-revascularization assessment of contractile function [55]. 31 coronary artery patients with anterior wall dysfunction and a mean left ventricular ejection fraction of $33 \pm 11\%$ were studied by exercise-redistribution-reinjection ^{201}Tl SPECT and by dynamic ammonia/FDG PET imaging during euglycemic hyperinsulinemic glucose clamp before revascularization. For assessing viability, echocardiography was performed at baseline and after revascularization. In this study, visual ^{201}Tl defect reversibility was present in 12/18 patients with (sensitivity 67%) and absent in 7/13 patients without viable myocardium (specificity 54%). Similar sensitivity and specificity were obtained with a quantitative index of ^{201}Tl uptake (> 50%) at reinjection. In the same study, the FDG/ammonia mismatch pattern had a sensitivity of 89% (16/18) and a specificity of 62% (8/13). Also, relative FDG uptake had a similar accuracy as compared to the mismatch pattern. Thus, FDG/flow PET imaging during glucose clamp had a better predictive accuracy for identification of viable myocardium than quantitative ^{201}Tl exercise-redistribution-reinjection imaging. Additional studies should address whether ^{201}Tl imaging and/or low dose dobutamine echocardiography should be performed as a first step in a sequential strategy involving PET imaging only as a second step viability test. (See also Chapters 14–18.)

References

1. Strauss HW, Harrison K, Langan JK et al. Thallium-201 for myocardial imaging. Relation of thallium-201 to regional myocardial perfusion. Circulation 1975; 51: 641–5.
2. Weich HP, Strauss HW, Pitt B. The extraction of thallium-201 by the myocardium. Circulation 1977; 56: 188–91.
3. Melin JA, Becker LC. Quantitative relationship between global left ventricular thallium uptake and blood flow: Effects of propranolol, ouabain, dipyridamole and coronary artery occlusion. J Nucl Med 1986; 27: 641–52.
4. Leppo JA. Myocardial uptake of thallium and rubidium during alterations in perfusion and oxygenation in isolated rabbit hearts. J Nucl Med 1987; 28: 878.
5. Moore CA, Cannon J, Watson DD et al. Thallium 201 kinetics in stunned myocardium characterized by severe postischemic systolic dysfunction. Circulation 1990; 81: 1622–32.
6. Sinusas AJ, Watson DD, Cannon JM Jr, Beller GA. Effect of ischemia and postischemic

dysfunction on myocardial uptake of technetium-99m-labeled methoxyisobutyl isonitrile and thallium-201. J Am Coll Cardiol 1989; 14: 1785–93.

7. Melin J, Becker L, Bulkley BH. Differences in thallium-201 uptake in reperfused and non reperfused myocardial infarction. Circulation Res 1983; 53: 414–19.

8. Chu A, Murdock RH, Cobb FR. Relation betwen regional distribution of Thallium 201 and myocardial blood flow in normal, acutely ischemic and infarcted myocardium. Am J Cardiol 1982; 50: 1141–4.

9. Khaw Ban A, Strauss W, Pohost GM et al. Relation of immediate and delayed thallium-201 distribution to localization of Iodine-125 antimyosin antibody in acute experimental myocardial infarction. Am J Cardiol 1983; 51: 1428–32.

10. Di Cola VC, Downing SE, Donabedian RK, Zaret BL. Pathophysiological correlates of thallium-201 myocardial uptake in experimental infarction. Cardiovasc Res 1977; 11: 141–6.

11. Sochor H, Schwaiger M, Schelbert HR et al. Relationship between Tl-201, Tc-99m (Sn) pyrophosphate and F-18 2-deoxyglucose uptake in ischemically injured dog myocardium. Am Heart J 1987; 114: 1066–78.

12. Chappuis F, Meier B, Belenger J et al. Early assessment of tissue viability with radioiodinated heptadecanoic acid in reperfused canine myocardium: Comparison with thallium-201. Am Heart J 1990; 119: 833–41.

13. Forman R, Kirk ES. Thallium-201 accumulation during reperfusion of ischemic myocardium: Dependence on regional blood flow rather than viability. Am J Caridol 1984; 54: 659–63.

14. Pohost GL, Zir L, Moore RH et al. Differentiation of transiently ischemic from infarcted myocardium by serial imaging after a single dose of thallium-201. Circulation 1977; 55: 294–302.

15. Grunwald AM, Watson DD, Hozgrefe HHJ et al. Myocardial thallium-201 kinetics in normal and ischemic myocardium. Circulation 1981; 64: 610–8.

16. Pohost GM, Okada RD, O'Keffe DD et al. Thallium redistribution in dogs with severe coronary artery stenosis of fixed caliber. Circulation Research 1981; 48: 439–46.

17. Melin JA, Wijns W, Keyeux A et al. Assessment of thallium-201 redistribution versus glucose uptake as predictors of viability after coronary occlusion and reperfusion. Circulation 1988; 77: 927–34.

18. Granato JE, Watson DD, Flanagan TL et al. Myocardial thallium-201 kinetics and regional flow alterations with 3 hours of coronary occlusion and either rapid reperfusion through a totally patent vessel or slow reperfusion through a critical stenosis. J Am Coll Cardiol 1987; 9: 109–18.

19. Granato JE, Watson DD, Flanagan TL et al. Myocardial thallium-201 kinetics during coronary occlusion and reperfusion: Influence of method of reflow and timing of thallium-201 administration. Circulation 1986; 73: 150–60.

20. Gewirtz H, Fischman AJ, Abraham S et al. Positron emission tomographic measurements of absolute regional myocardial blood flow permits identification of nonviable myocardium in patients with chronic myocardial infarction. J Am Coll Cardiol 1994; 23: 851–9.

21. Yamamoto Y, De Silva R, Rhodes CG et al. A new strategy for the assessment of viable myocardium and regional myocardial blood flow using ^{15}O-water and dynamic positron emission tomography. Circulation 1992; 86: 167–78.

22. Vanoverschelde JL, Melin JA, Bol A et al. Regional oxidative metabolism in patients after recovery from reperfused anterior myocardial infarction: Relation to regional blood flow and glucose uptake. Circulation 1992; 80: 1–11.

23. Vanoverschelde JL, Wijns W, Depré C et al. Mechanisms of chronic regional postischemic dysfunction in humans: New insights from the study of non-infarcted collateral dependent myocardium. Circulation 1993; 87: 1513–23.

24. Reimer KA, Jennings RB. The "wavefront phenomenon" of myocardial ischemic cell death. Transmural progression of necrosis within the framework of ischemic bed size (myocardium at risk) and collateral flow. Lab Invest 1979; 40: 633–44.

25. Jugdutt BI, Hutchins GM, Bulkley BM, Becker LC. Myocardial infarction in the conscious dog: Three-dimensional mapping of infarct, collateral flow and region at risk. Circulation 1979; 60: 1141–50.
26. Gewirtz H, Beller GA, Strauss HW et al. Transient defects of resting thallium scans in patients with coronary artery disease. Circulation 1979; 59: 707–13.
27. Berger BC, Watson DD, Burwell LR et al. Redistribution of thallium at rest in patients with stable and unstable angina and the effect of coronary artery bypass graft surgery. Circulation 1979; 60: 1114–25.
28. Iskandrian AS, Hakki AH, Kane SA et al. Rest and redistribution thallium-201 myocardial scintigraphy to predict improvement in left ventricular function after coronary artery bypass grafting. Am J Cardiol 1983; 51: 1312–6.
29. Mori T, Minamiji K, Kurogane H et al. Rest-injected thallium-201 imaging for assessing viability of severe asynergic regions. J Nucl Med 1991; 32: 1718–24.
30. Ragosta M, Beller GA, Watson DD et al. Quantitative planar rest-redistribution 201Tl imaging in detection of myocardial viability and prediction of improvement in left ventricular function after coronary bypass surgery in patients with severely depressed left ventricular function. Circulation 1993; 87: 1630–41.
31. Alfieri O, La Canna G, Giubbini R et al. Recovery of myocardial infarction. The ultimate target of coronary revascularization. Eur J Cardio-thorac Surg 1993; 7: 325–30.
32. Marzullo P, Parodi O, Reisenhofer B et al. Value of rest thallium-201/technetium-99^m sestamibi scans and dobutamine echocardiography for detecting myocardial viability. Am J Cardiol 1993; 71: 166–72.
33. Udelson JE, Coleman PS, Metherall J et al. Predicting recovery of severe regional ventricular dysfunction. Comparison of resting scintigraphy with ^{201}Tl and $^{99\,m}$Tc-Sestamibi. Circulation 1994; 89: 2552–61.
34. Lomboy CT, Schulman DS, Grill HP et al. Rest-redistribution thallium-201 scintigraphy to determine myocardial viability early after myocardial infarction. J Am Coll Cardiol 1995; 25: 210–7.
35. Dilsizian V, Perrone-Filardi P, Arrighi JA et al. Concordance and discordance between stress-redistribution and rest-redistribution Thallium imaging for assessing viable myocardium. Comparison with metabolic activity by positron emission tomography. Circulation 1993; 88: 941–52.
36. Gibson RS, Watson DD, Taylor GJ et al. Prospective assessment of regional myocardial perfusion before and after coronary revascularization surgery by quantitative thallium-201 scintigraphy. J Am Coll Cardiol 1983; 1: 804–15.
37. Sabia PJ, Powers ER, Ragosta M et al. Role of quantiative planar thallium-201 imaging for determining viability in patients with acute myocardial infarction and a totally occluded infarct-related artery. J Nucl Med 1993; 34: 728–36.
38. Yamamoto K, Asada S, Masuyama T et al. Myocardial hibernation in the infarcted region cannot be assessed from the presence of stress-induced ischemia: Usefulness of delayed image of exercise thallium-201 scintigraphy. Am Heart J 1993; 152: 33.
39. Cloninger KG, DePuey EG, Garcia EV et al. Incomplete redistribution in delayed thallium-201 single photon emission computed tomographic (SPECT) images: An overestimation of myocardial scarring. J Am Coll Cardiol 1988; 12: 955–63.
40. Kiat H, Berman DS, Maddahi J et al. Later reversibility of tomographic myocardial thallium-201 defects: An accurate marker of myocardial viability. J Am Coll Cardiol 1988; 12: 1456–63.
41. Yang LD, Berman DS, Kiat H et al. The frequency of late reversibility in SPECT thallium-201 stress-redistribution studies. J Am Coll Cardiol 1990; 15: 334–40.
42. Dilsizian V, Rocco TP, Freeman NMT et al. Enhanced detection of ischemic but viable myocardium by the reinjection of thallium after stress-redistribution imaging. N Engl J Med 1990; 323: 141–6.
43. Brunken RC, Modi FV, Hawkins RA et al. Positron emission tomography detects metabolic

viability in myocardium with persistent 24-hour single photon emission computed tomography 201-Tl defects. Circulation 1992; 86: 1357–69.

44. Ohtani H, Tamaki N, Yonekura Y et al. Value of thallium-201 reinjection after delayed SPECT imaging for predicting reversible ischemia after coronary artery bypass grafting. Am J Cardiol 1990; 66: 394–9.

45. Tamaki N, Ohtani H, Yamshita K et al. Metabolic activity in the areas of new fill-in after thallium-201 reinjection: Comparison with positron emission tomography using fluorine-18-deoxyglucose. J Nucl Med 1991; 32: 673–8.

46. Bonow RO, Dilsizian V, Cuocolo A, Bacharach SL. Identification of viable myocardium in patients with coronary artery disease and left ventricular dysfunction: Comparison of thallium scintigraphy with reinjection and PET imaging with ^{18}F-fluorodeoxyglucose. Circulation 1991; 83: 26–37.

47. Dilsizian V, Bonow RO. Differential uptake and apparent thallium-201 "washout" after thallium reinjection: options regarding early redistribution imaging before reinjection or after redistribution imaging after reinjection. Circulation 1992; 85: 1032–8.

48. Zimmermann R, Mall G, Rauch B et al. Residual ^{201}Tl activity in irreversible defects as a marker of myocardial viability. Clinicopathological study. Circulation 1995; 91: 1016–21.

49. Depré C, Vanoverschelde JL, Melin JA et al. Structural and metabolic correlates of the reversibility of chronic left ventricular ischemic dysfunction in humans. Am J Physiol 1995; 268: H1265–75.

50. Marin-Neto JA, Dilsizian V, Arrighi JA et al. Thallium reinjection demonstrates viable myocardium in regions with reverse distribution. Circulation 1993; 88: 1736–41.

51. Berman DS, Kiat H, Friedman JD et al. Separate acquisition rest thallium-201/stress technetium-99m sestamibi dual-isotope myocardial perfusion single-photon emission computed tomography: A clinical validation study. J Am Coll Cardiol 1993; 22: 1455–64.

52. Leon AR, Eisner RL, Martin SE et al. Comparison of single-photon emission computed tomographic (SPECT) myocardial perfusion imaging with thallium-201 and technetium-99m sestamibi in dogs. J Am Coll Cardiol 1992; 20: 1612–25.

53. Maublant JC, Marcaggi X, Lusson JR et al. Comparison between thallium-201 and technetium-99m methoxyisobutyl isonitrile defect size in single photon computed tomography at rest, exercise and redistribution in coronary artery disease. Am J Cardiol 1992; 69: 183–7.

54. Vanoverschelde JL, Marwick T, D'Hondt AM et al. Delineation of myocardial viability with low-dose dobutamine stress-echocardiography in patients with chronic ischemic left ventricular dysfunction. Circulation 1993; 88: 586.

55. Gerber BL, Vanoverschelde JL, Bol A et al. Comparison of Tl-201 SPECT and PET to predict viable myocardium in patients with ischemic left ventricular dysfunction. Eur J Nucl Med 1994; 21: 725.

56. Sansoy V, Glover DK, Watson DD et al. Comparison of thallium-201 resting redistribution with technetium-99m-sestamibi uptake and functional response to dobutamine for assessment of myocardial viability. Circulation 1995; 92: 994–1004.

57. Arnese M, Cornel JH, Salustri A et al. Prediction of improvement of regional left ventricular function after surgical revascularization. A comparison of low-dose dobutamine echocardiography with ^{201}Tl single photon emission computed tomography. Circulation 1995; 91: 2748–52.

58. Panza JA, Dilsizian V, Laurienzo JM et al. Relation between thallium uptake and contractile response to dobutamine. Implications regarding myocardial viability in patients with chronic coronary artery disease and left ventricular dysfunction. Circulation 1995; 91: 990–8

Corresponding Author: Dr Jacques A. Melin, Department of Nuclear Medicine, University of Louvain Medical School, Avenue Hippocrate 10/2580, B-1200 Brussels, Belgium

16. Assessment of myocardial viability before revascularization: Can sestamibi accurately predict functional recovery?

JAN H. CORNEL, AMBROOS E.M. REIJS, JOYCE POSTMA-TJOA and PAOLO M. FIORETTI

Introduction

The assessment of myocardial viability is an issue of considerable clinical relevance in the current era of thrombolytic therapy and coronary revascularization [1, 2]. The awareness of the potential of even severe regional and global dyssynergic myocardium to improve its functional state, has resulted in a search for the optimal diagnostic approach for its noninvasive assessment. The identification of myocardial regions with high and low probability of functional improvement after revascularization is of vital importance since this can be crucial for the decision of performing revascularization procedures in individual patients with multiple severe wall motion abnormalities.

Viability, defined as reversible myocardial dysfunction, may be caused by stunning or hibernation. Myocardial stunning is transient prolonged postischemic dysfunction that may occur after the restoration of normal flow [1]. Despite the absence of irreversible damage, mechanical dysfunction may persist after coronary reperfusion in different clinical scenarios such as after percutaneous transluminal coronary angioplasty, coronary artery bypass surgery or acute myocardial infarction with early reperfusion [3, 4]. Spontaneous recovery may occur within weeks and is dependent on the "area at risk", the duration of coronary occlusion and the presence and extent of collateral vessels [5]. In hibernating myocardium, chronic reduction in myocardial blood flow is thought to be matched by downregulation of the contractile cellular function [6, 7]. Successful coronary revascularization may lead to functional recovery of this chronic process. In contrast, myocardial necrosis and scar tissue formation do not lead to reversibility of contractile dysfunction. In individual patients, all types of reversible and irreversible contractile dysfunction may coexist with areas of normally contractile myocardium.

Recovery of function

Although normally contractile myocardium is obviously viable, a mixture of normal myocardium with scar or hibernating myocardium can both be present

C.A. Nienaber and U. Sechtem (eds): Imaging and Intervention in Cardiology. 249–258.
© 1996 Kluwer Academic Publishers.

Table 1. Factors influencing the recovery of left ventricular function after revascularization.

- Amount and degree of stunning (recent myocardial infarction, repetitive ischemia)
- Amount and degree of myocardial hibernation
- Presence and amount of myocardial scarring
- Graftable vessels
- Left ventricular plasty
- Completeness of revascularization
- Internal mammary arterial or vein graft
- Perioperative myocardial infarction
- Early graft closure
- Left ventricular dimensions
- Timing and method to assess regional left ventricular function
- Myocarditis/cardiomyopathy

in a hypokinetic myocardial region, but only that segment which hibernates may potentially improve after coronary revascularization. Thus accurate non-invasive methods are needed to discriminate between the different pathophysiologic mechanisms of hypo- or akinesis. Randomized trials in patients with coronary artery disease have indicated that coronary revascularization can lead to improved left ventricular function [8]. More recently it has been demonstrated that even in severe left ventricular dysfunction, ejection fraction can improve in selected patients [9]. These results implicate the potential to prolong survival as well as the quality of life in patients with left ventricular dysfunction. Thus patients with chronic advanced ischemic left ventricular dysfunction, even when elegible for heart transplantation, may improve after successful revascularization. Several factors may affect the outcome of such approach however (Table 1). It is conceivable that in patients with hibernating myocardium, repetitive episodes of superimposed stunning exist due to transient ischemia. Furthermore, not only the presence but more importantly the amount of myocardium in hibernation and the degree of myocardial scarring affect the outcome of revascularization.

Other factors mentioned in Table 1 and important to keep in mind are the success of revascularization and the preoperative left ventricular dimensions. Patients with severe left ventricular dilatation may be less likely to recover. Anyway, recovery of ventricular function may underestimate the real extent of myocardial viability due to sometimes inadequate restoration of regional myocardial blood flow. Various nuclear methods have received attention for the assessment of myocardial viability. This chapter focusses on the approach with technetium-99m labeled sestamibi as a perfusion agent to (1) distinguish hibernation (with or without superimposed stunning) from non-viable myocardium and (2) to predict functional recovery after coronary revascularization.

Properties of Tc-99m sestamibi

Sestamibi is a technetium-99m labeled myocardial perfusion agent, providing similar information as thallium-201 for the detection of coronary artery disease [10]. In comparison with thallium-201, sestamibi has the advantage of better imaging properties, particularly when single photon emission computed tomography (SPECT) is considered [11]. The gamma emission of technetium-99m sestamibi is higher (141 keV vs 68 to 80 keV) and its physical half life is shorter (6 vs 73 hours). Another difference between thallium-201 and sestamibi is the lower first pass extraction for sestamibi (40% vs 80%) [11, 12]. Although minimal myocardial redistribution occurs (<25% in 4 hours), the slow myocardial clearance of sestamibi compensates for its low first pass extraction [13]. The tissue uptake of sestamibi parallels coronary blood flow, with the exception of high flow conditions. Even under conditions of low coronary blood flow and in stunned myocardium, the myocardial uptake of sestamibi is comparable with that of thallium-201 [14]. Since the uptake of sestamibi is dependent on cell membrane integrity and mitochondrial function (membrane potential), it may from a cellular point of view also reflect myocardial viability [15].

While the use of sestamibi for myocardial perfusion is well accepted, its role for the assessment of myocardial viability is still controversial [2, 11, 16]. On the basis of these experiments, one may expect that sestamibi is comparable to thallium for the detection of viable, stunned myocardium, when myocardial perfusion has been restored after an ischemic episode. In contrast, thallium seems more suitable than sestamibi in the setting of hibernating myocardium, due to its properties to redistribute in a chronic low flow state [16]. In this condition, a sestamibi scan at rest is expected to show a perfusion defect, most likely underestimating the presence of viable myocardium. However, in the clinical setting stunned and hibernating myocardium often coexist and constitute a dynamic condition. Therefore, a distinction between the 2 syndromes is more theoretical than real in our daily clinical practice.

Sestamibi in chronic left ventricular dysfunction

Several recent publications describe the merit of sestamibi in the setting of chronic ischemic left ventricular dysfunction in order to distinguish viable myocardium from scar. There are two kinds of data available: first, comparative studies between sestamibi and other viability tracers like thallium-201 [17–24] or F-18 FDG using positron emission tomography [25, 26] and second, studies using the improvement of left ventricular wall motion after successful revascularization as a standard for myocardial viability [27–33].

Comparison of sestamibi with thallium-201

All studies comparing sestamibi and thallium-201 have reached similar conclusions, suggesting that myocardial regions with severely reduced sestamibi uptake at rest may contain viable tissue. Post-stress reinjection thallium imaging has been compared with sestamibi imaging at rest by different authors [17–19]. Cuocolo et al. [17] compared exercise-redistribution-reinjection with exercise-rest sestamibi (two day protocol) planar imaging in 20 patients with coronary artery disease and chronic left ventricular dysfunction (ejection fraction 30 ± 8%). Qualitative segmental analysis showed 122 myocardial segments (41%) with irreversible thallium uptake defects at redistribution. After thallium reinjection, in 57/122 of these segments (47%) tracer fill-in was noted. In contrast, 100/122 segments appeared as fixed defects (without reversibility) on the sestamibi images at rest. Furthermore, the resting sestamibi mean uptake score in the segments with perfusion defects was significantly worse compared to the reinjection thallium mean uptake score (5 point grading system).

Since quantitative analysis of SPECT images may improve diagnostic accuracy of comparative data, 26 patients with advanced chronic left ventricular dysfunction (mean ejection fraction 32 ± 6%) due to coronary artery disease, were studied with post-stress reinjection thallium as well as sestamibi SPECT at rest within 7 days [19]. The images were acquired 20 minutes after reinjection of 40 MBq of thallium-201 and 2 hours after intravenous administration of 370 MBq of sestamibi. All images were acquired using a single head rotating gamma camera with a low-energy, all purpose collimator. Thirty-two projections (180° scanning) were obtained with an acquisition time of 45 s/projection. Quantitative analysis was performed by circumferential profile analysis of six standardized short axis slices. The profiles were defined within the automatically detected endo- and epicardial boundaries. The normal limits for sestamibi and thallium were separately defined within 2 standard deviations of profiles (regional values) from a normal database. Perfusion defects were calculated by summing the areas below the lower limit of normal in the six short axis slices. The results, summarized in Table 2 and Figure 1, indicate that sestamibi uptake defects were systematically more severe compared to the reinjection thallium uptake defects (sestamibi = 1337 + 0.9 thallium; r = 0.74). This finding reinforces the idea that sestamibi may underestimate the extent of residual myocardial viability.

Table 2. Quantitative analysis of perfusion defect severity (unitless, mean ± standard deviation) using SPECT in 26 patients with chronic left ventricular dysfunction due to coronary artery disease: a comparison between sestamibi and thallium-201.

Sestamibi at rest	3627 ± 1587
Thallium reinjection	2553 ± 1309*

*p < 0.005 versus sestamibi.

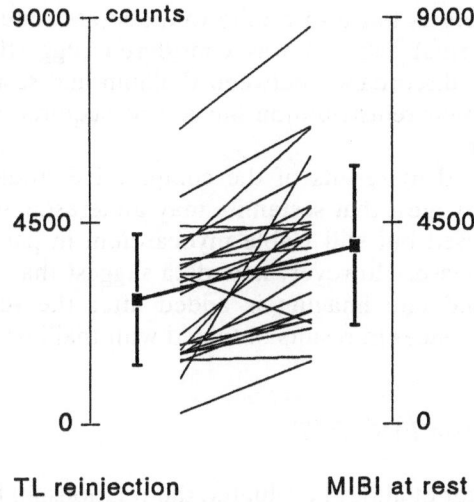

Figure 1. Graph which displays the comparison of quantitative analysis between the severity of uptake defects from resting sestamibi and post-stress reinjection thallium SPECT in 26 patients with chronic left ventricular dysfunction due to coronary artery disease. The data show a systematic overestimation of the defect severity by sestamibi across the whole range of defect sizes.

Several small studies recently compared sestamibi imaging at rest with rest-redistribution thallium imaging [20–24]. Cuocolo et al. [20] reported in 19 patients 48 segments with severe sestamibi perfusion defects. In 26/48 segments redistribution (4 hours) thallium revealed signs of viable tissue. These results are in agreement with other reports [21–24]. Taylor et al. [22] found in 32 patients 167 severe fixed defects (SPECT) with sestamibi, but 87 (52%) demonstrated thallium uptake on 24-hour redistribution imaging and thus suggested viable myocardium undetected by sestamibi. To circumvent the limitations of sestamibi, Maurea and coworkers [23, 24] reported the use of nitrates and delayed sestamibi imaging (redistribution). However, despite redistribution (5 hours) in 25% of the moderate to severe sestamibi uptake defects and similar results after nitrates, sestamibi still underestimates myocardial viability compared to rest-redistribution thallium in chronic coronary artery disease.

Recently, Dilsizian et al. [18] have compared the value of exercise/redistribution/reinjection thallium tomography with same day rest/exercise sestamibi tomography for the assessment of myocardial viability in 54 patients with a mean ejection fraction of 34 ± 14%. They found that 36% of the reversible thallium defects were determined to be irreversible on the stress/rest sestamibi studies. However the same authors found that the concordance between thallium and sestamibi increased from 75% to 93% if not only the reversibility of the perfusion defects but also a mild-to-moderate reduction in sestamibi (51 to 85% of normal activity) was considered suggestive of myocardial viability. Also, the discordance between thallium and sestamibi diminished if an additional 4-hour redistribution image was acquired after the injection of sestamibi at rest.

Thus, the concordant results of the comparative studies using different imaging protocols suggest that sestamibi may underestimate the presence of severely hypoperfused but still viable myocardium in patients with chronic coronary artery disease. However, new data suggest that when quantitative analysis is used and late imaging is added after the resting injection of sestamibi, the differences in results obtained with thallium and sestamibi are smaller.

Comparison with F-18 FDG PET

Recently, Altehoefer et al. [25] evaluated the relationship between sestamibi uptake at rest and glucose metabolism by FDG PET. They found, in a group of 111 patients with coronary artery disease and wall motion abnormalities, preserved glucose metabolism (FDG uptake >70%) in a substantial number of patients with reduced sestamibi uptake at rest (SPECT). Furthermore, of the myocardial segments with 31–70% of peak sestamibi uptake (moderate to severe defects) 13–61% were viable by PET criteria (Figure 2). On the other hand, sestamibi defects with ≤30% of peak activity are highly predictive for scar tissue (82%).

Thus, the severity of a given sestamibi perfusion defect may yield an indirect estimate of the likelihood of myocardial viability. Nevertheless, 30% of the patients had at least 1 viable segment with severely reduced uptake of sestamibi (<50% of peak activity). Similarly, Sawada and coworkers [26] showed in 20 patients (7 after recent myocardial infarction) that 50% of the moderate or severe sestamibi defects had preserved glucose metabolism (> 60% FDG uptake). They found no lower limit of sestamibi activity that excluded significant FDG uptake. Thus, sestamibi uptake clearly underestimates myocardial viability in comparison with FDG PET in patients with chronic coronary artery disease. These data are in agreement with the comparative data with various thallium imaging protocols as previously discussed. However regardless of the lower sensitivity of sestamibi for viable myocardium tracer uptake may still allow for correct prediction of functional recovery after successful revascularization. The extent of underestimation is of key importance since failure to detect limited amounts of viable myocardium may not have an impact on the outcome of revascularization.

Dilsizian et al. [18] have recently found in 25 patients that the agreement between same day rest/exercise sestamibi and PET imaging (FDG/blood flow matching) is greatly enhanced if an additional late redistribution imaging is acquired after the resting injection of sestamibi or if the severity of the sestamibi activity within the irreversible defects is taken in account. However,

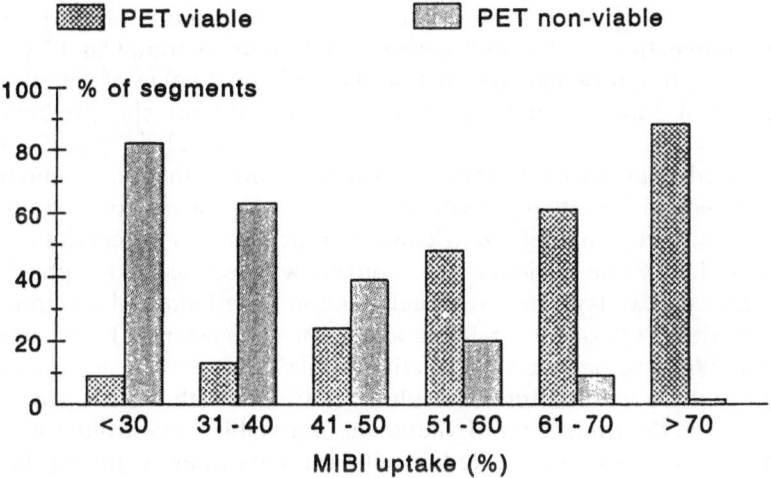

Figure 2. Results of the comparison between sestamibi uptake at rest and FDG PET derived from 111 patients with chronic coronary artery disease and wall motion abnormalities, from Altehoefer et al. [25]. It displays the percentage of viable (FDG uptake >70%) and nonviable (FDG uptake <50%) segments in relation to sestamibi defect severity. The sestamibi uptake, even when severely reduced (<50%), clearly underestimates the extent of viable myocardium when FDG PET is considered the "golden standard".

larger comparative studies are needed to answer the question to what myocardial extent sestamibi underestimates myocardial viability relative to the amount of myocardial scar (see also Chapters 1–4, 15 and 17).

Can sestamibi reliably predict functional recovery after revascularization?

The number of studies dealing with this topic is limited [27–33]. The results indicate, although small numbers of patients were studied, that sestamibi is not always a good indicator of functional recovery after revascularization. In particular, Maublant et al. [28] observed, in a group of 18 patients, that wall motion improved in 8 of 9 segments with a initial severe sestamibi defect 3 months after revascularization. Marzullo and coworkers [29] studied 14 patients with chronic coronary artery disease before and 3 months after revascularization. Sestamibi uptake at rest and planar rest-redistribution (16-hour) thallium-201 scans were acquired before revascularization. Compared to delayed redistribution thallium imaging, sestamibi uptake had a lower sensitivity (75 vs 86%) and specificity (84 vs 92%) to predict recovery of wall motion. Sciagrà et al. [31] reported their initial results with the use of an infusion of nitrates during tracer injection. They studied in 22 patients the recovery of function after revascularization with first-pass radionuclide ventriculography. They showed a predictive accuracy for sestamibi SPECT of 82%. This approach is of interest and confirms previous work by Galli and coworkers [32] and Maurea et al. [23] also using sestamibi and Medrano et al. [34] utilizing thallium reinjection. Zafrir and collegues [35] demonstrated in 18 patients with severe left ventricular dysfunction the additional value of simultaneous assessment of function and perfusion by sestamibi for the prediction of functional recovery. A recent study from Udelson et al. [33] performed a head-to-head comparison between rest-redistribution thallium tomography and rest injection of sestamibi (with imaging 1 hour post-injection), to predict the recovery of regional left ventricular dysfunction after successful revascularization. Thirty-one patients were studied with echocardiography before and on average 20 days after revascularization. Thallium and sestamibi had similar positive (75% for thallium and 80% for sestamibi) and negative (92% and 96%, respectively) predictive values for recovery of regional left ventricular dysfunction after revascularization. For both tracers, the "best" cut-off for the discrimination of viable and not viable myocardium was 60% of peak activity. These excellent results are somewhat surprising because sestamibi scintigraphy was acquired with no pre-medication of nitrates nor was late imaging performed [18]. These results, although very promising, should be viewed with some caution because of 1) the very short follow-up of 20 days after revascularization, and 2) the lack of information on the changes of global left ventricular function after revascularization (see also Chapters 1, 2, 9, 13 and 15).

Conclusion

Myocardial perfusion imaging may reflect viability, since tracer uptake requires adequate perfusion, cellular integrity and metabolic function. Technetium-99m is an excellent myocardial flow tracer, but from the data so far available it seems less suitable than thallium for the assessment of myocardial viability in chronic coronary artery disease. It tends to overestimate the extent of myocardial necrosis or scar.

However, since sestamibi possesses superior imaging properties, the underestimation of myocardial viability has lead to the development of alternative protocols. For the detection of viable myocardium, imaging 1 hour after sestamibi injection may not be optimal. The tracer is known to redistribute to a small degree, thus delayed imaging may enhance the detection of viable myocardium in severe perfusion defects [13, 18]. Furthermore, nitroglycerin administration before rest injection of sestamibi seems useful [23, 32] and also with the addition of functional data (first pass and/or gated imaging), revealing a complementary data set on function and perfusion, the proper identification of viability may be improved [27, 35]. Quantification of regional tracer uptake may also enhance the discrimination between viable and non-viable myocardium [18, 25, 27, 33]. However, even with quantitation, a significant amount of severe sestamibi defects still represent viable tissue [25, 29]. Finally, new methods for attenuation correction may reduce the number of artifacts, in particular false positive perfusion defects, in order to enhance diagnostic specificity.

Thus, although it seems that sestamibi SPECT with 1) quantification of the activity, 2) late imaging and 3) pre-medication with nitrates provides information on myocardial viability close to that of thallium and PET, further studies are needed to substantiate the usefulness of sestamibi for addressing the issue of viability. In particular we feel that the role of sestamibi for the prediction of functional recovery after revascularization has still to be defined in larger and possibly multicenter studies.

References

1. Bolli R. Myocardial 'stunning' in man. Circulation 1992; 86: 1671–91.
2. Dilsizian V, Bonow RO. Current diagnostic techniques of assessing myocardial viability in patients with hibernating and stunned myocardium. Circulation 1993; 87: 1–20.
3. Patel B, Kloner RA, Przyklenk K, Braunwald E. Postischemic myocardial "stunning": A clinically relevant phenomenon. Ann Intern Med 1988; 108: 626–8.
4. Bourdillon PDV, Broderick TM, Williams ES et al. Early recovery of regional left ventricular function after reperfusion in acute myocardial infarction assessed by serial two-dimensional echocardiography. Am J Cardiol 1989; 63: 641–6.
5. Sabia P, Powers ER, Ragosta M et al. An association between collateral blood flow and myocardial viability in patients with recent myocardial infarction. N Engl J Med 1992; 327: 1825–31.
6. Rahimtoola SH. A perspective on the three large multicenter randomized clinical trails of coronary bypass surgery for chronic stable angina. Circulation 1985; 72 (Suppl V): 123–35.
7. Braunwald E, Rutherford JD. Reversible ischemic left ventricular dysfunction: Evidence for the hibernating myocardium. J Am Coll Cardiol 1986; 8: 1467–70.
8. Alderman EL, Bourassa MG, Cohen LS et al. Ten-year follow-up of survival and myocardial infarction in the randomized coronary artery surgery study. Circulation 1990; 82: 1629–46.
9. Elefteriades JA, Tolis G, Levi E et al. Coronary artery bypass grafting in severe left ventricular dysfunction: Excellent survival with improved ejection fraction and functional state. J Am Coll Cardiol 1993; 22: 1411–7.
10. Kahn JK, McGhie I, Akers MS et al. Quantitative rotational tomography with Tl-201 and Tc-99m 2-methoxy-isobutyl-isonitrile: A direct comparison in normal individuals and patients with coronary artery disease. Circulation 1989; 79: 1282–93.
11. Liu P. New technetium 99 m imaging agents: Promising windows for myocardial perfusion and viability. Am J Card Imaging 1992; 6: 28–41.
12. Okada RD, Glover D, Gaffney T, Williams S. Myocardial kinetics of technetium-99m-hexakis-2-methoxy-2-methylpropyl-isonitrile. Circulation 1988; 77: 491–8.
13. Taillefer R, Primeau M, Costi P et al. Technetium-99m-sestamibi myocardial perfusion imaging in detection coronary artery disease: Comparison between initial (1-hour) and delayed (3-hour) postexercise images. J Nucl Med 1991; 32: 1961–5.
14. Sinusas AJ, Watson DD, Cannon Jr JM, Beller GA. Effect of ischemia and postischemic dysfunction on myocardial uptake of technetium-99m-labeled methoxyisobutyl isonitrile and thallium-201. J Am Coll Cardiol 1989; 14: 1785–93.
15. Beanlands RSB, Dawood F, Wen WH et al. Are the kinetics of technetium 99 m-methoxy isobutyl isonitrile affected by cell metabolism and viability? Circulation 1990; 82: 1802–14.
16. Bonow RO, Dilsizian V. Thallium-201 and technetium-99m sestamibi for assessing viable myocardium. J Nucl Med 1992; 33: 815–8.
17. Cuocolo A, Pace L, Ricciardelli B et al. Identification of viable myocardium in patients

with chronic coronary artery disease: Comparison of thallium-201 scintigraphy with reinjection and technetium-99m-methoxyisobutyl isonitrile. J Nucl Med 1992; 33: 505–11.

18. Dilsizian V, Arrighi JA, Diodati JG et al. Myocardial viability in patients with chronic coronary artery disease: Comparison of ^{99m}Tc-sestamibi with thallium reinjection and [^{18}F]fluorodeoxyglucose. Circulation 1994; 89: 578–87.

19. Cornel JH, Arnese M, Forster T et al. Potential and limitations of Tc-99m sestamibi scintigraphy for the diagnosis of myocardial viability. Herz 1994; 19: 19–27.

20. Cuocolo A, Maurea S, Pace L et al. Resting technetium-99m methoxyisobutylisonitrile cardiac imaging in chronic coronary artery disease: Comparison with rest-redistribution thallium-201 scintigraphy. Eur J Nucl Med 1993; 20: 1186–92.

21. Coleman PS, Metherall JA, Oao Q et al. Comparison of rest-redistribution thallium-201 uptake with resting sestamibi uptake in coronary artery disease (Abstr). J Nucl Med 1992; 33: 905.

22. Taylor AM, Merhige ME. Detection of myocardial viability: Sestamibi overestimates necrosis compared with thallium (Abstr). J Am Coll Cardiol 1993; 21: 283A.

23. Maurea S, Cuocolo A, Soricelli A et al. Resting technetium-99m mibi redistribution in patients with chronic coronary artery disease (Abstr). J Nucl Med 1994; 35: 114P.

24. Maurea S, Cuocolo A, Soricelli A et al. Nitrates improve the identification of viable myocardium by technetium-99m mibi spet imaging in chronic coronary artery disease (Abstr). J Nucl Med 1994; 35: 115P.

25. Altehoefer C, vom Dahl J, Biedermann M et al. Significance of defect severity in technetium-99m-MIBI SPECT at rest to assess myocardial viability: Comparison with fluorine-18–FDG PET. J Nucl Med 1994; 35: 569–74.

26. Sawada SG, Allman KC, Muzik O et al. Positron emission tomography detects evidence of viability in rest technetium-99m sestamibi defects. J Am Coll Cardiol 1994; 23: 92–8.

27. Rocco TP, Dilsizian V, Strauss HW, Boucher CA. Technetium-99m isonitrile myocardial uptake at rest: II. Relation to clinical markers of potential viability. J Am Coll Cardiol 1989; 14: 1678–84.

28. Maublant JC, Citron B, Lipiecki J et al. Predictive value of Tc-99m-sestamibi tomographic imaging as test for myocardial viability in hibernating myocardium (Abstr). J Am Coll Cardiol 1993; 21: 282A.

29. Marzullo P, Parodi O, Reisenhofer B et al. Value of rest thallium-201/technetium-99m sestamibi scans and dobutamine echocardiography for detecting myocardial viability. Am J Cardiol 1993; 71: 166–72.

30. Marzullo P, Sambuceti G, Parodi O. The role of sestamibi scintigraphy in the radioisotopic assessment of myocardial viability. J Nucl Med 1992; 33: 1925–30.

31. Sciagrà R, Bisi G, Santoro GM et al. Tc-99m-sestamibi nitrate imaging: Comparison of functional and perfusion changes in asynergic territories for the prediction of post-revascularization recovery (Abstr). J Nucl Med 1994; 35: 49P.

32. Galli M, Marcassa C, Silva P et al. Improvement of resting 99 mTc-sestamibi myocardial uptake by acute nitroglycerine administration (Abstr). J Am Coll Cardiol 1993; 21: 221A.

33. Udelson JE, Coleman PS, Metherall JHA et al. Predicting recovery of severe regional ventricular dysfunction. Comparison of resting scintigraphy with ^{201}thallium and ^{99m}Tc-sestamibi. Circulation 1994; 89: 2552–61.

34. Medrano R, Mahmarian JJ, Ashmore RF et al. The enhanced detection of myocardial viability with thallium-201 reinjection after nitroglycerine: A randomized, double blind, parallel, placebo controlled trail using quantitative tomography (Abstr). Circulation 1992; 86 (Suppl i): I-109.

35. Zafrir N, Vidne B, Bassevitch R, Lubin E. Extent of function-perfusion mismatch – a predictor for efficacy of coronary artery bypass grafting in patients with severe left ventricular dysfunction (Abstr). J Nucl Med 1994; 35: 126P.

Corresponding Author: Jan H. Cornel, Thoraxcenter, Room BA 350, University Hospital Rotterdam-Dijkzigt, Dr Molewaterplein 40, 3015 GD Rotterdam, The Netherlands

17. Assessment of viability in noncontractile myocardium before revascularization and prediction of functional recovery by PET

CHRISTOPH A. NIENABER

Introduction

The emergence of positron emission tomography (PET) in the clinical environment along with the synthesis of biologically active molecules and tracer kinetic principles has stimulated diagnostic in vivo tissue characterization in humans. While the concept of biological imaging has gained attraction for probing both the central nervous system and neoplastic tissues, current diagnostic benefit from PET is probably best defined in cardiovascular medicine.

PET imaging for myocardial viability

Positron emission tomography allows noninvasive assessment of myocardial metabolic processes and perfusion. Myocardial FDG (F-18-2 deoxyglucose) uptake by PET imaging is an established concept to identify myocardial viability, whereas the uptake of N-13 ammonia, O-15 oxygen or Rubidium-82 images myocardial perfusion. Furthermore it has been shown that the clearance of C11-acetate in normal and ischemic myocardium correlates closely with overall myocardial oxygen consumption (MVO_2) and may serve as an alternate marker of myocardial viability. In contrast to myocardial uptake of FDG the clearance of C11-acetate is independent of the overall substrate utilization and reflects the oxygen consumption eventually required for cell survival. The focus of this chapter is the impact of metabolic imaging with both FDG and C11-acetate on both the recovery of myocardial function and on clinical outcome after coronary revascularization by use of pharmaceutical, interventional and surgical means. Compared to conventional SPECT imaging PET exclusively allows the noninvasive interrogation of myocardial metabolic activity as well as quantification of myocardial blood flow and metabolic rates in humans, has better temporal and spatial resolution and enables true attenuation correction. Moreover, the family of positron emitting radiopharmaceuticals is growing with the demand to investigate various metabolic pathways. With PET evaluation of myocardial cell damage

C.A. Nienaber and U. Sechtem (eds): Imaging and Intervention in Cardiology, 259–277.
© 1996 *Kluwer Academic Publishers.*

after ischemic injury patients with acute and chronic ischemic heart disease may be better stratified for the most appropriate therapeutic intervention than with conventional radionuclide imaging.

Fluorine-18-fluoro-2-desoxyglucose (FDG) metabolism

FDG enters the myocardial cell from the blood proportional to the exogenous glucose concentration and is metabolized to FDG-6 phosphate by the hexokinase reaction. FDG-6 phosphate is not further metabolized via glycolysis, glycogen synthesis or the pentose phosphate shunt. Since the sarcolemma is largely impermeable for charged metabolites and myocardial dephosphorylation of FDG-6 phosphate is slow, FDG-6 phosphate remains trapped in the cytosol and accumulates with the exogenous glucose utilization [1]. In contrast to the brain with no glycogen synthesis, FDG uptake in the heart correlates with both glycolysis and glycogen synthesis. Since the rates of glycogen synthesis and utilization are in equilibrium the net accumulation of myocardial FDG-6-phosphate reflects the steady state extraction and phosphorylation rate of exogenous glucose [2, 3]. Thus, FDG kinetics as assessed by dynamic PET imaging may quantitatively reflect the rate of exogenous glucose utilization [4]. Under normoxic conditions myocardial glucose uptake is highest in the postprandial state when free fatty acid plasma levels are low.

Carbon 11-acetate metabolism

Whereas FDG uptake merely reflects the initial metabolic step of glucose metabolism, C11-acetate is a tracer to image allover cardiac oxidative metabolism [5]. Brown et al. have shown that the clearance of C11-acetate in normal and ischemic myocardium correlates closely with overall myocardial oxygen consumption [6]. Thus, C11-acetate clearance rate from the myocardium may be used as a quantitative index for myocardial oxygen consumption [7] since it is avidly extracted by the myocyte and bypasses glycolysis and beta-oxydation. Within the mitochondria, C11-acetate is converted to C11-acetyl-CoA, which enters the tricarboxylic acid cycle. C11-activity is cleared from the heart mainly in the form of C11-dioxide and traces substrate flux through the tricarboxylic acid cycle. Because the tricarboxylic acid cycle represents the final common metabolic pathway of cardiac oxydative metabolism, C11-acetate can be used to assess cardiac metabolism independent from overall substrate utilization [8]. New approaches for tracer kinetic modeling of C11-acetate take recirculation of C11-activity in form of C11-dioxide or bicarbonate into account and may eventually lead to absolute quantification of myocardial oxygen consumption [9].

Metabolic imaging of functionally impaired myocardium

Evidence of myocardial viability on the basis of myocardial perfusion, cell membrane integrity, and metabolic activity provides important diagnostic and prognostic information in patients with coronary artery disease and is likely to predict improvement of regional and global left ventricular function after revascularization. The downregulation of myocardial contractility represents a protective mechanism to maintain myocardial viability during regional reduction of myocardial blood flow [10, 11]. Residual metabolic activity is reflected by impaired oxidation of fatty acids and increased glycolytic flux [12]. Thus, during ischemic stress, the myocyte compensates for the loss of oxidative potential by shifting toward greater glucose utilization to generate high-energy phosphates. Subsequently PET imaging with FDG has been proposed for the identification of hibernating myocardium in chronic myocardial dysfunction caused by prolonged sublethal hypoperfusion in which myocytes remain viable but contractile function is chronically downregulated. Lack of FDG uptake in ventricular segments with reduced myocardial perfusion reflects myocardial scar tissue (Figure 1), while maintained FDG uptake identifies tissue viability in segments with reduced perfusion (Figure 2) [13]. In an alternate approach myocardial viability may be assessed by evidence of regional oxidative metabolism with C11-acetate imaging independent of both substrate availability and selection [14]. Decreases in C11-acetate clearance rate constants quantitatively describe the reduction of regional oxidative metabolism occurring in severe ischemia (Figure 3).

Myocardial viability in relation to contractile recovery and prognosis

Since patients with impaired left ventricular function benefit most from revascularization [15, 16], the differentiation of myocardial scar and hibernating myocardium is of major clinical importance. The extent of myocardial salvage and the amount of residual jeopardized myocardium are important clinical strata with prognostic impact to be addressed prior to interventions such as angioplasty and coronary artery bypass grafting. Regional FDG uptake has been shown to be predictive of functional recovery after myocardial revascularization (Table 1). Tillisch et al. [17] first demonstrated regional FDG uptake in the areas of reduced myocardial perfusion; this mismatch was in 75–85% predictive for recovery of wall motion after revascularization, while 78–92% of myocardial segments without metabolic activity in low flow areas did not recover despite revascularization. Interestingly, in 15–22% of regions FDG-PET may suggest tissue viability despite absence of functional recovery. Similar results were published by Tamaki [18] with a PET sensitivity and specificity for contractile recovery of 78% each as a result of bypass surgery; myocardial recovery in segments without metabolic activity was reported in

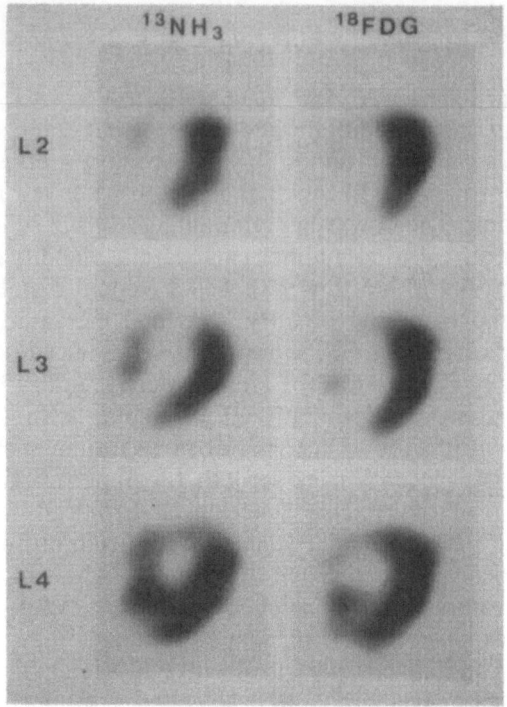

Figure 1. PET study of patient with previous anterior wall infarction shown in three horizontally oriented tomograms. The N13-ammonia study depicts a perfusion defect in the distal anterior wall and anterior septum accompanied by a corresponding defect in the FDG PET metabolic study. This match of both PET tracers is considered indicative of myocardial necrosis and irreversible damage confined to the perfusion territoryof the left anterior descending coronary artery (LAD).

22%. Similar results were reported by Nienaber et al. in patients with akinetic segments and FDG uptake undergoing PTCA [20].

Al-Aouar et al. [19] found that the predictive value for recovery of contractile function following revascularization in areas of reduced perfusion with preserved or increased FDG uptake was dependent on the degree of preoperative wall motion abnormality. Improvement of regional wall motion occurred in 75% of segments with akinesis or dyskinesis and relatively enhanced FDG uptake (to flow) preoperatively and even more often in hypokinetic segments. The absence of FDG uptake in regions of severe regional wall motion abnormality had a 90% predictive accuracy for no recovery of contractile function.

Conversely, predictive values of Tl-201-SPECT for functional recovery have been reported from 71 to 100% and for lack of recovery in the range of 63 to 100%. As shown in Table 2 SPECT tracers such as Tl-201 and to a lesser extent Tc-99m-MIBI may identify viability in roughly 40–50% of myocardial segments. However, more comparative data are needed to assess

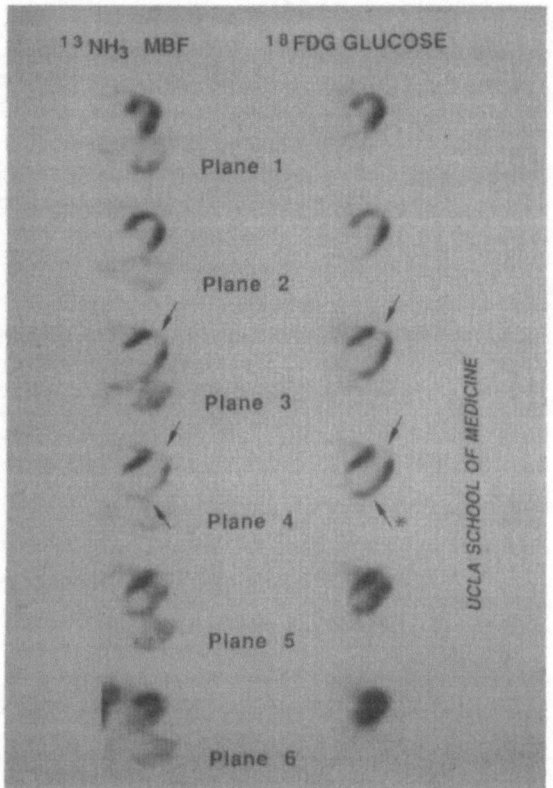

Figure 2. Combined PET blood flow/metabolism study of patient with clinical evidence of a previous anterior wall infarction and globally depressed left ventricular function. The N13-ammonia perfusion study reveals two perfusion defects; one is localized in the distal anterior wall (arrows) in planes 2 to 5, and a second perfusion defect is confined to the posterolateral aspects of teh left ventricular myocardium in planes 3 to 5 (arrows). The metabolic FDG PET study shows preserved FDG uptake (*) in the posterolateral region referred to as blood flow/metabolism mismatch indicating hibernating myocardium and reversibility of contractile dysfunction of the posterolateral segments. However, the anterior perfusion defect is matched with a corresponding lack of regional FDG uptake (arrow, planes 3 and 4) indicative myocardial scar in the anterior left ventricular segment.

whether the more expensive PET viability assessment is superior to reinjection Tl-201-SPECT imaging in predicting functional recovery after revascularization.

The temporal dissociation between recovery of regional blood flow, glucose metabolism and wall motion in ischemic human myocardium after coronary angioplasty (PTCA) was first examined in humans by serial PET and two-dimensional echocardiography before and 48 ± 20 hours after PTCA in patients with resting ischemic wall motion abnormalities [20]. Despite

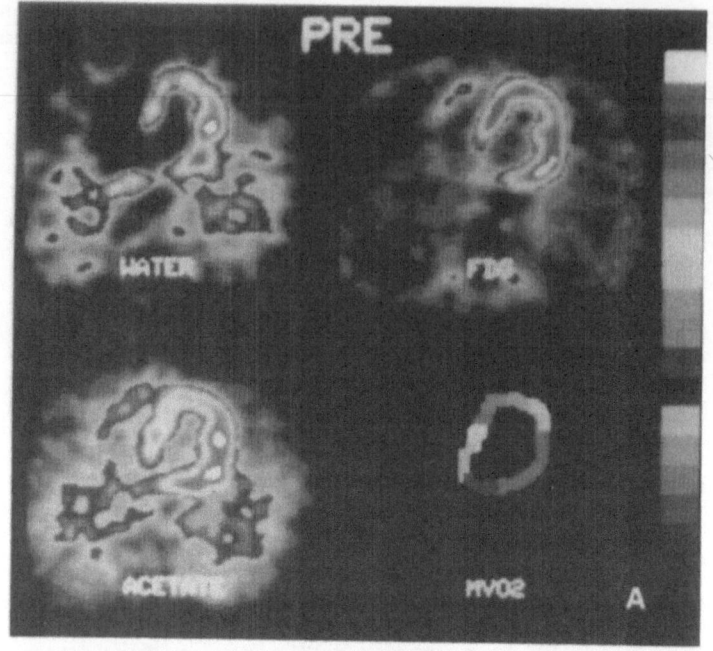

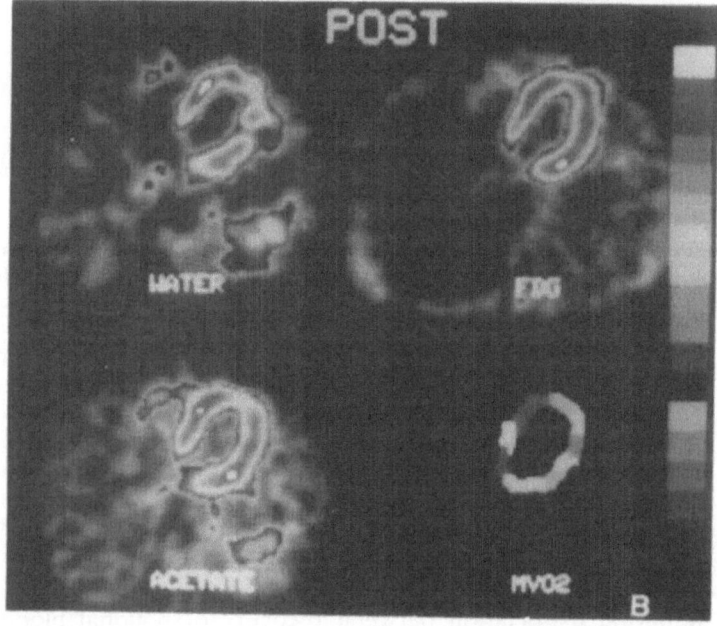

Table 1. Predictive values (in percent) of PET studies for functional improvement after success-ful coronary revascularization.

Source	N	Viable Functional improvement	Nonviable No functional improvement	Tracer
Tillisch [17]	17	85	92	FDG/NH^3
Tamaki [18]	22	78	78	FDG/NH^3
Nienaber [20]	12	93		FDG/NH^3
vom Dahl [56]	40	75	86	FDG/NH^3
Gropler [46]	32	73	78	FDG/H$_2$^{15}O
	32	82	88	Acetate/H$_2$^{15}O

Table 2. Comparative studies between Tl-201-/MIBI-SPECT and FDG-PET and percentage of fixed defects in SPECT that demostrate viability in FDG-PET.

Author	Patients	Fixed defects	Viable	Percent	SPECT tracer
Tamaki [57]	28	39	15	38	Tl-201
Brunken [40, 58]	26	101	47	47	Tl-201
Kiat [59]	21	122	74	61	Tl-201(24hrs.redist)
Dilsizian [60]	100	85	42	49	Tl-201(reinjection)
Ohtani [61]	24	32	15	47	Tl-201(reinjection)
Altehoefer [62]	46	167	38	23	Tc-99 m-MIBI

significant early improvement in blood flow, regional glucose metabolism and wall motion remained abnormal following PTCA, but revealed significant improvement after 67 ± 20 days. Quantitative measurements of enhanced regional glucose uptake relative to blood flow prior to PTCA were linearly related to the degree of *late* functional recovery. Thus, in patients with resting ischemic wall motion abnormalities undergoing PTCA, recovery of regional wall motion parallels normalization of glucose metabolism and is delayed relative to the early restoration of blood flow.

An illustrative case presenting with crescendo angina and large akinesis of the anterior wall is shown in Figure 4. PET revealed markedly reduced blood flow to the anterior wall and apex (Figure 4; left) which, as seen on the FDG images, was associated with regionally enhanced glucose utilization. Coronary angioplasty of a subtotal LAD occlusion restored blood flow to

←

Figure 3. (A) Myocardial perfusion, glucose metabolism and acetate uptake in a patient before myocardial revascularization (PRE) with evidence of viable tissue in the anterior left ventricular wall by preserved uptake of FDG whereas flow (O-15 water) is critically reduced. There is also a moderately reduced, but preserved acetate uptake in the perfusion territory of the LAD indicating a reduced Oxygen consumption (MVO$_2$) in the anterior wall relative to the normal posterolateral wall. (B) After successful revascularization both perfusion and glucose metabolism as well as acetate uptake appear normal. (For colour plate of this figure see **page 537**.)

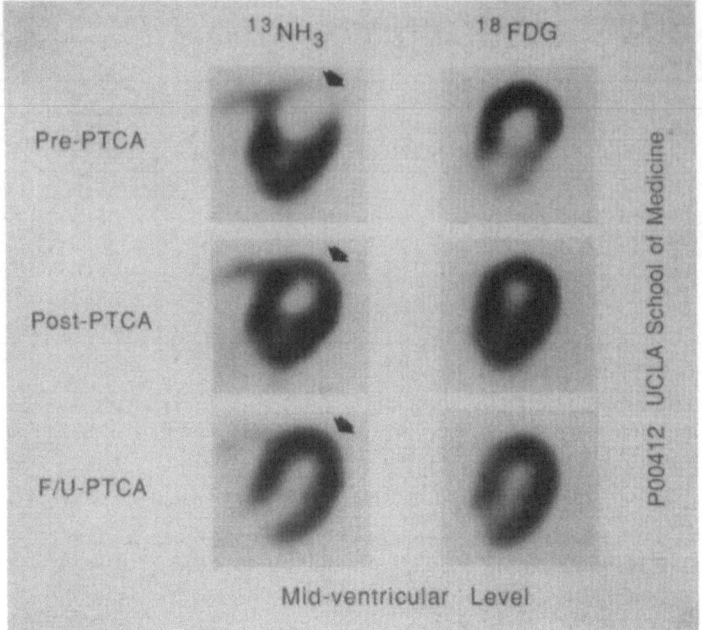

Figure 4. Serial sets of a representative mid-ventricular cross-sectional image of myocardial blood flow ($^{13}NH_3$ = N-13 ammonia) and glucose utilization (^{18}FDG glucose) obtained before (upper row) and three days (center row) and 67 days (lower row) after PTCA in a patient with akinesis of the anterior left ventricular wall. The pre-PTCA N-13 ammonia images reveal an extensive reduction in blood flow to the anterior and anteroseptal wall including the apex (arrow) which on the F-18 2-deoxyglucose images is associated with augmented glucose utilization. Because this patient was admitted acutely, the study was performed with the patient in fasted state, which explains the low glucose uptake in normally perfused myocardium. Three days after angioplasty (center row) blood flow to the anterior wall is markedly improved and perfusion to left ventricular myocardium is homogeneous (arrows). Glucose utilization in the LAD territory is still increased relative to blood flow to the anterior wall. At the time of the late follow-up study (lower row), both blood flow and glucose metabolism in the anterior wall have returned to normal.

the anterior wall as seen on the angiogram (Figure 5) and on a post-PTCA PET study (Figure 4; center); the mild decrease in N-13 activity indicated a slight residual flow deficit and some wall thinning. Glucose utilization at the time of the post-PTCA study continued to be increased relative to blood flow and wall motion of the anterior wall was still suppressed. When reexamined 76 days after PTCA, not only blood flow but, more importantly, glucose metabolism had returned to normal (Figure 4; right). At this time contraction of the anterior wall was markedly improved and paralleled by normalized global function; left ventricular ejection fraction was depressed at 32% prior to PTCA, remained abnormal at 34% early post-PTCA but improved to 62% at late follow-up.

The study by Nienaber et al. proved that segmental reduction in myocar-

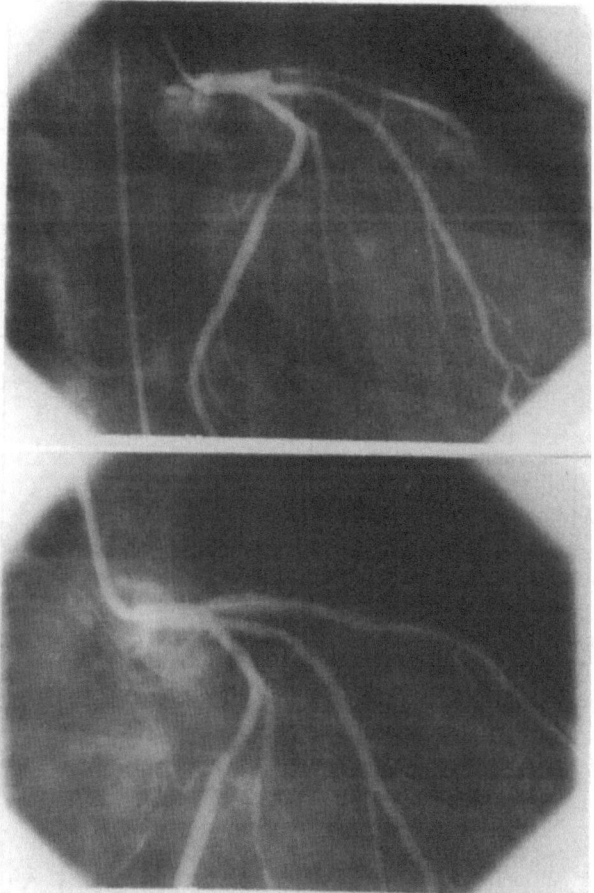

Figure 5. Corresponding coronary arteriograms obtained in the right anterior oblique projection before (upper image) and immediately after PTCA (lower image) in the patient shown in Figure 4 with anterior and apical akinesis. The LAD is subtotally occluded with only sluggish anterograde flow; after successful PTCA (lower image) the LAD is recanalized and normal anterograde flow is reestablished.

dial perfusion, metabolism and wall motion improved at different rates after revascularization [20]. Whereas myocardial perfusion recovered promptly after PTCA, wall motion in the entire group remained unchanged initially, but improved to almost normal contractile function late at follow-up with no further improvement in blood flow. Changes in the perfusion-metabolism mismatch were primarily related to improvement in perfusion early after revascularization, however, normalization of glucose metabolism and wall motion was documented (late) after six weeks. The relationship between preangioplasty perfusion-metabolism mismatch and the postangioplasty im-

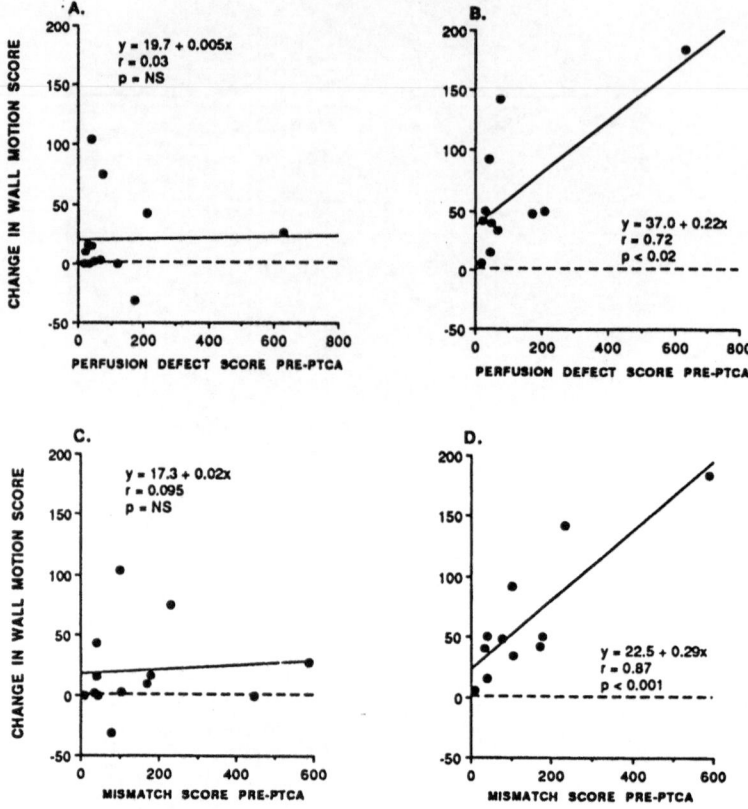

Figure 6. Comparison between the pre-existing blood flow metabolism mismatch score and the improvement in wall motion score from the pre-PTCA to the post-PTCA (left) and the F/U PTCA study (right). Improvement in wall motion at the time of the late follow-up study correlated linearly with the pre-existing blood flow metabolism mismatch score. The 13 data points on the left panel represent 13 dilated lesions and 13 perfusion territories in 12 patients. The 11 data points on the right panel pertain to 11 perfusion territories in 10 patients; two patients had to be excluded from follow-up (late) wall motion analysis due to early restenosis of the PTCA site.

provement in wall motion is shown in Figure 6. Changes in wall motion on the early postangioplasty studies were not related to the preangioplasty perfusion-metabolism mismatch score. However, there was a linear relation between the preangioplasty mismatch score and the functional improvement at follow-up. Although regional myocardial blood flow improved soon after PTCA, glucose utilization remained elevated suggesting an abnormal metabolic state early after PTCA. Two months after PTCA glucose utilization had eventually normalized relative to blood flow and myocardial dysfunction had significantly improved. This data confirm that a perfusion-metabolism mismatch on PET can correctly identify reversible dysfunction and demonstrate a temporal disparity between the recovery of segmental perfusion, metabolism and contractile function in previously hibernating myocardium (and possibly stunned) after successful PTCA. Importantly, the extent and severity of the perfusion-metabolism mismatch before PTCA appears to predict the magnitude of delayed improvement in wall motion [17, 18]. The results also shed more light on the concept of chronic functional and metabolic adaptation to persistent subcritical reductions in myocardial blood flow, referred to as "hibernating myocardium". Experimental evidence showed that an equilibrium of reduced oxygen supply and diminished demand with reversible impairment of contractile function can exist for some time [10, 11, 21]. Matzusaki et al. attained a sustained 37% reduction in segmental systolic function in response to a 56% reduction in blood flow to the endomyocardium over a 5 hour period [22]. In a swine model flow reduction to the endocardial layer by 53% was followed by a transient increase in anaerobic glycolysis as evidenced by lactate production, after which substrate metabolism remained oxidative [23]. Moreover, Opie et al. demonstrated enhanced glucose extraction and an increase in anaerobic glycolysis during sustained reductions in blood flow to small myocardial regions in dog experiments [24], consistent with the relatively increased FDG uptake in human hibernating myocardium.

Another mechanism that might explain a chronic alteration in segmental metabolism and contractile function are repetitive ischemic episodes induced by intermittent coronary occlusion and reperfusion; in an experimental setting this mechanism has been shown to result in severe impairment of contractile function referred to as "stunning" [25, 26]. In both ischemic and in "stunned" or post-ischemic myocardium, glucose utilization was found to be increased [27, 28]. A blood flow/metabolism mismatch in akinetic segments might therefore reflect "stunning" as a consequence of repeated episodes of acute ischemia alternating with periods of "reperfusion" in myocardial regions subtended by severely stenosed coronary arteries. It is possible that "stunning" dominates in patients with unstable or crescendo angina, whereas in the patients with stable coronary artery disease the blood flow metabolism mismatch may better correspond to "hibernation".

Changes in segmental blood flow, metabolism and function after angioplasty

The temporal dissociation between recovery of myocardial blood flow and regional myocardial function and the initial persistence of increased glucose utilization following PTCA is an important insight gained from PET and consistent with delayed recovery of contractile function following restoration of coronary blood flow after transient complete or partial coronary occlusions [22, 23, 25, 27] and compatible with augmented FDG uptake in post-ischemic myocardium [28]. Reperfusion after transient coronary occlusions is associated with an initial depression of fatty acid oxidation as evidenced by abnormal tissue clearance kinetics of C-11 palmitate and by segmentally enhanced uptake of FDG at 24 hours of reperfusion [29, 30]. Recent animal experimental studies suggested that the initial enhancement of F-18 2-deoxyglucose uptake is caused by an increase in anaerobic glycolysis [31]. The augmented release of lactate and the impairment in oxidative metabolism may reflect mitochondrial dysfunction as suggested from animal studies using C-11 acetate as a tracer of tricarbon acid cycle activity [29].

In hibernating myocardium early after revascularization exogenous glucose utilization remained elevated relative to blood flow and compared to reference tissue and regional rates of glucose utilization remained enhanced despite improvement in myocardial blood flow (24% prior to PTCA and by 29% early after PTCA) [20]. Differences in plasma substrate levels or substrate selection between serial studies were excluded and are unlikely to account for the persistent relative increase in glucose utilization immediately after PTCA, while regional blood flow at rest has already returned to normal. Flow reserve, however, may still be impaired as recently shown by subnormal myocardial uptake of Tl-201 during exercise within 9 days of PTCA which was eventually found normal at 3.3 months after PTCA [32]; microvascular "stunning" postulated by Bolli et al. may be one potential explanation [33].

The above temporal dissociation is also consistent with animal experiments [22, 27, 28, 34] as well as with late improvement in global left ventricular function observed in patients after PTCA [16, 35]. The delay in functional recovery, however, is at variance with recent findings by Cohen et al. [36] who noted immediate post-PTCA recovery of wall motion in myocardial segments supplied by the target vessel. Similarly, Sabbah et al. reported a 50% improvement in global left ventricular function within 24 to 48 hours after PTCA [37]. Because the latter two investigations examined symptomatic post-infarction patients, some of the improvements observed in these patients may have been due to the natural course after acute myocardial infarction and may not be attributed solely to PTCA. Catecholamine stimulation of post-ischemic myocardium or altered ventricular loading may be other reasons for early functional improvement. Differences in clinical presentation (stable/unstable angina) may also account for the reported variability in rates of recovery of contractile function.

Clinical implications

Restoration of coronary blood flow by PTCA resulted in a significant improvement of ischemic dysfunction, though full functional recovery is not observed until two months later. First, this study confirms that the blood flow/metabolism mismatch pattern by PET reliably and accurately identifies viable myocardium irrespective of functional impairment. Less sophisticated concepts have been used to identify reversibly injured myocardium such as contractile reserve by post-extrasystolic potentiation [38] or ventricular unloading by nitroglycerin [39]. However, sensitivity and specificity of these approaches are limited. Stress Tl-201 redistribution scintigraphy generally permits differentiation between irreversible and reversible injury but is limited when Tl-201 defects are fixed; identification of viability based on preserved metabolic activity is considered more accurate and reliable [40, 41, 58].

Secondly, the temporal disparity between recovery of myocardial blood flow and contractile function indicates that an early absence of functional improvement does not imply unsuccessful revascularization. Augmented glucose utilization early after PTCA is most likely reflecting effective substrate utilization as evidence of true tissue salvage. This observation is consistent with experimental findings where early evidence of metabolic activity in reperfused canine myocardium rather than restoration of myocardial blood flow predicted long term benefits of reperfusion [42]. Therefore, metabolic activity prior to revascularization accurately predicts the long term functional recovery of myocardium at risk.

Thirdly, the linear relationship between the pre-existing blood flow metabolism mismatch score (combining severity and extent of mismatch) on PET and the improvement in contractile function suggests that the magnitude of functional improvement can be predicted by imaging of blood flow and metabolism with PET [20]; this should prove clinically useful for deciding between interventional revascularization and conservative treatment in patients with severe coronary artery disease and regional or global left ventricular dysfunction, and also helpful to prognosticate the eventual functional outcome.

These results are supported by a study on patients with compromised left ventricular function prior to revascularization in whom the Michigan group reported a negative predictive value of 86% and positive predictive values from 40–75% depending on the severity of baseline wall motion abnormalities (personal communication). Moreover, Tamaki et al. [43] investigated 48 patients after myocardial infarction, 17 of which showed matched defects, whereas 31 patients demonstrated a mismatch in PET flow-metabolism imaging. At 2 year follow-up 39% of patients with PET mismatches and 6% of patients with matches had experienced cardiac events, defined as cardiac death, coronary artery bypass grafting or coronary angioplasty, or unstable angina. Various patterns of metabolic activity may be present in an infarct territory [44], especially after thrombolytic therapy; decreased metabolic activity in the infarct territory appears predictive for no subsequent improvement in function, whereas maintained FDG uptake is associated with a variable functional outcome. Failure of myocardium to recover despite evidence of metabolic activity was attributed to the lack of interventional therapy such as PTCA.

Similarly, Eitzman et al. [45] investigated 82 patients 40 of whom underwent successful revascularization; patients with PET evidence of hibernating myocardium who nevertheless did not undergo revascularization were more likely to experience either myocardial infarction, death, cardiac arrest or late revascularization for new symptoms (event rate 0.5; $p < 0.01$) than the patient group without evidence of viable myocardium in the risk area (event rate 0.139 or the subset with successful revascularization to viable tissue (event rate 0.12).

Alternative approach for the assessment of myocardial viability

Under normoxic conditions oxidative metabolism is a prerequisite for contractile function and the assessment of myocardial oxidative metabolism using C-11-acetate may be helpful to predict functional recovery after revascularization. In 16 patients Gropler et al. [46] showed that oxidative metabolism as assessed by C-11-acetate PET imaging was preserved in hibernating myocardium and a prerequisite for successful recovery of function after revascularization (Figure 3). The levels of oxidative metabolism were higher in patients with reversibly dysfunctional myocardium than in irreversibly dysfunctional myocardium; in their hands FDG uptake or regional perfusion did not reliably separate reversible from irreversible myocardial dysfunction.

Walsh et al. [47] demonstrated in patients after acute myocardial infarction that oxidative metabolism by C-11-acetate imaging was markedly diminished in infarcted segments and did not change appreciably over time. In contrast, reperfused myocardium in patients treated with thrombolysis showed gradual improvement in oxidative metabolism within 10 days after reperfusion. The depression of the C-11-acetate clearance ranged from severe in the central infarction to mild in the hypoperfused periinfarct zone delineated by flow imaging. Other authors showed that only measurements of oxidative metabolism by C-11-acetate differentiated reversibly dysfunctional (viable) myocardial segments from those that were irreversibly dysfunctional when compared to measurements of regional myocardial perfusion or overall glucose metabolism [48].

In a recent animal study Weinheimer et al. investigated the relationship between the recovery of oxidative metabolism after acute myocardial infarction and the recovery of contractile function after reperfusion. They demonstrated that prompt reperfusion is associated with more rapid and complete recovery of oxidative metabolism and myocardial function and that recovery of contractile function lags behind recovery of oxidative metabolism [14]. Regional oxygen consumption may thus be an independent marker for residual tissue viability and potentially useful for further stratification of therapeutic interventions.

Conversely, Vanoverschelde [49] demonstrated in 15 patients with acute myocardial infarction and reperfusion that C11-acetate kinetics did not differ between hypoperfused segments with and without flow/metabolism mismatches by FDG. These results are in conflict with previous findings [47, 48] and suggest that C-11-acetate does not provide additional information to that obtained from blood flow measurements. Before these conflicting results are clarified the clinical potential of C-11-acetate imaging remains unclear and speculative.

PET viability and cardiac transplantation

In patients with endstage ischemic cardiomyopathy cardiac transplantation is an accepted therapeutic strategy at many institutions. Due to donor shortage, only about 10% of patients eligible for cardiac transplantation undergo the operation. With the possibility of identifying hypoperfused but viable, i.e. salvageable myocardium, more aggressive coronary revascularization rather than cardiac transplantation in patients with progressive coronary artery disease and severe left ventricular dysfunction may be feasible [50]. Louie et al. [51] reported the clinical outcome of 207 patients initially proposed for cardiac transplantation, 22 of whom, however, underwent coronary artery revascularization based on the result of PET metabolic imaging; three year survival of the revasculated patients was $72 \pm 10\%$, similar to $73 \pm 6\%$ in the transplanted group. In 83% of these 22 patients the preoperative PET study showed a flow/metabolism mismatch indicating salvageable myocardium and left ventricular ejection fraction increased in these patients from 26 to 36% after revascularization. Two patients with no evidence of viability in the target area on the preoperative PET study subsequently had no improvement of contractile function after revascularization. Similar results were recently shown by Dreyfus et al. and underscore the usefulness of PET metabolic imaging to stratify potential heart transplant candidates for revascularization procedures [52].

Pitfalls in PET metabolic imaging

There are several factors potentially limiting the evaluation of regional tissue viability using PET with FDG or C-11-acetate. Accuracy of FDG as a marker for myocardial viability may suffer from regional differences in myocardial FDG uptake. Gropler et al. demonstrated less FDG accumulation in the interventricular septum versus the lateral wall [53]. In normals under fasting conditions C-11-acetate clearance rate constants are slightly higher in the septum compared to the lateral wall, suggesting higher oxygen consumption in this region. Furthermore delayed FDG uptake following reperfusion has been observed in animal studies and may complicate the metabolic evaluation of patients shortly after acute myocardial infarction [54]. Occasionally, FDG image quality is poor in patients with diabetes, but may be improved by insulin administration prior to FDG application [55]. Some patients studied soon after thrombolytic treatment and with heparin infusion show suppression of myocardial FDG uptake due to an elevation of plasma free-fatty acids [44]. High circulating catecholamine levels may also suppress myocardial glucose utilization because of their anti-insulin effect.

Conclusion

Combined perfusion and metabolic imaging using N-13-ammonia or O-15 water and FDG can accurately identify ischemically compromised myocardium and differentiate it from myocardial scars. The extent of myocardial salvage and the amount of residual jeopardized myocardium are important clinical questions to be addressed prior to further interventions like angioplasty, coronary artery bypass surgery or cardiac transplantation. Therefore viability studies using FDG alone matched with regional contractile function or in concert with a perfusion marker are useful in the identification of viable myocardium at risk and thus to select patients for revascularization. Maintained FDG uptake predicts functional recovery and the likelihood of further cardiac events after revascularization. In contrast to FDG, the kinetics of myocardial clearance of C-11-acetate are insensitive to the pattern of myocardial substrate use. Recovery of oxidative metabolism as assessed by C-11-acetate PET appears to precede and also to predict recovery of contractile function after revascularization in coronary artery disease and myocardial infarction. C-11-acetate, therefore, may be another tracer for the identification of tissue viability. Since PET is a highly expensive and sophisticated tool it should only be performed in well defined situations. At present PET studies are likely to improve the diagnostic information in patients with chronic advanced CAD with severely impaired left ventricular function. Moreover, coronary anatomy should be known prior to a PET viability study because only patients with an anatomy suitable for revascularization will eventually benefit from such an examination. Finally, in a clinical environment with limited access to PET it appears wise to perform metabolic imaging with PET in absence of reversible perfusion abnormalities on Tl-201 reinjection SPECT scans. (See also Chapters 3, 14–16 and 18.)

References

1. Gallagher BM, Folwer JS, Gutterson NI et al. Metabolic trapping as a principle of radiopharmaceutical design: Some factors responsible for the biodistribution of 18F-desoxy-2-fuoro-D-glucose. J Nucl Med 1978; 19: 1154–61.
2. Krivokapich J, Huang SC, Selin CE, Phleps ME. Fluorodesoxyglucose rate constants, lumped constant, and glucose metabolic rate in rabbit heart. Am J Physiol 1987; 252: H777–87.
3. Phelps ME, Huan SC, Hoffman EJ et al. Tomographic measurement of local glucose metabolic rate in humans with F-desoxy-2-fluoro-D-glucose: Validation of method. Ann Neurol 1979; 6: 371–38.
4. Gambhir SS, Schwaiger M, Huang SC et al. Simple noninvasive quantification method for measuring myocardial glucose utilization in humans employing positron emission tomography and fluorine-18-desoxyglucose. J Nucl Med 1989; 30: 359–66.
5. Buxton DB, Nienaber CA, Luxen A et al. Noninvasive quantitation of regional myocardial oxygen consumption in vivo with 1-C-11-acetate and dynamic positron emission tomography. Circulation 1989; 79: 134–42.

6. Brown M, Marshall DR, Sobel BE, Bergmann SR. Delineation of myocardial oxygen utilization with carbon-11-labeled acetate. Circulation 1987; 76: 687–96.
7. Armbrecht JJ, Buxton SR, Brunken RC et al. Regional myocardial oxygen consumption determined non-invasively in humans with 1-C-11-acetate and dynamic positron tomography. Circulation 1989, 80: 863–72.
8. Buxton DB, Schwaiger M, Nguyen A et al. Radiolabeled acetate as a tracer of myocardial tricarboxylic acid flux. Circ Res 1988; 63: 628–34.
9. Buck A, Hutchins GG, Westra P, Schwaiger M. Compartment model for delineation of myocardial C-11-acetate kinetics (Abstr). J Nucl Med 1990; 31: 777.
10. Rahimtoola SH. The hibernating myocardium (editorial). Am Heart J 1989; 117: 211–21.
11. Braunwald E, Rutherford JD. Reversible ischemic left ventricular dysfunction: Evidence for the "hibernating myocardium" (editorial). J Am Coll Cardiol 1986; 8: 1467–70.
12. Liedke AJ. Alterations of carbohydrate and lipid metabolism in the acutely ischemic heart. Progr Cardiovasc Dis 1981; 23: 321–36.
13. Marshall RC, Tillisch JH, Phelps ME et al. Effects and differentiation of resting myocardial ischemia in man with positron computed tomography, F18-labeled fluorodeoxyglucose and N13-ammonia. Circulation 1983; 67: 766–78.
14. Weinheimer CJ, Brown MA, Nohara R et al. Functional recovery after reperfusion is predicated on recovery of myocardial oxidative metabolism. Am Heart J 1993; 125: 939–49.
15. Detre K, Peduzzi P, Murphy M et al. Effect of bypass surgery on survival in patients in low- and high-risk subgroups delineated by the use of simple clinical variables. Circulation 1981; 63: 1329–38.
16. Kent KM, Bonow RO, Rosing DR et al. Improved myocardial function during exercise after successful percutaneous transluminal coronary angioplasty. N Engl J Med 1982; 306: 441–6.
17. Tillisch J, Brunken R, Marshall R et al. Reversibility of cardiac wall motion abnormalities predicted by positron tomography. N Engl J Med 1986; 314: 886–8.
18. Tamaki N, Yonekura Y, Yamashita K et al. Positron emission tomography using fluorine-18-deoxyglucose in evaluation of coronary artery bypass grafting. Am J Cardiol 1989; 64: 860–5.
19. Al-Aouar ZR, Eitzman D, Hepner A et al. PET assessment of myocardial tissue viability. The University of Michigan experience (Abstr) J Nucl Med 1990; 31: 801.
20. Nienaber CA, Brunken RC, Sherman CT et al. Metabolic and functional recovery of ischemic human myocardium after coronary angioplasty. J Am Coll Cardiol 1991; 18: 966–78.
21. Ratib O, Bidaut L, Nienaber C et al. Semiautomatic software for quantitative analysis of cardiac positron tomography studies. SPIE Medical Imaging II, International Society for Optical Engineering 1988; 914: 412–9.
22. Matsuzaki M, Gallagher KP, Kemper WS et al. Sustained regional dysfunction produced by prolonged coronary stenosis: Gradual recovery after reperfusion. Circulation 1983; 68: 170–182.
23. Fedele FA, Gewirtz H, Capone RJ et al. Metabolic response to prolonged reduction of myocardial blood flow distal to a severe coronary artery stenosis. Circulation 1988; 78: 729–35.
24. Opie LH, Owen P, Riemersma RA. Relative rates of oxidation of glucose and free fatty acids by ischemic and non-ischemic myocardium after coronary artery ligation in the dog. Eur J Clin Invest 1973; 3: 419–24.
25. Nicklas JM, Becker LC, Bulkley BH. Effects of repeated brief coronary occlusions on regional left ventricular function and dimension in dogs. Am J Cardiol 1985; 56: 473.
26. Braunwald E, Kloner RA. The stunned myocardium: Prolonged, postischemic ventricular dysfunction. Circulation 1982; 66: 1146–9.
27. Kloner RA, DeBoer LW, Darsee JR et al. Prolonged abnormalities of myocardium salvaged by reperfusion. Am J Physiol 1981; 241: 591H–9H.

28. Schwaiger M, Schelbert HR, Ellison D et al. Sustained regional abnormalities in cardiac metabolism after transient ischemia in the chronic dog model. J Am Coll Cardiol 1985; 6: 336–47.

29. Buxton DB, Schwaiger M, Vaghaiwalla Mody F et al. Regional abnormality of oxygen consumption in reperfusion with [1-^{11}C] acetate and positron emission tomography. Am J Cardiac Imaging (in press).

30. Schwaiger M, Schelbert HR, Keen R et al. Retention and clearance of C-11 palmitic acid in ischemic and reperfused canine myocardium. J Am Coll Cardiol 1985; 6: 311–20.

31. Schwaiger M, Neese RA, Araujo L et al. Sustained nonoxidative glucose utilization and depletion of glycogen in reperfused canine myocardium. J Am Coll Cardiol 1989; 13: 745–54.

32. Manyari DE, Knudtson M, Kloiber R, Roth D. Sequential thallium-201 myocardial perfusion studies after successful percutaneous transluminal coronary artery angioplasty: Delayed resolution of exercise-induced scintigraphic abnormalities. Circulation 1988; 77: 86–95.

33. Bolli R. Oxygen-derived free radicals and post-ischemic myocardial dysfunction ("stunned myocardium"). J Am Coll Cardiol 1988; 12:239–49.

34. Vatner SF. Correlation between acute reduction in myocardial blood flow and function in conscious dogs. Circ Res 1980; 47: 201–7.

35. De Feyter PJ, Suryapranata H, Serruys PW et al. Effects of successful percutaneous transluminal coronary angioplasty on global and regional left ventricular function in unstable angina pectoris. Am J Cardiol 1987; 60: 993–7.

36. Cohen M, Charney R, Hershman R et al. Reversal of chronic ischemic myocardial dysfunction after transluminal coronary angioplasty. J Am Coll Cardiol 1988; 12: 1193–8.

37. Sabbah HN, Brymer JF, Gheorghiade M et al. Left ventricular function after successful percutaneous transluminal coronary angioplasty for postinfarction angina pectoris. Am J Cardiol 1988; 62: 358–62.

38. Popio KA, Gorlin R, Bechtel D, Levine JA. Postextrasystolic potentiation as a predictor of potential myocardial viability: Preoperative analyses compared with studies after coronary bypass surgery. Am J Cardiol 1977; 39: 944–53.

39. Helfant RH, Pine R, Meister SG et al. Nitroglycerin to unmask reversible asynergy: Correlation with postcoronary ventriculography. Circulation 1974; 50: 108–19.

40. Brunken RC, Kottou S, Nienaber CA et al. PET detection of viable tissue in myocardial segments with persistent defects at Tl-201 SPECT. Radiology 1989; 172: 65–73.

41. Bonow RO, Dilsizian V, Cuocolo A, Bacharach SL. Identification of viable myocardium in patients with chronic coronary artery disease and left ventricular dysfunction. Comparison of thallium scintigraphy with reinjection and PET imaging with 18F-fluorodeoxyglucose. Circulation 1991; 83: 26–37.

42. Knabb RM, Bergmann SR, Fox KAA, Sobel BE. The temporal pattern of recovery of myocardial perfusion and metabolism delineated by positron emission tomography after coronary thrombolysis. J Nucl Med. 1987; 28: 1563–70.

43. Tamaki N, Yonekura Y, Yamasa K et al. Prognostic significance of augmented uptake of FDG on PET in areas of myocardial infarction (Abstr). J Nucl Med 1991; 32: 1039.

44. Schwaiger M, Brunken R, Grover-McKay M et al. Regional myocardial metabolism in patients with acute myocardial infarction assessed by positron emission tomography. J Am Coll Cardiol 1986; 8: 800–8.

45. Eitzman D, Al-Aouar Z, Kanter HL et al. Clinical outcome of patients with advanced coronary artery disease after viability studies with positron emission tomography. J Am Coll Cardiol 1992; 20: 559–65.

46. Gropler RJ, Geltman EM, Samapathkumaran K et al. Functional recovery after coronary revascularization for chronic coronary artery disease is dependent on maintenance of oxidative metabolism. J Am Coll Cardiol 1992; 20: 569–77.

47. Walsh MN, Geltman EM, Brown MA et al. Noninvasive estimation of regional myocardial

oxygen consumption by positron emission tomography with carbon-11 acetate in patients with myocardial infarction. J Nucl Med 1989; 30: 1798–808.

48. Gropler RJ, Siegel BA, Samapathkumaran K et al. Dependence of recovery of contractile function on maintenance of oxidative metabolism after myocardial infarction. J Am Coll Cardiol 1992; 19: 989–97.
49. Vanoverschelde JJ, Melin JA, Bol A et al. Regional oxidative metabolism in patients after recovery from reperfused anterior myocardial infarction: Relation to regional blood flow and glucose uptake. Circulation 1992; 85: 9–21.
50. Kron IL, Flanagan TL, Blackbourne LH et al. Coronary revascularization rather than cardiac transplantation for chronic ischemic cardiomyopathy. Ann Surg 1989; 210: 348–54.
51. Louie HW, Laks H, Milgalter E et al. Ischemic cardiomyopathy: Criteria for coronary revascularization and cardiac transplantation. Circulation 1991; 83 (Suppl): III 290–295.
52. Dreyfus GD, Duboc DD, Blasco A et al. Myocardial viability assessment in ischemic cardiomyopathy: Benefits from coronary revascularization. Ann Thoracic Surg 1994; 57: 1402–8.
53. Gropler RJ, Siegal BA, Lee KJ et al. Nonuniformity in myocardial accumulation of F-18–fluorodeoxyglucose in normal fasted humans. J Nucl Med 1990: 1749–56.
54. Hashimoto T, Kambara H, Fudo T et al. Non-Q wave versus Q wave myocardial infarction: Regional myocardial metabolism and blood flow assessed by positron emission tomography. J Am Coll Cardiol 1988; 12: 88–93.
55. Besozzi MC, Smith GT, Goodman MM et al. Improved clinical PET F-18–fluoro-deoxyglucose (FDG) imaging in diabetics following IV insulin injections (Abstr). J Nucl Med 1990; 30: 933.
56. vom Dahl J, Schwaiger M. Positronen-Emissions-Tomographie in der kardiologischen Diagnostik: Prinzipien und klinische Anwendungen. Schweiz Rundschau Med. 1992; 81: 1281–1289.
57. Tamaki N, Yonekura Y, Yamashita K et al. Relation of left ventricular perfusion and wall motion with metabolic activity in persistent defects on thallium-201 tomography in healed myocardial infarction. Am J Cardiol 1988; 62: 202–8.
58. Brunken RC, Mody VF, Hawkins RA et al. Positron emission tomography detects metabolic viability in myocardium with persistent 24-hour SPECT thallium-201 perfusion. defects. Circulation 1992; 86: 1357–69.
59. Kiat H, Berman DS, Maddahi J, Yang LD et al. Late reversibility of tomographic myocardial thallium-201 defects: An accurate marker of myocardial viability. J Am Coll Cardiol 1988; 12: 1456–63.
60. Dilsizian V, Rocco TP, Freeman NMT et al. Enhanced detection of ischemic but viable myocardium by reinjection of thallium after stress-redistribution. N Engl J Med 1990; 323: 141–6.
61. Othani H, Tamaki N, Yonekura Y et al. Value of thallium-201 reinjection after delayed SPECT imaging for predicting reversible ischemia after coronary bypass grafting. Am J Cardiol 1990; 66: 394–9.
62. Altehoefer C, Kaiser HJ, Dörr R et al. Fluorine-18 deoxyglucose PET for the assessment of viable myocardium in perfusion defects in Tc99 m-MIBI SPECT: A comparative study in patients with coronary artery disease. Eur J Nucl Med 1992; 19: 334–42.

Corresponding Author: Dr Christoph A. Nienaber, Department of Cardiology, University Hospital Eppendorf, Martinistrasse 52, D-20246, Hamburg, Germany

18. Assessment of viability in severely hypokinetic myocardium before revascularization and prediction of functional recovery: The role of echocardiography

LUC A. PIERARD

Introduction

Since the last decade, it is well established that persistent, severe myocardial dysfunction in patients with coronary artery disease does not always indicate myocardial necrosis and irreversible damage. The differentiation between viable and non viable tissue is thus of great clinical relevance in order to take an appropriate decision in the individual patient. Akinetic but viable myocardium may correspond to several different states that are important but difficult to be distinguished. The concepts of stunning and hibernation have been introduced [1, 2]; the terms are increasingly used; knowledge about their respective mechanisms has largely improved [3, 4] and several techniques have been studied for their identification [5]. These techniques can assess regional perfusion, membrane integrity, metabolism or contractility. There are several important questions to be answered in the clinical environment: Does this patient have viable myocardium? What is the extent of viable tissue? Does this patient require a revascularization procedure to improve his segmental function? Can I quantitatively predict the amount of functional recovery? What are the relative risks/benefits of the different therapeutic approaches? The answers to these questions are particularly crucial when global left ventricular function is severely depressed.

This chapter will review the role of echocardiography to assess viability and predict recovery in different clinical settings.

Myocardial states (Figure 1)

To achieve its goal of systolic contraction and active relaxation, the myocardium needs adequate energy supply from oxidative metabolism and is dependent on correct perfusion from sufficient coronary flow. Reduction in myocardial perfusion leads to ischemia which results in immediate loss of contraction [6]. There are several possible outcomes of myocardial ischemia [7]. If ischemia is severe, prolonged with total coronary occlusion and no residual

C.A. Nienaber and U. Sechtem (eds): Imaging and Intervention in Cardiology, 279–293.
© 1996 *Kluwer Academic Publishers.*

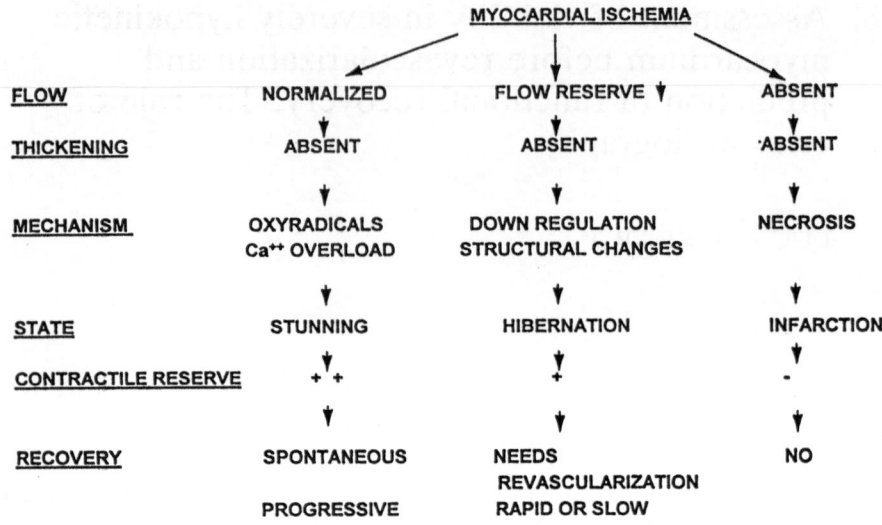

Figure 1. The different possible outcomes of myocardial ischemia.

flow, myocardial necrosis occurs and results in irreversible damage and scar formation. If ischemia is brief, ventricular dysfunction is immediately reversible and contractile recovery is rapid. If ischemia is longer, a period of postischemic dysfunction – stunning – is observed, despite complete normalization of flow. The duration of stunning may be long – several days – but functional recovery occurs spontaneously, without any intervention [8]. Myocardial dysfunction in stunned areas is associated with a decrease in oxidative metabolism and an impairment in fatty acids handling, induced by the transient reduction in oxygen delivery. However, stunned myocardium has a substantial metabolic and inotropic reserve. During inotropic stimulation by a catecholamine, regional myocardial thickening is largely increased with a concomitant increase in oxidative metabolism. This inotropic reserve can be used for therapeutic purposes, if left ventricular postischemic dysfunction causes hemodynamic instability. Experimental studies have demonstrated that functionally depressed but stunned myocardial regions may respond considerably, without adverse effects to beta-adrenergic agonists [9–11]. Functional reserve during inotropic stimulation can also be used for diagnostic purposes. However, optimal assessment of myocardial stunning requires the demonstration of flow-contraction mismatch – asynergy, despite normal flow – by simultaneous measurements of regional flow and thickening [12]. The diagnosis is thus frequently suggested retrospectively when spontaneous functional recovery has been demonstrated. However, the reversibility of a contractile abnormality does not necessarily imply myocardial stunning.

There is another possible outcome of myocardial ischemia. If some residual flow exists, regional contractile dysfunction that immediately follows the ischemic episode, can be matched to flow impairment. This time-dependent adjustment may lead to a steady state condition in which myocardial oxygen demand decreases and a delicate balance develops between reduced regional myocardial flow and function. This is called short-term hibernation. In experimental models of short-term hibernating myocardium, metabolic indexes of myocardial ischemia improve over time: lactate production gradually returns toward consumption during the ensuing hours [13]. In this model, inotropic reserve is also present and dobutamine administration increases regional contraction, but at the expense of metabolic recovery [4]. If the inotropic challenge is prolonged, maintenance of hibernation is disturbed, metabolically defined ischemia worsens and myocardial infarction develops [14]. These models are recent, but the term hibernation has been previously introduced from clinical evidence of functional recovery after late revascularization of asynergic areas [15]. This concept implies long-term hibernation during months or years. Down regulation of contractility is accompanied by histological abnormalities. The ultrastructural characteristics of the myocytes are loss of myofibrillar content, cellular swelling, accumulation of glycogen and abnormalities of the mitochondria [16]. Recent observations have demonstrated that some patients with chronic regional dysfunction, who had non-infarcted collateral-dependent asynergic myocardium with histological abnormalities had nearly normal resting flow, but a very limited flow reserve [17]. Thus, in contrast with stunned myocardium, hibernating myocardium needs an intervention to recover its function. Oxygen supply must improve; the intervention usually is a revascularization procedure: coronary angioplasty or bypass grafting.

Clinical settings

There are different clinical settings potentially associated with severely hypokinetic, but viable myocardium. Some of these clinical situations produce transient reversible ischemia followed by reperfusion; the ischemic insult may be regional in patients with variant or unstable angina, severe and prolonged exercise-induced ischemia or after percutaneous transluminal coronary angioplasty. Ischemia may be global in the case of cardiac surgery or cardiac transplantation. The development of stunning is thus likely in these conditions [18].

The two clinical situations in which the identification of viable and salvageable myocardium is most relevant are acute myocardial infarction and advanced coronary artery disease with impaired left ventricular function. The

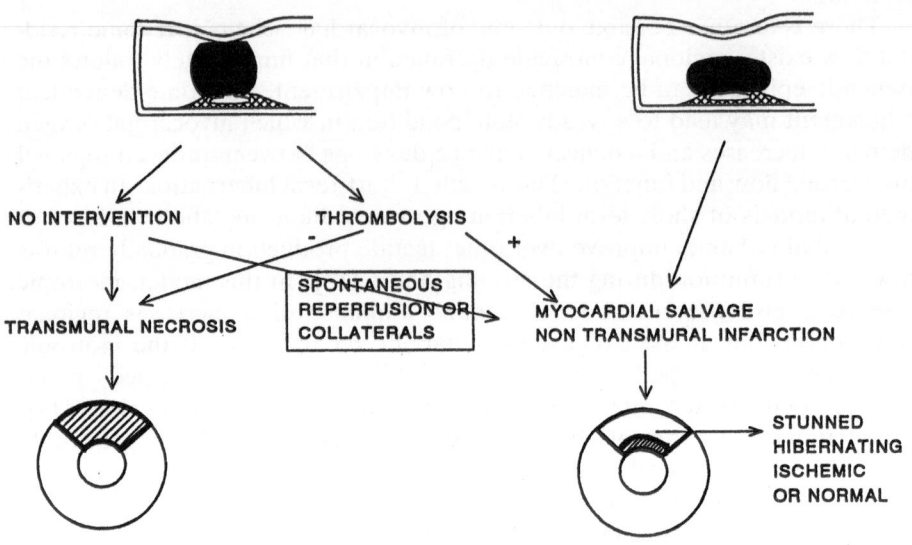

SUSTAINED CORONARY OCCLUSION   SUBTOTAL CORONARY OCCLUSION

Figure 2. Mechanisms of complete or incomplete infarction.

usefulness and limitations of echocardiography in these two settings must be presented separately.

Acute myocardial infarction

Incomplete infarction (Figure 2)

Acute myocardial infarction is caused in the majority of cases by the occurrence of coronary thrombosis. In the absence of collateral circulation, persistence of coronary occlusion more than a few hours is followed by complete, transmural necrosis of the affected area with a risk of cardiac rupture or infarct expansion and left ventricular remodeling. In contrast, the infarction may be incomplete if collateral circulation is recruitable when coronary thrombosis develops, if coronary artery obstruction remains incomplete or if spontaneous reperfusion occurs. In the interventional era, timely reperfusion is frequently the result of thrombolytic therapy or immediate angioplasty: the potentially transmural infarct is converted into a non transmural infarction. In this situation, there is a mixture of subendocardial necrosis and subepicardial salvage. The respective amount of necrotic and viable tissue is highly variable from patient to patient, depending on the rapidity of reperfusion, the quality of recovered flow and the severity of residual stenosis.

An incomplete infarction has two characteristics: functional recovery may occur, improving prognosis, but viable myocardium may be at jeopardy, with an increased risk of residual ischemia or recurrent cardiac events.

Functional recovery

Since early systematic coronary arteriography cannot be recommended after thrombolytic therapy [19], non-invasive techniques are important to distinguish between stunned, jeopardized and necrotic myocardium. Early assessment of regional contractility by echocardiography, radionuclide angiography or magnetic resonance imaging does not indicate the extent of myocardial salvage, because functional improvement is usually delayed for several days or even longer [20, 21]. The time course of functional recovery is controversial: some investigators suggested that most of the improvement occurred during the first 3 days [22] or the first 10 days [23]. Others found that functional recovery was modest in the first 3 days [24] and predominantly developed after hospital discharge [25].

It must be recognized that the absence of functional recovery in resting condition does not imply the absence of myocardial salvage: the remaining absence of thickening may be related to either a too important portion of necrosed endocardium or to a too critical residual coronary stenosis. Indeed, myocardial thickening at rest is largely dependent on the endocardial half of the ventricular segment [26]. When more than 20% infarct is present in a ventricular region, wall thickening is abolished at rest [27]. Thus, hypokinetic myocardium in baseline condition after acute myocardial infarction indicates that the transmural extent of necrosis is less than 20%. There is a threshold phenomenon and no difference in the degree of systolic thinning as the transmural extent of infarct increases from 21% to 100% [27].

The use of echocardiography: Advantages and limitations

Echocardiography is a widely available and relatively cheap technique which can be performed at the bedside. It provides real time visualization of myocardial thickening. Regional function can be monitored continuously during interventions. Storage and retrieval of images are improved since the development of digitization and similar views can be displayed simultaneously in a cine-loop format for comparing function at different times or before and during the infusion of a pharmacological agent. Echocardiography is however operator dependent: experience is required for correct recording and interpretation of images. Quantitation of regional myocardial thickening is accurate using M-mode echocardiography, but conventional M-mode can only be used in limited ventricular regions. Assessment of contractility in other segments not accessible to M-mode recording is only qualitative, leading to some subjectivity.

Dobutamine echocardiography after myocardial infarction

Myocardial viability

Postischemic, stunned myocardium has contractile reserve. A recent experimental model demonstrated that, in the absence of residual coronary stenosis, when subendocardial necrosis coexists with subepicardial stunning, the absolute degree of wall thickening during dobutamine indicates the extent of salvaged myocardium [28]. Furthermore, the dose of dobutamine needed to elicit maximal thickening is related to the amount of myocardial necrosis. In this experiment, there was no further increase in wall thickening at doses higher than 15 µg/kg/min [28].

We were the first to use low-dose dobutamine echocardiography for the identification of viable myocardium in patients with myocardial infarction after thrombolytic therapy: positron emission tomography (PET) was also performed for comparison [29]. Echocardiographic images were recorded in baseline conditions and during dobutamine infusion at 5 and 10 µg/kg/min. With PET, segmental perfusion and glucose uptake were measured at rest.

A group of patients had predominantly myocardial stunning: perfusion was normal with PET in the affected area and inotropic reserve was demonstrated with 5 or 10 µg/kg/min of dobutamine in akinetic segments. Spontaneous functional recovery was observed on the follow-up echocardiogram. Most of these patients had a non-Q wave infarction and non significant or moderate residual stenosis.

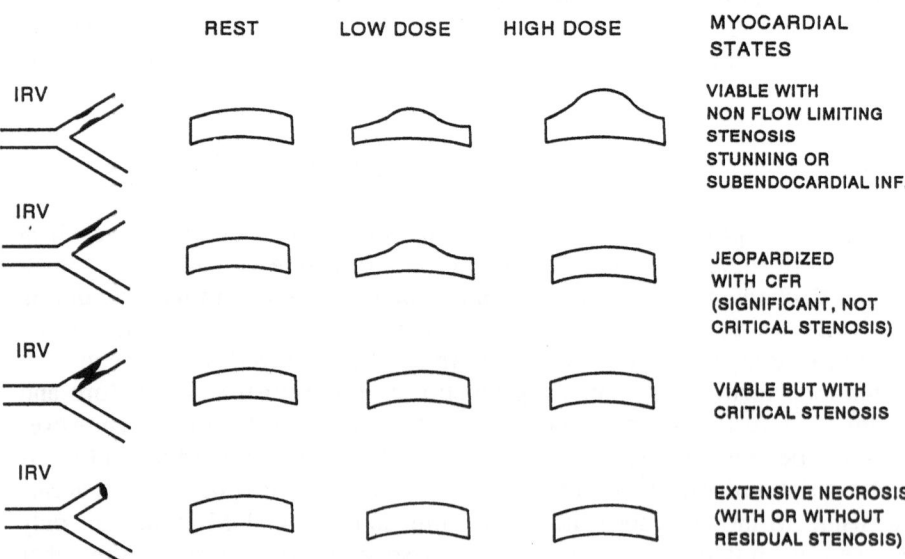

Figure 3. Dobutamine echocardiography after myocardial infarction. CFR = coronary flow reserve.

Another group of patients had akinetic segments, with decreased perfusion and high glucose uptake, indicating the presence of hibernating myocardium. Most patients, but not all, exhibited improvement in function with dobutamine infusion, but functional recovery was scarce. Loss of viability was confirmed in some patients by a follow-up PET study. It is also possible that some patients in this group who did not recover had a significant proportion of necrosis leading to absence of wall thickening at rest, but had viable myocardium in the outer layers with possible recruitment during exercise and prevention of left ventricular dilatation.

Finally, patients with concordant decrease in both perfusion and glucose utilization, indicating predominant necrosis, had no improvement with dobutamine and no functional recovery [29].

Our findings have been confirmed by other groups. Barilla et al. [30] studied patients with small infarcts and dobutamine responsive wall motion was sensitive for the assessment of postischemic dysfunction. Because most of their patients had critical coronary stenosis, functional recovery was significantly more frequent in those who underwent a revascularization procedure.

Smart et al. [31] found a lower dose of dobutamine (4 µg/kg/min) to be more sensitive in the detection of reversible dysfunction: it is probable that the higher dose used (20 or 40 µg/kg/min) in their study could have induced ischemia thus lowering the sensitivity.

Watada et al. [32] found an excellent correlation between the akinetic length ratios measured during dobutamine infusion (10 µg/kg/min) and in the late convalescent stage.

Jeopardized myocardium

It is important to differentiate stunned myocardium that can recover spontaneously, from jeopardized or hibernating myocardium that requires revascularization. Dobutamine echocardiography can also be used, but at increasing doses from 5 to 10, then 20, 30 and 40 µg/kg/min, with the addition of atropine (0.25 to 1 mg), if the increase in heart rate remains insufficient with dobutamine alone. Myocardial viability remains detectable at low dose during the early phase of the study, but contractility can deteriorate at a higher dose in the same segments or a normal adjacent zone. This biphasic pattern relates to a decrease in coronary flow reserve and indicates the presence of a significant residual stenosis of the infarct-related artery [33].

Sustained improvement, that is improvement in contractility till peak dose without deterioration suggests the presence of viable tissue, with non-flow limiting residual stenosis. The target heart rate – 85% of maximal heart rate – must be obtained in order to avoid false-negative results. In some patients, no improvement is observed at low dose of dobutamine in the affected segments, but abnormal wall thickening becomes apparent in adjacent segments at higher doses: this pattern is also suggestive of residual stenosis of the infarct-related artery. For instance, akinesis of the apical part of the septum and the anterior wall in basal conditions and inducible hypokinesis of the basal part with dobutamine suggest an incomplete infarction with a significant stenosis of the proximal left anterior descending artery. With high-dose dobutamine echocardiography, asynergy may also be identified at a distance of the infarct zone. We found that this observation indicates the presence of multivessel coronary artery disease with a sensitivity of 85%, a specificity of 88% and an overall accuracy of 87% [34].

In patients with a posterior infarction, when ischemia develops in adjacent segments, it is sometimes difficult to distinguish between ischemia within the infarct zone or in the territory of another vascular region without knowledge of the patient's coronary anatomy [35].

It must be recognized that persistence of akinesis in the affected region during a dobutamine test does not necessarily imply absence of residual viability. In the presence of a critical residual stenosis of the infarct-related vessel, when flow reserve is minimal, wall thickening may not increase despite significant amounts of viable myocardium. In our experience, contractile reserve is rare a few days after infarction, when the infarct-related artery is occluded, even when collaterals are visible at angiography. However, angiography is frequently performed several days or weeks after the acute event: collateral circulation observed at that moment is not representative of collateral function present during the first hours after the onset of infarction [36]. It is possible that collaterals were not recruitable for myocardial salvage but developed after the acute stage.

Other modes of stress echocardiography

Experimental data have demonstrated that the function of postischemic myocardium can be improved by an increase in coronary blood flow [37]. Picano et al. used the dipyridamole test in 22 patients after myocardial infarction and found a good concordance with delayed resting thallium scintigraphy for prediction of tissue viability [38]. In a subgroup of 15 patients, a significant functional recovery was found in 15 of 19 segments with and only 5 of 39 without dipyridamole-induced improvement (79 vs 13%, p < 0.01).

Improvement followed by worsening can also be found with dipyridamole, indicating that myocardium is viable but jeopardized [39].

Exercise echocardiography is theoretically another possible technique. Echocardiographic observation should however be made continuously during exercise for this purpose: however, this remains difficult. Post-exercise imaging is easier, but the biphasic response – improvement followed by deterioration – would indeed be missed by image recording limited to the post-exercise period. There are at present no published studies assessing the role of exercise echocardiography for identifying viable, but jeopardized myocardium.

Chronic coronary artery disease

Chronic ventricular dysfunction and possible recovery (Figure 4)

Functional recovery may occur after revascularization in patients with advanced coronary artery disease and left ventricular dysfunction [40]. The improved prognosis after bypass grafting is indeed highest in patients with triple-vessel disease and low ejection fraction [41]. This clinical observation led to the introduction of the term hibernating myocardium.

Although the exact mechanisms of hibernation are not yet fully understood [17], the issue of distinguishing between viable and fibrotic tissue has important implications for clinical decision making. This question is probably not very important when the main symptom is angina and when left ventricular dysfunction is moderate, but it is really crucial in patients with heart failure and low ejection fraction. Optimal evaluation should provide both high positive and high negative predictive value for recovery in order to select appropriately between revascularization and cardiac transplantation. However, in most patients, non contractile myocardium represents an admixture of areas in different states: scar, ischemia, stunning, hibernation or normal tissue. The relative amount of these different states is highly variable from patient to patient, from an area to another in the same patient and also probably from time to time in the same region. The problem is also com-

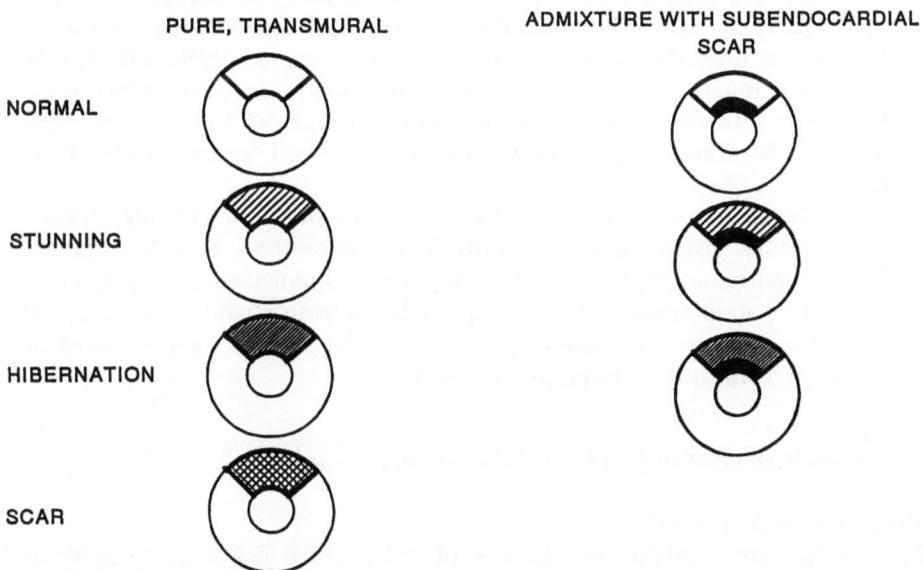

Figure 4. Possible states in a myocardial region. CRF = coronary flow reserve.

plicated by the absence of a gold standard. There is no imaging procedure which can serve as the best reference. Functional recovery after revascularization is frequently used for comparison and is indeed clinically essential, but it cannot be considered as a gold standard. Recovery of ventricular function depends on many factors: quality of the revascularization procedure, perioperative ischemia, recurrence of obstruction in native or graft vessels. The presence of necrotic endocardial layers prevents the recurrence of myocardial thickening in basal conditions, even when perfusion has improved in a large amount of viable epicardium. Furthermore, the time course of recovery may be highly variable: a too early assessment may underestimate the prevalence and degree of functional improvement [42].

Imaging techniques for identifying viability

Different imaging modalities are available for characterizing viable and salvageable tissue: they may provide informations on flow, membrane integrity, oxidative or glucose metabolism, and contractile reserve.

Thallium 201 scintigraphy has been extensively studied to assert the integrity of myocardial cell membranes, thus preserved viability. The classical stress and redistribution imaging has been shown to have a low sensitivity for this purpose. The accuracy has significantly improved by the introduction of new methodology: semi-quantitative analysis, reinjection of thallium after redistribution or resting scintigraphy with early and late imaging [5].

Metabolic imaging with PET has also emerged for identification of myocardial viability. Reversibly non-contractile tissue displays normal or increased ^{18}F fluorodeoxyglucose (FDG) uptake. Regions with a mismatch – reduced perfusion, but preserved FDG metabolism – contain predominantly viable cells [44] and functional recovery is frequently found after revascularization [45]. Patients with viable but compromised myocardium who were not treated by revascularization had an increased risk of subsequent severe cardiac event [46].

The assessment of contractile reserve in patients with chronic, severe coronary artery disease has been introduced more than 15 years ago by the use of ventriculography during epinephrine administration [47] or post-extrasystolic potentiation [48]. This approach has been abandoned during 10 years and is currently proposed by the echocardiographic measurement of contractile response to dobutamine infusion.

Dobutamine echocardiography in hibernating myocardium

Prediction of functional recovery

Few studies are available on the use of dobutamine echocardiography in patients with left ventricular dysfunction and chronic coronary artery disease, but the interest in this method is increasing. Three studies have assessed the accuracy of this technique in predicting improvement in systolic wall thickening after revascularization [49–51].

Cigarroa et al. [49] studied 49 patients with multivessel coronary artery disease and depressed left ventricular function (ejection fraction ≤ 45%). Contractile reserve during dobutamine stress echocardiography (from 5 to 20 µg/kg/min) was present in 24 patients. Successful revascularization was performed in 25 patients. Nine of 11 patients who improved wall thickening had contractile reserve (sensitivity 82%), whereas 12 of 14 patients who did not improve had no contractile reserve (specificity 86%).

La Canna et al. [50] selected 33 patients (22 with angina, 10 with dyspnea) scheduled for coronary artery bypass grafting. The dose of dobutamine was low (5 to 10 µg/kg/min). Before bypass surgery, 314 segments were akinetic. Dobutamine echocardiography predicted improvement in 178 of the 205 segments that recovered function after operation (sensitivity 87%) and identified 89 of the 109 segments that did not recover (specificity 82%).

Afridi et al. [51] performed dobutamine echocardiography using incremental doses of 2.5 to 40 µg/kg/min in 20 patients scheduled for coronary angioplasty. Four different responses were possible: no change in 39% of segments, sustained improvement in 18%, improvement at low dose and worsening at high dose in 20% and worsening alone in 15%. Combining worsening and biphasic responses resulted in a sensitivity of 74% and specificity of 73% for assessment of recovery of individual segments and 90% and 60%, respectively, for functional recovery of individual patients. The administration of low and high doses was essential, because the predictive value for recovery was highest in the presence of a biphasic response (72%), while sustained improvement had a predictive value (15%) as low as the "no change" response (13%).

Comparison with other imaging techniques
Several ongoing studies are designed to determine the relative value of different methods, including dobutamine echocardiography for the differentiation of viable myocardial tissue or scar. Published reports are scarce. Baer et al. [52] compared dobutamine transesophageal echocardiography (5 to 20 µg/kg/min) and FDG PET in 40 patients with chronic myocardial infarction. Dobutamine-induced systolic wall motion within basally akinetic region was observed in 21 (53%) of the 40 patients. In 210 (89%) of the 235 akinetic segments at rest, presence or absence of contractile reserve was concordant with normal or abnormal FDG uptake (≥ or < 50% of the maximal uptake in a region with normal wall motion).

To our experience, in chronic coronary artery disease, dobutamine-induced contractile reserve may be observed in the presence of different myocardial states, as determined by PET: hibernation, stunning or non transmural infarction. The two techniques are more complementary than redundant and should be integrated to coronary anatomy and clinical findings for appropriate decision making [53].

Conclusions

Echocardiography during an inotropic stimulation by dobutamine infusion is a new and promising tool for the evaluation of patients with severely hypokinetic myocardium after acute myocardial infarction or in a more chronic condition.

The observation of dobutamine-induced systolic wall thickening in basally akinetic areas is usually made at low dose of the drug. It implies that the myocardial segment is not transmurally necrotic or fibrotic. This response may however be seen in different situations: pure myocardial stunning – rare in the clinical arena – mixture of subendocardial necrosis and normal or stunned subepicardium, myocardial hibernation (isolated or associated with partial necrosis). The absence of improvement with dobutamine does not necessarily indicate the absence of any residual viable myocardium. The percentage of irreversible damage can exceed the possibility of inducing a detectable contractile reserve; flow reserve can be absent, because of critical coronary stenosis or ultrastructural alterations may be too important, with a loss of contractile material.

The observation of reworsening after early improvement is usually seen at high doses of dobutamine but can also be observed earlier. This pattern implies a state of hibernation and/or an abnormal coronary flow reserve. This information is essential for deciding a revascularization procedure but must be integrated with other informations provided by other available modalities. (See also Chapters 14–17.)

References

1. Braunwald E, Kloner RA. The stunned myocardium: Prolonged, post-ischemic ventricular dysfunction. Circulation 1982; 66: 1146–9.
2. Braunwald E, Rutherford JD. Reversible ischemic left ventricular dysfunction. Evidence for the "hibernating myocardium". J Am Coll Cardiol 1986; 8: 1467–70.
3. Bolli R. Mechanism of myocardial "stunning". Circulation 1990; 82: 723–38.
4. Schulz R, Guth BD, Pieper K et al. Recruitment of an inotropic reserve in moderately ischemic myocardium at the expense of metabolic recovery. A model of short-term hibernation. Circ Res 1992; 70: 1282–95.
5. Dilsizian V, Bonow RO. Current diagnostic techniques of assessing myocardial viability in patients with hibernating and stunned myocardium. Circulation 1993; 87: 1–20.
6. Vatner SF. Correlation between acute reductions in myocardial blood flow and function in conscious dogs. Circ Res 1980; 47: 201–7.
7. Kloner RA, Przyklenk K, Patel B. Altered myocardial states. The stunned and hibernating myocardium. Am J Med 1989; 86 (Suppl 1A): 14–22.
8. Heyndrickx GR, Millard RW, McRitchie RJ et al. Regional myocardial function and electrophysiological alterations after brief coronary artery occlusion in conscious dogs. J Clin Invest 1975; 56 : 978–85.
9. Bolli R, Zhu W, Myers ML et al. Beta-adrenergic stimulation reverses postischemic myocardial dysfunction without producing subsequent functional deterioration. Am J Cardiol 1985; 56: 964–8.

10. Ellis SG, Wynne J, Braunwald E et al. Response of reperfusion-salvaged, stunned myocardium to inotropic stimulation. Am Heart J 1984; 107: 13–9.
11. Becker LC, Levine JH, DiPaula AF et al. Reversal of dysfunction in postischemic stunned myocardium by epinephrine and postextrasystolic potentiation. J Am Coll Cardiol 1986; 7: 580–9.
12. Biessaux Y, Benoit T, Raskinet B et al. Is myocardial stunning frequent in unstable angina? Insight from simultaneous measurements of myocardial function and flow. Eur Heart J 1994; 15: 173 (Abstr Suppl).
13. Fedele FA, Gewirtz H, Capone RJ et al. Metabolic response to prolonged reduction of myocardial blood flow distal to a severe coronary artery stenosis. Circulation 1988; 78: 729–35.
14. Schulz R, Rose J, Martin C et al. Development of short-term myocardial hibernation. Its limitation by the severity of ischemia and inotropic stimulation. Circulation 1993; 88: 684–95.
15. Rahimtoola SH. A perspective on the three large multicenter randomized clinical trials of coronary bypass surgery for chronic stable angina. Circulation 1985; 72 (Suppl. V): V123–35.
16. Flameng W, Suy R, Schwarz F et al. Ultrastructural correlates of left ventricular contraction abnormalities in patients with chronic ischemic heart disease: Determinants of reversible segmental asynergy post-revascularization surgery. Am Heart J 1981; 102: 846–57.
17. Vanoverschelde JL, Wijns W, Depre C et al. Mechanisms of chronic regional postischemic dysfunction in humans. New insights from the study of noninfarcted collateral-dependent myocardium. Circulation 1993; 87: 1513–23.
18. Bolli R. Myocardial "stunning" in man. Circulation 1992; 86: 1671–91.
19. TIMI Study Group. Comparison of invasive and conservative strategies after intravenous tissue plasminogen activator in acute myocardial infarction. N Engl J Med 1989; 3201: 618–27.
20. Stack RS, Phillips HR III, Grierson DS et al. Functional improvement of jeopardized myocardium following intracoronary streptokinase infusion in acute myocardial infarction. J Clin Invest 1983; 72: 84–95.
21. Charuzi Y, Beeder C, Marshall LA et al. Improvement in regional and global left ventricular function after intracoronary thrombolysis: Assessment with two-dimensional echocardiography. Am J Cardiol 1984; 53: 662–5.
22. Bourdillon PDV, Broderick TM, Williams ES et al. Early recovery of regional left ventricular function after reperfusion in acute myocardial infarction assessed by serial two-dimensional echocardiography. Am J Cardiol 1989; 63: 641–6.
23. Zoghbi WA, Marian A, Cheirif JB et al. Time course of recovery of regional function following thrombolysis in acute myocardial infarction (TIMI): Preliminary observations for the TIMI trial phase II (Abstr). J Am Coll Cardiol 1990; 15: 233A.
24. Schmidt WG, Sheehan FH, Von Essen R et al. Evolution of left ventricular function after intracoronary thrombolysis for acute myocardial infarction. Am J Cardiol 1989; 63: 497–502.
25. Pfisterer M, Zuber M, Wenzel R et al. Prolonged myocardial stunning after thrombolysis: Can left ventricular function be assessed definitely at hospital discharge? Eur Heart J 1991; 12: 214–7.
26. Myers JH, Stirling MC, Choy M et al. Direct measurement of inner and outer wall thickening dynamics with epicardial echocardiography. Circulation 1986; 74: 164–72.
27. Lieberman AN, Weiss JL, Jugdutt BI et al. Two-dimensional echocardiography and infarct size: Relationship of regional wall motion and thickening to the extent of myocardial infarction in the dog. Circulation 1981; 63: 739–46.
28. Sklenar J, Ismail S, Villanueva FS et al. Dobutamine echocardiography for determining the extent of myocardial salvage after reperfusion. An experimental evaluation. Circulation 1994; 90: 1502–12.
29. Piérard LA, De Landsheere C, Berthe C et al. Identification of viable myocardium by

echocardiography during dobutamine infusion in patients with myocardial infarction after thrombolytic therapy: Comparison with positron emission tomography. J Am Coll Cardiol 1990; 15: 1021–31.

30. Barilla F, Gheorghiade M, Alam M et al. Low-dose dobutamine in patients with acute myocardial infarction identifies viable but not contractile myocardium and predicts the magnitude of improvement in wall motion abnormalities in response to coronary revascularization. Am Heart J 1991; 122: 1522–31.

31. Smart SC, Sawada S, Ryan T. Low-dose dobutamine echocardiography detects reversible dysfunction after thrombolytic therapy of acute myocardial infarction. Circulation 1993; 88: 405–15.

32. Watada H, Ito H, Oh H et al. Dobutamine stress echocardiography predicts reversible dysfunction and quantitates the extent of irreversible damaged myocardium after reperfusion of anterior myocardial infarction. J Am Coll Cardiol 1994; 24: 624–30.

33. Piérard LA. Comparison of approaches in the assessment of myocardial viability and follow-up of PTCA/CABG. Int J Cardiac Imag 1993; 9: 11–7.

34. Berthe C, Piérard LA, Hiernaux M et al. Predicting the extent and location of coronary artery disease in acute myocardial infarction by echocardiography during dobutamine infusion. Am J Cardiol 1986; 58: 1167–72.

35. Piérard LA, Sprynger M, Carlier J. Echocardiographic prediction of the site of coronary artery obstruction in acute myocardial infarction. Eur Heart J 1987; 8: 116–23.

36. Nitzberg WD, Nath HP, Rogers WJ et al. Collateral flow in patients with acute myocardial infarction. Am J Cardiol 1985; 56: 729–36.

37. Stahl LD, Aversano TR, Becker LC. Selective enhancement of function of stunned myocardium by increased flow. Circulation 1986; 74: 843–51.

38. Picano E, Marzullo P, Gigli G et al. Identification of viable myocardium by dipyridamole-induced improvement in regional left ventricular function assessed by echocardiography in myocardial infarction and comparison with thallium scintigraphy at rest. Am J Cardiol 1992; 70: 703–10.

39. Bolognese L, Rossi L, Sarasso G et al. Silent versus symptomatic dipyridamole-induced ischemia after myocardial infarction: Clinical and prognosis significance. J Am Coll Cardiol 1992; 19: 953–9.

40. Rahimtoola SH. The hibernating myocardium. Am Heart J 1989; 117: 211–21.

41. Alderman EL, Fisher LD, Litwin P et al. Results of coronary artery surgery in patients with poor left ventricular function (CASS). Circulation 1983; 68: 785–95.

42. Nienaber CA, Brunken RC, Sherman CD et al. Metabolic and functional recovery of ischemic human myocardium after coronary angioplasty. J Am Coll Cardiol 1991; 18: 966–78.

43. Ghods M, Pancholy S, Cave V et al. Serial changes in left ventricular function after coronary artery bypass: Implications in viability assessment. Am Heart J 1995; 129: 20–3.

44. Maes A, Flameng W, Nuyts J et al. Histological alterations in chronically hypoperfused myocardium. Correlation with PET findings. Circulation 1994; 90: 735–45.

45. Vom Dahl J, Eitzman DT, Al-Aouar ZR et al. Relation of regional function, perfusion and metabolism in patients with advanced coronary artery disease undergoing surgical revascularization. Circulation 1994; 90: 2356–66.

46. Eitzman D, Al-Aouar Z, Kanter HL et al. Clinical outcome of patients with advanced coronary artery disease after viability studies with positron emission tomography. J Am Coll Cardiol 1992; 20: 559–65.

47. Nesto RW, Cohn LH, Wynne J et al. Inotropic contractile reserve: A useful predictor of increased 5 year survival and improved postoperative left ventricular function in patients with coronary artery disease and reduced ejection fraction. Am J Cardiol 1982; 50: 39–44.

48. Popio KA, Gorlin R, Bechtel D, Levine JA. Postextrasystolic potentiation as a predictor of potential myocardial viability: Preoperative analyses compared with studies after coronary bypass surgery. Am J Cardiol 1977; 39: 944–53.

49. Cigarroa CG, De Filippi CR, Brickner ME et al. Dobutamine stress echocardiography

identifies hibernating myocardium and predicts recovery of left ventricular function after coronary revascularization. Circulation 1993; 88: 430–6.

50. La Canna G, Alfieri O, Giubbini R et al. Echocardiography during infusion of dobutamine for identification of reversible dysfunction in patients with chronic coronary artery disease. J Am Coll Cardiol 1994; 23: 617–26.

51. Afridi I, Kleiman NS, Raizner AE, Zoghbi WA. Dobutamine echocardiography in myocardial hibernation. Optimal dose and accuracy in predicting recovery of ventricular function after coronary angioplasty. Circulation 1995; 91: 663–70.

52. Baer FM, Voth E, Deutsch HJ et al. Assessment of viable myocardium by dobutamine transesophageal echocardiography and comparison with fluorine-18 fluorodeoxyglucose positron emission tomography. J Am Coll Cardiol 1994; 24: 343–53.

53. Piérard LA, Mélon P, De Landsheere C et al. Identification of hibernating myocardium: Comparison between low-dose dobutamine echocardiography and positron emission tomography. Acta Cardiologica 1994; 49: 506–7.

Corresponding Author: Dr Luc A. Pierard, Service de Cardiologie, CHU du Sart Tilman, B-4000 Liege, Belgium

19. Assessment of functional significance of the stenotic substrate by Doppler flow measurements

CHRISTIAN SEILER

Introduction

Imaging techniques currently used in the assessment of coronary stenoses include angiography, ultrasound, and angioscopy, all of which provide information on the degree of stenosis or morphologic appearance of the atherosclerotic lesion. However, angiographic appearance of stenotic lesions may provide misleading information regarding the functional significance of coronary stenosis, particularly in the presence of multiple lesions or diffuse atherosclerosis as frequently occurring in clinical coronary artery disease [1–6]. Newer imaging techniques such as intravascular ultrasound and angioscopy, are still largely experimental. It has been shown recently that Doppler crystal methodology has enabled cardiologists to estimate the functional impact of lesion severity on the capacity of a coronary artery to increase its flow under conditions of resistance vessel dilation [7]. Measurements made with the subselective Doppler catheter have been extensively validated [7, 8]. Such devices use a 20 MHz side- or tip-mounted Doppler crystal affixed to a 3F catheter with a zero-crossing technique to analyze Doppler signals. Lately, a 6 MHz subselective Doppler catheter has been developed which provides volume flow measurements independently of vessel size determination [9]. More recently, a device with an end-mounted 12 MHz Doppler crystal affixed to an 0.018 or 0.014 inch angioplasty-guidewire has been developed [10]. The determination of flow velocity at conditions of hyperemia and downstream from a lesion may provide misleading information on the functional significance of this stenosis since the microvascular, peripheral resistance – aside from stenosis severity – influences flow velocity distal to a given stenotic lesion. Furthermore, coronary flow velocity is only an indirect measure of flow, the variable to ultimately characterize adequacy of myocardial perfusion; flow is related to both velocity and coronary artery size which changes under varying conditions, and may be assessed by means of quantitative coronary angiography. Due to the fact that the coronary artery tree is a network of communicating branches in which vascular resistances in different vessel areas probably influence one another, the functional impact

C.A. Nienaber and U. Sechtem (eds): *Imaging and Intervention in Cardiology.* 295–310.
© 1996 *Kluwer Academic Publishers.*

of a particular stenotic lesion may also be influenced by the vascular resistance in adjacent myocardial areas.

The purpose of this report is to rewiev different Doppler techniques to assess the functional significance of coronary stenotic lesions, to describe shortcomings related to these techniques, and to outline possible ways to overcome these limitations.

Doppler theory

Coronary flow velocity is calculated from the Doppler frequency shift (which is the difference between the transmitted and returning frequency), using the following Doppler equation:

$$V = C(F_1 - F_0)/2F_0(\cos \Phi) \qquad (1)$$

where V = velocity of blood flow, F_0 = transmitting (transducer) frequency, F_1 = returning frequency, C = constant: speed of sound in blood, and Φ = angle of incidence.

Maximum velocity can be recorded provided the transducer beam is parallel to blood flow and Φ is zero, so that $\cos \Phi = 1$.

Furthermore, there is a direct relation between velocity and volumetric flow, where

flow = vessel area × velocity integral × heart rate

The differences or changes in Doppler coronary flow velocities, thus, can be used to represent changes in absolute coronary flow. Assuming a constant vessel diameter or determining vessel size by quantitative coronary angiography, flow rate can be calculated from multiplying vessel cross-sectional area (CSA), flow velocity integral (Vi), and heart rate:

$$\text{Flow} = \text{CSA} \times \text{Vi} \times \text{heart rate} \qquad (2)$$

If the interrogating angle is <20°, the velocity measurements will be within 5% of absolute values. The velocity integral can be easily measured in a 3-mm vessel by using a broad sample volume in the presence of a parabolic flow profile.

Intravascular Doppler ultrasound devices

Intravascular, catheter-based Doppler utrasound devices have been used to measure coronary flow reserve, and to calculate minimal stenosis area [7, 11–14]. Many improvements have been made since Benchimol [15] and Hartley and Cole [16, 17] introduced catheter-based Doppler systems in the 1970's.

Catheter-based devices are composed of piezoelectric crystals mounted at

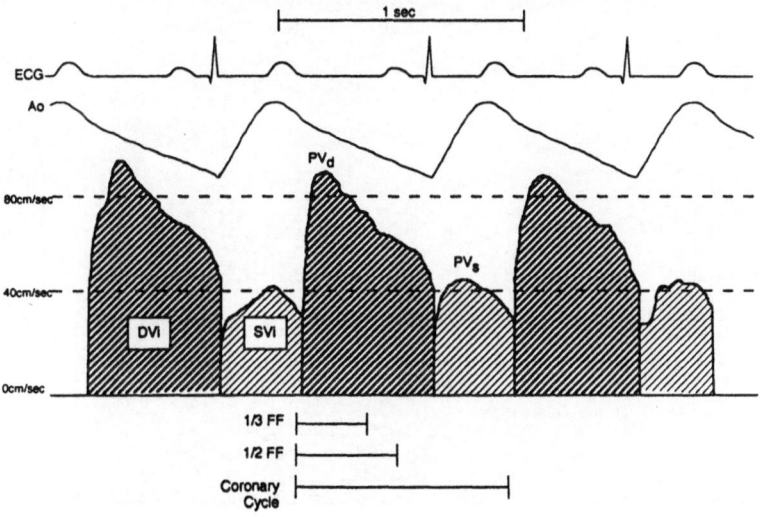

Figure 1. Schematic diagram of a normal coronary spectral Doppler flow velocity pattern obtained by means of a Doppler guidewire. Abbreviations: DVi = diastolic velocity integral; FF = flow fraction; PV_d = peak diastolic velocity; PV_s = peak systolic velocity; SVi = systolic velocity integral. (Reprinted with permission from Ofili EO et al. J Am Coll Cardiol 1993 [24].)

the tip or on the side of catheters as small as 3F [7, 18]. Most devices have a central lumen that can accommodate a standard 0.014 inch angioplasty guide wire to aid in subselective placement within the coronary artery tree. A device has been evaluated that uses a 1 mm ring-shaped transducer affixed to the tip of an angioplasty catheter [19]. Doppler velocity signals obtained by those catheter-based devices (Figure 1) are processed by a zero crossing technique. This technique provides an average velocity that approximates the peak velocity in the presence of non-stenotic or minimally narrowed vessels when a laminar flow pattern is preserved. However, with a significant stenosis, the coronary flow becomes turbulent and the true peak velocity cannot be accurately assessed by the zero crossing technique [14]. A catheter with a side-mounted transducer necessarily disturbs the flow velocity profile across the vessel in the sample volume because of the catheter shaft within the vessel at the point of interrogation. The shaft of a 1 mm diameter catheter upstream from a forward-directed ultrasound beam alters the flow velocity profile accross the vessel, depressing the peak velocity of blood flow in the sample volume [20]. Even at 1 mm in diameter ($\approx$3F), the Doppler catheters significantly alter blood flow. In small distal vessels, significant obstruction of the vessel by the catheter may occur, impeding baseline flow rate and

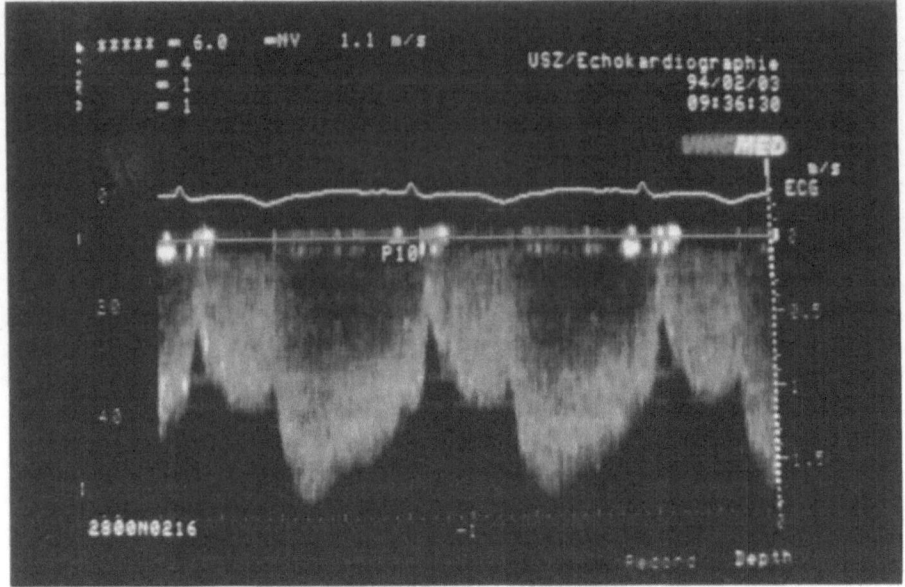

Figure 2. Normal coronary (continuous wave) spectral flow velocity pattern in the left anterior descending coronary artery obtained by a 3F Amplitude-Weighted-Mean-Velocity (AWMV) 6 MHz Doppler catheter.

inducing reactive hyperemia due to ischemia. A further limitation of conventionally used Doppler techniques is that only flow velocities and not volume flow is measured.

Recently, a 3F Doppler catheter has been developed which measures coronary blood flow volume independently from vessel cross-sectional area [9]. The ability of this device to obtain absolute volume flow measurements relates to the principle that in blood with normal content and distribution of red blood cells, the time integral of the amplitude-weighted mean blood flow velocity (AWMV) from continuous wave or pulsed wave Doppler spectra is directly related to absolute blood volume flow (Figure 2) [21]. In vitro validation of the AWMV-Doppler-catheter with a tip-mounted, circular 6 MHz crystal has provided fair correlations with directly measured volume flow (r = 0.84, variability for repeated measurements = 7.4%) [9]. Unfortunately, disadvantages related to the size of the catheter are not eliminated with the AWMV-catheter.

To obviate size-related limitations of current Doppler flow velocity techniques, a 12 MHz Doppler transducer mounted on a 0.018 inch (0.46 mm) or even 0.014 inch angioplasty guide wire (Flowire®, Cardiometrics, Mountain View, CA) has recently been developed and validated [10, 22]. The combination of a high pulse repetition frequency (up to 90 kHz) and a sampling depth of 5 mm permits recording of coronary flow velocities up to 4 m/s without aliasing [10]. The forward directed ultrasound beam with 25° divergence angle samples a large (although not as large as with the 6 MHz AWMV-cath) portion of the flow profile. The velocity signals are processed by fast Fourier transformation and all representative velocities within the ultrasound beam are displayed in a spectral format. The instantaneous spectral peak velocity measurement provides a relatively position-insensitive characterization of the velocity in an artery, and it is an accurate correlation of absolute flow provided that the vessel diameter remains constant [10]. However, there are several specific limitations related to the Doppler flow guidewire. The Doppler guidewire has to be manipulated for optimization of signal strength by using the gray scale signal amplitude and peak velocity as indicators of proper positioning within the vessel. In tortuous coronary segments or if the guide wire tip is preformed into a significant curve, extensive manipulation may be required to point the transducer away from the vessel wall and into the flow stream [22]. Occasionaly, vessel wall artifact cannot be avoided and the guide wire must be repositioned into an alternative segment of the vessel. In large vessels in which the guide wire is angled, the ultrasound beam may not intersect the true maximal flow velocity, and errors in reproducibility of Doppler velocity measurements occur.

Coronary flow velocity parameters and patterns in normal coronary arteries

It has been noted that coronary flow at rest may be similar in normal and abnormal arteries. Coronary vasodilatory reserve, first introduced conceptually by Coffman and Gregg more than 30 years ago [23], is the calculated ratio of hyperemia to baseline mean velocity (or rather absolute flow). Several coronary vasodilating agents as well as physical exercise have been used to challenge the coronary system by increasing flow and exaggerating differences in flow (and velocity) beyond stenotic lesions. The coronary vasodilator reserve based on Doppler velocity measurements in humans without coronary atherosclerosis has been found to be approximately 2.5 and similar in all three coronary arteries [24]. From data obtained in experimental animal models, coronary vasodilatory reserve has been correlated with angiographic lesion severity and this concept has been proposed to identify patients with physiologically significant lesions [1]. However, abnormal flow reserve is seen not only with epicardial stenosis, but also in situations where the coronary microcirculation is impaired, such as diabetes, hypertension, myocardial infarction, and cardiomyopathy [25].

To assess normal flow velocity, Ofili and coworkers [24] performed simultaneous flow velocity measurements using the Doppler flow-guidewire technique in angiographically normal, proximal and distal coronary arteries (Figure 3 and Table 1). The diastolic velocity integral at baseline was significantly

Zero Cross Catheter Coronary Flow Velocity at Baseline and after Maximal Hyperemia

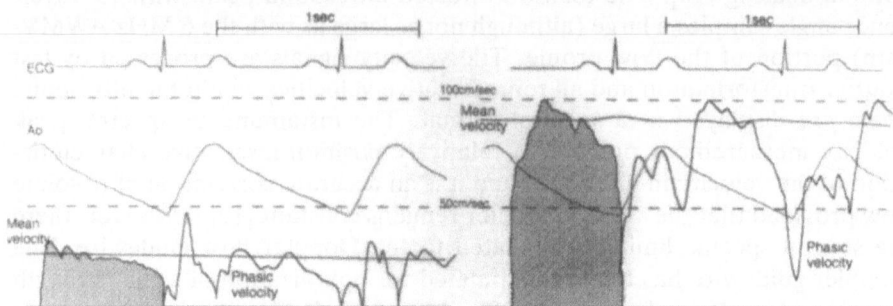

Figure 3. Zero cross catheter coronary flow velocity in a patient with normal coronary arteries at baseline (left) and after maximal hyperemia (right). (Reprinted with permission from Ofili EO et al. J Am Coll Cardiol 1993 [24].)

higher for the proximal left anterior compared with the proximal right coronary arteries. With hyperemia, mean velocity, peak diastolic velocity, and diastolic velocity integral were significantly higher in the proximal left anterior descending coronary artery compared with the proximal left circumflex and right coronary arteries. Proximal and distal mean velocity in each of the main three coronary arteries was not significantly different at baseline and

Table 1. Velocity parameters at baseline and with hyperemia in individual coronary arteries. (Reprinted with permission from Ofili EO et al. J Am Coll Cardiol 1993 [24].)

	Baseline			Hyperemia[a]		
	LAD	LCX	RCA	LAD	LCX	RCA
Proximal						
Peak D vel (cm/sec)	49 ± 20	40 ± 15	37 ± 12	104 ± 28[b]	79 ± 10	72 ± 13
Mean vel (cm/sec)	31 ± 15	25 ± 8	26 ± 7	66 ± 18[b]	50 ± 14	48 ± 13
D vel int (cm/sec)	18 ± 11[c]	13 ± 5	11 ± 4	37 ± 15[b]	27 ± 9	22 ± 9
1/3 FF (%)	45 ± 4[c]	44 ± 5	40 ± 5	44 ± 5	43 ± 6	41 ± 4
D/S	2.0 ± 0.5[c]	1.8 ± 0.7	1.5 ± 0.5	2.0 ± 0.5	1.9 ± 0.6	1.9 ± 0.8
Distal						
Peak D vel (cm/sec)	35 ± 16	35 ± 8	28 ± 8	70 ± 17	71 ± 22	67 ± 16
Mean vel (cm/sec)	23 ± 11	21 ± 6	21 ± 9	45 ± 12	45 ± 12	42 ± 9
D vel int (cm/sec)	13 ± 9	10 ± 3	8 ± 5	9 ± 6	11 ± 8	9 ± 2
1/3 FF (%)	46 ± 2	45 ± 9	39 ± 6	45 ± 3	42 ± 7	40 ± 9
D/S	2.4 ± 0.8 [c]	2.1 ± 0.8	1.4 ± 0.3	2.2 ± 1.0	1.9 ± 0.8	1.6 ± 0.3

[a]All 3 coronary arteries had significantly higher absolute velocity parameters during hyperemia (p < 0.001).
[b]Left anterior descending (LAD) versus left circumflex (LCX) and right coronary artery (RCA).
[c]LAD versus RCA.
D = diastolic; D/S = peak diatolic to peak systolic; D vel int = diastolic flow velocity integral; 1/3 FF = one-third flow fraction; Vel = velocity.

with hyperemia although there was a tendency to persistently lower distal than proximal velocities.

Thus, a small Doppler device which can be placed at different locations of decreasing vascular bedsize without obstructing the coronary flow is essential for the assessment of flow velocities in coronary artery trees. Secondly, flow velocities appear not to be preserved in the entire coronary artery tree as previously suggested [26]. Finally, flow velocities obtained at given locations in the coronary artery tree seem to be directly related to the amount of myocardium supplied from these points. This is in agreement with physical principles underlying the anatomic structure of the coronary artery tree [6]. According to one of these principles, that of minimum viscous energy dissipation of the blood circulating through the coronary tree, the cross-sectional area (CSA) of a coronary artery at any given point in the coronary artery tree is related to blood flow rate (F) as follows:

$$CSA = K \times F^{2/3} \tag{3}$$

where K is a constant ($= 0.004$). F is directly proportional to the blood-supplied myocardial mass, and – via the continuity equation – it is related to blood flow velocity as shown in Equation (2). Combining Equations (2) and (3), the coronary flow velocity integral decreases with decreasing coronary artery size as follows:

$$V_i = K' \times HR^{-1} \times CSA^{1/2} \tag{4}$$

It has been shown in animals [27] and in humans [28, 29] that the coronary artery size is directly, curvilinearly and closely related to the myocardial mass supplied by this artery.

In their investigation of normal coronary artery flow velocities in humans, Ofili et al. [24] found that all three coronary arteries showed a predominant diastolic pattern in both proximal and distal arterial segments (Figures 2 and 3). This pattern was less marked in the right coronary artery, which had a significantly lower peak diastolic-to-systolic flow velocity ratio compared with the left anterior descending coronary artery. This less marked diastolic predominant pattern may be due to a relatively unimpeded right coronary systolic flow as a result of the lower right than left ventricular contractile force.

Assessment of coronary artery stenoses

Coronary artery pulsed Doppler catheters and intraoperatively placed coronary artery probes have been used to measure the blood flow velocity in diseased human epicardial coronary arteries and to assess coronary vasodilator reserve. Utilizing the Doppler guidewire technique, there have been a few clinical studies investigating the behavior of coronary flow reserve, and of different flow velocity variables and patterns (see also Figure 3) pre- and immediately post-coronary-angioplasty [12, 22, 24]. Since one of the major clinical implications of accurate and reproducible functional assessment of coronary artery stenoses by any of the aforementioned methods (and by quantitative coronary angiography) consists of predicting and evaluating the effect of coronary angioplasty (PTCA) immediately after the procedure, it will subsequently be focused on parameters obtained by Doppler flow measurements for the assessment of changing stenotic lesions following PTCA.

Coronary flow reserve

Some studies [30, 31] have demonstrated poor correlation of flow reserve with angiographic indexes of stenosis severity. Investigations [11, 19, 32] using Doppler coronary artery catheters to perform subselective flow reserve measurements after angioplasty have produced inconsistent results. Wilson et al. [11] reported that although papaverine-induced flow reserve increased acutely from a mean of 2.0 ± 0.1 before angioplasty to 3.6 ± 0.3 after successful angioplasty, the range of flow reserves after angioplasty was widespread (2.5 to 7.5). Studies from the same laboratory [33] documented a good correlation between angiographic degree of stenosis and coronary flow reserve before angioplasty. However, no correlation between coronary flow reserve and percent area stenosis or minimal cross-sectional area was observed after angioplasty. Kern et al. [12] reported that angioplasty did not significantly increase basal but papaverine-induced hyperemic coronary artery flow velocity. Thus, papaverine-induced flow reserve remained only minimally improved after angioplasty and significantly lower than in normal vessel segments. Measurement of coronary flow reserve several weeks after angioplasty has yielded a more consistent relation between flow reserve and residual angiographic stenosis [11]. However, such data on late improvement in flow reserve do not provide the information needed for decision-making during the angioplasty procedure. Explanations of this dissociation between angiographic improvement after angioplasty and coronary flow reserve include inaccuracies in angiographic assessment of stenosis severity, effects of collateral circulation to the affected vessel, drugs that may limit vasodilator response, abnormalities of autoregulation due to long-standing ischemia, release of local factors that affect coronary vasomotor tone, alteration of smooth muscle vasomotor tone due to mechanical trauma, and a parallel increase in baseline and hyperemic flow that would obscure any change in flow reserve [22, 34–36].

Assessment of stenosis severity by the continuity equation

Data obtained by using coronary artery Doppler catheters to assess stenosis severity have included measurement of ratios of post-stenotic jet velocity/normal coronary artery velocity [14]. These ratios may be used to quantify the percent area stenosis by means of the continuity equation. However, although the percent cross-sectional area stenosis and minimal cross-sectional area derived from Doppler guidewire measurements in humans were significantly correlated with the corresponding angiographic measurements, with this approach a good Doppler signal could be achieved in only 16% of cases [37]. Possible explanations for the difficulty to obtain adequate Doppler signals within a stenosis include reduced echointensity of the blood due to diminished erythrocyte-rouleaux formation at increased blood flow shear rates [38], and difficulty in orientating the Doppler sample volume in the narrowed tapering segment immediately proximal to the lesion.

Absolute flow velocity parameters

Recently, Segal and coworkers [22] provided evidence that, in the absence of any significant change in distal coronary artery diameter, time-averaged peak velocity increased significantly by 84% in the distal coronary artery after successful angioplasty. These increases in basal flow after angioplasty may explain the absence of significant changes in the flow ratio after angioplasty because both basal and hyperemic flow have been shown to increase in this study. Smaller percent changes of 20% have been noted in proximal average peak velocity [22]. Flow in proximal coronary artery segments may not be reflective of flow in distal vessels [39]. Extramural coronary arteries may act as capacitance vessels, with forward systolic flow in proximal segments and reverse systolic flow in distal branches [40]. In accordance with such models of the coronary circulation, discrepancies between instantaneous proximal coronary artery inflow and distal coronary artery outflow may be anticipated and have been documented [22] illustrating the importance of flow velocity measurements performed distal to the site of the coronary artery stenosis. Furthermore, absolute flow velocity parameters are not preserved throughout the coronary artery tree, and are closely related to the amount of myocardial mass supplied by the point within the coronary artery tree where velocity is determined [6]; therefore and even in the case of velocity measurements distal to the site of the coronary artery stenosis, they may not be suitable for describing the functional significance of coronary artery stenotic lesions.

Phasic flow velocity patterns and diastolic/systolic velocity ratio

The demonstration in closed chest humans of phasic coronary artery flow waveforms in the distal coronary artery beyond a significant stenosis with the Doppler flow guide wire has confirmed the intraoperative findings of Kajiya et al. [41, 42]. With a significant (>70%) diameter stenosis, diastolic flow components are significantly reduced, whereas systolic flow components are less affected (Figure 4). It has been shown [22] that after angioplasty,

**Schematic of a Doppler Guidewire Velocity Spectrum Proximal and Distal
of a Coronary Artery Stenosis Before and After PTCA**

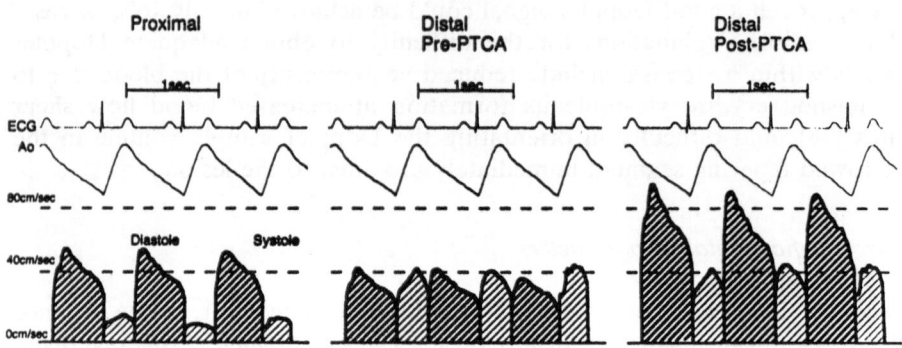

Figure 4. Schematic of Doppler guidwire velocity spectrum (maximal hyperemia) proximal and distal of a coronary artery stenosis before and after coronary angioplasty. Left: proximal flow velocity is normal. Middle: distal flow velocity before PTCA is diminished (proximal/distal ratio >1.7) with a loss of phasic flow pattern (equal systolic and diastolic flow integrals, diastolic/systolic flow velocity ratio <1.2). Right: Normalization of the distal flow velocity after PTCA. (Reprinted with permission from Kern MJ et al. Am J Cardiol 1993 [44].)

diastolic flow velocity increased significantly whereas systolic flow velocity increased less (Figure 4).

Several investigators [1, 43] documented a reduction in the diastolic/systolic coronary flow ratio in animal models with artificial coronary artery stenoses. Similarly, studies [41, 42] on diseased human left anterior descending coronary arteries during bypass surgery using an 80-channel pulsed Doppler probe revealed a marked reduction in diastolic flow velocity and unchanged systolic flow velocity during graft occlusion. Segal et al. [22] documented a significant difference in distally measured mean diastolic/systolic flow velocity ratio between normal and significantly stenosed coronary arteries of 1.8 ± 0.5 versus 1.3 ± 0.5, respectively ($p < 0.01$). After angioplasty, mean diastolic/systolic flow velocity ratio increased to 1.9 ± 0.6, representing a significant ($p < 0.01$) + 46% change from values before angioplasty. In the same study [22], mean diastolic/systolic flow velocity ratios measured proximal to the coronary stenosis have not been documented to show similar abnormalities. Kern et al. [44] examined differences in flow velocity ratios accross stenotic lesions to correlate flow parameters with measured translesional pressure gradients to assess the utility of flow velocity to characterize the hemodynamic significance of lesions. In this study, a strong correlation between translesional pressure gradients and the ratios of the proximal/distal total flow velocity integral ($r = 0.8$, $p < 0.001$) has been

Pressure Gradient-Flow Velocity Relation for Different Degrees of Experimentally Induced Coronary Constrictions in Dogs

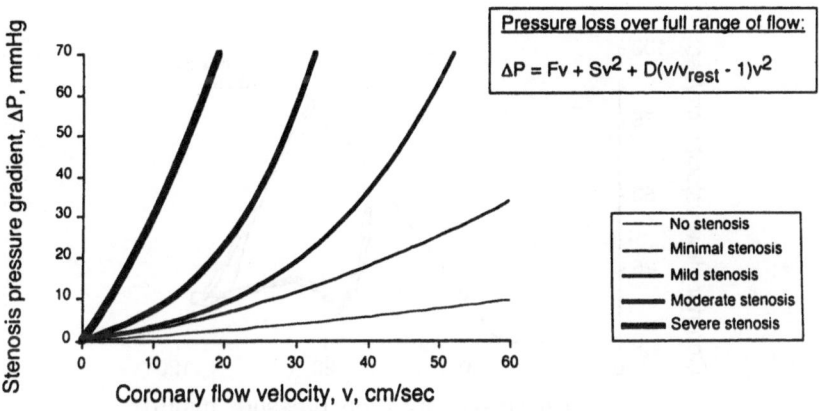

Figure 5. Pressure gradient/velocity relation for different degrees of stenosis severity. The equation to the right of the plot describes the pressure loss over full range of flow due to increasing stenosis severity (increasing thickness of the depicted pressure/velocity curves). The coefficients are hydraulic coefficients of friction (F), of fluid separation (S), and of augmented worsening of the pressure gradient/velocity relation during vasodilation (D). (Adapted with permission from Gould KL. Circ Res 1978 [48].)

demonstrated. Proximal/distal total flow velocity integral ratios >1.7 have been shown to be associated with translesional gradients of >30 mmHg.

Translesional pressure gradient/flow velocity relation

Miniaturization of flow velocity and pressure sensors with guidewire technology now permits the application of methodologic approaches previously limited to the experimental animal laboratory [45–47]. Both experimental and clinical studies have indicated that the slope of the instantaneous hyperemic pressure gradient/diastolic, distal peak flow velocity relation (Figure 5) yields a reproducible and accurate assessment of the physiologic significance of coronary stenoses [45–49]. The *simultaneous* measurement of the instantaneous pressure gradient and distal flow velocity is essential and provides a relation characterizing the hemodynamic properties of the stenosis independently of the instantaneous microvascular resistance since its influence on both variables of the pressure gradient/velocity relation is similar. The pressure gradient/velocity relation (Figure 5) due to increasing stenosis severity over a range of coronary flows has been described to fit the following equation [48]:

Instantaneous Hyperemic Diastolic Flow Velocity / Coronary Driving Pressure Relation

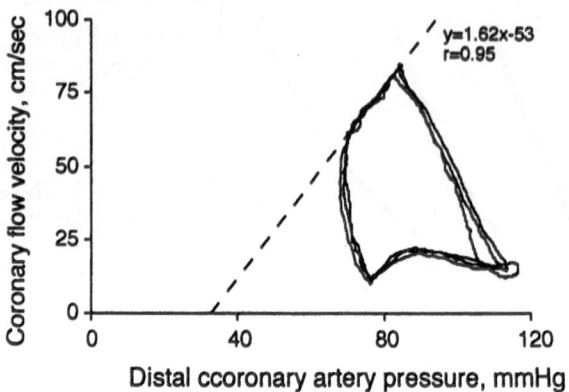

Figure 6. Coronary flow velocity/pressure loops during maximal hyperemia in 3 consecutive sinus beats. During mid-late diastole, a linear relation is observed with an extrapolated zero-flow pressure of 37 mmHg. (Reprinted with permission from Serruys PW et al. Am J Cardiol 1993 [45].)

$$\Delta P = Fv + Sv^2 + D(v/v_r - 1)v^2$$

where F, S and D denote hydraulic, stenosis-specific coefficients of fluid layer friction (F), poststenotic blood flow separation (S) and increased worsening of the pressure gradient/velocity relation during vasodilation (D); v and v_r indicate distal diastolic flow velocity at maximum hyperemia and at resting conditions, respectively.

In addition to the pressure gradient/velocity relation the instantaneous flow velocity/coronary driving pressure relation has been proposed for the functional characterization of the stenosis severity [45, 49] and for the analysis of the characteristics and functional integrity of coronary flow resistance. Flow velocity/pressure loops (Figure 6) during maximal hyperemia show a linear relation during mid- to late-diastole with an extrapolated value for zero-flow pressure which reflects the microvascular resistance provided that flow velocity is measured distal to a stenotic lesion.

A prerequisite for a widespread clinical application of these indexes is the assessment of the reproducibility and the identification of the normal and pathologic range in a large patient population [47]. Furthermore, the functional impact of stenotic lesions in adjacent vascular areas on these relations needs to be determined. Experimental data indicate [50] that certain stenosis combinations proximal and distal of a coronary artery bifurcation lead to branch steal in one of the branches distal to the bifurcation (daughter branch,

B_2). Branch steal describes the phenomenon that during the ascent of flow to short-term, maximal hyperemia in the parent (B_0) and one daughter branch (B_1), there is a decrease of flow in B_2 relative to the maximum in B_0 and B_1 which will be reached after that in B_2. Thus, not only the instantaneous microvascular resistance but also the functional significance of coronary stenoses in parallel or in series with the one under investigation may influence its functional impact on myocardial perfusion. Therefore, in order to definitely assess functional significance of a particular stenotic lesion and the effect of its dilation on the perfusion of adjacent myocardial areas, an estimate of the functional interrelation of all the stenotic lesions within the coronary artery tree is needed. However, since the simultaneous, guidewire-based intracoronary measurement of pressure/velocity relations at several stenoses is not achievable, quantitative coronary angiographic assessment of the entire coronary artery tree including all stenotic lesions still has to provide an estimate of their respective functional influence [6]. (See also Chapters 6, 7, 19, 21 and 22.)

Summary

The angiographic appearance and even quantitative evaluation of coronary lesions may provide misleading information regarding the physiologic significance of coronary stenosis, particularly in the setting of multiple stenoses or diffuse atherosclerosis. Information on coronary blood flow velocity determined by means of Doppler techniques provides functional data complementary to the morphologic data obtained from angiography. Early Doppler ultrasound catheters provided an accurate measure of coronary blood flow velocity, but were limited by relatively large diameters (3F) and, thus, determinations of only proximal coronary artery physiology. A recently developed, intracoronary Doppler-tipped angioplasty guidewire is an important technical advance over earlier catheter techniques, and permits examination of coronary flow velocity both proximal and distal to coronary obstructions. Several coronary flow velocity parameters obtained by Doppler techniques have been evaluated as predictors of lesion significance and outcome after revascularization procedures. Measurements performed distal (as opposed to proximal) to the coronary stenosis appear to be more reliable for the assessment of the functional impact of a stenosis. Coronary flow reserve measurements are of limited utility immediately following angioplasty, regardless of whether measurements are obtained proximal or distal of a stenosis. Absolute flow velocity parameters are closely related to the amount of myocardial mass supplied by the point within the coronary artery tree where velocity is determined; therefore, they are not preserved throughout the coronary tree and, thus, not suitable for describing the functional significance of coronary artery stenotic lesions. Flow velocity ratios such as the proximal-to-distal mean velocity ratio may reflect more reliably the functional significance of a stenosis by providing information comparable to the trans-stenotic pressure gradient. Determination of the instantaneous hyperemic pressure gradient/distal flow velocity relation obtained by velocity and pressure sensors with guidewire technology, probably provides reproducible and accurate assessment of flow parameters independent of microvascular resistance, and may more precisely characterize the physiologic significance of coronary stenoses.

Acknowledgements

Dr Rolf Jenni, University Hospital Zurich, Switzerland, is acknowledged for his contribution (Figure 2) and suggestions in the preparation of this manuscript.

References

1. Gould KL, Lipscomb K, Hamilton GW. Physiologic basis for assessing critical coronary artery stenosis. Am J Cardiol 1974; 33: 87–94.
2. Harrison DG, White CW, Hiratzka LF et al. The value of lesion cross-sectional area determined by quantitative coronary angiography in assessing the physiologic significance of proximal left anterior descending coronary arterial stenosis. Circulation 1984; 69: 1111–9.
3. Wilson RF, Marcus ML, White CW. Prediction of physiologic significance of coronary arterial lesion geometry in patients with limited coronary artery disease. Circulation 1987; 75: 725–32.
4. Klocke FJ. Measurement of coronary blood flow and degree of stenosis: current clinical implications and continuing uncertainties. J Am Coll Cardiol 1983; 1: 31–41.
5. Marcus ML, White CW. Coronary flow reserve in patients with normal coronary angiograms. J Am Coll Cardiol 1985; 6: 1254–6.
6. Seiler C, Kirkeeide RL, Gould KL. Basic structure-function relations of the epicardial coronary vascular tree. Basis of quantitative coronary arteriography for diffuse coronary artery disease. Circulation 1992; 85: 1987–2003.
7. Wilson RF, Laughlin DE, Holida MD et al. Transluminal subselective measurement of coronary blood flow velocity and vasodilator reserve in man. Circulation 1985; 72: 82–92.
8. White CW, Marcus ML, Wilson RF. Methods of measuring coronary flow in humans. Prog Cardiovasc Dis 1988; 31: 79–94.
9. Jenni R, Ritter M, Vieli A et al. Assessment of coronary flow using amplitude weighted mean velocity: In vitro validation of a new intravascular Doppler system. Eur Heart J 1993; 14: 327 (Abstr).
10. Doucette JW, Corl D, Payne H et al. Validation of a Doppler guide wire for intravascular measurement of coronary artery flow velocity. Circulation 1992; 85: 1899–1911.
11. Wilson RF, Johnson MJ, Marcus ML et al. The effect of coronary angioplasty on coronary flow reserve. Circulation 1988; 76: 873–85.
12. Kern MJ, Deligonul U, Vandormael M et al. Impaired coronary vasodilator reserve in the intermediate post coronary angioplasty period: Analysis of coronary artery flow velocity indexes and regional cardiac venous efflux. J Am Coll Cardiol 1989; 13: 860–72.
13. McGinn AL, White CW, Wilson RF. Interstudy variability of coronary flow reserve: Influ-

ence of heart rate, arterial pressure, and ventricular preload. Circulation 1990; 81: 1319–30.

14. Johnson EL, Yock PG, Hargrave VK et al. Assessment of severity of coronary stenoses using a Doppler catheter: Validation of a method based on the continuity equation. Circulation 1989; 80: 625–35.

15. Benchimol A, Stegall HF, Gartlan JL. New method to measure phasic coronary blood flow velocity in man. Am Heart J 1971; 81: 93–101.

16. Hartley CJ, Cole JS. An ultrasonic pulsed Doppler system for measuring blood flow in small vessels. J Appl Physiol 1974; 37: 626–9.

17. Cole JS, Hartley CJ. The pulsed Doppler coronary artery catheter: Preliminary report of a new technique for measuring rapid changes in coronary artery flow velocitiy in man. Circulation 1977; 56: 18–25.

18. Sibley DH, Millar HD, Hartley CJ, Whitlow PL. Subselective measurement of coronary blood flow velocity using a steerable Dopper catheter. J Am Coll Cardiol 1986; 8: 1332–40.

19. Serruys PW, Juillière Y, Zijlstra F et al. Coronary blood flow velocity during percutaneous transluminal coronary angioplasty as a guide for assessment of the functional result. Am J Cardiol 1988; 61: 253–9.

20. Tadaoka S, Kagiyama M, Hiramatsu O et al. Accuracy of 20 MHz Doppler catheter coronary artery flow velocimetry for measurement of coronary blood flow velocity. Cathet Cardiovasc Diagn 1990; 19: 205–13.

21. Jenni R, Ritter M, Eberli F et al. Quantification of mitral regurgitation with amplituide-weighted mean velocity from continuous wave Doppler spectra. Circulation 1989; 79: 1294–9.

22. Segal J, Kern MJ, Scott NA et al. Alterations of phasic coronary artery flow velocity in humans during percutaneous coronary angioplasty. J Am Coll Cardiol 1992; 20: 276–86.

23. Coffman JD, Gregg DE. Reactive hyperemia characteristics of the myocardium. Am J Physiol 1960; 199: 1143–9.

24. Ofili E, Kern MJ, Labovitz AJ et al. Analysis of coronary blood flow velocity dynamics in angiographically normal and stenosed arteries before and after endolumen enlargement by angioplasty. J Am Coll Cardiol 1993; 308–16.

25. Strauer B. The significance of coronary flow reserve in clinical heart disease. J Am Coll Cardiol 1990; 15: 775–83.

26. Caro CG, Pedley TJ, Schroter RC, Seed WA. Flow in pipes and around objects. In: Caro CG, Pedley TJ, Schroter RC, Seed WA, editors. The mechanics of the circulation. New York: Oxford University Press, 1978: 44–78.

27. Seiler C, Kirkeeide RL, Gould KL. Measurement from arteriograms of regional myocardial bed size distal to any point in the coronary vascular tree for assessing anatomic area at risk. J Am Coll Cardiol 1993; 21: 783–97.

28. Hutchins GM, Bulkley BH, Miner MM, Boitnott JK. Correlation of age and heart weight with tortuosity and caliber of normal human coronary arteries. Am Heart J 1977; 94: 196–202.

29. Vieweg WVR, Alpert JS, Hagan AD. Caliber and distribution of normal coronary arterial anatomy. Cathet Cardiovasc Diagn 1976; 2: 269–80.

30. White CW, Wright CB, Doty DB et al. Does visual interpretation of the coronary arteriogam predict the physiologic importance of a coronary stenosis? N Engl J Med 1984; 210: 819–24.

31. Harrison DG, White C, Hiratzka LF et al. The value of lesion cross-sectional area determined by quantitative coronary angiography in assessing the physiologic significance of proximal left anterior descending coronary arterial stenosis. Circulation 1984; 69: 1111–9.

32. Kern MJ, Presant S, Deligonoul U et al. The effects of coronary angioplasty on nitroglycerin-induced augmentation of regional myocardial blood flow. J Intervent Cardiol 1988; 1: 121–30.

33. Wilson RF, Laughlin DE, Ackell PH et al. Transluminal, subselective measurement of

coronary artery blood flow velocity and vasodilator reserve in man. Circulation 1985; 72: 82–92.

34. Furchgott RF, Zawadzki JV. The obligatory role of endothelial cells in the relaxation of arterial smooth muscle by acetylcholine. Nature 1980; 288: 373–6.

35. Ludmer PL, Selwyn AP, Shook TL et al. Paradoxical vasoconstriction induced by acetylcholine in atherosclerotic coronary arteries. N Engl J Med 1986; 315: 1046–51.

36. Waller BF. Early and late morphological changes in human coronary arteries after percutaneous transluminal coronary angioplasty. Clin Cardiol 1983; 6: 363–72.

37. Di Mario C, Meneveau N, Gil R et al. Maximal blood flow velocity in severe coronary stenoses measured with a Doppler guidewire. Limitations for the application of the continuity equation in the assessment of stenosis severity. Am J Cardiol 1993; 71 (Suppl): 54D–61D.

38. Yuan YW, Shung KK. Ultrasonic backscatter from flowing whole blood. I: Dependence on shear rate and hematocrit. J Acoust Soc Am 1988; 84: 52–8.

39. Chillan WM, Marcus ML. Effects of coronary and extravascular pressure on intramyocardial and epicardial blood velocity. Am J Physiol 1985; 248: H170–8.

40. Lee J, Chambers DE, Akizuki S, Downey JM. The role of vascular capacitance in the coronary arteries. Circ Res 1984; 55: 751–762.

41. Kaijya F, Ogasawara Y, Tsujioka K et al. Evaluation of human coronary blood flow with an 80 channel 20 MHz pulsed Doppler velocimeter and zero-cross and Fourier transform methods during cardiac surgery. Circulation 1986; 74 (Suppl III): III–53–60.

42. Kaijya F, Ogasawara Y, Tsujioka K et al. Analysis of flow characteristics in post-stenotic regions of the human coronary artery during bypass graft surgery. Circulation 1987; 76: 1092–100.

43. Furuse A, Klopp EH, Brawley RK, Gott VL. Hemodynamic determinations in the assessment of distal coronary artery disease. J Surg Res 1975; 19: 25–33.

44. Kern MJ, Donohue TJ, Aguirre FV et al. Assessment of angiographically intermediate coronary artery stenosis using the Doppler flowire. Am J Cardiol 1993; 71 (Suppl): 26D–33D.

45. Serruys PW, Di Mario C, Meneveau N et al. Intracoronary pressure and flow velocity with sensor-tip guidewires: a new methodologic approach for assessment of coronary hemodynamics before and after coronary interventions. Am J Cardiol 1993; 71: 41D–53D.

46. Gould KL. Interactions with the distal coronary vascular bed. In: Gould KL, editor. Coronary artery stenosis. New York: Elsevier, 1991: 31–9.

47. Gould KL. Phasic pressure-flow and fluid-dynamic analysis. In: Gould KL, editor. Coronary artery stenosis. New York: Elsevier, 1991: 40–52.

48. Gould KL. Pressure-flow characteristics of coronary stenoses in unsedated dogs at rest and during coronary vasodilation. Circ Res 1978; 43: 242–53.

49. Mancini GBJ, Cleary RM, DeBoe AF et al. Instantaneous hyperemic flow-versus-pressure slope index. Microsphere validation of an alternative to measures of coronary reserve. Circulation 1991; 84: 862–70.

50. Seiler C, Kirkeeide RL, Gould KL. Stenoses at coronary artery bifurcations: Direct in vivo demonstration of coronary branch steal during hyperemia. Eur Heart J 1995; 16 (Suppl): 170 (Abstr).

Corresponding Author: Dr Christian Seiler, Department of Internal Medicine, University Hospital, Freiburgstrasse, CH-3010 Berne, Switzerland

20. Angiographic assessment of immediate success and the problem (definition) of restenosis after coronary interventions

DAVID P. FOLEY and PATRICK W. SERRUYS

Introduction

Despite the recent technological advances in medical imaging which have facilitated ultrasonographic and angioscopic imaging of the coronary vessel wall and lumen, which are described in other areas of this book, coronary angiography is still the universal routine clinical imaging technique both for guiding and assessing acute results of coronary interventions, as well as for evaluating long term restenosis. In this chapter, we discuss the angiographic assessment of [1] success of coronary interventions in the immediate term and [2] especially in the long term, with specific emphasis on evolving methodological approaches to defining restenosis.

Assessment of immediate interventional success

The antithesis of success is of course failure, and 2 distinct categories of acute interventional failure may be considered:

(i) Abrupt vessel closure

When occurring in the catheterization laboratory, this event obviously does not present a problem in recognition. The reported incidence of acute coronary artery occlusion during or after balloon angioplasty has varied, depending on the definition of time interval, i.e. whether in the catheterization laboratory, or during the first 24 hours, or the in-hospital period, from 2% to 10% [1–4]. Although the sometimes catastrophic consequences of acute vessel closure initially restricted application of PTCA to centres with on-site surgical standby, increased operator experience and angioplasty equipment, as well as the development of perfusion balloon catheters and increasing availability and proven value of bail-out stent implantation (as well as portable devices for percutaneous extracorporeal circulatory support), allow performance of percutaneous interventions in centres without actual on-site surgical back-up

C.A. Nienaber and U. Sechtem (eds): Imaging and Intervention in Cardiology, 311–340.
© 1996 *Kluwer Academic Publishers.*

[5]. Nevertheless, despite its decreasing frequency and improved manageability, acute closure remains the major cause of in-hospital morbidity and mortality associated with percutaneous angioplasty. The mechanisms of abrupt coronary artery occlusion are multifactorial and include, in various combinations depending on circumstances, 1) vasoconstriction or frank spasm of comparatively undiseased segments adjacent to a treated lesion, 2) elastic recoil following dilatation, 3) platelet adhesion and aggregation with ensuing intracoronary thrombus formation, 4) sub-intimal or mural haemorrhage and 5) mechanical obstruction due to large intimal dissection and/or extruded atheromatous material [4, 6–9].

It is rarely possible to accurately distinguish between these mechanisms by angiography (Figure 1) and it is, in fact, likely that each individual case of

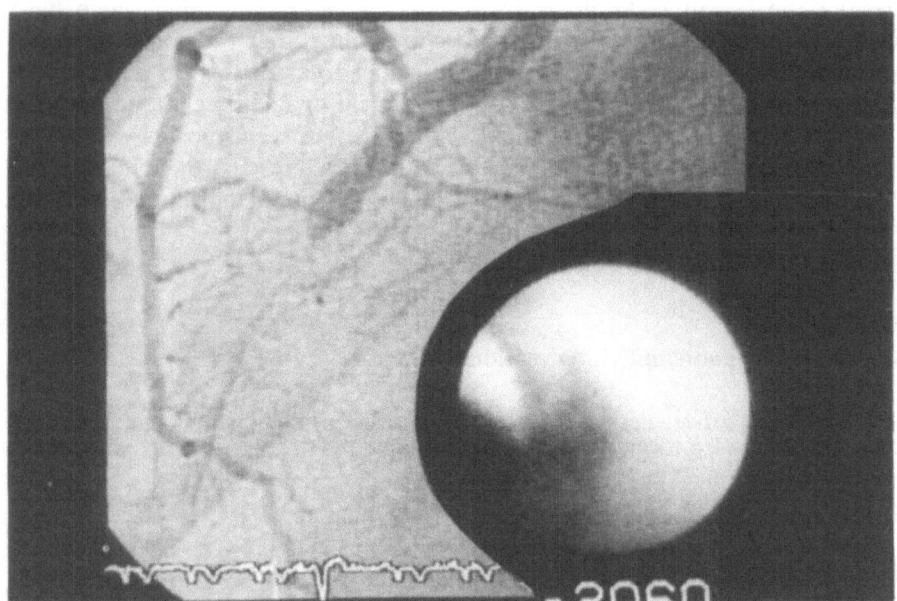

Figure 1. Example of the uncertainty of the precise cause of acute coronary occlusion during balloon angioplasty by angiography (left anterior oblique projection), which may be clarified by intracoronary angioscopy. Balloon dilatation of a proximal right coronary artery lesion resulted in the angiographic appearance shown, whereby it is appreciated that although the vessel is now completely occluded, there is no specific sign of the presence of intimal dissection or intracoronary thrombus. Angioscopy performed shortly after occlusion showed complete occlusion of the lumen by a red thrombus (seen here occupying the entire lower left quadrant of the angioscopic field, below the bright white appearance of the guidewire, which has been positioned across the stenosis), with no significant intimal dissection, except for some small superficial intimal disruptions which cannot be appreciated in this still picture and are a characteristic postangioplasty angioscopic feature. (For colour plate of this figure see **page 538**.)

acute closure is precipitated and maintained by a combination of these factors. Angiographic studies have been unable to determine the cause in 50% of cases [4]. Based on current knowledge of the mechanisms of balloon angioplasty provided by intravascular ultrasound [10, 11], occlusive dissection after dilatation would appear to account for the vast majority of abrupt coronary artery occlusion. Intracoronary angioscopy studies have confirmed the frequency of intimal dissection after balloon dilatation and have also shown that non-occlusive thrombus accompanies intimal dissection in most cases [12] and occlusive thrombus may itself be the primary cause of closure in 20% of instances [13]. Although acute coronary occlusion during PTCA is unpredictable in the individual patient, gender (female), symptomatic status (unstable angina) and severity, extent and complexity of coronary artery lesions, as well as location in angulated coronary segments, have been shown to be important pre procedural factors [1–7, 14].

Introduction of directional, extraction and rotational atherectomy, laser balloon and excimer laser angioplasty, despite increasing the applicability of percutaneous recanalization, have not overcome the problem of acute vessel closure. Although the development of perfusion balloons allowing prolonged inflation time provided considerable respite from the threat of acute closure during angioplasty, bail-out stent implantation, as a permanent scaffold, has presented the greatest single advance in the treatment of acute vessel occlusion after angioplasty. Nevertheless, although acute and sub-acute stent occlusion has undergone a reduction in frequency since the earliest reports, it remains a well documented reality in 0.4–30% of cases, depending on whether implantation was elective, or for the emergency relief of acute occlusion after failed PTCA [15–20]. Thrombosis within the stent has traditionally been believed to be the main culprit of such acute (or sub-acute) stent occlusion, but the use of coronary angioscopy after acute or sub-acute stent occlusion has suggested that occlusive coronary dissection may be the predominant cause in some patients [21]. Such information, as well as extensive intravascular ultrasound studies after intervention, highlights the inability of coronary angiography to effectively or reliably distinguish between thrombus and dissection in cases of acute coronary occlusion after failed intervention. Large studies will be required to precisely define the causative mechanisms of acute occlusion after various therapeutic interventions, as well as to objectively determine the role of angioscopy in individual cases, to facilitate tailoring of appropriate management strategies. Since practitioners are already reporting that angioscopic findings influence therapeutic strategy during routine intervention, its application to management of acute closure may ultimately become widely practiced, particularly if management reconsiderations as a consequence of the specific information provided are found to actually influence acute and long term clinical outcome.

Thus, although angiographic recognition of the occurrence of acute vessel closure is elementary, the information provided by angiography is too crude to allow identification of specific causology, so that more sophisticated intra-coronary imaging techniques must be employed to facilitate appropriate individual management strategies.

(ii) Sub-optimal acute interventional results

Visual qualitative assessment of angiogram

Traditionally, visual angiographic assessment has been the cornerstone of clinical practice, in determining the need for coronary intervention or surgery and for interactively judging the most difficult aspect of intervention, as with many medical treatments – when to stop. Although it is difficult to disbelieve what our eyes tell us, the unreliability of visual interpretation of the cine angiogram, even by experienced eyes, is now well recognized, leading to significant overestimation of lesion severity pre-PTCA and underestimation of residual narrowing post intervention (Figures 2 and 3). Some years ago, a simple clinical quantitative angiographic study from our group [22] explored the reliability of visual estimates of coronary artery stenosis in the 90% range, asking the clinically relevant question: "does the 90% stenosis actually exist?". The conclusion was, excluding lesions where the anterograde blood flow was TIMI grade I or occasional cases with TIMI grade 2 flow (ie. sub-total or "functional" occlusions), authentic 90% diameter stenoses probably do not exist. In this study, interventionalists were asked to estimate the percent diameter stenosis of and TIMI grade blood flow through the target lesion before balloon angioplasty. Blood flow was again recorded after guide-wire insertion across the target lesion. The likelihood of flow reduction or occlusion after insertion of the guidewire was predicted on the basis of the visual estimation of stenosis severity (% diameter stenosis) and the quantitatively measured vessel size (interpolated reference diameter) and was compared with actual blood flow. For example, if the observer estimated a 90% diameter stenosis and the vessel diameter was quantitatively measured at 3 mm, the residual lumen diameter, according to the visual estimate would be 0.3 mm. Introduction of a 0.018 inch guidewire (0.48 mm) should thus cause total occlusion of the vessel and this stenosis grading by the observer was classified as a "predicted occlusion". While observers frequently provided estimates of stenosis severity corresponding with "predicted occlusion", actual occlusion or flow reduction by one or more TIMI grades

---

→

Figure 2. (a, b) Angiogram, in the left anterior oblique projection, depicting a proximal stenosis in the right coronary artery pre-intervention. It is probably fair to state that most of us who were clinically trained to evaluate angiograms would estimate this stenosis in the region of 90% diameter stenosis for practical purposes. Figure 2b shows the automated analysis of this segment by the CAAS system, whereby a 70% diameter stenosis is measured, which corresponds to a 91% area stenosis. This illustrates the points that we do tend to visually overestimate severe stenoses and that perhaps this is because we see the area stenosis but call it diameter stenosis.

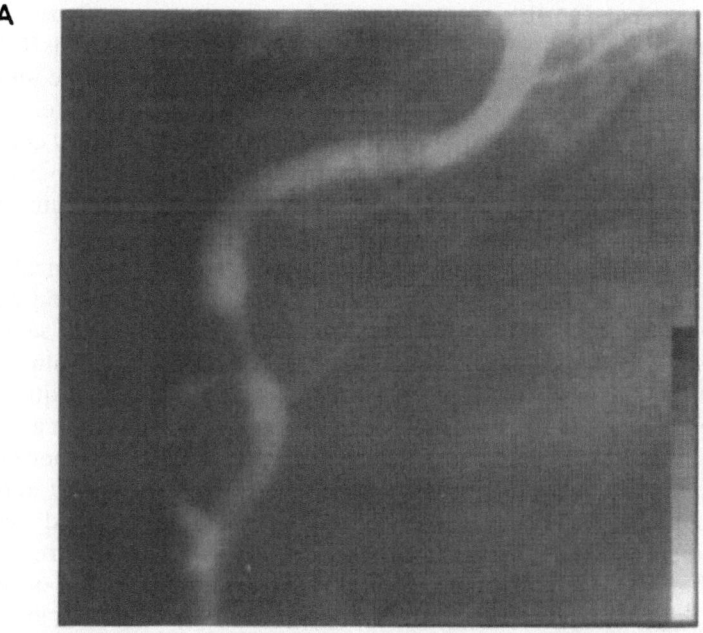

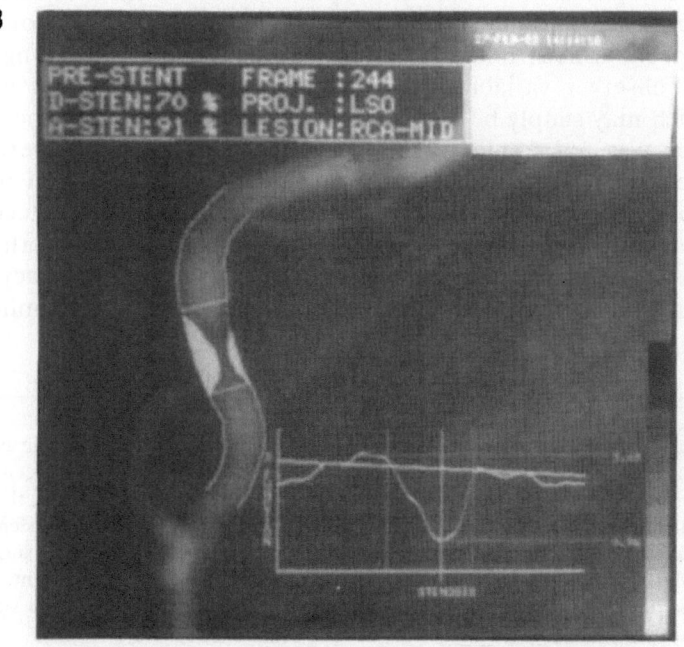

rarely occurred. In all cases where guide wire insertion across the target lesion caused flow reduction, baseline flow had been classified as TIMI grade 1 or occasional grade 2. Thus, it could be concluded that where anterograde blood flow is "normal", lesion severity never reaches a diameter stenosis of 90%. Accordingly, angiographic evaluation systems which allow classification of lesions of such severity, do not reflect actual lesion dimensions, will describe lesions which are not physiologically possible and are thus unsuitable for important studies.

Extensive experience with serial quantitative analysis in clinical trials has shown that among 1445 lesions, excluding TIMI 1 and 0 flow, only 5% were measured at greater than 74% diameter stenosis and the most severe lesion was 86% [23]. To clinicians unfamiliar with QCA, these values for pre-angioplasty "critical" lesions may appear low, but in fact, a quantitatively measured percent diameter stenosis of 74% corresponds with an area stenosis of approximately 93% [23] (see Figure 2, for example). Furthermore, fluid dynamic principles would indicate that the pressure gradient required to maintain blood flow across lesions of 80% or greater would actually be physiologically impossible [23]. Fleming et al. [24] have interestingly suggested that visual overestimations of percent diameter stenosis of moderate-severe coronary lesions arise due to the observer "seeing" the area stenosis but calling it diameter stenosis (Figure 2).

The large intra-and inter-observer variation [25, 26], and lack of correlation with pathological [27] and physiological [28] findings of visually evaluated coronary cine-angiograms are now well recognized. The reproducibility of visual lesion assessment is influenced by the severity of the coronary stenosis, so that, in general, lesions between 20–70% diameter obstruction by visual assessment (so called "mild-moderate" lesions) have a wider range of intra and inter observer variability than stenoses less than 20% or more than 70%, which may simply be a fundamental human limitation, since observer experience was not found to influence this finding [29]. Nevertheless, it may be considered somewhat reassuring that a brief period of training in quantitative angiographic analysis using an automated edge detection technique can considerably improve visual estimation of stenosis severity towards agreement with quantitative measurements [24, 30]. The accuracy of visual lesion assessment of coronary cine-angiograms is thus most limited in the

---

→
Figure 3. (a, b) Post Palmaz-Schatz stent implantation angiogram (in the same projection as Figure 2) of the coronary segment depicted in Figure 2. The plain angiogram seems to show a virtually normalized segment, compared with the previous angiogram. However, the automated detection algorithm, shown in Figure 3b, actually detects a 28% diameter stenosis (which corresponds with a 48% area stenosis), which may come as a considerable surprise to the physician who believes he has just implanted and fairly optimally deployed a stent. In addition, this example illustrates the type of post-stent angiographic result which must be striven for, to really optimize deployment and reduce a stenosis to 0% range.

A

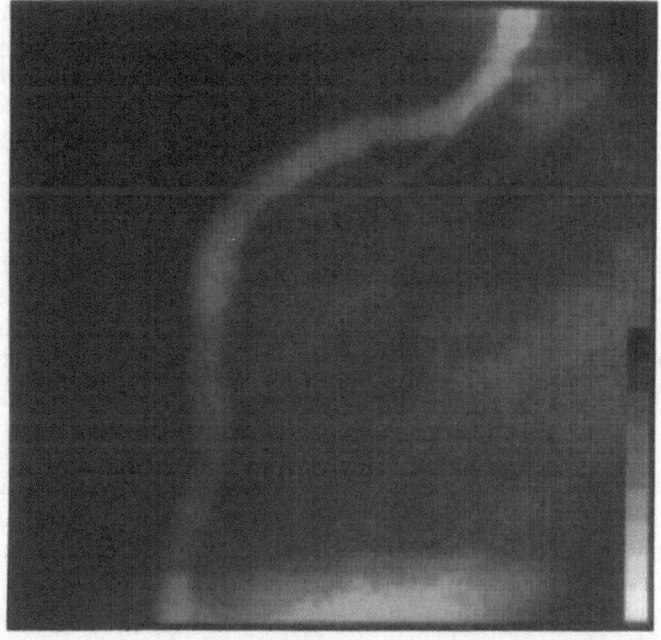

B

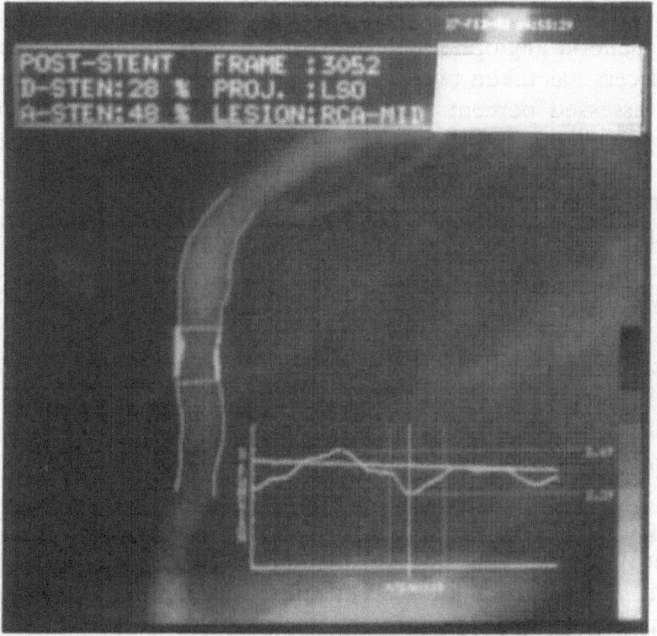

range of "intermediate severity", which are frequently observed after balloon angioplasty and at follow up, and in which minor luminal changes may have major haemodynamic consequences. While resting coronary blood flow is not altered until an obstruction of at least 85% of the diameter is present, maximal coronary flow is already diminished by obstructions as small as 30%, and marked impairment of coronary flow reserve (CFR) occurs with progressive diameter stenosis above 70% [31]. A recent report, where visual interpretation of coronary arteriograms was compared with quantitative coronary arteriographic assessment, confirmed earlier findings that: 1) visual estimates of "moderately" severe stenosis were up to 30% higher than actual percent diameter stenosis, 2) visual estimates diagnosed significantly more three-vessel disease, 3) visual interpretation significantly overestimated initial lesion severity and underestimated stenosis severity after angioplasty [24, 28].

These limitations make visual assessment an unacceptable measurement technique for multicentre clinical investigations of biological agents or new devices aimed at improving early and/or late results of intervention, in order to ultimately guide clinical practice. Over the last decade, it has become increasingly appreciated that objective independent evaluation is mandatory to guarantee the reliability and integrity of final results and conclusions of such trials. However, a logistic problem in randomized angioplasty trials is caused by the need to stratify patients immediately after intervention as procedural success or not, so that only patients with so called "successful" intervention may be randomized to receive "anti-restenosis" therapy of some kind. Thus, an immediate declaration must be made by the interventionalist, as to success or not, without access to an independent authority. In clinical trials of balloon angioplasty to date, the angiographic approach to defining acute success has taken two forms, a requirement for a certain reduction in visually assessed percent diameter stenosis, usually a reduction by 20%, and/or, achievement of post-procedural percent stenosis of less than some specific cut-off point, usually 50% diameter stenosis, but some earlier trials used 60% as the cut point (Table 1). Even in trials currently in progress, in which the primary angiographic end-point is evaluated by an off-line angiographic core laboratory using automated quantitative analysis, this apparently crude definition of immediate success is still applied, for the fundamental reason that no superior approach, which is easily applicable and satisfactorily reproducible, is yet universally available to all potential investigators.

Technical aspects of quantitative angiography post-angioplasty

Post-angioplasty angiograms frequently demonstrate luminal haziness and irregularity and varying degrees of contrast extravasation or dissection. In addition, luminal irregularities and filling defects may be visible to the observer and it has been demonstrated by intravascular angioscopy and ultra-

Table 1. Previously and currently employed angiographic criteria for primary success of PTCA.

Author (ref.)	Year	Diameter gain at PTCA (%)	Residual diameter post-PTCA (%)	Other criteria
Gruentzig et al.	1983	≥20	–	Elimination of symptoms
Holmes et al.	1984	≥20	–	No in-hospital CABG
Kent et al.	1984	≥20	–	Absence of MI, death, CABG during hospitalization
Faxon et al.	1984	≥ 20	–	
Faxon et al.	1984	≥ 40	–	
O'Neill et al.	1984	–	–	Increase in CFR ≥ 1.2 gradient ≤25% of MAP
Meier et al.	1984	≥20	–	Functional improvement
Corcos et al.	1985	≥20	≤60%	
Levine et al.	1985	≥20	–	No complications (unspecified)
Mata et al.	1985	≥20	≤60%	
Kaltenbach et al.	1985	≥20		
Wijns et al.	1985	–	≤50%,	With good run-off and filling of the distal vessel. Elimination of symptoms
Serruys et al.	1985	–	≤50%	Mean pressure gradient across the stenosis, normalized for MAP ≤ 0.2
Leimgruber et al.	1986	≥20	–	Absence of MI, CABG, in-hospital death
Bertrand et al.	1986	≥20	–	No complications (unspecified)
Vandormael et al.	1987	≥30	≤50%	No in-hospital complications and functional improvement
Myler et al.	1987	≥35	≤50%	Gradient less than 15 mm Hg + absence of major in-hospital complications
Guiteras Val et al.	1987	≥20	–	Without procedure-related complications
de Feyter et al.	1988	–	≤50%	Transstenotic gradient index reduced to < 0.30 + Relief of acute ischemic symptoms, no death or CABG
Halon et al.	1989	≥20	≤50%	
Quigley et al.	1989	–	≤50%	No major in-hospital complications
Renkin et al.	1990	≥20	≤50%	
Rupprecht et al.	1990	≥20	≤50%	No major in-hospital complications
Serruys et al.	1991	–	<50%	
CARPORT	1991	–	<50%	No major immediate cardiac events
MERCATOR	1992	–	<50%	No major immediate cardiac events

Table 1. Continued.

Fischman et al.	1992	–	<50%	Tissue retrieval, no major cardiac complication
Roubin et al.	1992	–	<50%	
Popma et al.	1993	–	<50%	Tissue retrieval, no ischemic in-hospital complications
CAVEAT	1993	–	<50% (goal of < 20%)	
CCAT	1993	–	≤50%	(angiographic success)
			≤50%	No major in-hospital complications
AMRO	1994	–	<50%	No immediate major cardiac complications
BENESTENT	1994	–	<50%	No immediate major cardiac complications
STRESS	1994	–	<50%	No immediate major cardiac complications
BOAT	1994	–	<20%	
BENESTENT II	1994	–	<20%	No immediate major cardiac complications
EUROCARE	1994	–	<20%	+tissue retrieval
MUSIC	1994	IVUS definition of optimal stent deployment		

CABG = coronary artery bypass graft; CFR = coronary flow reserve; MAP = mean aortic pressure; MI = myocardial infarction; CARPORT = Coronary Artery Restenosis Prevention On Repeated Thromboxane-antagonism; MERCATOR = Multicentre European Research trial with Cilazapril after Angioplasty to prevent Transluminal Obstruction and Restenosis; CAVEAT = Coronary Angioplasty versus Excisional Atherectomy Trial; CCAT = Canadian Coronary Atherectomy Trial; AMRO = AMsterdam-ROtterdam (randomized trial of excimer laser coronary angioplasty versus balloon angioplasty (ELCA) in native primary coronary artery lesions); BENESTENT = BElgium NEtherlands STENT (randomized comparison of Palmaz-Schatz stent implantation versus balloon angioplasty in native primary coronary artery disease); STRESS = STent REStenosis Study (randomized comparison of Palmaz-Schatz stent implantation versus balloon angioplasty in native primary coronary artery disease); BOAT = Balloon angioplasty versus Optimal Atherectomy Trial. EUROCARE = EUROpean Carvedilol Atherectomy Restenosis Evaluation; MUSIC = Multicentre UltraSound In Coronary arteries.

sound that intraluminal flaps and thrombus may be present, but not angiographically detectable [10–12]. Furthermore, balloon dilatation has been shown to distort luminal geometry to a non-circular configuration [6, 10, 11]. Many investigators have listed these angiographically evident and invisible morphological changes as potential contributors to the known deterioration in quantitative angiographic measurement reliability after balloon angioplasty [32–35]. For example, if an intimal dissection is opacified by contrast during angiography, it may be identified as the true luminal contour by an automated edge detection algorithm, leading to an overestimation of the true luminal dimension or, on the other hand, the observer may correct the automatically detected borders, excluding the dissection (Figure 4). In this case, because of the subjectivity of the interaction by the observer, reproducibility of the findings, which is one of the principle strengths of automated quantitative analysis, is lost. In addition, it cannot be consistently interpreted from visual inspection of the angiogram at what exact level the true vessel lumen is traversed or compromised by the apparent dissection and the true luminal diameter may be underestimated. Since there is no objective information available as to what approach is correct in handling these cases, a decision taken by the Angiographic Committee of the MERCATOR trial that the automated edge detection algorithm should not be corrected in its automatic tracing of the vessel contours in the region of an apparent dissection [36], has been consistently retained as routine practice at our core laboratory. This empirical approach allows the algorithm to include a dissection if there is no separation from the true lumen – separation by 2 pixels or more (thus approximately 0.1–0.15 mm in real terms, depending on the magnification mode used) would be sufficient for the algorithm to exclude the dissection from the vessel lumen. In this context, the use of videodensitometry instead of edge detection analysis, would not solve the problem, mainly due to the inherent limitations of this analytical approach – whereby the density of the opacified segment is compared between the "stenosis" and a selected "normal reference", based on the assumption of a relationship between contrast density and luminal area, which may be altered or lost at each step involved in the acquisition, storage, transfer and analysis of images. To handle a contrast extravasation for example, the contrast opacified dissection plane either would be included in the densitometric profile, leading to overestimation of the true luminal cross sectional area, or, if not included, would have to be subtracted by the programme, to obtain a net cross-sectional videodensitometric profile of the target segment, which would be likely to underestimate the true luminal cross sectional area (Figure 5, for example). The previously mentioned study from our group investigating the potential applicability of single view angiography for quantitative analysis [34], found that the variability of measurements obtained from orthogonal views of the mid-segment of the right coronary artery (theoretically the easiest segment

---

→

Figure 4. (a, b) Example of the difficulty in post angioplasty quantitative angiographic analysis presented by the presence of contrast extravasation in the region of the target stenosis. In this case, a type B dissection is evident post-PTCA of a distal circumflex lesion (right anterior oblique projection). If the automated analysis algorithm is allowed to follow the contours it detects, the analysis in Figure 4a is obtained, with inclusion of the extravasation as part of the lumen. The measured minimal luminal diameter is 2.53 mm and the reference diameter is 3.14 mm, giving a percent diameter stenosis of 19%. On the other hand, if minor observer correction at the proximal end of the stenosis directs the algorithm to ignore the extravasation, the detected contours obtained are as shown in Figure 4b, with a measured minimal luminal diameter of 1.34 mm and a reference diameter of 3.07 mm, giving a 56% diameter stenosis. Videodensitometric analysis in Figure 4a is not quite in parallel with the edge detection curve, since the contrast density is inhomogeneous. However, this analysis also includes the extravasation and does not help to indicate whether or not the so-called dissection contributes to the vessel lumen or not.

A

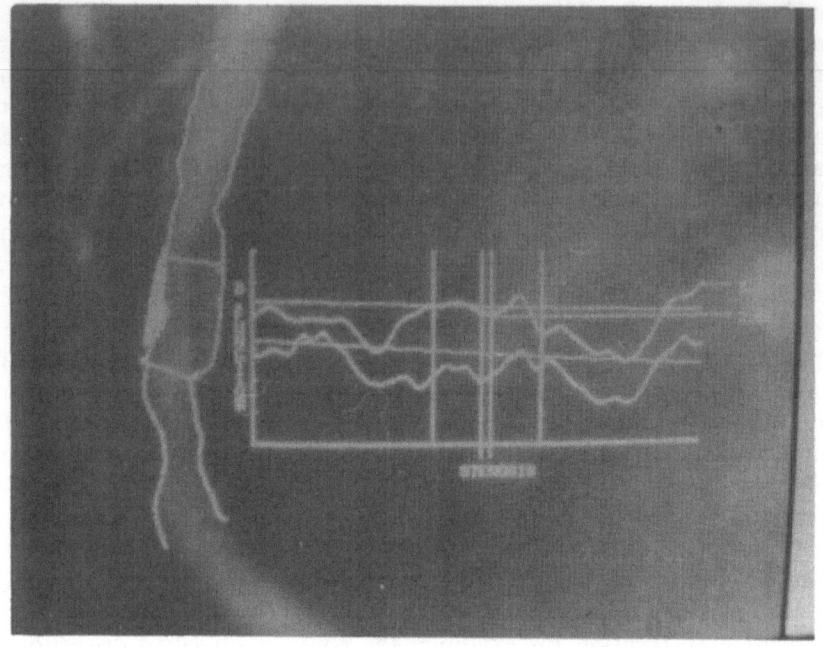

B

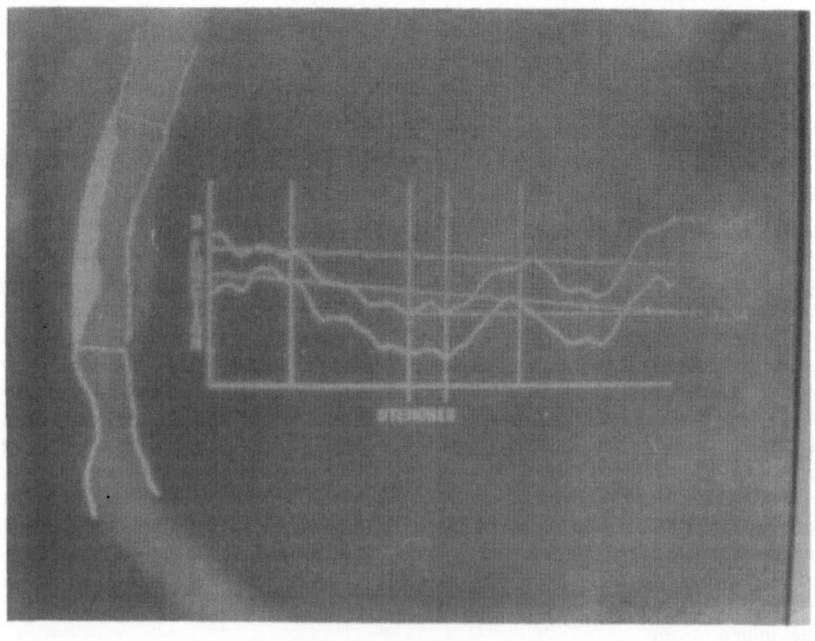

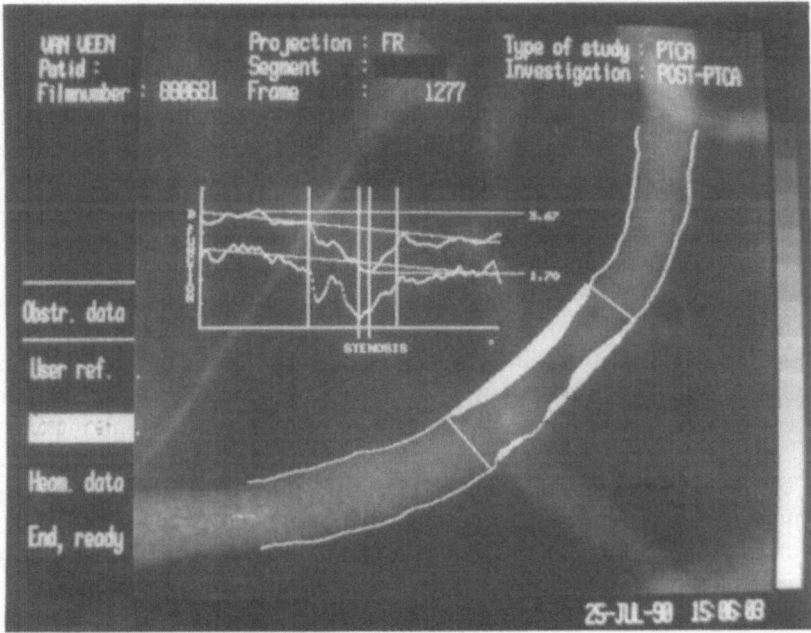

Figure 5. Quantitative analysis of a distal circumflex lesion post angioplasty in the left superior oblique projection to illustrate the difficulty frequently encountered in using videodensitometry to measure coronary stenoses. The edge detection algorithm provided the upper of the 2 curves shown, with a "dip" at the minimal luminal diameter, which is shown as 1.70 mm. The lower curve actually "dips" almost to the X axis at the point of the MLD, indicating an extremely severe stenosis. This is due to excessive background subtraction, on account of a sidebranch passing behind the target stenosis, which has not affected the edge detection process, as the sidebranch crosses at an extremely acute angle, so it is ignored by the algorithm. Thus, a typical post-PTCA result (MLD of 1.70 mm is in the region of the mean observed in 4 major restenosis prevention trials [86]) would have been classified as a total occlusion by automated videodensitometry – illustrating the need for optimal conditions for reliable application of this measurement approach.

for which to obtain optimal orthogonal images) was too great to recommend routine use of a single projection, for both edge detection and videodensitometry or an average of measurements obtained by each approach. However, it was noteworthy that while the agreement between orthogonal views deteriorated from pre to post-PTCA, this was less marked for videodensitometry than for edge detection. We hypothesized that this could be due to the fallacious assumption of a circular morphology for edge detection calculations and the independence of videodensitometric measurements from luminal morphology. An additional interesting finding in this study was that the deterioration in agreement between orthogonal measurements by edge detection was independent of the presence or absence of visible dissection, which would seem to indicate that, on balance, the presence of angiographically visible dissection in approximately 35% of lesions post-PTCA [37], does not unduly skew the results of edge detection analysis, compared with "non-dissected cases".

In a 24-hour follow-up angiographic study of 106 patients after successful balloon angioplasty, no difference in mean minimal luminal diameter or cross sectional area was found from immediately post-PTCA to 24 hours [38]. This finding indicated that there is no phenomenon of delayed elastic recoil of the dilated lesion in the first 24 hours after PTCA and that angiography immediately post-PTCA is indeed suitable for quantitative analysis in clinical trials, without the need for further repeat angiography 24 hours later for that purpose. In addition, the standard deviation of the mean difference in minimal luminal diameter from post-PTCA to 24 hours could be used to delineate the post-PTCA measurement variability of the CAAS system, which was found to be 0.20 mm and must be considered to be eminently acceptable, in view of the previous description of potential pitfalls of post-PTCA angiographic analysis. Based on our previously published concept of using the measurement variability of the analysis system as a categorical cut-off criteria for confirmation of a definite change in measured luminal dimensions over time, using these data, the post-PTCA measurement variability of the CAAS system could be stated as 0.40 mm (two standard deviations of the mean difference in repeated measurements). A change greater than this figure from post-PTCA to subsequent angiography could therefore, with 95% confidence, be considered as a definite "real" change and could not be explained merely by measurement variability of the system. Other investigators have also reported on the findings of 24-hour follow up studies using automated quantitative angiography, with generally similar findings [39–41].

Single or multiple angiographic projections

A considerable source of variation in approach to quantitative coronary angiographic measurement arises from differences of opinion regarding the use of a single angiographic projection in which the stenosis appears "worst" pre intervention (and repeating measurements from that same projection post intervention and at follow up), or alternatively using multiple projections identically repeated at all phases of intervention and taking the mean of measurements from these so called "multiple matched projections". Our group has always advocated the latter approach in an attempt to provide a 3 dimensional perspective of the target lesion [32, 33], which is of particular relevance when it is remembered that approximately 70% of coronary artery stenoses are eccentric rather than concentric in morphological profile [42]. In addition, a number of studies from our group have suggested that changes in the luminal area of an artery, produced by the mechanical disruption of its internal wall as a result of balloon angioplasty, cannot be assessed accurately from the detected contours of the vessel from a single plane angiographic view [32, 34]. Significant differences in luminal dimensional measurements emerge from quantitative angiographic analysis of single or multiple projections [43]. Even combining information derived from videodensitometry (which does not require the frequently erroneous assumption of a circular cross section) with data provided by automated edge detection, does not provide acceptably precise luminal area or diameter measurements when only a single angiographic projection is used [34]. Use of multiple projections (at least 2 orthogonal or near orthogonal for the right coronary artery and at least 3 separated by at least 30° for left coronary artery) identically repeated pre and post intervention has consequently been routinely and vigorously applied to multicentre interventional trials in which our institution has played a co-ordinating role [16, 19, 36, 44–47]. Other groups and a number of large important interventional trials, on the other hand, have employed and continue to apply, single "worst view" as the basis for quantitative measurements [17, 18, 48–56], with in our view, the attendant danger of potentially erroneous or misleading results. In fact, a recent post-hoc exploratory study of the CAVEAT trial [57] revealed that had multiple angiographic projections instead of the single worst view approach been used to report the findings of CAVEAT, a marginally significant (p = 0.045) angiographic benefit, in terms of minimal luminal diameter at follow up, of DCA over PTCA would have been found (1.50 mm for DCA compared with 1.40 mm for PTCA), whereas in the reported results the difference in MLD at follow up (1.35 mm for DCA and 1.23 mm for PTCA) was not significant (p = 0.076). In addition, the overall restenosis rates for balloon angioplasty and atherectomy (48% and 42%, respectively) would have been much lower than was initially reported (57% and 50%, respectively), although no significant difference between the groups would have been found. The conclusion of this exploration, like previous conclusions from our own studies [34, 43] is that such comparative findings carry definite implications for comparisons between different angiographic studies. Although, intuitively, a multiple (matched) view approach would seem superior, in providing tomographic images, it is likely that to objectively and independently determine the most reliable of these approaches in the clinical setting, comparison of each approach with measurement series obtained by high quality intracoronary ultrasound would be required. Definitions of acute success and also assessment of late "restenosis" will be affected, to a greater or lesser degree, by whether a single or multiple angiographic projections are used.

Definition of acute success based on objective measurements

(i) On-line quantitative coronary angiography
The rapidly increasing availability of on-line automated and semi-automated quantitative angiographic analysis packages with all modern digital acquisition systems, puts this powerful measurement tool in the hands of virtually all interventionalists. Consequently, many multicentre randomized interven-

tional trials currently in progress or in the planning stages have begun to require an on-line quantitative definition of immediate interventional success. Increasing use of stent implantation and directional atherectomy as primary devices for coronary revascularization has led to the emergence of the "bigger is better" maxim [54–56, 58] so that previously acceptable angiographic definitions for interventional success (Table 1) may soon become obsolete. Accordingly, the criteria for "sub-optimal" acute results must logically change in parallel. In the ongoing BOAT, BENESTENT II and EURO-CARE trials, to name but a few, the target for acute procedural success will be a diameter stenosis <20% post intervention, using on-line quantitative angiography.

The appropriateness, at least in the acute term, of this apparently aggress-ive attitude to coronary intervention has been supported by objective evi-dence provided by intracoronary ultrasound guidance of stent implantation. It has been shown that angiographic monitoring frequently does not provide adequate information, in regard to optimization of the acute interventional result, in a considerable proportion of cases [59]. This evidence has been so clinically convincing that many experienced interventionalists now routinely employ the so-called "Swiss-kiss" procedure after stent deployment in order to optimize expansion, even when the post-deployment angiographic appear-ance seems satisfactory. Studies using intracoronary ultrasound guidance to optimize the acute result of stent implantation have also reported a strikingly low incidence of acute and sub-acute stent thrombosis, despite the absence of routine post procedural anti-coagulation, a practice which has concomitantly dramatically reduced the rate of bleeding complications [60]. This develop-ment, if confirmed in larger randomized studies, will represent a giant leap forward for coronary intervention and carries the far-reaching implication that stent implantation, when feasible and in favourable morphological con-ditions, may become the "golden fleece" for percutaneous recanalization. However, enthusiasm must be tempered somewhat for the time being until the long term results of such therapeutic improvisation have been established. Although both the BENESTENT and STRESS trials reported the first de-monstration in a randomized clinical trial of a convincing reduction in ex-pected angiographic "restenosis rates" and clinical events through Palmaz–Schatz stent implantation compared with balloon angioplasty, because of the need for anticoagulation, the incidence of "major bleeding" was significantly greater among stented patients [18, 19]. Moreover, although stented lesions demonstrated significantly greater minimal luminal diameter at follow up angiography in both trials, the degree of angiographic luminal renarrowing during 6 months follow up was significantly greater in stented lesions. Accord-ingly, restenosis must still be considered to represent at least the "fly in the ointment" or "blot on the landscape" for coronary angioplasty, if not quite the Achilles' Heel – which, historically, proved to be a fatal flaw. While the search for the "magic bullet" to prevent restenosis continues and intensi-fies, some major evolutional changes in the angiographic methods for evaluation and definition of restenosis have unfolded in recent years and are described in the next section.

(ii) Physiological parameters

As a consequence of the progressively widening acceptance of quantitative angiography as the gold standard for angiographic measurement of stenosis severity, on-line quantitative analytic packages have been built in to modern digital angiographic imaging equipment. The reliability of some of these packages compared with off-line analysis of cinefilm has already been demonstrated to be acceptable. Using experimentally validated haemodynamic equations, automated quantitative angiographic systems can provide extensive physiological parameters on a stenotic coronary segment. Theoretical pressure-flow relationships constructed using the quantitative measurements of stenosis dimensions have been reported to correctly identify the presence of critical lesions with high sensitivity and specificity [31, 61–66]. Recently, adaptation of angioplasty guide wires to allow intracoronary doppler and pressure measurement has facilitated validation of these theoretical pressure-flow relationships in the clinical setting of the catheterization laboratory [64]. A number of studies have additionally reported accurate evaluation of short, medium and long term functional results of interventions using coronary flow reserve measurement by digital angiography [63, 65, 66]. However, in unselected patients, coronary flow reserve, measured in this manner, was not found to improve immediately after apparently successful angioplasty and showed only a minor improvement at 24 hours [67]. These conflicting results were believed to be simply due to the principal fundamental limitation of coronary flow reserve measurement, namely variability due to the influence of a number of unquantifiable confounding factors (such as diffuse coronary disease, microvascular disease, prior myocardial infarction, myocardial hypertrophy, collateral blood flow, tachycardia, hypertension etc.).

Currently an international multicentre clinical trial is in progress to evaluate the comparability of quantitative angiography and changes in coronary blood flow measured by doppler wire before and after balloon angioplasty (DEBATE – Doppler Evaluation of Balloon Angioplasty Trial End-points). In other chapters of this book, the use of doppler wire and of intra-coronary pressure measuring devices, which have led to the development of novel physiological measurements (such as stenosis flow reserve and fractional flow reserve) for the quantification of coronary stenosis severity and of the results of intervention, will be described in detail. Application of these techniques to the evaluation of angiographically "moderate" appearing stenoses appears to present a major advance and this is indeed an expanding and exciting area, but further studies are required to determine the ultimate place of these measurement devices in coronary investigation and therapy outside highly specialised centres.

Angiographic definition of restenosis

Recurrence of stenosis, luminal renarrowing or "restenosis" after initially successful angioplasty appears to be an inherent consequence of obligatory injury to the coronary vessel wall during intervention. In the approximately 30–50% of patients who experience recurrence of anginal symptoms or ischemia or an actual major adverse cardiac event (MACE, ie. cardiac death, myocardial infarction, bypass graft surgery or reintervention) in the 6 months after apparently successful angioplasty, "restenosis" has traditionally been attributed with responsibility for this considerable attenuation of the potential longterm benefit of the procedure. However, it is now well known that clinical events and recurrence of symptoms and/or ischemia after successful angioplasty are not always a direct consequence of renarrowing of a previously treated lesion, but may be secondary to incomplete initial revascularization or deterioration/progression in other untreated lesions [68]. Likewise, it has been shown that a considerable degree of renarrowing may develop at the site of a successful intervention without precipitating either anginal complaints or adverse cardiac events [69]. Consequently, to identify patients with actual lesion recurrence, it must be concluded that an objective method of measurement would be necessary. Because of the widespread use of coronary angiography as the guiding tool for coronary disease management, clinicians logically made use of the angiogram to detect and define lesion recurrence or restenosis after successful angioplasty.

Restenosis – a binary event or continuous process?

Since clinical decision making is essentially a binary practice, whereby a patient either has or does not have a disease and receives or does not receive therapy, it was legitimate to define the occurrence of restenosis along similar lines. Accordingly, an angiographically described lesion of 50% diameter stenosis or more at a follow up angiogram became considered to represent clinical restenosis. This apparently arbitrary cut-point was actually founded on good scientific evidence, being based on physiological experimental studies which demonstrated that when coronary vessel diameter is reduced to 50% or less, coronary flow reserve becomes impeded [31]. This definition of restenosis was not universally accepted, however, and a number of other angiographic definitions were introduced by investigators, to depict the concept of some degree of deterioration in stenosis severity since angioplasty. The National Heart Lung and Blood Institute published 4 different definitions of angiographic restenosis. Over the intervening decade, for various reasons, perhaps primarily because none of these definitions could be shown to really reflect clinical status, a proliferation of other definitions became used, some reflecting recurrence of a "severe" stenosis, others indicating deterioration of a certain degree or a combination of these and some including a definition of a successful acute result (Table 2).

Table 2. Definitions of the occurrence of angiographic restenosis which have been applied in clinical studies.

1. Diameter stenosis ⩾ 50% at follow up
2. Diameter stenosis ⩾ 70% at follow up
3. Diameter stenosis ⩾ 50% at follow up, where diameter stenosis immediately post-PTCA was < 50%
4. Diameter stenosis ⩾ 70% at follow up, where diameter stenosis immediately post-PTCA was < 50% (NHLBI II)
5. Diameter stenosis > 50% at follow up with > 10% deterioration in diameter stenosis since PTCA, where diameter stenosis was < 50% post-PTCA and a gain of > 10% was achieved at PTCA
6. Loss ⩾ 30% diameter stenosis from post PTCA to follow up (NHLBI 1)
7. Loss during follow up of at least 50% of the initial gain at PTCA (NHLBI 4).
8. Loss ⩾ 20% diameter stenosis from post PTCA to follow up
9. Return to within 10% of the pre-PTCA diameter stenosis (NHLBI 3)
10. Area stenosis ⩾ 85% at follow up
11. Loss ⩾ 1 mm^2 in stenosis area from post PTCA to follow up
12. Loss ⩾ twice the long term lesion measurement variability of the quantitative angiographic measurement system:
    (i) loss ⩾ 0.72 mm in minimal luminal diameter (MLD) from post-PTCA to follow-up
    (ii) loss ⩾ 0.50 mm in MLD from post-PTCA to follow-up
    (iii) loss ⩾ 0.40 mm in MLD from post-PTCA to follow-up

PTCA = percutaneous transluminal coronary angioplasty; NHLBI = National Heart, Lung, and Blood Institute of the United States.

With the introduction of automated quantitative angiography providing actual coronary dimensional measurements [70, 71], it was possible to derive more objective indices of restenosis, using the long term measurement variability of the analysis system as the cut-off point for "real" or "significant" luminal deterioration [72], instead of an arbitrary percentage stenosis measurement. More importantly, however, the use of quantitative analysis in large patient populations enabled considerable conceptual advances in the understanding of and approach to restenosis. During 1988, 2 separate independent studies employing serial monthly angiography in consecutive patient groups undergoing successful coronary angioplasty demonstrated renarrowing at the site of angioplasty to be a gradual time-related phenomenon, which appeared to reach a zenith at 4–6 months [73, 74] and developed to some degree in virtually all treated lesions. Application of a number of commonly used angiographic definitions of restenosis to these patients was associated with widely differing results. Moreover, patients defined as having restenosis by some definitions were categorized as not having restenosis by others. Accordingly, it was concluded that such definitions must be considered to be of very dubious and limited clinical relevance in identifying specific risk factors for development of restenosis. Indeed the relevance of attempting to apply binary criteria to describe the long term angiographic results of angioplasty in a treated patient population became subject to serious questioning.

To determine the actual distribution of luminal change from initially successful balloon angioplasty to 6 month angiographic follow up, quantitative angiographic measurements from 1445 patients were examined by our group and a virtually normal Gaussian plot was observed [23]. Similar findings were independently reported by Kuntz and colleagues in patients treated by stent implantation and directional atherectomy [75]. This would immediately suggest that "restenosis" is, in fact, fundamentally a normally distributed process (and not a binary event, as had been the clinical belief which was supported by a clinical investigation in a large patient population [76]). Such findings are not really all that surprising, since the underlying pathobiological processes as have been elegantly summarized and described by Forrester [77] constitute essentially the normal healing response to acute physical injury. These angiographic findings, moreover, not only make good biological sense, but also carry considerable implications for design of clinical trials investigating the effect of pharmacological agents and new interventional devices for prevention of restenosis. Statistical calculation of the sample size required to demonstrate a desired treatment effect, assuming that restenosis is a continuous phenomenon, may lead to as much as 250% reduction in total patient numbers, compared with assumption of restenosis as a categorical event [78]. Accordingly, most recent clinical interventional trials have employed this approach and have reported ultimate angiographic findings according to the mean change in minimal luminal diameter from immediately after angioplasty to follow up angiography, compared between the treatment groups [44–46]. Nevertheless, undoubtedly motivated by clinical demands, many trials have focused primarily on a binary clinical approach to the angiographic definition of restenosis [48, 49], while recent studies adopt a more comprehensive approach reporting findings from both perspectives [19, 20, 52, 53].

As with all aspects of medical research, a balance must be maintained between scientific objectivity and integrity and practical clinical relevance when approaching this now perennial problem of defining restenosis. While quantitative angiography, enabling objective and reproducible coronary luminal measurement, is becoming rapidly more widespread (through the advent of dedicated on-line systems as part of new digital angiographic acquisition systems and the mandatory employment of quantitative angiography in all modern "restenosis prevention trials" and "new device trials"), it seems unlikely that the pragmatic binary clinical view of restenosis will be replaced with the apparently esoteric and less practical scientific perspective of a continuous phenomenon which, de facto, can have no "cut-off" point or definition. It is inescapable, however, that true progress in this area can only be made through the adoption of such a scientific approach [58, 79].

Quantifying restenosis in clinical studies and trials – importance of measuring the angiographic outcome and the restenosis process

According to current philosophy, it is appreciated that there are essentially two interwoven aspects of the late result of coronary intervention which must be considered [58, 79]. On the one hand, there is the outcome, which is to say, the clinical status of the patient. From the anatomical viewpoint, the diameter of an epicardial vessel at its narrowest point is what actually dictates coronary blood flow capacity to the myocardium, so measurement of this diameter (the "minimal luminal diameter") in a treated vessel in the follow up angiogram may be considered to reflect the late outcome of a particular intervention for a particular patient or group of patients. On the other hand, the extent of luminal encroachment or renarrowing occurring from immediately after the intervention to the check-up angiogram may be considered to convey the degree of new tissue growth and vessel remodelling. Measurement of this aspect of the late result, as the *change* in minimal luminal diameter from post intervention to follow up, will reflect the therapeutic effectiveness of a supplementary pharmaco-biological agent or device in restricting the processes which contribute to renarrowing of the treated vessel segment. Thus both the process of restenosis (angiographically conveyed by the loss in minimal luminal diameter) and the late outcome (conveyed by the minimal luminal diameter at follow up) need to be measured in order to provide a complete picture of the consequences of a particular coronary intervention. Because these 2 end-points are fundamentally opposite, two equally correct but apparently contradictory perspectives began to emerge from clinical research in recent years, based on preferential focus on one or other end-point [58, 79]. On the basis of the direct linear relationship observed between luminal gain at intervention and luminal loss during follow up and the finding that luminal gain is the most powerful determinant of luminal loss [80–84] the somewhat cryptic, "the more you gain, the more you lose" adage emerged [79]. At the same time, based on the positive linear relationship observed between post procedural luminal diameter and the luminal diameter at follow up and the finding that the post procedural luminal diameter was the greatest predictor of the follow up luminal diameter [54, 56], the "bigger is better" aphorism was propagated [58] and was immediately attractive to clinicians in its essential simplicity. At first glance, these hypotheses appear to be fundamentally contradictory, but each is an equally valid and relevant interpretation of comprehensive investigations of extensive quantitative angiographic data. As a consequence of the attendant confusion caused to clinicians by these enigmas, metaphorical reference has been made in recent editorials on this controversial area [58, 79], to "the doughnut" and "the hole", whereby the doughnut reflects the neointimal hyperplastic process and the hole is the patent lumen ultimately remaining at the end, a simple metaphor first introduced by Schwartz et al. in their seminal experimental investigation of the injury/neointimal response relationship [85]. Also, the analogy of income taxation has been used to illustrate the value of increasing luminal gain (gross income) in order to maximize minimal luminal diameter at follow up (net take home income) despite the attendant increasing luminal loss (total tax paid). The enigma may also be encapsulated by observations on a drinking glass containing water to the half-way mark; is it half empty or half full? Ultimately, the final message emerging from these seemingly semantic, but fundamentally relevant methodological debates, is that in clinical restenosis studies, it is of central importance to measure both the process of restenosis, to determine whether the agent under investigation had a restraining or inhibitory effect, as well as the ultimate clinical/angiographic outcome, to determine whether the long term outcome is actually improved as a consequence of the treatment or device being tested.

Does the choice of device influence late results? New statistical approaches to evaluation of angiographic restenosis

The real dilemma remaining now for interventional cardiologists, with widespread clinical application of stent implantation, directional and rotational atherectomy and laser angioplasty, is whether there is a niche in clinical practice for appropriate application of each of these devices, or whether there is in reality an ideal interventional device which should thus be preferentially used. Results of observational studies evaluating new devices compared with historical angioplasty results are difficult to interpret, since directional atherectomy and stent implantation are inherently more applicable to larger coronary vessels than balloon angioplasty, which may lead to biased evaluation, since late results are known to be beneficially influenced by larger vessel size [54, 86]. Randomized trials of balloon angioplasty with directional atherectomy have been largely inconclusive thusfar [52, 53], but new trials employing the strategy of optimization of the acute result are ongoing. As previously mentioned, the first real suggestion of improvement in late interventional results using a new device has been provided by the results of randomized comparisons of Palmaz-Schatz stent implantation with balloon angioplasty, demonstrating significant advantage of stent implantation in terms of acute and 6 month clinical and angiographic results [19, 20]. Further hope for continued improvement has been provided through rigorous application of the "bigger is better" philosophy to stent implantation by availing of the practical on-line guiding possibilities of intracoronary ultrasound [59]. Optimization of the acute luminal result in this manner may obviate the need for stringent anticoagulation regimes, the complications of which have considerably contributed to scepticism on the real place of stent implantation as first line revascularization therapy in coronary artery disease [19, 20].

Despite continuing clinical focus on angiographic binary "restenosis rate", there has been a progressive shift away from simple statistical comparisons using the binary "restenosis" end-point in clinical studies in recent years. More sophisticated statistical approaches, using multiple logistic regression analysis, were initially applied in 1991 to determine predictors of binary restenosis [48, 49]. Since then, the assumption of a continuous distribution of angiographic luminal measurements has become fundamental to evaluation of restenosis, in order to improve our understanding of the interplay of the multiplicity of clinical, angiographic morphological, angioplasty procedural and quantitative luminal dimensional factors associated with luminal renarrowing. Accordingly, using multiple linear regression analysis, we and others have reported that the greatest determinant of luminal loss is luminal gain and that the most powerful predictor of a larger luminal diameter at follow up angiography is the acute post procedural result [51, 54, 56, 80–86]. However, whereas others have reported that it is the acute result of intervention which is important and that the device used for intervention is essentially irrelevant [54, 56], we have found significant differences between devices in the renarrowing response to luminal increase (independently of the acute post procedural result, the coronary vessel size, pre procedural stenosis severity and lesion location), a finding which would suggest inherent device specific properties in provocation of restenosis [87–89]. Our recent finding, also using multiple linear regression modelling, of a beneficial influence of larger vessel size on late angiographic results [86], may partly explain the perceived benefit of stent implantation and directional atherectomy over balloon angioplasty, since these devices are preferentially applied to lesions in larger coronary vessels. The question of inherent device specific effects on the restenosis process and late angiographic outcome now needs to be addressed in detail in ongoing trials and to be firmly resolved to facilitate clinical decision making in choosing appropriate devices for intervention.

Further statistical approaches applied to the evaluation of quantitative angiographic data include spline modelling to investigate the possibility of "non-linear" associations between luminal increase at intervention and subsequent renarrowing. Conflicting reports have been presented as preliminary findings of such investigations [90, 91] and no conclusive findings have yet been published to challenge the currently accepted view of a linear relationship between gain and loss. The fundamental hypothesis of a generally Gaussian distribution for luminal changes during follow up has likewise come under some recent scrutiny in a large patient group with quantitative angiographic follow up after successful balloon angioplasty [92]. Although the ultimate findings are not yet published, there is an intimation of a bimodal distribution pattern suggesting 2 distinct lesion populations in terms of luminal renarrowing. This would indeed be a complete turnaround in terms of concepts of restenosis, although not a complete return to the "binary" view of restenosis (since both apparent lesion populations are reported to display an approximately "normal distribution"). However, further comment on this investigation would be inappropriate in the absence of finalized and verified data. Suffice it to state that the concept of angiographic restenosis continues to rapidly evolve, is far from final resolution and the last word has most certainly not be written.

New frontiers in restenosis prevention – the era of optimization: but what about chronic recoil and vessel remodelling?

Whatever the future holds in respect of "restenosis definition" and statistical approaches to evaluation of the effect of devices and pharmaco-biological agents, it is evident that we are definitely entering the era of optimization of the acute interventional result. "Poor Old Balloon Angioplasty" cannot optimize the acute interventional result due to the inevitable phenomenon of acute elastic recoil [9]. Similarly, excimer laser angioplasty and rotation abrasion virtually always require adjunctive balloon angioplasty to provide satisfactory acute results. Stent implantation can completely prevent acute elastic recoil [93] and directional atherectomy can considerable ameliorate recoil [94], but each of these devices provokes, on average, considerably more intimal luminal renarrowing than is usual after balloon angioplasty [19, 20, 51–53, 75, 79]. A further confounding factor is introduced into the restenosis equation through recent evidence, which points toward a greater than recognised contribution of vascular remodelling to long term luminal renarrowing [95–98]. Accordingly, "optimal angioplasty", by atherectomy and particularly by stent implantation, may merely be "shifting the goalposts" in "restoring the Glagovian [99–101] balance" in the diseased coronary artery. Intracoronary ultrasound is developing rapidly and is already being employed to evaluate acute results and to investigate mechanisms of intervention and predictors of restenosis (PICTURE (Post Intra-Coronary Treatment Ultrasonic Result Evaluation)) and will be used to establish optimal acute results and to evaluate late results in some upcoming clinical interventional trials (eg. OARS (Optimal Atherectomy Restenosis Study), BOAT (Balloon angioplasty versus Optimal Atherectomy Trial), EUROCARE (EUROpean Carvedilol Atherectomy Restenosis Evaluation), MUSIC (Multicentre Ultra-Sound In Coronary arteries)). Large serial studies using this imaging technique will be required to ultimately clarify the hyperplastic and rheological/-remodelling components of the restenosis phenomenon.

Although optimal angioplasty represents an exciting advance in practical intervention and may produce considerably improved overall long term results [54, 56, 84, 87], it seems unlikely to present the ultimate answer to the problem of restenosis. Trials of pharmaco-biological agents in tandem with new device intervention will undoubtedly proliferate in the coming years, to deal with the principle aspects of restenosis, by capitalizing on the physical and mechanical properties of these devices for acutely maximizing the coronary lumen (and perhaps inhibiting chronic recoil and promoting favourable vessel remodelling), by concomitantly attempting to reducing the long term intimal hyperplastic process. Exciting prospects include progress with increasingly sophisticated devices for local intramural drug delivery, coating of endoluminal stents for sustained local release of anti-thrombotic, anti-proliferative or other agents and bio-degradable stents. Whatever the component parts of the restenosis process and whatever the ingredients of the "magic bullet" may be, it seems clear that high quality angiography, with off-line quantitative analysis at dedicated core-laboratories, is still the most *universally* useful and applicable tool for serial evaluation of the results of coronary intervention and of the impact of new therapies in large patient populations.

References

1. Ellis SG, Roubin GS, King SB III et al. Angiographic and clinical predictors of acute closure after native vessel coronary angioplasty. Circulation 1988; 77: 372–79.
2. Detre KM, Holmes DR, Holubkov R et al., coinvestigators of the NHLBI PTCA Registry. Incidence and consequences of periprocedural occlusion: The 1985–1986 NHLBI PTCA Registry. Circulation 1990; 82: 739–50.
3. de Feyter PJ, van den Brand M, Laarman GJ et al. Acute coronary artery occlusion during and after percutaneous transluminal coronary angioplasty. Frequency, prediction, clinical course, management and follow-up. Circulation 1991; 83: 927–36.
4. Lincoff AM, Popma JJ, Ellis SG et al. Abrupt vessel closure complicating coronary angioplasty: Clinical, angiographic and therapeutic profile. J Am Coll Cardiol 1992; 19: 926–35.
5. Reifart N, Preusler W, Storger H et al. Outcome of 10,000 coronary interventional procedures without on-site surgical backup (Abstr). Circulation 1993; 88: I-217.
6. Block PC, Myler RK, Stertzer S et al. Morphology after transluminal angioplasty in human beings. N Engl J Med 1981; 305: 382–5.
7. Waller BF. "Crackers, Breakers, Stretchers, Drillers, Scrapers, Shavers, Burners, Welders and Melters".The future treatment of atherosclerotic coronary artery disease? A clinical-morphologic assessment. J Am Coll Cardiol 1989; 13: 969–87.
8. Fischell TA, Derby G, Tse TM, Stadius ML. Coronary artery vasoconstriction routinely occurs after percutaneous transluminal coronary angioplasty. A quantitative arteriographic analysis. Circulation 1988; 78: 1323–34.
9. Rensing BJ, Hermans WRM, Beatt KJ et al. Quantitative angiographic assessment of elastic recoil after percutaneous transluminal coronary angioplasty. Am J Cardiol 1990; 66: 1039–44.
10. Tenaglia AN, Buller CE, Kisslo KB et al. Mechanisms of directional atherectomy and balloon angioplasty as assessed by intracoronary ultrasound. J Am Coll Cardiol 1992; 20: 685–91.
11. Braden GA, Herrington DM, Downes TR et al. Qualitative and quantitative contrasts in the mechanisms of lumen enlargement by coronary balloon angioplasty and directional coronary atherectomy. J Am Coll Cardiol 1994; 23: 40–8.
12. Den Heyer P, Foley DP, Escaned J et al. Angioscopic versus angiographic detection of intimal dissection and intracoronary thrombus. J Am Coll Cardiol 1994; 23: 649–55.
13. Jain SP, White CJ, Collins TJ et al. Etiologies of abrupt occlusion at PTCA: Angioscopic morphology. J Am Coll Cardiol 1993; 21: 484A.
14. Hermans WR, Foley DP, Rensing BJ et al., on behalf of the Carport and Mercator Study groups. Usefulness of quantitative and qualitative angiographic lesion morphology and clinical characteristics in predicting major adverse cardiac events during and after native coronary balloon angioplasty. Am J Cardiol 1993; 72: 14–20.
15. Sutton JM, Ellis SG, Roubin GS et al. Major clinical events after coronary stenting: The multicentre registry of acute and elective Gianturco-Roubin stent placement. Circulation 1994; 89: 1126–37.
16. Serruys PW, Strauss BH, Beatt KJ et al. Angiographic follow-up after placement of a self-expanding coronary artery stent. N Engl J Med 1991; 324: 13–7.
17. Carrozza JP Jr., Kuntz RE, Levine MJ et al. Angiographic and clinical outcome of intracoronary stenting: Immediate and long term results from a large single-center experience. J Am Coll Cardiol 1992; 20: 328–37.
18. Schatz RA, Baim DS, Leon M et al. Clinical experience with the Palmaz-Schatz coronary stent. Initial results of a multicenter study. Circulation 1991; 83: 148–61.
19. Serruys PW, Macaya C, de Jaegere P et al., for the Benestent study group. A comparison of balloon angioplasty and Palmaz-Schatz stent implantation in patients with coronary artery disease. N Engl J Med 1994; 331: 489–95.

20. Schatz RA, Penn IM, Baim DS et al., for the STRESS investigators. A randomized comparison of coronary artery stent placement and balloon angioplasty in the treatment of coronary artery disease. N Engl J Med 1994; 331: 496–501.

21. Den Heyer P, van Dijk RB, Twisk SP, Lie KI. Early stent occlusion is not always caused by thrombosis. Catheter Cardiovasc Diagn 1993; 29: 136–40.

22. Danchin N, Juilliere Y, Beatt KJ et al. Visual assessment of coronary artery stenoses: Is the 90% diameter stenosis an invalid concept? Eur Heart J 1988; 9 (Abstr Suppl): 0406.

23. Rensing BJ, Hermans WR, Deckers JW et al. Luminal narrowing after percutaneous transluminal coronary balloon angioplasty follows a near Gaussian distribution. A quantitative angiographic study in 1445 successfully dilated lesions. J Am Coll Cardiol 1992; 19: 939–45.

24. Fleming RM, Kirkeeide RL, Smalling RW, Gould KL. Patterns in visual interpretation of coronary angiograms as detected by quantitative coronary angiography. J Am Coll Cardiol 1991; 18: 945–51.

25. DeRouen TA, Murray JA, Owen W. Variability in the analysis of coronary arteriograms. Circulation 1977; 55: 324–8.

26. Meier B, Gruentzig AR, Goebel N et al. Assessment of stenoses in coronary angioplasty: Inter- and intraobserver variability. Int J Cardiol 1983; 3: 159–69.

27. Arnett EN, Isner JM, Redwood DR et al. Coronary artery narrowing in coronary heart disease: Comparison of cineangiographic and necropsy findings. Ann Int Med 1979; 91: 350–6.

28. White CW, Wright CB, Doty DB et al. Does visual interpretation of the coronary arteriogram predict the physiologic importance of a coronary stenosis? N Engl J Med 1984; 310: 819–24.

29. Beaumann GJ, Vogel RA. Accuracy of individual and panel visual interpretations of coronary arteriograms: Implications for clinical decisions. J Am Coll Cardiol 1990; 16: 108–13.

30. Danchin N, Juilliere Y, Foley DP, Serruys PW. Visual versus quantitative assessment of the severity of coronary artery stenoses: Can the angiographer's eye be re-educated? Am Heart J 1993; 126: 594–600.

31. Gould KL, Lipscomb K, Hamilton GW. Physiologic basis for assessing critical coronary stenoses: Instantaneous flow response and regional distribution during coronary hyperemia as measures of coronary flow reserve. Am J Cardiol 1974; 33: 87–94.

32. Serruys PW, Reiber JHC, Wijns W et al. Assessment of percutaneous transluminal coronary angioplasty by quantitative coronary angiography: Diameter versus densitometric area measurements. Am J Cardiol 1984; 54: 482–8.

33. Reiber JHC, Serruys PW. Quantitative Coronary Angiography. In: Marcus ML, Schelbert HR, Skorton DJ, Wolf Gl, editors. Cardiac imaging, a companion to Braunwalds heart disease. New York: Saunders, 1991: 211–80.

34. Escaned J, Foley DP, Haase J et al. Quantitative coronary angiography during coronary angioplasty with a single angiographic view: A comparison of automated edge-detection and videodensitometric techniques. Am Heart J 1993; 126: 1326–33.

35. Sanz ML, Mancini J, LeFree MT. Variability of quantitative digital subtraction angiography before and after percutaneous transluminal coronary angioplasty. Am J Cardiol 1987; 60: 55–60.

36. The Mercator Study Group. Does the new angiotensin converting enzyme inhibitor cilazapril prevent restenosis after percutaneous transluminal coronary angioplasty? The results of the Mercator study: A multicentre randomized double-blind placebo-controlled trial. Circulation 1992; 86: 100–11.

37. Hermans WRM, Rensing BJ, Foley DP et al. "Therapeutic dissection" and the occurrence of restenosis. A quantitative angiographic analysis in 778 lesions after successful angioplasty. J Am Coll Cardiol 1992; 20: 767–80.

38. Foley DP, Deckers J, van den Bos AA et al. Is there a need for repeat coronary angio-

graphy 24 hours after successful balloon angioplasty, to evaluate early luminal deterioration and facilitate quantitative analysis. Am J Cardiol 1993; 72: 1342–48.

39. Hanet C, Wijns W, Michel X, Schroeder E. Influence of balloon size and stenosis morphology on immediate and delayed elastic recoil after percutaneous transluminal coronary angioplasty. J Am Coll Cardiol 1991; 18: 506–11.

40. Hanet C, Michel X, Schroeder E, Wijns W. Lack of detectable delayed elastic recoil during the first 24 hours after coronary balloon angioplasty (Abstr). Eur Heart J 1992; 13 (Abstr Suppl): 2228.

41. Lablanche JM on behalf of the FACT Investigators. Recoil twenty four hours after coronary angioplasty: A computerized angiographic study (Abstr). J Am Coll Cardiol 1993; 21: 35A.

42. Thomas AC, Davies MJ, Dilly S et al. Potential errors in the estimation of coronary arterial stenosis from clinical arteriography with reference to the shape of the coronary arterial lumen. Br Heart J 1986; 55: 129–39.

43. Foley DP, Rodenberg L, Hermans WR, Deckers JW. Coronary luminal measurements from multiple "matched" angiographic projections compared with single "worst" projection. Circulation 1993; I-641 (Abstr).

44. Serruys PW, Rutsch W, Heyndrickx GR et al. Prevention of restenosis after percutaneous transluminal coronary angioplasty with thromboxane A2 receptor blockade. A randomized, double blind, placebo controlled trial. Circulation 1991; 84: 1568–80.

45. Faxon DP, on behalf of the MARCATOR investigators. Angiotensin converting enzyme inhibition and restenosis: The final results of the MARCATOR trial. Circulation 1992: 86: I-53 (Abstr).

46. Serruys PW, Klein W, Thijssen JPG et al. Evaluation of Ketanserin in the prevention of restenosis after percutaneous transluminal coronary angioplasty: A multicentre randomized double-blind placebo-controlled trial. Circulation 1993; 88: 1588–601.

47. Foley DP, Bonnier H, Jackson G et al., on behalf of the FLARE study group. Prevention of restenosis after coronary balloon angioplasty: Rationale and design of the FLuvastatin Angioplasty REstenosis (FLARE) trial. Am J Cardiol 1994; 73: 50D–61D.

48. Hirshfeld JW, Schwartz SS, Jugo R et al., and the M-Heart Investigators. Restenosis after coronary angioplasty: A multivariate statistical model to relate lesion and procedural variables to restenosis. J Am Coll Cardiol 1991; 18: 647–56.

49. Bourassa MG, Lesperance J, Eastwood C et al. Clinical, physiologic, anatomic, and procedural factors predictive of restenosis after percutaneous transluminal coronary angioplasty. J Am Coll Cardiol 1991; 18: 368–76.

50. Popma JJ, Califf RM, Topol EJ. Clinical trials of restenosis following angioplasty. Circulation 1991; 84: 1426–37.

51. Popma JJ, De Cesare N, Pinkerton CA et al. Quantitative analysis of factors affecting late lumen loss and restenosis after directional atherectomy. Am J Cardiol 1993; 71: 552–7.

52. Topol EJ, Leya F, Pinkerton CA et al., for the CAVEAT study group. A comparison of directional atherectomy with coronary angioplasty in patients with coronary artery disease. N Engl J Med 1993; 329: 221–7.

53. Adelman AG, Cohen EA, Kimball BP et al. A comparison of directional atherectomy with balloon angioplasty for lesions of the left anterior descending coronary artery. N Engl J Med 1993; 329: 228–33.

54. Kuntz RE, Safian RD, Carroza JP et al. The importance of acute luminal diameter in determining restenosis after coronary atherectomy or stenting. Circulation 1992; 86; 1827–35.

55. Kuntz RE, Hinohara T, Robertson GC et al. Influence of vessel selection on the observed restenosis rate after endoluminal stenting or directional atherectomy. Am J Cardiol 1992; 70: 1101–8.

56. Kuntz RE, Gibson CM, Nobuyoshi M, Baim DS. Generalized model of restenosis after conventional balloon angioplasty, stenting and directional atherectomy. J Am Coll Cardiol 1993; 21: 15–25.

57. Lincoff AM, Keeler GP, Berdan LG et al., for the CAVEAT investigators. "Worst view" angiographic analysis in CAVEAT provided a "worst case" scenario of restenosis rates and vessel luminal diameters (Abstr). Circulation 1994; 90: I-60.

58. Kuntz RE, Baim DS. Defining coronary restenosis. Newer clinical and angiographic paradigms. Circulation 1993; 88: 1310–23.

59. Nakamura S, Colombo A, Gaglione A et al. Intracoronary ultrasound observations during stent implantation. Circulation 1994; 89: 2026–34.

60. Colombo A, Hall P, Almagor Y et al. Results of intravascular ultrasound guided coronary stenting without subsequent anticoagulation. J Am Coll Cardiol 1994: 335A.

61. Klocke FJ. Measurements of coronary blood flow and degree of stenosis. Current clinical implications and continuing uncertainties. J Am Coll Cardiol 1983; 1: 31–41.

62. Kirkeeide RL, Gould KL, Parsel L. Assessment of coronary stenoses by myocardial perfusion imaging during pharmacologic coronary vasodilation. Validation of coronary flow reserve as a single integrated functional measure of stenosis severity reflecting all its geometric dimensions. J Am Coll Cardiol 1986; 7: 103–13.

63. Zijlstra F, Fioretti P, Reiber JHC, Serruys PW. Which cineangiographically assessed anatomic variable correlates best with functional measurements of stenosis severity? A comparison of quantitative analysis of the coronary cineangiogram with measured coronary flow reserve and exercise/redistribution Thallium-201 scintigraphy. J Am Coll Cardiol 1988; 12: 686–91.

64. Di Mario C, Krams R, de Feyter PJ, Serruys PW. Slope of the instantaneous hyperemic diastolic coronary flow velocity-pressure relation: A new index for the assessment of the physiological significance of coronary stenosis in humans. Circulation 1994; 90: 1215–25.

65. Zijlstra F, den Boer A, Reiber JHC et al. The assessment of immediate and long-term functional results of percutaneous transluminal coronary angioplasty. Circulation 1988; 1: 15–24.

66. Hodgson JM, Riley RS, Most AS, Williams DO. Assessment of coronary flow reserve using digital angiography before and after successful percutaneous transluminal coronary angioplasty. Am J Cardiol 1987; 60: 61–5.

67. Laarman, GJ, Serruys PW, Suryapranata H et al. Inability of coronary blood flow reserve measurements to assess the efficacy of coronary angioplasty in the first 24 hours in unselected patients. Am Heart J 1991; 122: 631–8.

68. Califf RM, Ohman EM, Frid DJ et al. Restenosis: The clinical issues. In: Topol EJ, editor. Textbook of interventional cardiology. Philadelphia: W.B. Saunders, 1990: 363–94.

69. Laarman GJ, Luijten HE, van Zeyl LG et al. Assessment of "silent" restenosis and long-term follow-up after successful angioplasty in single vessel coronary artery disease: The value of quantitative exercise electrocardiography and quantitative coronary angiography. J Am Coll Cardiol 1990; 16: 578–85.

70. Brown BG, Bolson E, Frimer M, Dodge HT. Quantitative coronary arteriography. Estimations of dimensions, haemodynamic resistance and atheroma mass of coronary artery lesions using the arteriograms and digital computation. Circulation 1977; 55: 329–37.

71. Reiber JHC, Booman S, Tan HS et al. A cardiac image analysis system. Objective quantitative processing of angiocardiograms. Proc Comp Cardiol 1978: 239–42.

72. Reiber JHC, Serruys PW, Kooijman CJ et al. Assessment of short-, medium-, and long-term variations in arterial dimensions from computer assisted quantitation of coronary cineangiograms. Circulation 1985; 71: 280–8.

73. Serruys PW, Luijten HE, Beatt KJ et al. Incidence of restenosis after successful coronary angioplasty: A time-related phenomenon. A quantitative angiographic study in 342 consecutive patients at 1, 2, 3 and 4 months. Circulation 1988; 77: 361–71.

74. Nobuyoshi M, Kimura H, Nosaka H et al. Restenosis after successful percutaneous transluminal coronary angioplasty: Serial angiographic follow-up of 299 patients. J Am Coll Cardiol 1988; 12: 616–23.

75. Kuntz RE, Safian RD, Levine MJ et al. Novel approach to the analysis of restenosis after the use of three new coronary devices. J Am Coll Cardiol 1992; 19: 1493–9.

76. King SB III, Weintraub WS, Tao X et al. Bimodal distribution of diameter stenosis 4 to 12 months after angioplasty: Implications for definitions and interpretation of restenosis. J Am Coll Cardiol 1991; 17: 345A (Abstr).
77. Forrester JS, Fishbein M, Helfant R, Fagin J. A paradigm for restenosis based on cell biology: Clues for development of new preventive therapies. J Am Coll Cardiol 1991; 17: 758–69.
78. Serruys PW, Rensing BJ, Luijten HE et al. Restenosis following coronary angioplasty. In: Meier B, editor. Interventional cardiology, Toronto, Lewiston, New York, Bern, Gottingen, Stuttgart: Hogrefe and Huber, 1990: 79–115.
79. Serruys PW, Foley DP, Kirkeeide RL, King SB III. Restenosis Revisited – insights provided by quantitative coronary angiography. Am Heart J 1993; 126: 1243–67.
80. Rensing BJ, Hermans WR, Vos J et al., on behalf of the Carport Study group. Quantitative angiographic risk factors of luminal narrowing after coronary balloon angioplasty using balloon measurements to reflect stretch and elastic recoil at the dilatation site. Am J Cardiol 1992; 69: 584–91.
81. Rensing BJ, Hermans WRM, Vos J et al. on behalf of the Coronary Artery Restenosis Prevention on Repeated Thromboxane Antagonism (CARPORT) study group. Luminal narrowing after percutaneous transluminal coronary angioplasty. A study of clinical, procedural and lesional factors related to long term angiographic outcome. Circulation 1993; 88: 975–85.
82. Hermans WRM, Rensing BJ, Foley DP et al., on behalf of the MERCATOR study group. Patient, lesion and procedural variables as risk factors for luminal re-narrowing after successful coronary angioplasty: A quantitative analysis in 653 patients with 778 lesions. J Cardiovasc Pharmacol 1993; 22: S45–S57.
83. de Jaegere P, Serruys PW, Bertrand M et al. Angiographic predictors of recurrence of restenosis after Wiktor stent implantation in native coronary arteries. Am J Cardiol 1993; 72: 165–70.
84. Umans VA, Robert A, Foley DP et al. Clinical, histologic and quantitative angiographic predictors of restenosis following directional coronary atherectomy: A multivariate analysis of the renarrowing process and late outcome. J Am Coll Cardiol 1994; 23: 49–58.
85. Schwartz RS, Huber KC, Murphy JG et al. Restenosis and the proportional neointimal response to coronary artery injury: Results in a porcine model. J Am Coll Cardiol 1992; 19: 267–74.
86. Foley DP, Melkert R, Serruys PW. The influence of coronary vessel size on the renarrowing process and late angiographic outcome after successful balloon angioplasty. Circulation 1994; 90: 1239–51.
87. Umans VA, Keane D, Foley DP et al. Optimal use of directional coronary atherectomy is required to ensure long-term angiographic benefit: A study with matched procedural outcome after atherectomy and angioplasty. J Am Coll Cardiol 1994; 24: 1652–9.
88. Foley DP, Keane D, Serruys PW. Does the method of transluminal coronary revascularization influence restenosis? A comparison of balloon angioplasty, atherectomy and stents. Br J Clin Pract 1995; 49: 7–15.
89. Foley DP, Serruys PW. Restenosis after percutaneous intervention: Is there a device specificity? In: Topol E and Serruys PW, editors. Current review of interventional cardiology. Philadelphia: Current Medicine, 1995; 236–58.
90. Kuntz RE, Foley DP, Keeler GP et al. on behalf of the CAVEAT investigators. Relationship of acute luminal gain to late loss following directional atherectomy or balloon angioplasty in CAVEAT. Circulation 1993: I-495 (Abstr).
91. Foley DP, Melkert R, Umans VA et al. Is the relationship between luminal increase and subsequent renarrowing linear or non-linear in patients undergoing coronary interventions? J Am Coll Cardiol 1994; 23: 302A.
92. Lehmann KG, Melkert R, Serruys PW. Contributions of frequency distribution analysis to the understanding of coronary restenosis. Circulation 1994; 90: I-59 (Abstr).
93. Haude M, Erbel R, Issa H, Meyer J. Quantitative analysis of elastic recoil after balloon

angioplasty and after intracoronary implantation of balloon-expandable Palmaz-Schatz stents. J Am Coll Cardiol 1993; 21: 26–34.

94. Kimball BP, Bui S, Cohen EA et al. Comparison of acute elastic recoil after directional atherecomy versus standard balloon angioplasty. Am Heart J 1992; 124: 1459–66.

95. Kovach JA, Mintz GS, Kent KM et al. Serial intravascular ultrasound studies indicate that chronic recoil is an important mechanism of restenosis following transcatheter therapy (Abstr). J Am Coll Cardiol 1993; 21: 484A.

96. Kakuta T, Currier JW, Haudenschild CC et al. Differences in compensatory vessel enlargement, not intimal formation, account for restenosis after angioplasty in the hypercholesterolemic rabbit. Circulation 1994; 89: 2809–15.

97. Post MJ, Borst C, Kuntz RE. The relative importance of arterial remodelling compared with intimal hyperplasia in lumen renarrowing after balloon angioplasty. A study in the normal rabbit and the hypercholesterolemic Yucatan micropig. Circulation 1994; 89: 2816–21.

98. Isner JM. Vascular remodelling. Honey, I think I shrunk the artery. Circulation 1994; 89: 2937–41.

99. Glagov S. Intimal hyperplasia, vascular remodelling and the restenosis problem. Circulation 1994; 89: 2888–92.

100. Glagov S, Weisenberg E, Zarins CK et al. Compensatory enlargement of human atherosclerotic coronary arteries. N Engl J Med 1987; 316; 1371–5.

101. Losordo DW, Rosenfield K, Kaufman J et al. Focal compensatory enlargement of human coronary arteries in response to progressive atherosclerosis: In vivo documentation using intravascular ultrasound. Circulation 1994; 89: 2570–8.

Corresponding Author: Prof. Patrick W. Serruys, Erasmus University Ee 2332, PO Box 1738, 3000 DR Rotterdam, The Netherlands

21. Immediate evaluation of percutaneous transluminal coronary balloon angioplasty success by intracoronary Doppler ultrasound

MICHAEL HAUDE, DIETRICH BAUMGART, GUIDO CASPARI, JUNBO GE and RAIMUND ERBEL

Introduction

Percutaneous transluminal coronary angioplasty has achieved a dominant role for the treatment of patients with coronary artery disease. In several European countries and the US the number of angioplasty procedures has exceeded the number of coronary artery bypass graft operations [1, 2].

The success of this procedure is evaluated by an improvement of the stenotic luminal narrowing as assessed by angiography. Different definitions of residual stenosis, however, can be applied to post-angioplasty angiographic results. Most common in PTCA, post-procedural success is defined as less than 50% diameter residual stenosis as judged by eye-balling of the operator. More recently, on-line digital angiographic quantification techniques allow the immediate calculation of residual stenosis dimensions after PTCA in a more objective fashion by utilizing computer-based automatic edge detection [3, 4]. Nevertheless, these parameters reflect only morphologic changes of luminal narrowing but do not provide information on the functional improvement of coronary flow, nor predict procedure-related complications or long-term restenosis.

In order to evaluate the functional significance of a coronary stenosis and of a residual post-angioplasty stenosis, Andreas Grüntzig, the inventor of the PTCA technique, and others utilized the transstenotic pressure gradient [5–9], and documented a clear reduction of transstenotic pressure gradient by a successful PTCA procedure. Nevertheless, this technique came out of fashion since these measurements were not always reliable [10]. Moreover, the physiologic value of these measurements, even these obtained with the smallest catheters, were questioned, since the catheter itself impedes flow in the coronary arterial lumen.

These limitations prompted investigators to use blood flow measurements for the functional assessment of angioplasty results.

Since coronary flow (F) is defined as [11]:

$$F = \text{vessel volume} \cdot \text{flow velocity integral} \cdot \text{heart rate}$$

C.A. Nienaber and U. Sechtem (eds): Imaging and Intervention in Cardiology. 341–358.
© 1996 *Kluwer Academic Publishers.*

with vessel volume = vessel length · vessel cross-sectional area there is a direct relation between flow velocity and volumetric flow. Assuming no significant changes in vessel length and heart rate between two flow measurements, vessel area can be substituted by vessel cross-sectional area, and flow is primarily related to this cross-sectional area and the flow velocity integral.

Coronary flow velocity can be calculated from the Doppler frequency shift, which is the difference between the transmitted and returning frequency, using the Doppler equation [12]:

$$V = \frac{c \cdot (F_1 - Fo)}{2 \cdot F_0 \cdot (\cos \phi)}$$

with C = constant: speed of sound in blood, V = blood flow velocity, F_0 = transmitting frequency, F_1 = returning frequency; and ϕ = angle of incidence.

Maximum velocity can be recorded when the transducer ultrasound is parallel to blood flow and ϕ is zero, so that $\cos \phi = 1$. If the interrogating angle is >0 but <20°, the velocity measurements will be within 5% of the absolute values. The velocity integral can be measured in smaller vessels by using a broad sample volume in the presence of a parabolic flow profile [12].

Doppler catheters

Until recently, coronary flow velocities were measured by Doppler catheters, the smallest being about 3 F in diameter [13, 14]. Because of their size, the application of these Doppler catheters was limited to the proximal and middle part of coronary arteries and frequently did not allow the passage through a coronary stenosis to measure distal flow velocity. Another point of concern was that these Doppler catheters processed velocity signals by zero-crossing analysis resulting in potential for overestimation of true peak velocities in the presence of turbulent flow or motion artifact [15].

The Doppler angioplasty wire

More recently, a steerable guidewire (175 cm long, 0.018 or 0.014 in diameter) steerable guidewire became available that was equipped with a 12 MHz transducer at its distal tip (Figure 1, Flowire™, Cardiometrics; Mountain View, CA, USA). The low profile of this wire permits the device to be advanced beyond a coronary stenosis to the distal part of the vessel with no significant flow limitations [16]. Furthermore, the Flowire™ can be used as a guidewire for balloon angioplasty catheters and, thereby, permits continuous recording of blood flow velocity before, during and after PTCA without

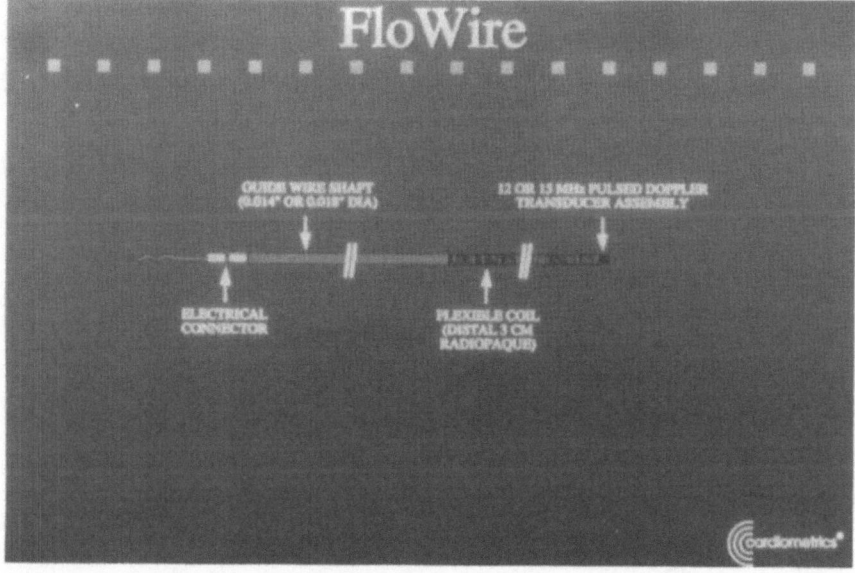

Figure 1. Doppler coronary flow wire (Flowire™, Cardiometrics, Mountain Vew, CA, USA) for continuous monitoring of intracoronary flow velocity.

repositioning of the device, which was necessary with previous Doppler catheters [17, 18]. Flow velocity signals from Doppler guidewires are processed on-line by fast Fourier transform with spectral display. Several velocity parameters can be calculated by analysis of the spectral waveform and have been found to correlate with absolute coronary flow measurements in both in vitro and in vivo validation studies [16]. The Doppler spectrum is digitized and the following parameters are derived (Figure 2):
- peak diastolic flow velocity (PVd)
- peak systolic flow velocity (PVs)
- integral of the diastolic velocity (DVi)
- integral of the systolic velocity (SVi)
- first 1/3 flow fraction
- first 1/2 flow fraction
- diastolic to systolic peak velocity
- diastolic to systolic velocity integral
- proximal to distal mean velocity

The continuously digitized Doppler spectrum can be recorded on a S-VHS video recorder and a video printer allows hard-copy documentation of certain measurement intervals.

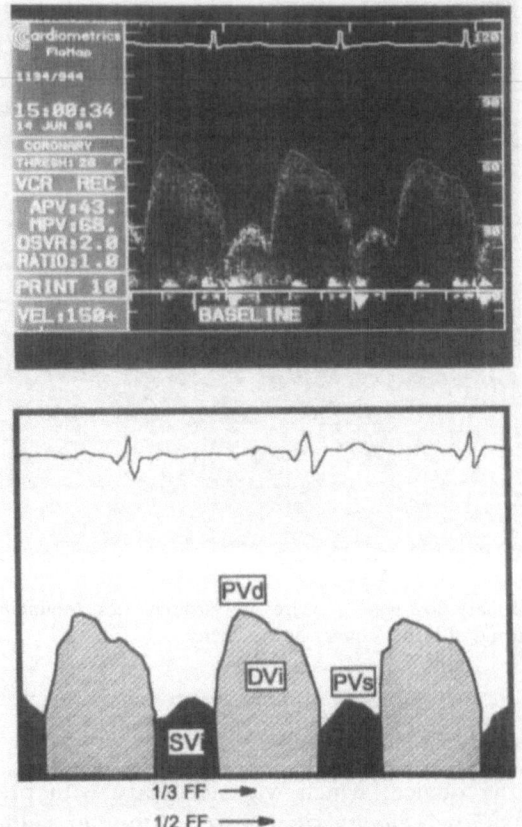

Figure 2. Intracoronary Doppler flow velocity profile as obtained by the Flowire™ and derived parameters. DVi = diastolic velocity integral, PVd = diastolic peak velocity, PVs = systolic peak velocity, SVi = systolic velocity integral, 1/3 FF = first third flow fraction, 1/2 FF = first half flow fraction.

The concept of coronary flow reserve

Baseline coronary flow at resting conditions may be similar in normal and abnormal arteries, while hyperemia induces differences in flow in arteries without stenoses as compared to stenotic arteries [19–22]. Therefore, several coronary vasodilating agents, such as dipyridamole, papaverine [23], adenosine [24] or contrast medium [25], have been administered to increase coronary flow and exaggerate differences in flow and flow velocity beyond stenotic lesions. When coronary flow velocity parameters are recorded at baseline and hyperemia, coronary vasodilatory reserve can be calculated as the ratio of hyperemia to baseline velocity [21, 22]. The Flowire™ system software allows recordings of phasic and hyperemic flow velocity profiles and derived parameters as well as a trend recording with a decreased temporal resolution to identifiy peak flow velocity ratio (Figure 3).

Coronary flow velocity during balloon angioplasty

Doppler flow velocity profiles proximal and distal to the target lesion were recorded in 25 patients with single vessel coronary artery disease without collateral supply of the stenotic vessel before and after a successful balloon angioplasty procedure. Measurements were performed at baseline and during hyperemia by intracoronary administration of 8 to 10 mg papaverine or 12 to 18 μg adenosine. Patients baseline and angiographic characteristics are presented in Table 1.

A representative angiographic example is shown in Figure 4; minimal luminal diameter of a stenosis in the left anterior descending artery increased from 1.23 mm (59.5%) to 2.40 mm (32.6%) by three inflations of a 3.0 mm balloon catheter for 60 s with an inflation pressure of 8 atm. In this patient pre-interventional Doppler flow velocity recordings proximal to the stenotic vessel segment documented adequate hyperemic response with a coronary flow velocity ratio of 2.8 (Figure 4). While advancing the Doppler flow wire through the stenosis to the distal part of the vessel, a marked acceleration of flow velocity was recorded within the stenosis (Figure 5). Flow velocity recordings distal to the stenosis documented a markedly reduced hyperemic response with a flow velocity ratio of 1.39 (Figure 6).

During balloon angioplasty, antegrade flow velocity was discontinued, while retrograde collateral flow velocity was recorded although no collaterals were visualized angiographically (Figure 7, top panel). After a one minute dilatation period, balloon deflation was followed by reactive hyperemia (Figure 7, bottom panel).

The post-angioplasty Doppler flow velocity measurements document a subsequent pronounced hyperemic response to intracoronary adenosine with a Doppler flow velocity ratio of 4.63 (Figure 8, right upper and lower panels). During pull back of the Doppler angioplasty guide wire through the residual stenosis to the proximal vessel segment, no change in Doppler flow velocity was recorded. In the proximal vessel segment, hyperemic response to intracoronary adenosine resulted in an improved coronary flow velocity ratio of 4.05 which was almost similar to that measured distal to the residual stenosis, and was markedly increased compared to the pre-angioplasty result (Figure 9).

Monitoring distal baseline and hyperemic flow velocity before and after PTCA

The unique advantage of the flow wire is that crossing of tight stenoses is easy, which then allows recording of distal flow velocity. It was documented

baseline

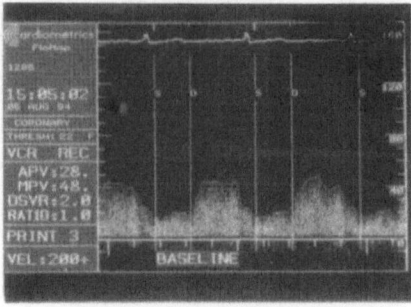

hyperemia

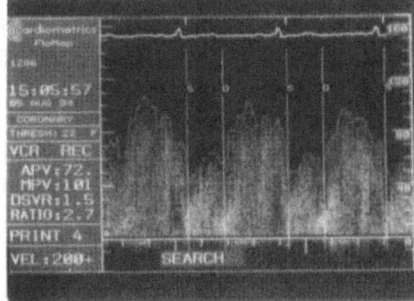

trend

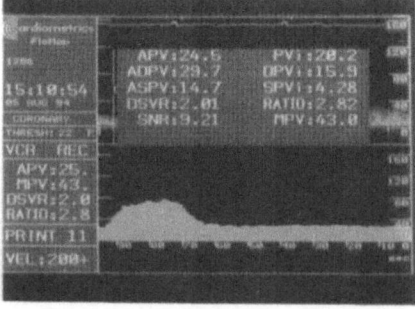

Figure 3. Intracoronary Doppler flow velocity profiles before (baseline) and during hyperemia induced by intracoronary injection of adenosine and trend analysis to depict the duration of hyperemic response recorded in the proximal segment of the left anterior descending artery.

that a successful angioplasty procedure primarily improves distal hyperemic flow velocity and, thereby, flow velocity ratio (Figure 10). Nevertheless, 17 of 25 patients with a mean residual stenosis diameter of 2.18 ± 0.45 mm ($28 \pm 22\%$) had coronary flow velocity ratios below 2.8, which was the cut-

Table 1. Baseline demographic and angiographic data of 25 patients with single coronary artery disease without angiographic evidence of collaterals who underwent successful balloon angioplasty (PTCA) with monitoring of coronary flow velocity by the Flowire™.

Demographic parameters	
Male/female	21 (84%)/4 (16%)
Age (yr)	56 ± 12
Systemic hypertension	10 (40%)
Diabetes mellitus	2 (8%)
Cigarette smoking	14 (56%)
Cholesterol > 200 mg/dl	16 (64%)
Obesity	10 (40%)
Angina pectoris	
CCS I	3 (12%)
CCS II	10 (40%)
CCS III	10 (40%)
CCS IV	2 (8%)
Previous MI	0
Previous PTCA	7 (28%)
Target lesion	
LAD	15 (60%)
LCx	3 (12%)
RCA	7 (28%)

Angiographic parameters	
MLD before PTCA (mm)	1.05 ± 0.41
MLD after PTCA (mm)	2.27 ± 0.43
Dref before PTCA (mm)	3.04 ± 0.50
Dref after PTCA (mm)	3.07 ± 0.48
Lesion length (mm)	14 ± 8
Eccentric lesion	8 (32%)
Calcified lesion	8 (32%)
Angiographic collaterals	None
Balloon/artery ratio	0.98 ± 0.08

CCS = Canadian Cardiovascular Society, Dref = reference diameter, MI = myocardial infarction, LAD = left anterior descending artery, LCx = left circumflex artery, MLD = minimal luminal diameter, RCA = right coronary artery

off level for flow velocity ratios in normal vessels. These findings persisted over a recording period of 10 to 15 minutes after the final balloon deflation [26–28]. The average residual stenosis of about 30% after balloon angioplasty despite adequate matching of the balloon size was a result of elastic recoil. Intimal tears and dissections producing flow limiting flaps, and local thrombus formation, and persisting changes in vasomotor response to hyperemia in the distal microvasculature are possible explanations for this finding. Moreover, persistent abnormal coronary perfusion despite an acceptable angiographic post-PTCA result has been reported in unclear perfusion studies (see Chapter 23).

before PTCA

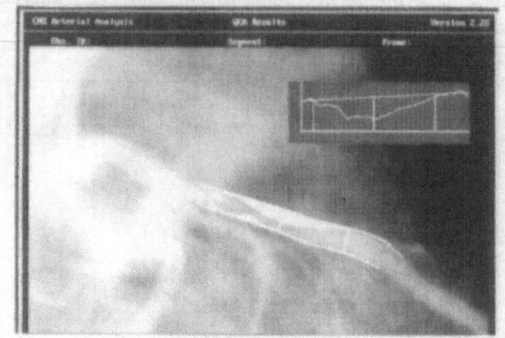

MLD: 1.23 mm   Dref: 3.03 mm   %-MLD: 59.5%
MCA: 1.19 mm²   Aref: 7.21 mm²   %-MCA: 83.5%

after PTCA

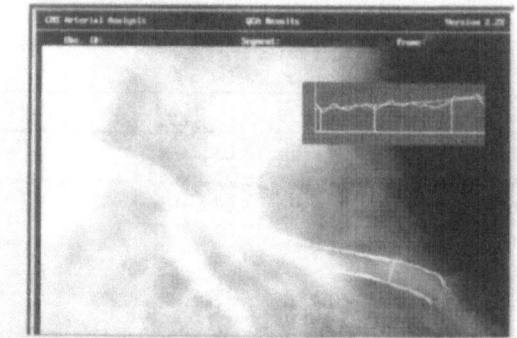

MLD: 2.40 mm   Dref: 3.10 mm   %-MLD: 32.6%
MCA: 4.52 mm²   Aref: 7.54 mm²   %-MCA: 40.1%

Figure 4. Quantitative coronary angiography of a stenosis in the left anterior descending artery before and after coronary balloon angioplasty (PTCA). Aref = reference vessel cross- sectional area, Dref = reference vessel diameter, MCA = minimal cross-sectional area, MLD = minimal luminal diameter.

Relationship between proximal and distal flow velocity changes before and after PTCA

In normal coronary arteries without angiographic documentation of stenotic segments, distal mean velocity is similar to proximal mean flow velocity [17, 29, 30]. In contrast, stenotic vessel segments presented a significantly increased ratio of proximal to distal mean flow velocity (1.93 ± 0.64 before angioplasty versus 1.18 ± 0.16 after successful angioplasty versus 1.07 ± 0.09

proximal to stenosis

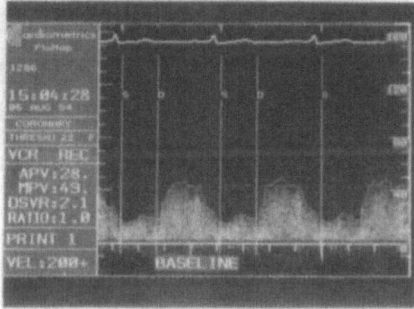

in stenosis

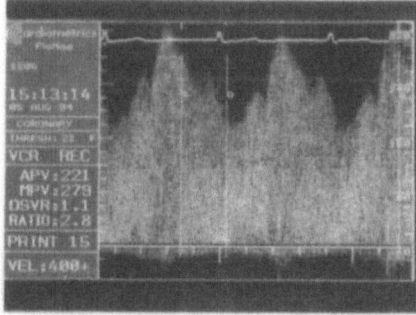

distal to stenosis

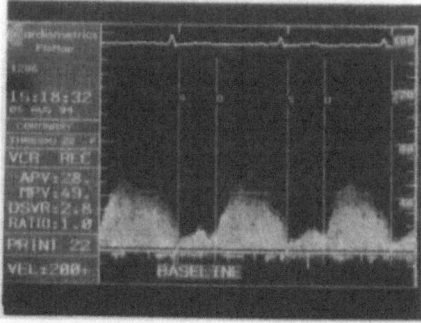

Figure 5. Doppler flow velocity recordings while advancing the Flowire™ through the coronary stenosis.

in 18 reference vessel segments without stenoses; Figure 11). Similar results have been reported by other authors [17, 18]. The major difference in flow velocity between proximal and distal vessel segments of stenotic coronary arteries was measured during hyperemia. During pharmacologically induced

baseline

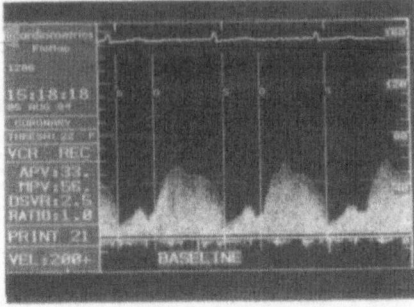

hyperemia

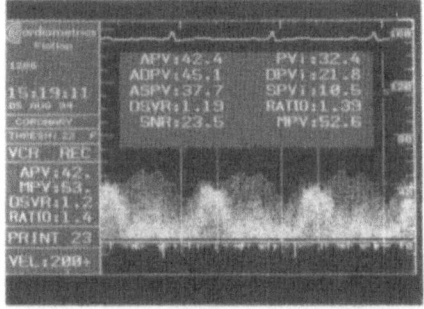

trend

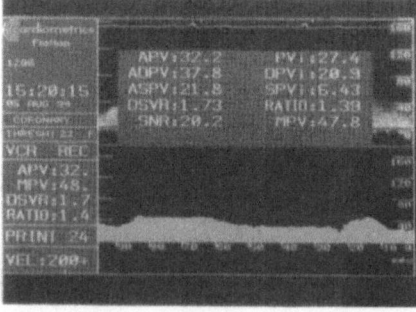

Figure 6. Doppler flow velocity recordings distal to the target stenosis at baseline and during hyperemia after intracoronary injection of adenosine.

hyperemia coronary flow increased significantly more in the proximal vessel segment than in the segment distal to the stenosis (Table 2). After a successful angioplasty procedure, both proximal and distal flow velocities and flow velocity ratios became similar during baseline and hyperemic measurements.

collateral flow
during PTCA

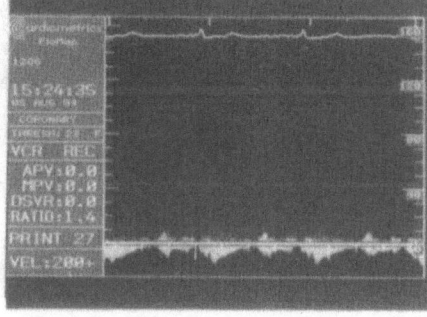

reactive hyperemia
after balloon deflation

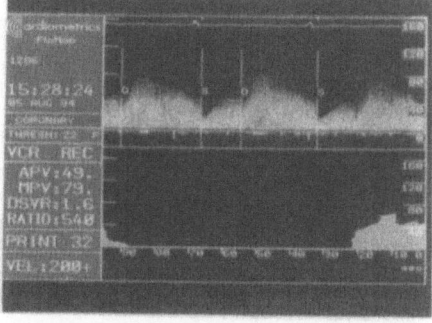

Figure 7. Doppler flow velocity recordings during balloon occlusion with negative flow velocity direction representing retrograde collateral flow and reactive hyperemia after balloon deflation.

Diastolic to systolic phasic flow velocity patterns before and after PTCA

Epicardial coronary arteries show a diastolic predominant flow pattern in both the proximal and distal coronary segments with a normal diastolic to systolic mean flow ratio of 1.5 or more [17]. In the above mentioned studies, this value decreased to 1.4 ± 0.6 distal to significant coronary stenoses, while after successful balloon angioplasty a ratio of 1.9 ± 0.8 was calculated (Figure 12). The distal diastolic to systolic peak flow velocity ratio increased from 2.3 ± 0.8 to 3.0 ± 1.1 (Figure 12). In contrast to coronary flow reserve, which is usually not measured within the normal range immediately after a successful angioplasty procedure, the normalization of diastolic to systolic

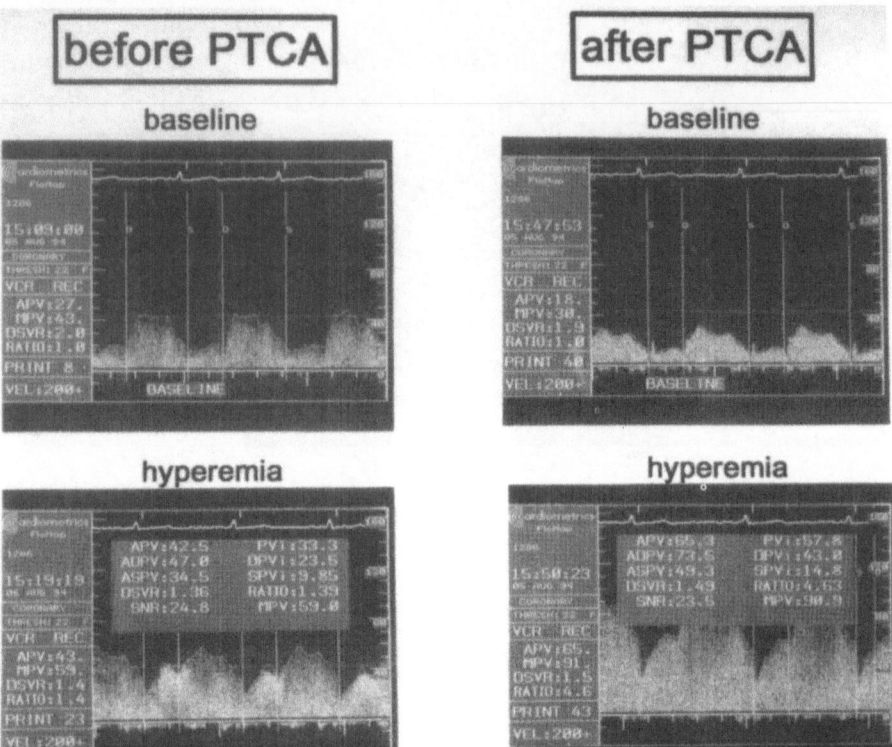

Figure 8. Doppler flow velocity recordings distal to the target stenosis at baseline and during hyperemia after intracoronary injection of adenosine before and after successful balloon angioplasty.

post-stenotic flow velocity ratios after successful angioplasty was noted within 10 to 15 minutes, as described by others [18]. In contrast, proximal diastolic to systolic mean velocity ratios were similar before and after balloon angioplasty (1.9 ± 0.7 vs 2.0 ± 0.6; n.s.). In conclusion distal flow velocity measurements provide more information about the functional result of an angioplasty procedure compared to proximal measurements. A potential reason for this might be that proximal flow velocity in a vessel segment without proximal stenosis is not influenced so much by a distal flow limiting target stenosis as distal flow velocity in the vessel segment distal to that target lesion.

Evaluation of collateral flow velocity during PTCA

The Doppler wire allows continuous recording of distal flow velocity during PTCA. Donohue et al. reported about retrograde collateral flow velocity

baseline

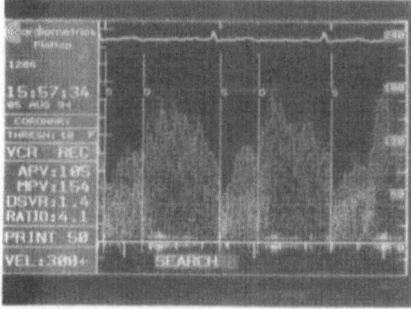

hyperemia

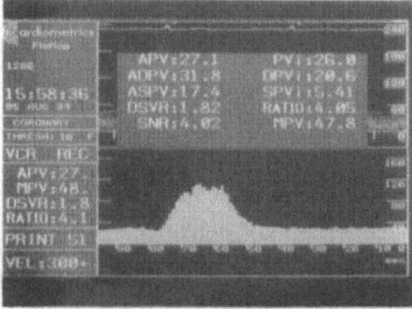

trend

Figure 9. Doppler flow velocity recordings proximal to the target stenosis at baseline and during hyperemia after intracoronary injection of adenosine after successful balloon angioplasty

monitoring during balloon insufflation [31]. In a patient population without angiographically detectable collaterals, retrograde collateral flow velocity during balloon occlusion was detected in 12 of 25 patients with a mean flow velocity of 11 ± 8 cm/s starting 25 ± 8 s after balloon insufflation. These 12 patients presented no angina nor ECG changes during the dilatation period

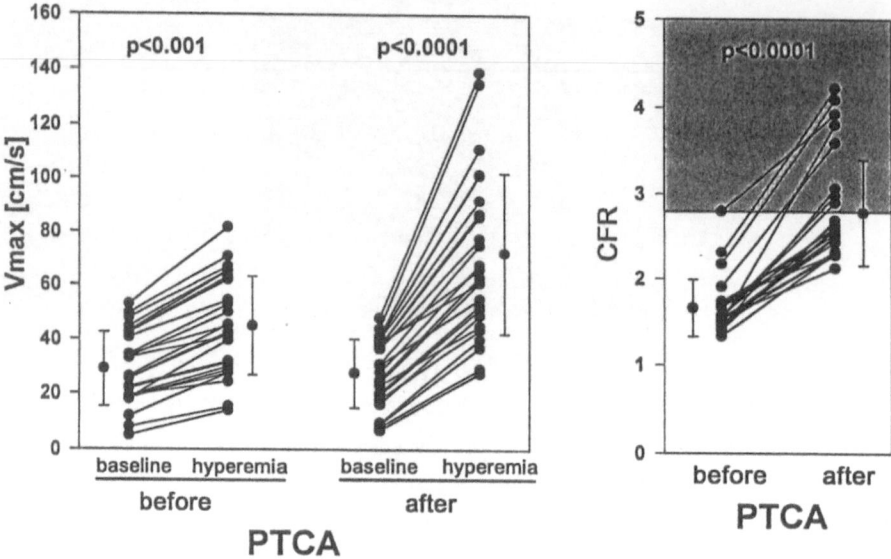

Figure 10. Maximum flow velocity (Vmax) at baseline and during hyperemia and coronary flow velocity ratios (CFR) measured before and after successful coronary balloon an gioplasty (PTCA).

of 60 to 90 s. Thus, the Doppler wire identifies recruitable collaterals during angioplasty which are not identified angiographically. The use of the Doppler angioplasty flow wire is likely to permit the evaluation of ischemic responses to hemodynamic and pharmacological perturbations of the collateral coronary circulation in patients.

Limitations of the flow velocity monitoring by Doppler flow wires

Despite the ease of application in daily use, the Doppler flow wire has some limitations. As with other ultrasound-based techniques, accurate peak velocity measurements can only be obtained when the transducer is placed as near as parallel to blood flow as possible. The broad beam spread (27°) minimizes the position-dependent component of signal acquisition, which makes most wire positions satisfactory for detecting the highest flow velocity. Nevertheless, in large and tortuous vessel segments, considerable manipulation may be required to achieve satisfactory Doppler signals (see also Chapter 17).

Monitoring coronary flow velocity using a Doppler guidewire is a technique, which can be easily incorporated into interventional procedures. Measurements distal to stenotic vessel segments are more predictive of lesion significance and of procedural success than those made proximal to the lesion.

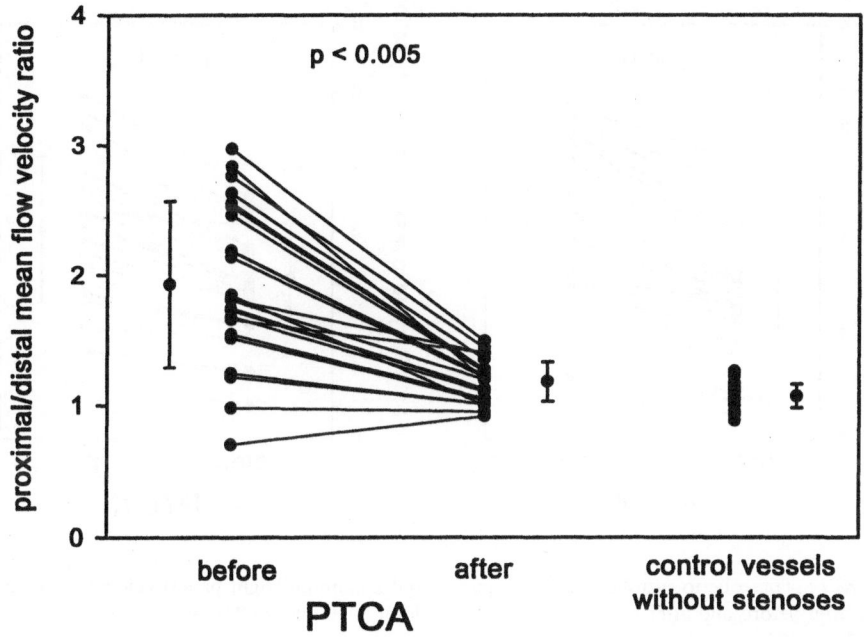

Figure 11. Proximal to distal mean flow velocity ratio before and after successful PTCA in 25 patients with single vessel disease compared to the results obtained from 18 control vessels without stenoses.

Table 2. Baseline and hyperemic maximum flow velocities and flow velocity ratios (CFR) before and after successful coronary balloon angioplasty (PTCA) in 25 patients.

	Before PTCA			After PTCA		
	Proximal	Distal	p value	Proximal	Distal	p value
Baseline	38 ± 16 cm/s	29 ± 14 cm/s	0.04	34 ± 17 cm/s	28 ± 13 cm/s	n.s.
Hyperemia	82 ± 26 cm/s	45 ± 18 cm/s	<0.001	88 ± 28 cm/s	72 ± 30 cm/s	0.06
CFR	2.2 ± 0.42	1.7 ± 0.33	<0.001	2.6 ± 0.66	2.7 ± 0.62	n.s.

n.s. = no statistical difference.

Measurements of distal flow velocity, average peak velocity, phasic diastolic to systolic relationships or mean diastolic to systolic flow velocity ratio are complementary parameters to measurements of coronary flow velocity reserve and appear to reflect functional improvement immediately following coronary interventions. Further experimental and clinical trials are needed to establish the clinical usefulness of these parameters.

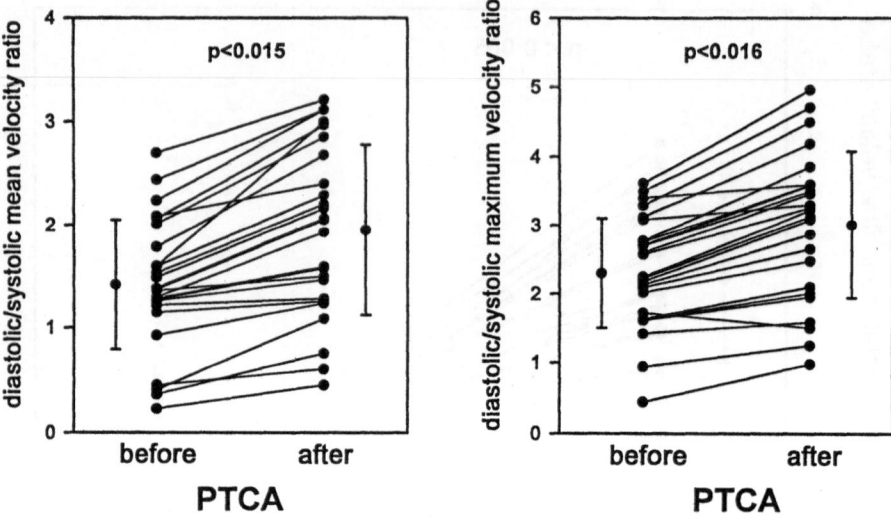

Figure 12. Diastolic to systolic mean (left panel) and maximum (right panel) velocity ratios as measured before and after successful coronary balloon angioplasty (PTCA).

References

1. Unger F. European survey on open heart surgery interventional cardiology PTCA in 1991. Report of the Institute for Cardiac Survey of the European Academy of Sciences and Arts. Salisburgi MCMII: Academia Scientiarum et Artium Europaea, 1991: 7–126.
2. Ryan TJ, Bauman WB, Kennedy JW et al. Guidelines for percutaneous transluminal coronary angioplasty, a report of the American College of Cardiology/ American Heart Association task force on assessment of diagnostic and therapeutic cardiovascular procedures (committee on percutaneous transluminal coronary angioplasty). J Am Coll Cardiol 1993; 7: 2033–54.
3. Reiber JHC. An overview of coronary quantitation techniques as of 1989. In: Reiber JHC, Serruys PW, editors. Quantitative coronary arteriography. Dordrecht: Kluwer Academic Publishers, 1991: 55–132.
4. Sanz Ml, Mancini GBJ, Lefree MT et al. Variability of quantitative digital substraction coronary angiography before and after percutaneous transluminal coronary angioplasty. Am J Cardiol 1987; 60: 55–60.
5. Grüntzig AR, Senning A, Siegenthaler WE. Nonoperative dilatation of coronary-artery stenosis: Percutaneous transluminal coronary angioplasty. N Engl J Med 1979; 301: 61–8.
6. Leibhoff R, Bren G, Katz R et al. Determinants of transstenotic gradients observed during angioplasty: An experimental model. Am J Cardiol 1983; 52: 1311–7.
7. Peterson RJ, King SB III, Fajman WA et al. Relation of coronary artery stenosis and pressure gradient to exercise induced ischemia before and after coronary angioplasty. J Am Coll Cardiol 1987; 10: 253–60.
8. Hodgson JM, Reinert S, Most AS et al. Prediction of long-term clinical outcome with final translesional pressure gradient during coronary angioplasty. Circulation 1986; 74: 563–6.
9. Anderson HV, Roubin GS, Leimgruber PP et al. Measurement of transstenotic pressure

gradient during percutaneous transluminal coronary angioplasty. Circulation 1986; 73: 1223–30.

10. Serruys PW, Wijns W, Reiber JHC et al. Values and limitations of transstenotic pressure gradients measured during percutaneous coronary angioplasty. Herz 1985; 10: 337–42.

11. Hatle L, Angelsen B. Flow velocity and volumetric principle. In: Hatle L, Angelsen B, editors. Doppler ultrasound in cardiology. Philadelphia: Lea & Febiger, 1985: 14–28.

12. Cole JS, Hartley CJ. The Doppler coronary artery catheter: Preliminary report of a new technique for measuring rapid changes in coronary artery flow velocity in man. Circulation 1977; 56: 18–25.

13. Hartley CJ, Cole JS. An ultrasonic pulsed Doppler system for measuring blood flow in small vessels. J Appl Physiol 1974; 37: 626–30.

14. Kern MJ, Courtois M, Ludbrook P. A simplified method to measure coronary blood flow velocity in patients: Validation and application of a new Judkins style Doppler tipped angiographic catheter. Am Heart J 1990; 120: 1202–8.

15. Di Mario C, Roelandt JRTC, de Jaegere P et al. Limitations of the zero-crossing detector in the analysis of intracoronary Doppler. A comparison with fast Fourier analysis of basal, hyperemic and transstenotic blood flow velocity measurements in patients with coronary artery disease. Cathet Cardiovasc Diagn 1993; 28: 56–64.

16. Doucette JW, Coral TD, Payne HM et al. Validations of a Doppler guidewire for in travascular measurement of coronary artery flow velocity. Circulation 1992; 85: 1899–1911.

17. Ofili EO, Labovitz AJ, St Vrain JA et al. Analysis of coronary blood flow dynamics in angiographically normal and stenosed arteries before and after endoluminal enlargement by angioplasty. J Am Coll Cardiol 1993; 21: 308–16.

18. Segal J, Kern MJ, Scott NA et al. Alterations of phasic coronary artery flow velocity in man during percutaneous coronary angioplasty. J Am Coll Cardiol 1992; 20: 276–86.

19. Gould KL, Kirkeeide RL, Buchi M. Coronary flow reserve as a physiologic measure of stenosis severity. J Am Coll Cardiol 1990; 15: 459–74.

20. Strauer B. The significance of coronary reserve in clinical heart disease. J Am Coll Cardiol 1990; 15: 775–83.

21. Wilson RF, Laughlin DE, Ackell PH et al. Transluminal, subselective measurement of coronary artery blood flow velocity and vasodilator reserve in man. Circulation 1985; 72: 82–92.

22. Klocke FJ. Measurements of coronary blood flow and degree of stenosis: Current clinical implications and continuing uncertainties. J Am Coll Cardiol 1983; 1: 31–41.

23. Wilson RF, White CW. Intracoronary papaverine: An ideal coronary vasodilator for studies of the coronary circulation in conscious humans. Circulation 1986; 73: 444–51.

24. Wilson RF, Wyche K, Christensen BV et al. Effects of adenosine on human coronary arterial circulation. Circulation 1990; 82: 1595–1606.

25. Zijlstra F, Reiber JC, Juiliere Y et al. Normalization of coronary flow reserve by percutaneous transluminal coronary angioplasty. Am J Cardiol 1988; 61: 55–60.

26. Hodgson JM, Williams DO. Superiority of intracoronary papaverine to radiographic contrast for measuring coronary flow reserve in patients with ischemic heart disease. Am Heart J 1987; 114: 704–10.

27. Wilson RF, Johnson MR, Marcus ML et al. The effect of coronary angioplasty on coronary flow reserve. Circulation 1988; 77: 873–85.

28. Kern MJ, Deligonul U, Vandormael M et al. Impaired coronary vasodilator reserve in the immediate postcoronary angioplasty period: Analysis of coronary artery flow velocity indexes and regional cardiac venous efflux. J Am Coll Cardiol 1989; 13: 860–72.

29. Johnson El, Yock PG, Hargrave VK et al. Assessment of severity of coronary stenoses using a Doppler catheter: Validation of a method based on the continuity equation. Circulation 1989; 80: 625–35.

30. Nakatani S, Yamagishi M, Tamai J et al. Quantitative assessment of coronary artery stenosis by intravascular Doppler catheter technique: Application of the continuity equation. Circulation 1992; 85: 1786–91.

31. Donohue TJ, Kern MJ, Aguirre FV et al. Assessing the hemodynamic significance of coronary artery stenoses: Analysis of translesional pressure – flow velocity relationships patients. J Am Coll Cardiol 1993; 22: 449–58.

Corresponding Author: Dr Michael Haude, Cardiology Department, University of Essen, Hufel-andstrasse 55, D-45122 Essen, Germany

22. Evaluation of the effect of new devices by intravascular ultrasound

DIRK HAUSMANN, PETER J. FITZGERALD and PAUL G. YOCK

Introduction

During recent years, a variety of second-generation techniques became available for catheter treatment of symptomatic coronary disease. In contrast to balloon angioplasty, these devices are designed for the reduction of plaque mass (directional, rotational and TEC atherectomy, laser angioplasty) or to maintain vessel geometry (stents). The ability of the second-generation devices to accomplish these goals mainly depends on vessel and lesion morphology. It is logical that optimal visualization of the target lesion is even more essential for the efficacy of these techniques than for balloon angioplasty. efficacy and safety of the new catheter devices is one of the most challenging clinical applications of intravascular ultrasound (IVUS) imaging [1]. In contrast to conventional angiography, IVUS provides a cross-sectional view of the lumen and plaque; thus, it has the potential to better characterize vessel geometry as well as extent, location and composition of the plaque (Figures 1 and 2). Initial experience with IVUS imaging during the clinical use of second-generation devices suggests that IVUS may be a helpful tool to optimize these interventions (see also Chapters 21, 22 and 25).

Directional atherectomy

The unique design of catheters for directional coronary atherectomy (DCA) allows selective removal of plaque. Based on previous angiographic experience, DCA is primarily used for debulking eccentric, non-calcified lesions in proximal, non-tortuous vessel that are large enough to house the DCA device.

Mechanisms of DCA

IVUS imaging during DCA has been helpful in further elucidating the physical mechanisms of DCA (Figure 3). Tenaglia et al. [2] compared IVUS

C.A. Nienaber and U. Sechtem (eds): Imaging and Intervention in Cardiology. 359–377.
© 1996 *Kluwer Academic Publishers.*

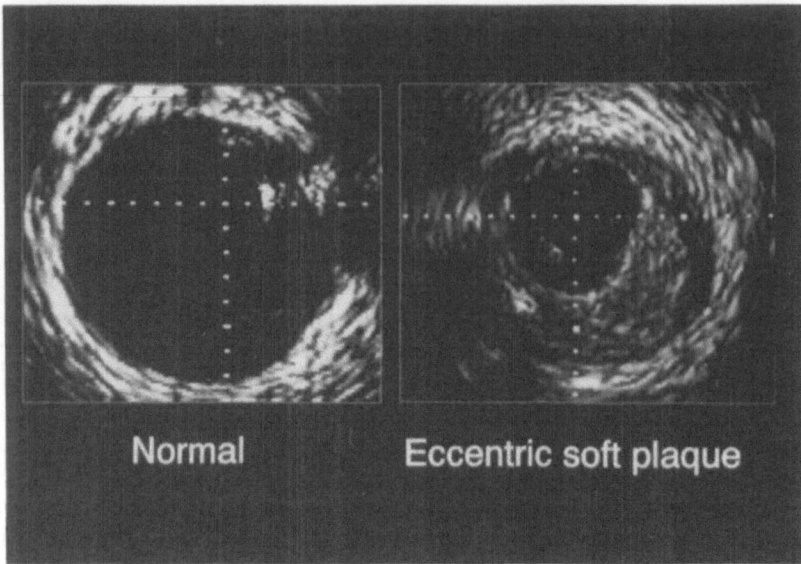

Figure 1. Intravascular ultrasound (IVUS) images of normal and atherosclerotic coronary arteries. Left: Normal IVUS image of the left main coronary artery. The inner echolucent area represents the vessel lumen bordered by the echogenic adventitia. Media and intima cannot be seen on the IVUS scan of normal coronary arteries with current catheters. Right: IVUS image of a diseased coronary artery. The vessel lumen is obstructed by eccentric soft plaque (inner echogenic layer). The media is echolucent and appears as a dark band between plaque and adventitia.   Calibration = 0.5 mm.

findings in patients after DCA or balloon angioplasty. Although both techniques resulted in comparable minimal lumen diameters, the total vessel area (area of lumen and plaque) was enlarged only after angioplasty; furthermore, dissections occurred more frequently after angioplasty than after atherectomy (50 vs 7%). It was concluded from these findings that plaque removal is in fact the major mechanism for lumen gain after DCA whereas vessel stretching and creation of neolumen by dissections are more important during balloon angioplasty [2].

Braden et al. [3] compared IVUS findings before and after DCA. Overall, reduction of plaque cross-sectional area was significant (14.3 ± 0.8 vs 10.5 ± 0.7 mm^2; $p < 0.001$) and represented the sole mechanism of lumen gain in 60% of patients. However, a significant increase in total vessel area (16.7 ± 0.8 vs 17.5 ± 0.8; mm^2; $p < 0.02$) was found after DCA; vessel stretching was even the sole mechanism for lumen improvement in 12% and was combined with plaque reduction in 28% of patients. In the subgroup of concentric lesions, the incidence of vessel stretching was highest: in 30% of patients stretching was the major mechanism of lumen enlargement and in 40% both stretching and plaque reduction contributed to lumen gain. Simi-

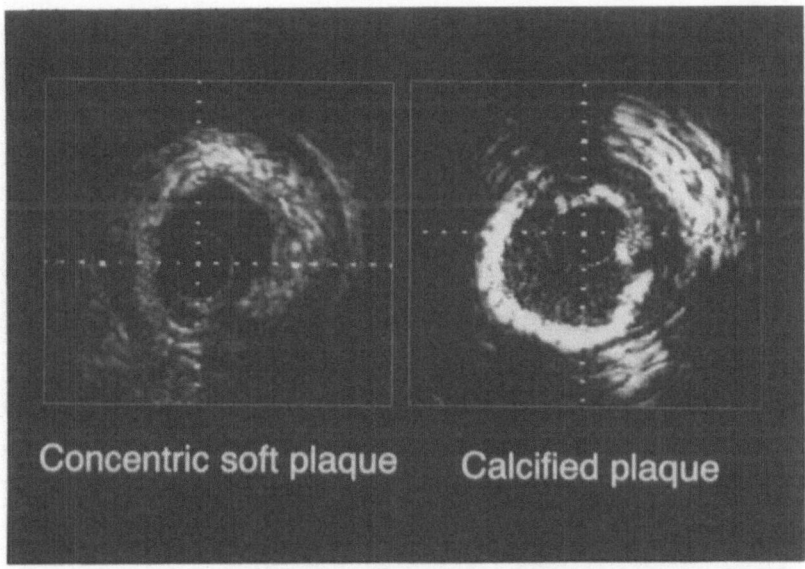

Figure 2. Intravascular ultrasound (IVUS) images of atherosclerotic coronary arteries. Left: IVUS image of a concentric, noncalcific plaque (inner echogenic layer). The media is echolucent and appears as a dark band between plaque and adventitia. Right: IVUS image of a calcified plaque. The calcium appears as a dense, echogenic structure surrounding the majority of the vessel lumen ("napkin ring"). Calcium deposits result in shadowing of the peripheral portion of the plaque between 4 and 12 o'clock. Calibration = 0.5 mm.

larly, Nakamura et al. [4] observed during IVUS imaging that 41% of the lumen gain after DCA was due to vessel stretching and only 59% to plaque removal. From these studies [3, 4] it appears that vessel stretching by DCA is more frequently observed than commonly anticipated, especially in concentric lesions.

Lesion calcification

Calcification of the plaque is among the most important factors determining the success of DCA. With the trend to perform transcatheter therapies also in older patient populations as well as in patients with multi-vessel disease, the incidence of plaque calcification is constantly increasing. However, conventional contrast angiography is often unable to detect the presence and extent of calcium; finally, it provides absolutely no information about the location of the calcium in the plaque (deep or superficial).

By using IVUS imaging, Mintz et al. [5] found significant lesion calcification in as many as 76% of candidates scheduled for transcatheter therapy of coronary disease; in contrast, fluoroscopy detected plaque calcification in only 48% of these patients (p < 0.001). One quadrant of calcification was

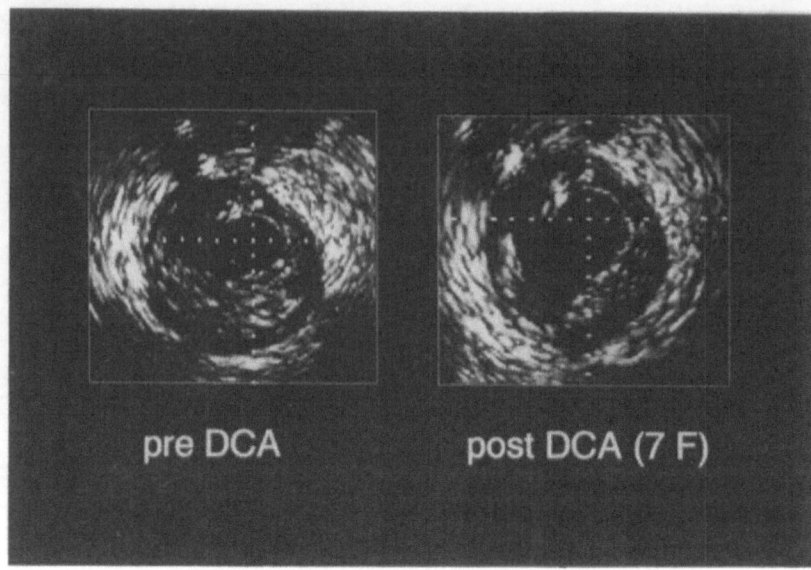

Figure 3. Intravascular ultrasound (IVUS) imaging before and after directional coronary atherectomy (DCA). Left: Prior to DCA, ultrasound imaging shows eccentric soft plaque. Right: After DCA, a distinct cut into the plaque can be seen. Despite angiographically successful DCA with only minimal residual plaque a significant amount of residual plaque remains. Calibration = 0.5 mm.

found in 26% of the patients and >2 quadrants in 50% of the patients; the calcification was located superficial in the plaque in 38%, deep in 12% and both superficial and deep in 28% of the patients.

The amount of residual plaque after DCA is clearly related to the extent of plaque calcification. In patients undergoing IVUS imaging after DCA, Popma et al. [6] found larger residual plaque by IVUS in lesions with >2 quadrant calcium (16.9 ± 4.8 mm^2) than in those with <2 quadrants or no calcium (11.9 ± 4.6 and 12.6 ± 5.5 mm^2; $p < 0.001$). In addition to the pure presence of calcium in the plaque, the exact location of calcium in the plaque also affects the procedural results. In a study by Fitzgerald et al. [7], the effect of DCA was compared in lesions with no calcium, superficial calcium and in those with calcium localized deep in the plaque as assessed by pre-procedural IVUS imaging. The weight of the tissue retrieved by DCA was significantly less ($p < 0.001$) in lesions with superficial calcium (10.3 ± 5.8 mg) than in lesions with deep calcium (19.7 ± 6.9 mg) or non-calcified lesions (22.5 ± 7.2 mg). Similarly, the vessel lumen after DCA was smallest in the lesions with superficial calcium. These findings are in agreement with observations by de Lezo et al. [8] that plaque reduction after DCA is greater in echolucent than in echogenic plaques (76 ± 21 vs

$60 \pm 18\%$; $p < 0.05$); however, this group found that despite better acute lumen gain in plaque characterized as echolucent by IVUS the restenosis rate was lower in echogenic plaque.

As known from experimental studies and from clinical experience, IVUS imaging confirmed that DCA removes no or only little calcium from the plaque [4]. However, preliminary observations indicate that DCA might be more efficient in debulking calcified lesions when combined with prior rotational atherectomy or laser angioplasty ("device synergy") [9, 10].

Residual plaque

Assessing the amount and location of residual plaque during DCA is important for the decision to end the procedure, upsize the device, change the cutting direction, change to another device or continue with the same device. Although contrast angiography can demonstrate the improvement in vessel lumen after DCA, it is limited in assessing the precise amount and location of residual plaque. Due to compensatory enlargement of the vessel at the site of plaque growth, major parts of the atheroma are usually located outside the vessel contour that is defined by the angiographically normal reference segment. Furthermore, angiographically normal reference segments may already have disease occupying up to 30–40% of the potential vessel cross-sectional area and this may further obscure intramural atheroma at the lesion site.

Since the primary goal of DCA is removal of plaque and IVUS has the advantage of visualizing the atherosclerotic plaque directly, this technique is ideal for measuring plaque before and after atherectomy [1]. Using IVUS imaging, it has been shown that excellent angiographic results after DCA still have large amounts of residual plaque [6] (Figures 3, 4). In one study, only 20% of the total plaque mass present before the intervention was removed by DCA [4]. It is our experience that in most cases the use of IVUS during DCA results in more aggressive plaque debulking as compared to angiographic assessment alone.

Orientation of the DCA device

The extent and accuracy of plaque removal may both be important factors for the degree of restenosis after DCA. Large amounts of residual plaque combined with injury to the normal vessel wall may lead to a higher incidence of restenosis at follow-up. It has been shown that without IVUS guidance approximately 50% of the DCA cuts extend at least into the media and that 30% reach the adventitia [11]. Directing of the DCA device into the area of maximal plaque may be critically important, especially when highly eccentric lesions are treated. However, angiography has 2 major limitations in identifying the location and amount of maximal plaque. First, due to the large amount of atheroma outside the vessel lumen contour, conventional angio-

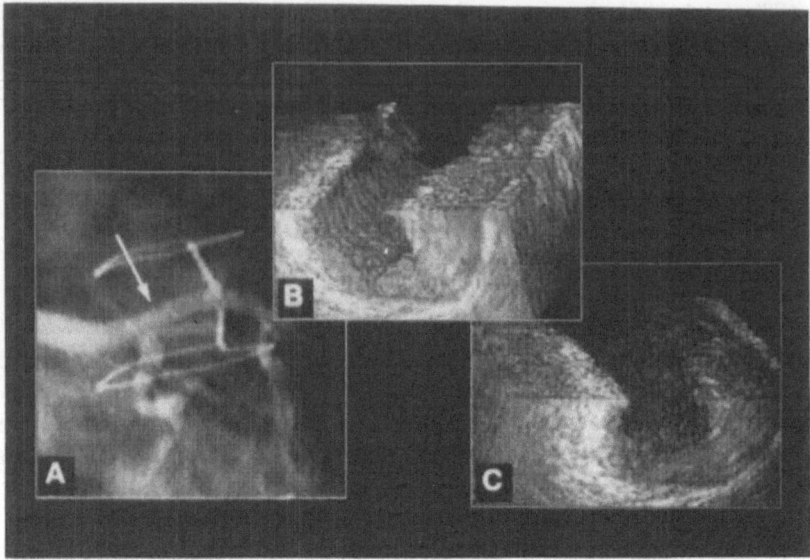

Figure 4. Intravascular ultrasound (IVUS) imaging after directional coronary atherectomy (DCA). A: Angiography shows only minimal residual stenosis at the site of DCA (arrow). B and C: Three-dimensional reconstruction of IVUS images obtained from the region of DCA show large amounts of residual eccentric plaque.

graphy may not depict maximal plaque accumulation. Second, even when the maximal plaque is correctly identified on the angiogram it is often difficult to correctly direct the atherectomy device into this area because angiography provides no rotational orientation.

Currently, IVUS is the only technique to provide rotational orientation in vessels [12]. When IVUS is used for orientation of the atherectomy housing, a branch near the target lesion should be identified and the angle to the area of maximal plaque should be determined. Using the angiographic pattern of the branches, the optimal direction of the DCA device into the area of maximal plaque accumulation can be selected [12]. For example, in the left anterior descending artery, the angle between the maximal plaque and the diagonal branches can be used to orient the atherectomy device.

Combined imaging/DCA catheter

Current IVUS catheter design requires that the DCA catheter is removed to allow imaging. Since information from the ultrasound scan is helpful before, during and after the procedure, frequent changes of catheters are necessary. It is logical that the perspective of combined imaging/therapeutic catheters is attractive to many interventionalists. Such devices have been developed in recent years [13]. One prototype catheter has been tested in vitro and in animal experiments. An image out of the open housing is provided, so that the target lesion can be evaluated before cutting. Initial results suggest that medial injury can be reduced by this device [13]. A commercially available combined atherectomy/imaging device is currently entering clinical testing.

Rotational atherectomy (PTRA)

Experimental studies have shown that the PTRA burr is deflected by soft plaque while it effectively removes fibro-calcific and calcified atheroma resulting in a sharp lumen-wall interface [14]. Previous observations based on angiography suggested that PTRA may be especially useful in calcified and/or ostial lesions as well as in lesions with complex morphology. Due to the small size of the burrs (1.0–2.5 mm) such lesions in small vessels are ideal targets for PTRA. Even with a higher proportion of more complex lesions, the results of PTRA with regard to procedural success, complications and restenosis are very similar to balloon angioplasty [15].

Mechanism of rotational atherectomy

The physical effects of PTRA were studied by Mintz et al. [16] using IVUS imaging in 28 consecutive patients. Most lesions (79%) were calcified with a mean calcification arc of 160 ± 126 degrees. Following rotablation therapy, the lumen-intima interface was very distinct (more than usually seen in native plaque) and circular, especially in highly calcified lesions. Deviations from cylindrical geometry occurred only in areas of soft plaque or superficial tissue disruption of calcified plaque. Despite angiographic completion of the procedure an average of 54% plaque area remained in the vessels. Interestingly, the lumen after PTRA measured by IVUS was slightly larger than the largest burr used (1.19 ± 0.19 fold the largest burr size). This may be explained by non-axial movement of the burr or by vasoconstriction during PTRA. Dissections occurred after PTRA in 43% of cases but were usually restricted to the surface of the residual plaque. Experimental studies showed microfissures created at the contact zone of the burr and hard tissue. These fissures cannot be detected by IVUS, probably because of limited resolution of the technique combined with the strong acoustic reflection ("blooming") from the sharp lumen-intima interface.

Kovach et al. [17] performed IVUS imaging with quantitative measurements in 48 lesions (46 patients) before and after PTRA. After rotational atherectomy, lumen area increased (1.8 ± 0.9 vs 3.9 ± 1.1 mm^2), plaque + media area decreased (15.7 ± 4.1 vs 13.0 ± 4.7 mm^2), the extent of calcification was reduced and 26% of lesions showed local dissection (usually originating *within* a calcified deposit). After adjunct balloon angioplasty, total vessel area increased due to vessel stretching (16.7 ± 4.8 vs 18.8 ± 5.6 mm^2), plaque + media remained unchanged and 77% of lesions had dissections usually located *adjacent* to calcified plaque [17]. Thus, the primary mechanism of PTRA appears to be selective ablation of hard atherosclerotic plaque without arterial expansion. Adjunct angioplasty results in arterial expansion of non-calcified plaque elements [17]. In soft plaque, however, the vessel lumen after rotational atherectomy is often not ideally round and is also smaller than the largest burr size used. This may be due to less effective plaque ablation because of deflection of the burr (differential cutting).

In a preliminary study, Koschyk et al. [18] performed IVUS before and after PTRA as well as after adjunct balloon angioplasty with low pressures (3 atm, 60 sec) in 13 lesions and observed an average lumen gain after rotational atherectomy of 29% and an additional gain of 31% after angioplasty. In 12 of the 13 lesions the lumen enlargement by angioplasty was concentric and dissections were not observed in any of the lesions. PTRA reduced wall thickness and increased the lumen area; thus, according to the rule of Laplace, adjunct balloon angioplasty after PTRA can use low inflation pressures to obtain a similar wall stress as high pressure balloon angioplasty without prior PTRA.

Combination with other transcatheter techniques

The largest rotational burr is 2.5 mm in diameter and requires a 10 French guiding catheter; in addition, the largest burr tip used is usually 70 to 80% of the reference vessel diameter. In particular in large vessels, PTRA has therefore to be combined with other techniques to obtain sufficient lumen size. Most centers used conventional balloon angioplasty as the adjunct to PTRA.

The experience with PTRA and adjunct DCA is still limited. In a series of 9 patients, Mintz et al. [10] performed serial IVUS measurements before and after these procedures in large coronary arteries. Target lesions calcification was 271 ± 92 degrees before and 210 ± 120 degrees after PTRA ($p < 0.05$) and further decreased to 163 ± 122 degrees after adjunct DCA. Total vessel area was unchanged after PTRA and after DCA; in contrast, lumen area was increased and plaque + media area was decreased by both techniques. In contrast to the experience with DCA alone, the combined use of PTRA and DCA resulted in distinct cuts into areas of calcified plaque [10]. Obviously, PTRA renders the lesion susceptible to plaque removal by DCA (synergistic effect); DCA as an adjunct to PTRA causes more plaque removal and less "Dotter" effect than DCA alone. The authors [10] concluded that in selected cases DCA should be considered as an alternative to adjunct balloon angioplasty following PTRA.

Rotational atherectomy may also be considered when adequate stent deployment is required in lesions with fibro-calcific plaque. Goldberg et al. [19]

performed IVUS in 43 patients scheduled for stent placement; fluoroscopy showed lesion calcification in none of the patients whereas IVUS revealed calcium in 20 (47%) patients. Patients with calcified lesions by IVUS underwent PTRA (burr size: 1.75 ± 0.23 mm) prior to stent placement. Following stent placement, IVUS documented a round and symmetric lumen with well-expanded struts in all patients. However, despite prior rotational atherectomy final lumen cross-sectional area was significantly smaller in patients with calcified as compared to non-calcified plaque (7.5 ± 1.8 vs 9.0 ± 2.0 mm; $p < 0.05$). Thus, IVUS imaging indicates that although stents can be placed in calcified lesions following PTRA the degree of stent expansion may still be limited by rigid plaque [19].

Guidance of PTRA

It is our experience that guidance of PTRA by IVUS imaging frequently results in the application of larger burrs earlier in the procedure because the amount of residual plaque is underestimated by contrast angiography. When the target lesion is still significantly calcified following PTRA with a large amount of residual plaque, repeat ablation using a larger burr size seems to be prudent although this may slightly increase the risk of complications. The use of balloon angioplasty (especially with inflation pressures ≥ 4 atm) in lesions with significant calcification after PTRA may carry the risk of major dissections. On the other hand, lesions without evidence of calcium following PTRA may be successfully treated by conventional balloon angioplasty. Low pressure balloon angioplasty should then be used to limit the wall stress in the residual plaque (Figure 5).

However, the most important impact of IVUS imaging with regard to PTRA is the identification of plaque calcification *prior* to the procedure. Due to the high incidence of plaque calcification not adequately visualized by conventional angiography, IVUS imaging in patients scheduled for balloon angioplasty and DCA often leads to a change in strategy in favor of PTRA (see also Chapters 21 and 25).

Stents

Angiography, although previously considered as the gold standard of arterial imaging, does not provide all of the information which would be of value to completely, accurately and safely guide stent placement. In general, there is a need to know more about the nature of the underlying lesion than angiography can provide, to better visualize the stent and determine completeness of expansion and to see details of intimacy of stent/vessel wall contact; furthermore, details of intra-stent luminal pathology is required to plan optimal secondary intra- or peri-stent interventions [20]. Several studies have

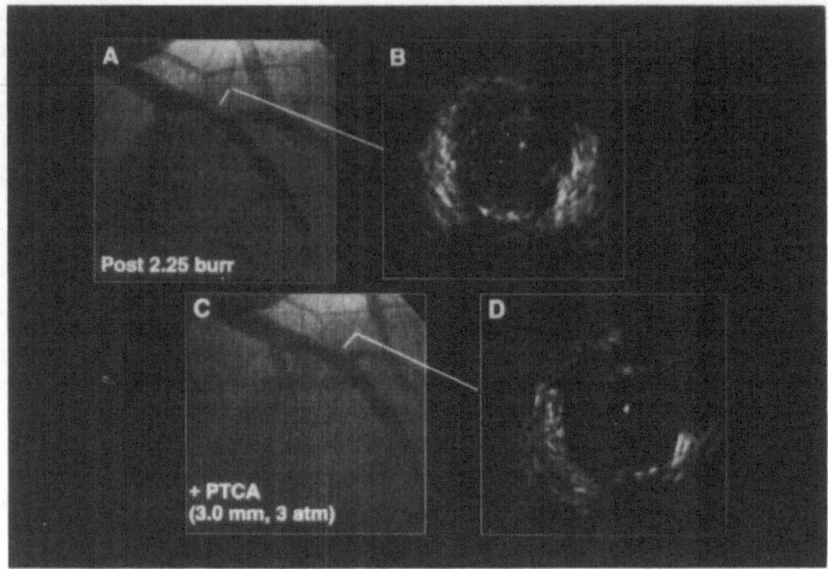

Figure 5. Intravascular ultrasound (IVUS) imaging during rotational atherectomy (PTRA). A:
Following PTRA with a 2.25 mm burr, angiography shows moderate residual stenosis in the
mid portion of the left anterior descending artery. B: The ultrasound scan following PTRA with
a 2.25 mm burr directly demonstrates a significant plaque residual. As often observed after
PTRA, the lumen/plaque interface is unusually distinct and the lumen shape is circular. C:
Adjunct balloon angioplasty (3.0 mm, 3 atm) was performed to improve the lumen gain; subsequent angiography shows only minimal residual stenosis. D: IVUS imaging after adjunct balloon
angioplasty confirms further lumen gain without major dissection of the plaque. The amount of
plaque, however, was unchanged by angioplasty.

shown that angiography overestimates the vessel size after stent placement
[21, 22] and is incapable of precisely visualizing the details of the stent.

The guidance of stent placement is one of the most important applications
of intracoronary ultrasound in device assessment. While the metal struts of
stents are usually not radiopaque their echoreflective appearance creates a
distinct appearance on the ultrasound scan; hence, the struts can easily be
differentiated from the vessel wall (Figure 6). The various types of endovascular stents have a typical appearance on the ultrasound scan and are described in detail elsewhere [20]. Understanding the typical appearance of
different types of endovascular stents on the ultrasound scan is essential to
recognize suboptimal results after stent placement. Experimental studies
with histologic validation have shown that IVUS measurements of stent
dimensions are very accurate [23]. Optimal stent/vessel size ratio can be
provided by clear and accurate imaging of the location, shape and degree of
arterial pathology [23].

Mintz et al. [24] pioneered the use of timed pullback of IVUS catheters

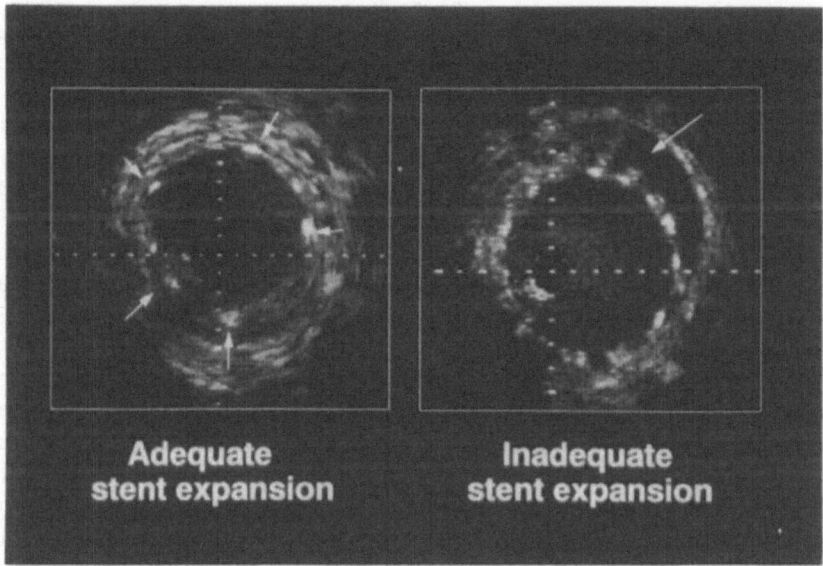

Figure 6. Intravascular ultrasound (IVUS) imaging after stent placement. Left: With optimal stent placement, IVUS imaging shows that the metal struts (arrows) of the stent are apposed to the vessel wall and that the in-stent lumen is symmetric. Right: Although the stent is expanded symmetrically, IVUS imaging detects incomplete apposition of the struts to the wall (arrow). The metal struts in this part of the vessel are fully exposed to blood. Calibration = 0.5 mm.

for 3-dimensional reconstruction of arterial segments. In vitro and human in vivo studies have shown that IVUS images can be used to reconstruct the spatial geometry of endovascular stent [24]. Furthermore, these authors advised the IVUS user that reconstruction of stents should be one of the tests of imaging systems designed to perform 3-dimensional reconstruction because of the known appearance of stents.

The mechanism of restenosis in stents can also be diagnosed using IVUS. The metal struts provide a marker for the original lumen border; thus, intimal hyperplasia and mechanical compression of the stent can be differentiated. Based on IVUS findings, neointimal proliferation (predominantly within the first 3 months) seems to be the major factor contributing to in-stent restenosis.

Guidance of stent deployment

Soon after the introduction of stents into the arena of interventional devices, occasional case reports documented that IVUS imaging may be helpful to identify inadequate stent expansion despite optimal angiographic results [25] (Figure 6). Prior to stent placement, IVUS appears to be useful to measure the true vessel size (vessel size without plaque) more accurately than angiography for more precise balloon size selection. Animal experiments have shown that IVUS accurately identifies undersizing of stents relative to the vessel and overlapping of the stent [26]. Schrywer et al. [27] reported a case with a parallel tract dissection after balloon angioplasty of a restenosis lesion in the right coronary artery. IVUS was used to identify the true lumen and the length of the dissection; the patient subsequently underwent successful stenting of the artery. Furthermore, IVUS studies have shown that the larger lumen gain with stent implantation in combination with balloon angioplasty as compared to balloon angioplasty alone is probably due to more vessel expansion [28].

Nakamura and colleagues [21] recently reported their observations from IVUS imaging during Palmaz-Schatz stent insertion in 63 consecutive patients (65 lesions treated). Although all patients had a satisfactory angiographic result, 52 (80%) patients showed inadequate stent expansion and required further dilatations. In these 52 patients, angiographic lesion diameter was 3.12 ± 0.47 mm after the first and 3.61 ± 0.49 mm after final balloon dilatation; the balloon size was 3.7 ± 0.3 for the initial and 4.1 ± 0.4 mm for the final dilatations. Inflation pressures were 11.1 ± 1.9 atm during the first and 12.0 ± 2.6 atm during the final dilatations [21]. It was possible to improve stent underexpansion in all cases with repeated balloon dilatation using larger balloons or higher pressures. Vessel rupture occurred in one patient in whom a balloon was used that was 1.5 mm larger than the distal reference vessel [21].

In the same study [21] IVUS measurements showed that the actual cross-sectional lumen area at the tightest point of the stented segment ranged between 50 and 75% of the expected value (based on balloon size) after the first dilatation and between 61 and 71% after the final dilatation. The minimum lumen diameter within the stented segment was 2.7 ± 0.4 mm after the first dilatations and increased to 3.1 ± 0.5 mm after the final dilatations. An important manifestation of stent underexpansion was that the lumen cross-sectional area was smaller than the distal reference lumen [21]. Despite angiographically satisfactory results, IVUS shows that in the majority of cases the stented lumen areas are substantially below the values for the proximal or distal reference segment (media to media). These authors concluded that IVUS imaging is useful during stent insertion because it helps to detect stent underexpansion and incomplete apposition of the struts with the vessel wall; furthermore, IVUS enables the interventionalist to choose an appropriately sized balloon to maximize lumen area [21].

As with other interventional devices, combined imaging/therapeutic catheters have been used for stent placement. Mudra et al. [22] used a combined imaging/balloon angioplasty catheter for stent placement in 21 patients. Minimal luminal diameter was overestimated by quantitative angiography compared to IVUS measurements mainly due to eccentric lumen shape or incomplete vessel wall attachment. Further stent expansion based on IVUS findings resulted in an additional 25% lumen gain.

Stent deployment without anticoagulation

Acute and subacute coronary thrombosis occurs in 3–25% of patients after emergent stent placement. Consequent anticoagulation with heparin, Coumadine and platelet inhibitors is therefore necessary. This, on the other hand, can lead to severe bleeding complications and also significantly prolongs the hospital stay. It appears logical that minimizing the exposure of metal struts to the blood (by full stent expansion) may also diminish the risk of thrombosis. It is generally accepted that proper stent placement without in- or outflow obstruction is important to limit acute and subacute stent thrombosis, and possibly also restenosis.

Based on their experience in this area, Colombo and coworkers [21, 29] developed the following criteria for optimal stent placement guided by IVUS imaging: 1) The stent should be fully apposed to the wall; 2) lumen symmetry index (ratio of minimal/maximal lumen diameter) should be ≥0.7; and 3) the stented lumen area should be ≥60% of the reference vessel area (average of proximal and distal vessel area, media to media). Several multi- and single-center studies are currently undertaken to further evaluate the use of IVUS during stent placement [29].

Using these IVUS-derived criteria, Colombo et al. [29] studied 191 patients undergoing Palmaz-Schatz stenting (including only 3% after dissection or acute closure) in 219 lesions (97% native coronary arteries). The 164 patients with optimal stent placement (according to IVUS criteria) were subsequently treated only with Ticlopidine 250 mg bid for 2 months (no heparin or Coumadin). No episodes of acute or subacute stent thrombosis or bleeding complications occurred during a follow-up of 41–153 days (mean 91 days) [29]. In more recent preliminary work, Colombo and colleagues have emphasized using the average of the proximal and distal reference *lumen* areas as the target value for stent expansion. In summary, it appears that the potential thrombogenicity of metallic stents can be substantially diminished by full stent expansion by high pressure and large balloon sizes to optimize in-stent diameter and flow [29]. Clearly, the aggressive use of larger balloons/higher pressure must be tempered with the risk of vessel rupture.

Laser angioplasty

Clinical experience with IVUS imaging during laser angioplasty is still limited. Schrywer et al. [30] studied 9 patients following excimer laser angioplasty and subsequent balloon angioplasty in coronary arteries. Intima disruptions were more frequent but dissections occurred less frequently compared to balloon angioplasty alone. Substantial residual plaque with little evidence for major atheroma debulking was found. These authors therefore concluded from this preliminary study that effects of laser angioplasty may be acoustic shockwaves that facilitate subsequent balloon dilatation. In a series of 6 patients undergoing excimer laser angioplasty followed by DCA, Mintz et al. [9] performed IVUS to monitor the results of these procedures. The arc of lesions calcification was unchanged after laser angioplasty, but decreased after adjunct DCA. Total vessel area was unchanged and extent of plaque decreased after laser angioplasty. After adjunct DCA, total vessel area still remained unchanged whereas plaque extent further decreased; atherectomy cuts were noted even in heavily calcified lesions. It was concluded from this study in a limited number of patients, that excimer laser angioplasty reduces plaque mass and appears to render the calcified plaque susceptible to the DCA device [9].

Other centers [31] reported that the amount of coronary plaque following excimer laser angioplasty is unchanged to that prior to balloon angioplasty. In addition, the amount of plaque is similar in patients with excimer laser and adjunct balloon angioplasty compared to patients with balloon angioplasty alone [31]. This has led to the speculation that reducing plaque mass is not the primary mechanism of this technique.

Again, the combination of a therapeutic laser catheter with diagnostic IVUS imaging in the same catheter has great practical appeal and thus a catheter (9F) combining laser angioplasty and simultaneous IVUS imaging capabilities was recently introduced [32]. This prototype catheter allows ultrasound imaging during laser ablation. Laser pulses are usually accompanied by the appearance of scattered echogenic material inside the vessel which adversely affects IVUS imaging of the plaque; however, IVUS imaging is possible immediately after ablation. The appearance of spontaneous echo contrast is most likely caused by the release of microparticulated matter by the laser discharges, or by creation of microbubbles of gas. IVUS with this prototype combined device was not useful in directing the laser ablation but allowed lumen measurements without changing catheters [32].

In an experimental study, White et al. [33] performed IVUS guidance of Holmium-YAG laser angioplasty in occlusions of canine vessels. IVUS enabled concentric initial recanalization of the occlusions although vessel perforations occurred in this study. Aretz et al. [34] showed the feasibility of a catheter combining IVUS imaging and Holmium-YAG laser angioplasty in an in vivo canine model. In a clinical case also using Holmium-YAG laser coronary angioplasty, Itoh et al. [35] speculated that the effect of this device is not only the direct ablation of plaque but also the "Dotter" effect by the catheter itself.

Transcutaneous extraction atherectomy (TEC)

Transcutaneous extraction catheters (TEC) use 2 cutting blades with a central lumen attached to a vacuum bottle; this design allows cutting of plaque and sucking the material from vessels. This technique is preferentially used to treat total occlusions in peripheral arteries. IVUS imaging may be helpful to elucidate the exact mechanism of this therapy.

Tobis et al. [31] reported a study with TEC atherectomy used in conjunction with balloon angioplasty of superficial femoral arteries. Again, IVUS after TEC atherectomy showed large amounts of residual plaque despite satisfactory angiographic results. With 2.7 mm TEC atherectomy, only an 11% reduction in plaque area was observed; however, the major lumen gain was achieved by adjunct balloon dilatation with plaque fracture and separation of the torn ends [31]. Most important, IVUS imaging has shown that these devices are quickly deflected from hard plaque and take the path of least resistance, usually between internal elastic membrane and the plaque itself; this may carry a substantial risk of media or adventitia perforation. The device reenters the true lumen when the plaque becomes thinner at a more distal segment [31].

Limitations of IVUS imaging

IVUS has the ability to provide accurate, high-resolution images of the vessel cross-section in the majority of patients and enables the user to obtain morphologic and geometric information not accesible by conventional angiography. Nevertheless, several limitations of the technique have to be considered:

- With eccentric position of the IVUS catheter the vessel wall segments with the least favorable angle of interrogation show approximately 30% reduction in backscatter when compared to a centered catheter position [36]. This may lead to misinterpretation of plaque composition and errors in plaque and lumen measurements. Non-orthogonal catheter position also causes geometric distortion of the vessel [37, 38].
- Air bubbles in the housing of mechanical systems may attenuate image quality and can be the source for image misinterpretation. Failure to achieve a precise rotation can result in non-uniform rotational distortion of the image.
- Calcium deposits or thick fibrous tissue cause shadowing of underlying structures that can be misinterpreted as dissections; furthermore, the outer border of the plaque can not be identified in these areas. Finally, dense tissue, especially calcium deposits, causes multiple echos by reverberation.
- Echogenicity of blood is relatively high during IVUS imaging with 20–30 MHz. Since blood backscatter intensity is a function of flow velocity the differentiation of lumen and wall may be difficult in areas of low blood

flow, such as dissections. In these cases, delineation of the vessel wall may be facilitated by injecting saline (negative contrast) or echocontrast agents (positive contrast) [39].

- IVUS has limitations for the differentiation between thrombus and soft plaque when 20–30 MHz transducers are used.
- The ultrasound scan yields virtually no overview over the coronary tree and the longitudinal orientation in the vessel from the images alone is often difficult. Fluoroscopic control of the catheter position and correlation to side branches has to be performed. The use of a constant pullback may be useful starting from a clearly defined point in the vessel which has been documented by angiography; 3D-reconstruction may also be helpful for better spatial orientation.
- During IVUS imaging, the position of the imaging catheter relative to the vessel is affected by axial and longitudinal translation. Furthermore, systolic/diastolic changes in vessel dimensions have to be considered for lumen measurements.
- In mechanical systems, the guide wire causes shadowing of a certain part of the ultrasound image. Electronic systems and newer mechanical systems (where the wire is temporarily moved out of the imaging plane) have no wire artifact. Near field artifacts can be a source of misinterpretation with all IVUS catheters, especially when the catheter is directly adjacent to the vessel wall [38].
- IVUS systems have a lower limit of resolution with regard to the axial, lateral and out-of-plane direction; this depends on the type of system used and also on the actual distance from the transducer.
- Differentiation of fibrous and non-calcified plaque may be impossible in certain patients. Backscatter of the plaque strongly depends on the gain settings and the angle of incidence of the ultrasound beam.
- Since IVUS catheters are stiff in the region of the imaging element, advancing the catheter can be a problem when curved segments or tight stenoses have to be crossed, especially when surface calcium is present; crossing such lesions may cause a certain amount of "Dottering" effect. With the development of IVUS catheter with a diameter of approximately 1 mm, even distal or tortuous segments can be reached and tight lesions can be crossed in most cases.
- Intracoronary IVUS imaging may cause acute complications in a small number of patients. Incidence, type and causes of such complications were analyzed in a study of 2207 patients undergoing IVUS imaging in 28 international centers [40]: Major complications occurred in 8 (0.4%) patients (5 myocardial infarction, 3 emergency bypass surgery) undergoing IVUS for diagnostic reasons (1 patient) or during interventions (7 patients). Minor complications were observed in 15 (0.7%) patients (8 dissections, 4 acute occlusion, 1 embolism, 1 thrombus, 1 arrhythmia); 3 of these patients were studied for diagnostic reasons and 12 during interventions.

In addition, 3% of all patients showed vessel spasm during IVUS imaging (see also Chapters 21, 22 and 25).

Conclusion

In contrast to balloon angioplasty, second-generation devices for transcatheter treatment of symptomatic coronary disease are designed for the reduction of plaque mass or to maintain vessel geometry. Currently, selection of the optimal therapeutic strategy is based primarily on angiographic criteria, such as location, length, calcification and morphology of the lesion, vessel size and tourtousity. Despite some limitations IVUS may be helpful to optimize these interventions by better characterizing the target lesion before, during and after these procedures. Although other factors than morphology of the target lesion have to be considered for the interventional strategy (DCA limited to large, non-tortuous vessels, suboptimal lumen gain by PTRA in large vessels, etc.) better characterization of the lesion by IVUS may result in a better rationale for device selection. Despite the advantages of IVUS imaging, it has to be remembered that a clinical benefit from the additional use of IVUS has not been shown yet in a randomized trial format. Several multicenter studies are currently underway to evaluate this issue.

The overall input of IVUS imaging on the strategy during transcatheter procedures can be best explained by a recent report of the Washington Heart Center [41]: Among nearly 700 lesions, IVUS findings resulted in change of procedural strategy in 44% of patients. A change from transcatheter to surgical therapy occurred in 2% and change in device selection (type, size) in 25% of patients. Furthermore, IVUS findings of lesions severity were considered because of equivocal angiographic data in 16% of patients. Perhaps most interesting of all, the frequency of change in strategy increased significantly with greater operator experience.

References

1. Yock PG, Fitzgerald PJ, Sudhir K et al. Intravascular ultrasound imaging for guidance of atherectomy and other plaque removal techniques. Int J Card Imaging 1991; 6: 179–89.
2. Tenaglia AN, Buller CE, Kisslo KB et al. Mechanisms of balloon angioplasty and directional coronary atherectomy as assessed by intracoronary ultrasound. J Am Coll Cardiol 1992; 20: 685–91.
3. Braden GA, Herrington DM, Downes TR et al. Qualitative and quantitative contrasts in the mechanism of lumen enlargement by coronary balloon angioplasty and directional coronary atherectomy. J Am Coll Cardiol 1993; 23: 40–8.
4. Nakamura S, Mahon DJ, Yang J et al. Intravascular ultrasound imaging before and after directional atherectomy (DCA). Circulation 1993; 88 (Suppl): I–502 (Abstr).
5. Mintz GS, Douek P, Pichard AD et al. Target lesion calcification in coronary artery disease: An intravascular ultrasound study. J Am Coll Cardiol 1992; 20: 1149–55.

6. Popma JJ, Mintz GS, Satler LF et al. Clinical and angiographic outcome after directional coronary atherectomy. A qualitative and quantitative analysis using coronary arteriography and intravascular ultrasound. Am J Cardiol 1993; 72: 55E–64E.

7. Fitzgerald PJ, Mühlberger VA, Moes NY et al. Calcium location within plaque as a predictor of atherectomy tissue retrieval: An intravascular ultrasound study. Circulation 1992; 86 (Suppl I): I–516 (Abstr).

8. De Lezo JS, Romero M, Medina A et al. Intracoronary ultrasound assessment of directional coronary atherectomy: Immediate and follow-up findings. J Am Coll Cardiol 1993; 21: 298–307.

9. Mintz GS, Pichard AD, Kent KM et al. Transcatheter device synergy: Preliminary experience with adjunct directional coronary atherectomy following high-speed rotational atherectomy or excimer laser angioplasty in the treatment of coronary artery disease. Cathet Cardiovasc Diagn 1993; 1: 37–44.

10. Mintz GS, Pichard AD, Popma JJ et al. Preliminary experience with adjunct directional coronary atherectomy after high-speed rotational atherectomy in the treatment of calcific coronary artery disease. Am J Cardiol 1993; 71: 799–804.

11. Garrat KN, Holmes DR, Bell MR et al. Restenosis after directional coronary atherectomy: Differences between primary atheromatous and restenosis lesions and influence of subintimal tissue resection. J Am Coll Cardiol 1990; 16: 1665–71.

12. Kimura BJ, Fitzgerald PJ, Sudhir K et al. Guidance of directed coronary atherectomy by intracoronary ultrasound imaging. Am Heart J 1992; 124: 1365–9.

13. Yock PG, Fitzgerald PJ, Sykes C et al. Morphologic features of successful coronary atherectomy determined by intravascular ultrasound imaging. Circulation 1990; 82 (Suppl III): III–676 (Abstr).

14. Hansen DD, Auth DC, Hall M, Ritchie JL. Rotational endarterectomy in normal canine coronary arteries: Preliminary report. J Am Coll Cardiol 1988; 11: 1073–7.

15. Ellis SG, Popma JJ, Buchbinder M et al. Relation of clinical presentation, stenosis morphology and operator technique to the procedural results of rotational atherectomy and rotational atherectomy-facilitated angioplasty. Circulation 1994; 89: 882–92.

16. Mintz GS, Potkin BN, Keren G et al. Intravascular ultrasound evaluation of the effect of rotational atherectomy in obstructive atherosclerotic coronary artery disease. Circulation 1992; 86: 1383–93.

17. Kovach JA, Mintz GS, Pichard AD et al. Sequential intravascular ultrasound characterization of the mechanisms of rotational atherectomy and adjunct balloon angioplasty. J Am Coll Cardiol 1993; 22: 1024–32.

18. Koschyk D, Terres W, Chen C, Hamm CW. Mechanismus der Lumenvergrößerung nach Rotablation und anschließender PTCA mit niedrigen Drücken – Untersuchung mit intravaskulärem Ultraschall. Z Kardiol 1994; 83 (Suppl 1): 12 (Abstr).

19. Goldberg SL, Hall P, Almagor Y et al. Intravascular ultrasound guided rotational atherectomy of fibro-calcific plaque prior to intracoronary deployment of Palmaz-Schatz Stents. J Am Coll Cardiol 1994; (Suppl) 290A (Abstr).

20. Slepian MJ. Application of intraluminal ultrasound imaging to vascular stenting. Int J Card Imaging 1991; 6: 285–311.

21. Nakamura S, Colombo A, Gaglione A et al. Intracoronary ultrasound observations during stent implantation. Circulation 1994; 89: 2026–34.

22. Mudra H, Klauss V, Blasini R et al. Intracoronary ultrasound guidance of stent deployment leads to an increase of luminal gain not discernible by angiography. J Am Coll Cardiol 1994; Suppl; 71A (Abstr).

23. Cavaye DM, Tabbara MR, Kopchok GE et al. Intraluminal ultrasound assessment of vascular stent deployment. Ann Vasc Surg 1991; 5: 241–6.

24. Mintz GS, Pichard AD, Satler LF et al. Three-dimensional intravascular ultrasonography: Reconstruction of endovascular stents in vitro and in vivo. J Clin Ultrasound 1993; 21: 609–15.

25. Deaner ANS, Cubukcu AA, Rees MR. Assessment of coronary stent by intravascular ultrasound. Int J Cardiol 1992; 36: 124–6.
26. Tenaglia AN, Kisslo K, Kelly S et al. Ultrasound guide wire-directed stent deployment. Am Heart J 1993; 125: 1213–6.
27. Schryver TE, Popma JJ, Kent KM et al. Use of intracoronary ultrasound to identify the "true" coronary lumen in chronic coronary dissection treated with intracoronary stenting. Am J Cardiol 1992; 69: 1107–8.
28. Burckhard-Meier C, Albrecht D, Kaspers S et al. Mechanismen der Lumenzunahme bei PTCA und Stent-Implantation: Vergleichende Untersuchung mit intrakoronarem Ultraschall. Z Kardiol 1994; 83 (Suppl 1): 139 (Abstr).
29. Colombo A, Hall P, Almagor Y et al. Results of intravascular ultrasound guided coronary stenting without subsequent anticoagulation. J Am Coll Cardiol 1994; (Suppl); 335A (Abstr).
30. Schrywer TE, Garrand TJ, Mintz GS et al. Intravascular ultrasound assessment of high risk lesions after excimer laser coronary angioplasty. J Am Coll Cardiol 1992; 19 (Suppl); 223A (Abstr).
31. Tobis JM, Mahon DJ, Goldberg SL et al. Lessons from intravascular ultrasonography: Observations during interventional angioplasty procedures. J Clin Ultrasound 1993; 21: 589–607.
32. Duda SH, Huppert PE, Kreis A et al. Ultrasound-monitored laser angioplasty: Preliminary clinical results. Cardiovasc Intervent Radiol 1993; 16: 89–92.
33. White RA, Kopchok GE, Tabbara MR et al. Intravascular ultrasound guided holmium: YAG laser recanalization of occluded arteries. Lasers Surg Med 1992; 12: 239–45.
34. Aretz HT, Gregory KW, Martinelli MA et al. Ultrasound guidance of laser atherectomy. Int J Card Imaging 1991; 6: 231–7.
35. Itoh A, Miyazaki S, Nonogi H et al. Angioscopic and intravascular ultrasound imagings before and after percutaneous holmium-YAG laser coronary angioplasty. Am Heart J 1993; 125: 556–8.
36. DiMario C, Madretsma S, Linker D et al. The angle of incidence of the ultrasonic beam: A critical factor for the image quality in intravascular ultrasonography. Am Heart J 1993; 125: 442–8.
37. Chae JS, Brisken AF, Maurer G, Siegel RJ. Geometric accuracy of intravascular ultrasound imaging. J Am Soc Echo 1992; 5: 577–87.
38. Finet G, Maurincomme E, Tabib A et al. Artifacts in intravascular ultrasound imaging: Analyses and implications. Ultrasound Med Biol 1993; 19: 533–47.
39. Hausmann D, Sudhir K, Mullen WL et al. Contrast-enhanced intravascular ultrasound: Validation of a new technique for delineation of the vessel wall surface. J Am Coll Cardiol 1994; 23: 981–7.
40. Hausmann D, Fitzgerald PJ, Daniel WG et al. and the SAFETY of ICUS Study Group. Safety of Intracoronary Ultrasound: A multicenter, multicatheter registry in 1837 Patients. Circulation 1993; 88 (Part 2): I–549. (Abstr).
41. Mintz GS, Pichard AD, Kent KM et al. The influence of pre-intervention intravascular ultrasound imaging on subsequent transcatheter treatment strategies. Circulation 1993; 88 (Suppl): I–597 (Abstr).

Corresponding Author: Dr Dirk Hausmann, Department of Cardiology, Division of Internal Medicine, Hannover Medical School, Konstanty-Gutschow-Str. 8, 30625 Hannover, Germany

23. Can restenosis after coronary angioplasty be predicted by scintigraphy?

ELIZABETH PRVULOVICH and RICHARD UNDERWOOD

Introduction

Percutaneous transluminal coronary angioplasty (PTCA) was first performed by Grüntzig in 1977 [1]. In the last decade it has proved to be an effective method of revascularising the myocardium in selected patients with coronary artery disease. Initially performed mainly in patients with single vessel coronary disease, it is now used in multivessel disease, bypass graft stenoses, and total coronary artery occlusions.

A logical part of any intervention in medicine is to assess the effect of that intervention from studies of anatomy or function before and after the procedure. Myocardial perfusion scintigraphy has the ability to visualise abnormal perfusion directly and to relate its site to the known coronary anatomy. It can therefore be used to confirm the success of the intervention, to detect unexpected complications, and to assess recurrence of symptoms objectively from changes in the pattern of perfusion. It may also provide a method of predicting restenosis.

When considering the role of myocardial perfusion scintigraphy it should be remembered that coronary arteriography provides anatomical information and perfusion imaging provides functional information, and that it is not always possible to predict the result of one test from the other.

Documentation of improved myocardial perfusion

Myocardial perfusion scintigraphy has been used to demonstrate improved regional perfusion after angioplasty. Using planar thallium imaging, Verani and colleagues [2] showed that uptake in regions supplied by stenotic coronary arteries averaged 49% of that in normal myocardium. After angioplasty uptake in the same areas increased to 71%, and 68% of areas with initial perfusion defects had returned to normal. Further objective evidence of improved myocardial perfusion after angioplasty was provided by DePuey and colleagues [3] who used tomography to demonstrate perfusion abnor-

C.A. Nienaber and U. Sechtem (eds): Imaging and Intervention in Cardiology, 379–385.
© 1996 *Kluwer Academic Publishers.*

malities in 93% of patients before angioplasty, and improvement in 76% of patients one to two days after angioplasty.

Although myocardial perfusion during stress clearly improves after successful angioplasty, residual defects are frequently seen early after successful dilatation. Several authors have noted relatively poor agreement between angiographic and scintigraphic determinants of coronary perfusion at this time [3, 4].

Manyari and colleagues [4] studied 43 patients who underwent angioplasty for single vessel coronary disease. Exercise perfusion imaging was performed before angioplasty and at mean times afterwards of 9 days, 3.3 months, and 6.6 months. Coronary angiography between 6 and 9 months documented coronary patency in all patients. Myocardial perfusion in the distribution of the dilated artery improved progressively until 3 months but thereafter no improvement was seen.

Haemodynamic studies support scintigraphic evidence of progressive improvement in regional myocardial perfusion after angioplasty. In a recent study [5], quantitative coronary angiography was compared with intracoronary Doppler assessment of coronary flow reserve in 31 patients immediately after and at a mean of 7.7 months after angioplasty. Immediately after successful angioplasty, coronary flow reserve did not correlate significantly with residual stenosis, and in 55% of patients coronary flow reserve was improved but remained abnormal. Only later was a significant relationship seen and, in the absence of restenosis, coronary flow reserve was eventually normal in all patients (see also Chapter 22).

Detection of complications

Myocardial perfusion imaging can be used to detect procedural complications such as myocardial infarction and side-branch occlusion which are not always detected angiographically or by monitoring cardiac enzymes. If a previously reversible thallium defect becomes fixed after angioplasty this suggests that myocardial damage has occurred.

Assessment of the target lesion

Myocardial perfusion imaging has a unique role in the evaluation and management of patients with multivessel disease. Often angioplasty in these patients is staged, with the most severe stenosis being dilated first and further vessels being considered if symptoms persist or there is evidence of reversible ischaemia in another territory. Perfusion imaging is an effective method of identifying the lesion which is most significant functionally [6], and repeated imaging after angioplasty may reveal residual ischaemia in the same territory or in another territory and may be used to guide further procedures.

Breisblatt and colleagues [7] used exercise thallium imaging in 85 patients with multivessel disease to identify the most significant stenosis and the need for a further procedure after this lesion had been dilated. All lesions were technically suitable for angioplasty and the magnitude of the reversible perfusion defect was used to define the target lesion. Before angioplasty, thallium imaging identified the target lesion in 93% of patients. One month later, two groups had been identified by repeat imaging: 47 patients with no evidence of ischaemia in a different territory, and 38 patients with ischaemia at a distance. One year later, 17% of the first group and 79% of the second group had undergone further angioplasty for recurrent symptoms.

Restenosis after angioplasty

Angioplasty has a high primary success rate, and the appearance of the coronary arteriogram is improved in between 80 and more than 90% of patients. Unfortunately, restenosis after an initially successful procedure is a problem. Reported rates of restenosis vary because there are many definitions with little standardisation of method, timing, and rate of late arteriography. Restenosis occurs in up to 50% of patients within the first six months [8], with the majority of recurrence being evident between 1 and 3 months [9].

Restenosis can be detected by the recurrence of symptoms, by electrocardiography, by noninvasive imaging, and by coronary arteriography. Frequent arteriograms are costly and are not without risk. Symptoms are an unreliable indicator because many patients are asymptomatic despite restenosis. In a recent study by Hecht and colleagues [10] only 34% of patients with restenosis had chest pain during treadmill exercise. Interpretation of symptoms after angioplasty can also be difficult, and up to 50% of patients with chest pain do not have restenosis [11]. The choice of test for the detection and prediction of restenosis therefore lies between exercise electrocardiography and myocardial perfusion imaging.

Exercise electrocardiography is safe, widely available and inexpensive but it is of limited value for detecting restenosis. It is difficult to apply in many patients with an abnormal electrocardiogram at rest, and when it is applicable wide variations in sensitivity have been reported [12–15]. Bengtson and colleagues [13] performed exercise electrocardiography and coronary angiography 6 months after angioplasty in 303 patients. The sensitivity and specificity of the exercise electrocardiogram for the detection of restenosis was 60% and 69%, with positive and negative predictive accuracies of 61% and 84%, respectively. Laarman [14] and Marie [15] reported much lower sensitivities of 25% and 24% respectively.

Other reasons for the poor detection rate of restenosis by exercise electrocardiography include its inability to detect coronary occlusion with good collateral supply and its low sensitivity for the detection of single vessel coronary disease. Even when the test is abnormal, the difficulty in localising areas of ischaemia means that it is difficult to distinguish restenosis from progression or unmasking of disease in other sites.

Myocardial perfusion imaging and restenosis

Residual perfusion defects are frequent after successful angioplasty but they generally normalise 3 to 4 months later, and it is sensible to defer imaging for the detection of restenosis for some time. Perfusion imaging is certainly effective in detecting restenosis. Hecht and colleagues [10] studied 116 patients and demonstrated that tomographic thallium imaging could both detect restenosis and differentiate it from progression of disease in other arteries. Imaging was 86% sensitive, specific and accurate for the detection of restenosis and the results were similar after single and multiple vessel angioplasty and after complete or partial revascularisation. Significant stenoses in arteries which were not dilated were detected with a sensitivity of 91%, a specificity of 84% and an accuracy of 85%. In all, 81% of such stenoses were detected. Importantly, in a later study [16] the same group demonstrated that perfusion imaging was equally sensitive, specific and accurate in detecting restenosis in asymptomatic and symptomatic patients.

Myocardial perfusion imaging is therefore accurate in predicting recurrent ischaemia and restenosis. Although no therapy has yet successfully prevented restenosis, identification of patients with a high likelihood of restenosis would allow more appropriate follow-up. Wijns and colleagues [17] performed planar thallium imaging one month after successful angioplasty in 91 patients, and angiography was performed at 6 months, or earlier if symptoms recurred. Reversible ischaemia was predictive of recurrence of angina in 66% and of restenosis in 74% of patients. The positive and negative predictive values for restenosis were 74% and 83% respectively. In contrast, the exercise electrocardiogram was not predictive of recurrent angina or stenosis.

Breisblatt and colleagues [18] have reported convincingly the value of myocardial perfusion imaging. One hundred twenty-one patients underwent serial imaging in the first year after successful angioplasty, and those who developed symptoms and an abnormal scan were referred for coronary angiography. Reversible ischaemia in the territory of the dilated artery was seen in 26 (25%) of 104 asymptomatic patients 4 to 6 weeks after angioplasty. Of these, 22 (86%) had clinical and angiographic evidence of restenosis at 6 months as did 25 (96%) at one year. 87% of patients with eventual restenosis were predicted by perfusion imaging 4 to 6 weeks after angioplasty. In contrast, patients with a normal scan at 3 to 6 months, with or without associated symptoms, had a very low likelihood of restenosis. Interestingly, thallium imaging performed earlier than 1 month was not predictive of restenosis. Seven of a separate group of 15 patients without symptoms had reversible perfusion defects 1 to 2 weeks after angioplasty, but by 4 to 6 weeks the images in 4 of these 7 had normalised. The 3 patients in whom the images did not normalise later developed symptoms and restenosis.

Several groups have studied very early perfusion imaging after angioplasty but the results are generally not as good as the studies using later imaging. For instance, Hardoff and colleagues [19] imaged at 12 to 24 hours and they identified 52% of patients with later restenosis. Miller and colleagues [20] imaged at 2 weeks and they showed that delayed thallium clearance, reversible ischaemia, and a pressure gradient across the lesion after angioplasty of more than 20 mm Hg identified patients with a fourfold greater risk of restenosis and clinical events at one year. However, only 24% of patients with reversible ischaemia eventually restenosed in this study.

In contrast, Jain and colleagues [21] used tomographic imaging after oral dipyridamole in 53 patients 3 days after successful angioplasty. Of 14 patients with continuing reversible abnormalities, 10 (71%) had restenosed by 21 months, but only 3 (12%) patients without such abnormalities restenosed. It is possible that vasodilation is more effective than dynamic exercise at predicting restenosis early after the procedure but these results require confirmation.

Asymptomatic ischaemia after angioplasty

Whether repeated angiography should be performed in an asymptomatic patient with reversible ischaemia after angioplasty is controversial, but the answer obviously depends upon whether further intervention can reduce the risk of events. Patients with restenosis and silent ischaemia certainly have defects of similar extent and severity as patients who are symptomatic [16], and silent ischaemia in the setting of myocardial infarction or unstable angina carries an increased risk of events [22, 23]. Angioplasty can abolish silent ischaemia [24], but whether this reduces the risk of future events is not known. Repeat angioplasty in silent restenosis would be justified if restenosis *per se* increased the risk of acute events based on the lesion, and if intervention reduced the risk of these events. Until such evidence is available, most clinicians are reluctant to repeat angiography and angioplasty in the absence of symptoms, and any further investigation except formal assessment of symptoms by exercise testing is probably not indicated. The cost-efficacy of such exercise testing incorporating either electrocardiography or myocardial perfusion scintigraphy remains to be established.

Conclusion

Myocardial perfusion imaging can assess the success of angioplasty in terms of myocardial perfusion, it can identify the need for intervention in other arteries, and it can detect complications of the procedure. If delayed for a sufficient interval to allow transient haemodynamic abnormalities to resolve (6 weeks), it is accurate in detecting restenosis that has already occurred and in predicting future restenosis and the recurrence of symptoms. Routine perfusion imaging after intervention is therefore logical if the patient continues to have symptoms, and such symptoms are perhaps best assessed objectively by formal exercise testing. Such exercise testing can easily be coupled with perfusion imaging but the cost-efficacy of such as policy has not been established. In the absence of symptoms, the need for routine perfusion imaging depends upon whether the prognosis of silent restenosis and ischaemia is improved by further intervention. Randomised studies to answer this question are not available.

References

1. Grüntzig AR, Senning A, Siegenthaler WE. Nonoperative dilation of coronary artery stenosis: Percutaneous transluminal angioplasty. N Engl J Med 1979; 301: 61–8.
2. Verani MS, Tadros S, Raizner AE et al. Quantitative analysis of thallium-201 uptake and washout before and after transluminal coronary angioplasty. Int J Cardiol 1986; 13: 109–24.
3. DePuey EG, Roubin GS, Cloninger KG et al. Correlation of transluminal coronary angioplasty parameters and quantitative thallium-201 tomography. J Invasive Cardiol 1988; 1: 40–50.
4. Manyari DE, Knudtson M, Kloiber R, Roth D. Sequential thallium-201 myocardial perfusion studies after successful percutaneous transluminal coronary angioplasty: Delayed resolution of exercise induced scintigraphic abnormalities. Circulation 1988; 77: 86–95.
5. Wilson RF, Johnson MR, Marcus ML et al. The effect of coronary angioplasty on coronary flow reserve. Circulation 1988; 77: 873–85.
6. Scholl JM, Chaitman BR, David PR et al. Exercise electrocardiography and myocardial scintigraphy in the serial evaluation of the results of percutaneous transluminal coronary angioplasty. Circulation 1982; 66: 380–90.
7. Breisblatt WM, Barnes JV, Weiland F, Spaccavento LJ. Incomplete revascularisation in multivessel percutaneous transluminal coronary angioplasty: The role for stress thallium-201 imaging. J Am Coll Cardiol 1988; 11: 1183–90.
8. Nobuyoshi M, Kimura T, Nosaka H et al. Restenosis after successful percutaneous transluminal coronary angioplasty: Serial angiographic follow-up of 229 patients. J Am Coll Cardiol 1988; 12: 616–23.
9. Serruys PW, Luijten HE, Beatt KJ et al. Incidence of restenosis after successful coronary angioplasty: A time related phenomenon. A quantitative angiographic study in 342 consecutive patients at 1, 2, 3 and 4 months. Circulation 1988; 77: 361–71.
10. HS Hecht, Shaw RE, Bruce TR et al. Usefulness of tomographic thallium-201 imaging for detection of restenosis after percutaneous transluminal coronary angioplasty. Am J Cardiol 1990; 66: 1314–8.
11. Holmes DR, Vlietstra RE, Smith HC et al. Restenosis after percutaneous transluminal coronary angioplasty (PTCA): A report from the PTCA registry of the National Heart, Lung and Blood Institute. Am J Cardiol 1984; 53: 77C–81C.
12. Honan MB, Bengtson JR, Pryor DB et al. Exercise treadmill testing is a poor predictor of anatomic restenosis after angioplasty for acute myocardial infarction. Circulation 1989; 80: 1585–94.
13. Bengtson JR, Mark DB, Honan MB et al. Detection of restenosis after elective percutaneous

transluminal coronary angioplasty using the exercise treadmill test. Am J Cardiol 1990; 65: 28–34.

14. Laarman G, Luijten HE, Louis GPM et al. Assessment of "silent" restenosis and long-term follow-up after successful angioplasty in single vessel coronary artery disease: The value of quantitative exercise electrocardiography and quantitative coronary angiography. J Am Coll Cardiol 1990; 16: 578–85.

15. Marie PY, Danchin N, Karcher G et al. Usefulness of exercise SPECT-thallium to detect asymptomatic restenosis in patients who had angina before coronary angioplasty. Am Heart J 1993; 126: 571–7.

16. Hecht HS, Shaw RE, Chin HL et al. Silent ischaemia after coronary angioplasty: Evaluation of restenosis and extent of ischaemia in asymptomatic patients by tomographic thallium-201 exercise imaging and comparison with symptomatic patients. J Am Coll Cardiol 1991; 17: 670–7.

17. Wijns W, Serruys PW, Reiber JHC et al. Early detection of restenosis after successful percutaneous transluminal coronary angioplasty by exercise-redistribution thallium scintigraphy. Am J Cardiol 1988; 55: 357–61.

18. Breisblatt WM, Weiland FL, Spaccavento LJ. Stress thallium-201 imaging after coronary angioplasty predicts restenosis and recurrent symptoms. J Am Coll Cardiol 1988; 12: 1199–1204.

19. Hardoff R, Shefer A, Gips S et al. Predicting late restenosis after coronary angioplasty by very early (12 to 24 h) thallium-201 scintigraphy: Implications with regard to mechanisms of late coronary restenosis. J Am Coll Cardiol 1990; 15: 1486–92.

20. Miller DD, Liu P, Strauss HW et al. Prognostic value of computer-quantitated exercise thallium imaging early after percutaneous transluminal coronary angioplasty. J Am Coll Cardiol 1987; 10: 275–83.

21. Jain A, Mahmarian JJ, Borges-Neto S et al. Clinical significance of perfusion defects by thallium-201 single photon emission tomography following oral dipyridamole early after coronary angioplasty. J Am Coll Cardiol 1988; 11: 970–6.

22. Theroux PM, Waters DD, Halpen C et al. Prognostic value of exercise testing soon after myocardial infarction. N Engl J Med 1979; 301: 341–5.

23. Weiner DA, Ryan TJ, McCabe CH et al. Significance of silent myocardial ischaemia during exercise testing in patients with coronary artery disease. Am J Cardiol 1987; 59: 725–9.

24. Stone GW, Spaude S, Ligon, Hartzler GO. Usefulness of percutaneous transluminal coronary angioplasty in alleviating silent myocardial ischaemia in patients with absent or minimal painful myocardial ischaemia. Am J Cardiol 1989; 64: 560–4.

Corresponding Author: Prof S.R. Underwood, National Heart & Lung Institute, Royal Brompton Hospital, Sydney Street, London SW3 6NP, UK

24. Evaluation of immediate and long-term results of intervention by echocardiography: Can restenosis be predicted?

ALBERT VARGA and EUGENIO PICANO

Introduction

Coronary artery revascularization with either coronary artery bypass surgery or percutaneous transluminal coronary angioplasty is an effective therapeutic procedure in the management of properly selected patients with coronary artery disease [1, 2]. For patient selection and assessment of procedure efficacy, a functional evaluation of stenosis is mandatory. As stated by Andreas Grüntzig at the dawn of the angioplasty era [3], "imaging postcatheterization permits evaluation of the physiologic significance of an observed lesion – to determine the potential effect of dilatation on perfusion distal to the lesion". In addition, a preangioplasty imaging evaluation "provides a baseline for noninvasive post-angioplasty monitoring of the procedure success. As with the patient who has undergone bypass surgery, subjective symptoms are usually a good guide, but are not sufficient for the longitudinal evaluation of the procedure" [3].

Several methods have been proposed for the physiologic evaluation of revascularization results, including stress electrocardiography, radionuclide ventriculography, and nuclear perfusion scintigraphy, combined with either exercise or exercise-independent pharmacological stress [4]. Recently, stress echocardiography testing was proposed as a cost-effective method for the diagnosis of coronary artery disease [5]. It is a relatively new technique which combines cardiovascular stress with echocardiographic imaging in the diagnosis of coronary artery disease. It is based on the proved hypothesis that stress-induced ischemia will result in regional wall motion abnormalities that can be detected by two dimensional echocardiography. The technique has received a tremendous interest in recent years, for both scientific and economic reasons. Consistent scientific evidence has documented that the transient regional dyssynergy has an accuracy which is substantially better than ECG changes and chest pain, and at least comparable with perfusion deficits detectable by perfusion scintigraphy – regardless of the type of associated stress (exercise, or dobutamine, or dipyridamole, or adenosine) [5]. In the present era of "health care rationing", the interest on stress

C.A. Nienaber and U. Sechtem (eds): Imaging and Intervention in Cardiology, 387–399.
© 1996 Kluwer Academic Publishers. Printed in the Netherlands.

echocardiography is steadily increasing given the mounting pressure of cost-containment [6]. As an additional advantage in the revascularized patient, who needs repeating serial testing before and at various intervals after revascularization, echocardiography employs "patient-" and "enviroment-friendly" nonionizing energy, ideal for sequential evaluations.

Suitability of stress echocardiography to assess the effects of revascularization procedures

From the theoretical point of view, a diagnostic test should fulfill some prerequisites in order to be suitable for studying the immediate or delayed responses to various forms of therapy. These basic requisites are: 1) high short term reproducibility and 2) possibility to stratify a positive response so that the stress-induced ischemia can be graded and the effects of therapy can be quantified. Stress echocardiography has shown excellent short-term reproducibility [5]. In addition, the diagnosis of myocardial ischemia by stress echocardiography is not made after a binary (yes or no) response, but rather according to a complex stratification along spatial and temporal coordinates [5]. During stress echocardiography, the anatomic and functional impairment is proportional to the area subtended by a system with three coordinates representing the circumferential (horizontal) extension of ischemia (x axis), the transmural (vertical) extent of ischemia (y axis), and the duration of the "ischemia-free" stress time (z axis) (Figure 1). Both the transmural and the circumferential extent of ischemia can be combined in the Wall Motion Score Index, which provides an integrated, semiquantitative and computer-independent estimation of the severity and extent of the dyssynergy [5]. The ischemia-free stress time (i.e., the time from onset of stress by exercise or drug infusion to development of a regional asynergy) is conceptually similar to exercise time – i.e., the time from onset of exercise to development of 0.1 mV of ST segment depression. Not only physical, but also pharmacological tests (such as dobutamine or dipyridamole) allow titrating the stress response in the time domain with lower drug load being associated to greater functional severity of coronary stenoses [5].

Goals of stress echocardiography in revascularized patients

The practical impact of stress echocardiography in assessing revascularization procedures has been shown by several groups, with various types of stresses – physical, electrical, pharmacological – both in coronary artery bypass surgery [7–12], and in coronary angioplasty [13–29]. The main tasks of physiologic testing in revascularization can be summarized as follows (Table 1):
• Anatomic identification of disease and geographic localization, with physi-

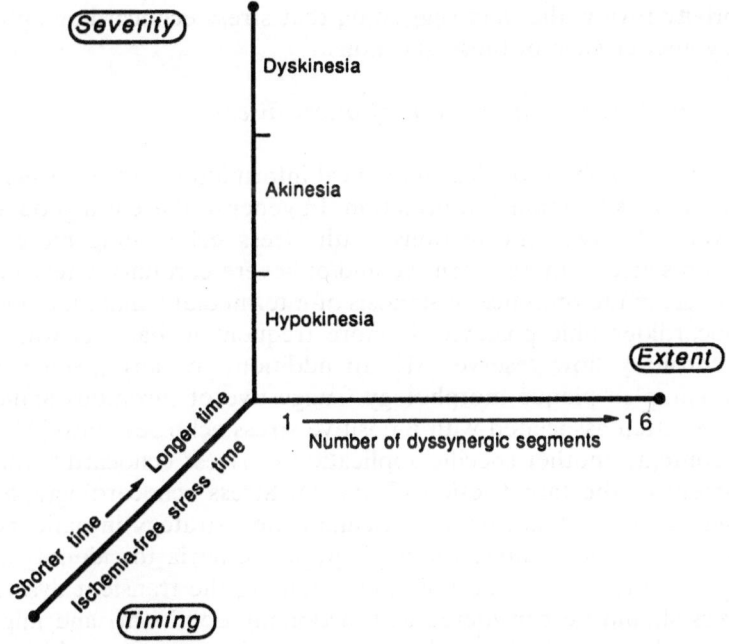

Figure 1. Space and time coordinates of the ischemic response during stress echocardiography: x axis, the number of segments into which the left ventricle is divided; y axis, the severity of dyssynergy that is correlated to the degree of coronary flow impairment; z axis, the ischemia-free stress time. (Reprinted, by permission, from [6].)

Table 1. Goals of stress echocardiography in patients undergoing revascularization.

1. *Anatomic coronary disease identification*
   A. Physiologic assessment of stenosis of intermediate anatomic severity
   B. Identification of target lesion in multivessel disease
2. *Risk stratification in early uncomplicated acute myocardial infarction*
3. *Identification of myocardial viability*
4. *Documentation of improved myocardial function*
5. *Detection of complications*
6. *Identification of restenosis or graft occlusion or disease progression*

ologic assessment of stenosis of intermediate anatomic severity and identification of target lesion in multivessel disease;
- Risk stratification to identify patients more likely to benefit, in terms of survival, from revascularization procedures;
- Identification of myocardial viability in regions with dyssynergy at rest;
- Documentation of improved myocardial function;
- Detection of complications;
- Identification of restenosis.

We will briefly review the data suggesting that stress echocardiography can successfully answer each of these questions.

Assessment and localization of coronary artery disease

Coronary arteriography provides anatomical information and stress echocardiography provides functional information. In general, there is a good agreement between the two informations, with stress echo being more often positive in presence of more extensive and/or severe coronary artery disease [30]. However, in the presence of stenosis of intermediate anatomic severity, stress echocardiographic positivity is more frequent in patients with more impaired coronary flow reserve [31]. In addition, for any given stenosis severity, a complex plaque morphology (suggestive of thrombus and/or ulcers) is more often associated with a positive stress echo response [32].

In this context, another specific application of stress echocardiography is the assessment of the target lesion (Table 1). Stress echocardiography can be especially useful in tailoring a revascularization strategy in patients with multivessel disease, integrating the angiographic criteria for identifying the ischemia-producing vessel. The lesion determining the transient dyssynergy during stress should be considered as functionally dominant, and might be the target of the first dilatation [15]. After angioplasty, a positive stress echocardiogram can be of help in separating patients with persistent positivity in the territory of the dilated coronary artery or with positivity in the territory fed by the less diseased coronary vessel [15]. In the first case, the angioplasty was ineffective, or stenosis recurred in the dilated vessel. In the second case, both stenosed vessels had a significant reduction in regional flow reserve before angioplasty, and stress echocardiography, which is stopped at the appearance of a regional dyssynergy, localized only the more diseased vessel. The correction of the stenosis in the most diseased artery can unmask as functionally dominant the artery that originally was less stenosed.

Risk stratification

The importance of risk stratification should be taken into account when assessing the indication to coronary revascularization, especially in asymptomatic patients in whom the main aim of the revascularization procedure may be to improve prognosis. Data from stress echo multicenter trials EPIC (Echo Persantine International Cooperative) [33] and EDIC (Echo Dobutamine International Cooperative) studies [34] strongly suggest that the prognostic outlook is not synonymous with "destiny" and a dramatic change in the natural history can be achieved by properly targeted interventions strategically oriented by results of physiologic testing. In patients evaluated early after an acute uncomplicated myocardial infarction, an impressive beneficial effect of revascularization on survival is only detectable in patients with a positive stress echo test [33]; a revascularization performed in asymptomatic patients with negative stress echo tests has no beneficial effects on reinfarction and cardiac death [33].

Identification of myocardial viability

Both low-dose dobutamine [35] and dipyridamole [36] have the potential to recognize asynergic but viable myocardium by recruiting an inotropic reserve, although with different underlying mechanisms. The receptor target is $\beta1$ adrenergic receptor for dobutamine, and A2 adenosine receptor for dipyridamole. The cellular target is the myocyte for dobutamine and the vascular smooth muscle cell for dipyridamole. In patients with preserved global left ventricular function, the identification of viability at an intermediate stage is necessary to separate jeopardized myocardium – showing a "biphasic" response (akinesia at rest; improvement at inotropic phase; akinesia at peak stress) – from necrotic tissue – showing a monotonous, steady response (akinesia at rest; akinesia at low dose; akinesia at peak stress) (Figure 2). In patients with severely depressed left ventricular function, the documentation of viability might represent an indication to a coronary revascularization – even selective, when viability is documented only in certain coronary territories. For this latter application, however, stress echocardiography has been inadequately validated to date [37].

Documentation of improved myocardial function

According to the conceptual framework outlined in Figure 1, it is also easy to assess the results of the revascularization procedure – which can be completely successful, with disappearance of inducible ischemia (Figure 3), or partially successful, with persisting inducible ischemia (Figure 4). The timing of postangioplasty stress echo varies widely, ranging from 24 hours to 1 week in the various studies [13–29]. All these studies demonstrated a comparable reduction in stress echo positivity rates, ranging from 70 to 100% pre and 10 to 30% post-angioplasty.

McNeill et al. [20] studied 28 patients before and after successful elective coronary angioplasty. The initial studies were performed 1 day before and the second ones within 3 days (mean 1.3) after angioplasty. The frequency of dobutamine-induced new wall motion abnormalities decreased from 20 (71%) before to 4 (14%) after angioplasty. Before angioplasty, wall motion score index (an indicator of left ventricular wall motion, an increase of which indicates impaired wall motion due to myocardial ischemia) increased from 1.06 to 1.23 at peak stress, but there was no significant increase in this index in the study after angioplasty.

Broderick et al. of the Indianapolis group [16] evaluated 36 patients with exercise-echocardiography. Twenty-five patients (69%) had provokable ischemia before, and 14 (38%) after angioplasty. The peak wall motion score index was 1.48 ± 0.47 before, and fell to 1.37 ± 0.50 after angioplasty

REGIONAL FUNCTION DURING PHARMACOLOGICAL STRESS
- 5 different patterns -

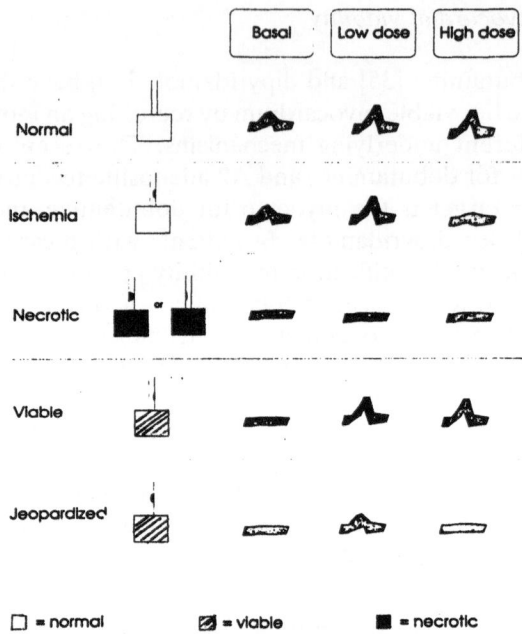

Figure 2. Schematic representation of different mechanical patterns during pharmacological stress echocardiography, as a function of the condition of the basally asynergic zone (viable versus necrotic) and of the anatomy of the infarct-related vessel (patent versus stenotic). Necrotic tissue (third row) shows unchanged function throughout the test, regardless of the underlying anatomic condition of the infarct-related vessel. Viable tissue (fourth row) shows an early functional recovery. A critical stenosis in a different remote vessel is detected as a new dyssynergy in a region with normal function at rest, remote from the infarcted zone. In jeopardized myocardium (fifth row), there is an early functional recovery; at a later stage, however, there may be a marked worsening (and/or an extension) of the regional functional impairment if a significant stenosis is present in the infarct-related vessel. (Reprinted, by permission, from [6].)

(p < 0.001), suggesting that the induced dyssynergy – even when still present following angioplasty – was less severe and extensive in comparison with the pre-angioplasty control.

In a joint venture of the Pisa CNR and Milan-Niguarda Hospital [15], dipyridamole stress echo was performed in 74 consecutive patients before and after angioplasty. The stress echo test was positive in 58 patients before and in only 16 after the procedure (92 vs 25%, p < 0.01). In the 16 patients with positive DET, before and after angioplasty, dipyridamole-time increased from 5.6 ± 2.2 before to 7.3 ± 2.4 minutes immediately after the procedure

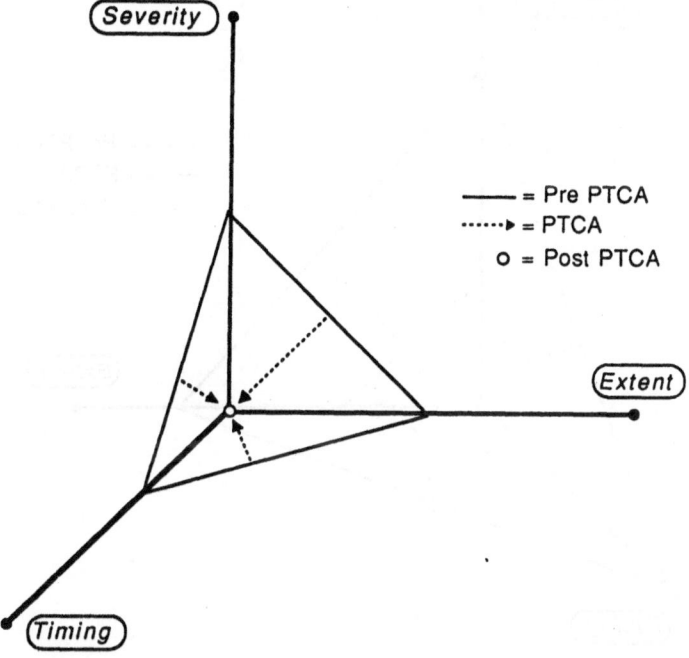

Figure 3. A completely successful PTCA: following the intervention, the stress-echo test becomes completely negative – ideally placed at the origin of the system of coordinates localizing the stress-induced ischemia.

(p < 0.05). In these same 16 patients, the number of dyssynergic segments decreased from 6.8 ± 2.4 before to 4.7 ± 1.3 after the procedure (p < 0.01).

The possible physiologic benefit exerted by revascularization on the regional coronary reserve appears to be the most likely explanation for the improvement in stress test results. A persistently positive stress test after angioplasty has an unfavorable prognostic implication, placing the patient in a subset at high risk for recurrence of symptoms [19]. The limited or even the total lack of improvement in the test response after angiographically successful angioplasty may have several explanations. The residual stenosis may be anatomically "insignificant" and still haemodynamically important because there is a poor correlation between percent lumen reduction and regional flow reserve, particularly very early after angioplasty. Alternatively, there may be an early restenosis of a vessel in the very first few days after angioplasty that could be a nonsignificant stenosis at the immediate follow-up angiography after angioplasty. In addition, although restenosis is a heterogeneous syndrome, it may actually reflect residual stenosis, which may be difficult to recognize on post-PTCA angiograms because of the apparent

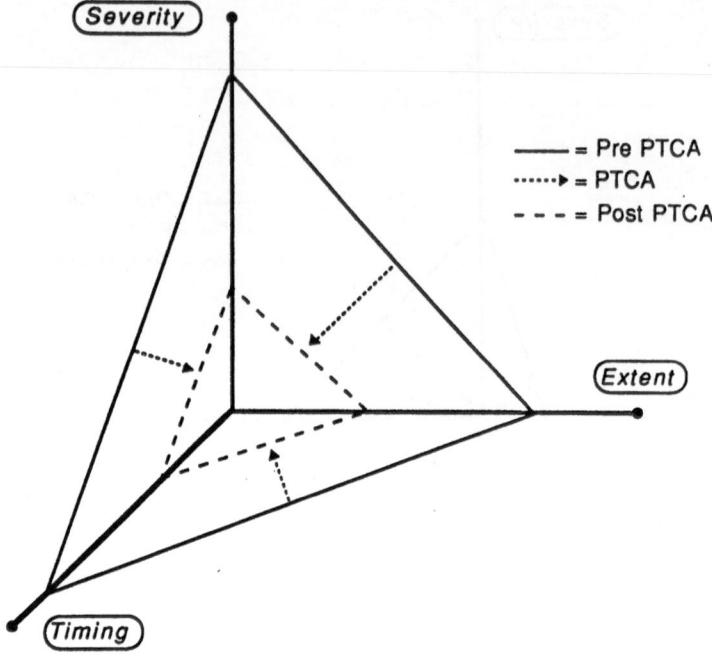

Figure 4. A partially successful PTCA. The severity of the ischemic response is proportional to the area of the triangle whose vertices are placed on the coordinates of ischemia. The area obviously "shrinks" following intervention, but the test remains positive, suggesting a primary failure, or an incomplete revascularization, or an early restenosis.

improvement in luminal dimensions secondary to extravasation of contrast into the media to the plaque, with fissuring and dissection.

Detection of complications

Resting echocardiography – without any stress – can be used to detect procedural complications such as myocardial infarction and side branch occlusion which are not always detected angiographically or by monitoring cardiac enzymes. If a previously reversible transient dyssynergy becomes fixed after angioplasty this suggests that myocardial damage has occurred. On the other hand, if a region previously dyssynergic at rest shows improvement, the functional recovery can be attributed to a previously "hibernating" region whose baseline perfusion has been restored by angioplasty [35–37].

Restenosis after angioplasty

Angioplasty has a high primary success rate, and the appearance of the coronary arteriogram is improved between 80 and more than 90% of patients, but restenosis occurs in up to 30% of patients within the first six months. The capacity of prospectively predict restenosis on the basis of clinical and angiographic variables remains limited. Exercise electrocardiography has a limited accuracy, although the negative predictive value of a maximal negative ECG in an asymptomatic patient with single vessel disease and normal resting ECG is high [38]. Perfusion imaging is certainly effective in predicting restenosis [4]. The diagnostic and predictive accuracy of studies performed in the post-angioplasty period can be summarized by stating that the negative predictive value of a normal myocardial perfusion study is excellent, whereas the positive predictive value of an abnormal study early (<2 weeks) after angioplasty in an asymptomatic population is limited [38].

Stress echocardiography has proved effective in detecting restenosis. Merstes et al. performed bicycle stress echocardiography in an unselected series of 86 patients at an average of 6.5 months after a revascularization procedure [25]. They found a sensitivity of 83% and a specificity of 85% for stress echocardiography detection of significant coronary artery disease – due to either stenosis progression or restenosis.

Pirelli et al. evaluated 50 asymptomatic patients with ST segment depression during maximal exercise testing 3 months after successful coronary angioplasty with dipyridamole echocardiography showing a good sensitivity (75%) and excellent specificity (90%) for the detection of restenosis [27].

Stress echocardiography appears also suitable for immediate assessment of efficacy of revascularization, achieved with either bypass surgery or coronary angioplasty. The practical relevance of this information is especially important for angioplasty. The group with the largest experience in the field of stress echocardiography for early evaluation of angioplasty results is certainly the one of Miodrag Ostojic and coworkers, in Beograd [39–41]. Their policy has been to systematically perform stress echo before and after intervention, thus obtaining an ideal baseline (each patient serving as his or her own control). If the stress echo remains positive after the intervention, this indicates primary failure or early restenosis: they recommend that coronary angiography be repeated and, if this finding is questionable, that coronary intravascular ultrasound be performed, when suitable. In this way restenosis can be usually accurately detected and treated [41]. This is consistent with recent studies showing that a dipyridamole-MIBI SPECT positivity, early after an angiographically successful angioplasty, can be at least partially explained with a higher plaque burden detected by intracoronary ultrasound [42].

Comparison between stress echo and myocardial perfusion imaging early after percutaneous transluminal coronary angioplasty

A few data are available on the head-to-head comparison between perfusion and stress echo testing after angioplasty. In a preliminary report, Marwick et al. described a direct comparison of dobutamine stress perfusion scintigraphy and echocardiography in 26 patients within 24 hours of PTCA and they showed residual stress perfusion defects in 5 patients (19%), only one of whom had abnormal function by stress echocardiography [22]. At 1 month after angioplasty, Fioretti et al. found concordant exercise echo and thallium-201 SPECT results in 17 out of 19 patients [21]. At a later stage (3 months from angioplasty) in the follow-up [27], Pirelli et al. performed a direct comparison of dipyridamole echo and exercise thallium scintigraphy and showed a similar sensitivity (75 vs 83%) and specificity (96 vs 84%) for angiographically assessed restenosis [27]. More data are clearly needed at this time to assess the relative merits of perfusion imaging versus stress echo in the early detection of restenosis.

Limitations of stress echocardiography

Obviously, stress echocardiography requires an acceptable acoustic window in resting conditions and specialized personnel for the performance and interpretation of the test. It has been suggested that the learning curve to reach the plateau of diagnostic accuracy is no more than 100 studies, and in expert hands stress echocardiography is highly reliable and reproducibile [43]. Furthermore, stress echocardiography cannot be effectively used to assess the results of angioplasty in those patients in whom the test was negative before the procedure; however, in patients in whom state of the art protocols are applied (with high dose dipyridamole or dobutamine with atropine coadministration), a stress echo negativity at maximal drug dose makes questionable the indication to revascularization. It is also obvious that exercise ECG stress testing – whenever feasible and interpretable – remains the first line test for assessing the physiologic meaning of coronary stenosis and for evaluating test results. However, it has feasibility problems, it is certainly less accurate in coronary disease identification and stratification, and its positive predictive power is particularly poor for restenosis detection. The highest incremental value of stress echocardiography is achieved in patients with non diagnostic or ambiguous exercise ECG stress test results.

Conclusions

Stress echocardiography can play a role in the management of patients undergoing revascularization. Before revascularization, stress echocardiography allows the localization of the site and extent of myocardial ischemia and underlying coronary artery disease. Stress echo results also help identify asymptomatic patients who will benefit more from revascularization in terms of survival. Moreover, stress echocardiography usefully integrates the angiographic criteria for identifying the ischemia producing vessels in multivessel disease, as well as for the physiologic assessment of stenosis of intermediate severity. Pharmacological stress echocardiography offers, in one sitting, reliable information on resting function and myocardial viability: two critical issues that should integrate inducible ischemia in assessing the indication to revascularization. Stress echocardiography positivity soon after angiographically successful angioplasty identifies patients with primary failure or early restenosis who are at a high risk for recurrence of symptoms. When symptoms recur after revascularization, or even in asymptomatic patients, stress echocardiography reliably identifies coronary restenosis. Systematic application of stress echocardiography for the functional evaluation of patients before and after catheter-based revascularization has a tremendous potential to save both lives and health care money, and it is an easy guess into the future that a tighter interplay between cath-lab and echo-lab will certainly help the cardiologists to use the revascularization tools in a more strategic fashion – on the basis of the physiological targets identified by stress echo results.

References

1. Grüntzig AR, Senning A, Siegenthaler WE et al. Non-operative dilatation of coronary artery stenosis: Percutaneous transluminal angioplasty. N Eng J Med 1979; 301: 61–68.
2. Kirklin JW, Akins CW, Blackstone EH et al. ACC/AHA task force report. Guidelines and indications for coronary artery by pass graft surgery. A report of the American College of Cardiology/American Heart Association task force on assessment of diagnostic and therapeutic cardiovascular procedures (subcommittee on coronary artery bypass graft surgery). J Am Coll Cardiol 1991; 17: 543–89.
3. Bloomfield ME, Gruntzig AR, Stertzer SH. Thallium-201 myocardial imaging and coronary angioplasty: Synergistic diagnostics. DuPont-New England Nuclear Medical Products Monograph no. 15C585A-2358. N. Billerica MA: DuPont, May 1984: 18–23.
4. Prvulovich E, Underwood R. Can restenosis after coronary angioplasty be predicted by scintigraphy? In: Nienaber CA, Sechtem U, editors. Imaging and intervention in cardiology. Dordrecht, Kluwer Academic Publishers, 1996.
5. Picano E. Stress echocardiography. From pathophysiological toy to diagnostic tool. Circulation 1992; 85: 1604–12.
6. Picano E. Stress echocardiography, 2nd ed. Heidelberg: Springer Verlag, 1994.
7. Sawada SG, Judson WE, Ryan T et al. Upright bycicle exercise echocardiography after coronary artery bypass grafting. Am J Cardiol 1989; 64: 1123–9.
8. Biagini A, Maffei S, Baroni M et al. Early assessment of coronary reserve after bypass surgery by dipyridamole transesophageal echocardiographic stress test. Am Heart J 1990; 120: 1097–101.
9. Bongo AS, Bolognese L, Sarasso G et al. Early assessment of coronary artery bypass graft patency by high-dose dipyridamole echocardiography. Am J Cardiol 1991; 67: 133–6.
10. La Canna G, Alfieri O, Giubbini R et al. Echocardiography during infusion of dobutamine for identification of reversibility dysfunction in patients with chronic coronary artery disease. J Am Coll Cardiol 1994; 23: 617–26.
11. Crouse LJ, Vacek JL, Beauchamp GD et al. Exercise echocardiography after coronary bypass grafting. Am J Cardiol 1992; 70: 572–6.
12. Bjoernstad K, Aakhus S, Lundbom J et al. Digital dipyridamole stress echocardiography in silent ischemia after coronary artery bypass grafting and/or after healing of acute myocardial infarction. Am J Cardiol 1993; 72: 640–6.

13. Labovitz AJ, Lewen M, Kern MJ et al. The effects of succesful PTCA on left ventricular function: Assessment by exercise echocardiography. Am Heart J 1989; 117: 1003–8.

14. Massa D, Pirelli S, Gara E et al. Exercise testing and dipyridamole echocardiography test before and 48 h after succesful coronary angioplasty: Prognostic implications. Eur Heart J 1989; 10 (Suppl) G): 13–7.

15. Picano E, Pirelli S, Marzilli M et al. Usefulness of high dose dipyridamole echocardiography test in coronary angioplasty. Circulation 1989; 80: 807–15.

16. Broderick T, Sawada S, Armstrong WF et al. Improvement in rest and exercise-induced wall motion abnormalities after coronary angioplasty: An exercise echocardiographic study. J Am Coll Cardiol 1990; 15: 591–9.

17. Aboul-Enein H, Bengston JR, Adams DB et al. Effect of the degree of effort on exercise echocardiography for the detection of restenosis after coronary artery angioplasty. Am Heart J 1991; 122: 430–7.

18. Pirelli S, Danzi GB, Alberti A et al. Comparison of usefulness of high dose dipyridamole echocardiography and exercise electrocardiography for detection of asyptomatic restenosis after coronary angioplasty. Am J Cardiol 1991; 67: 1335–8.

19. Pirelli S, Massa D, Faletra F et al. Exercise electrocardiography versus dipyridamole echo-cardiography testing in coronary angioplasty. Early functional evaluation and prediction of angina recurrence. Circulation 1991; 83: III38–41.

20. McNeill AT, Fioretti PM, Al-Said SM et al. Dobutamine stress echocardiography before and after coronary angioplasty. Am J Cardiol 1992; 69: 740–5.

21. Fioretti PM, Pozzoli MM, Ilmer B et al. Exercise echocardiography versus thallium-201 SPECT for assessing patients before and after PTCA. Eur Heart J 1992; 13: 213–9.

22. Marwick T, Baudhuin T, Willemart W et al. Differential alteration of regional left ventricu-lar function and perfusion responses to cardiac stress early after coronary angioplasty. Eur Heart J 1992; 13 (Suppl): 404.

23. Hoffmann R, Kleinhans E, Bexten M et al. Transesophageal pacing echocardiography for identification of patients with restenosis after percutaneous transluminal coronary angiopla-sty. Circulation 1992; 19: 54A.

24. Akosah KO, Porter TR, Simon R et al. Ischemia-induced regional wall motion abnormality is improved after coronary angioplasty: Demonstration by dobutamine stress echocardio-graphy. J Am Coll Cardiol 1993; 21: 584–9.

25. Mertes H, Erbel R, Nixdorff U et al. Exercise echocardiography for the evaluation of patients after nonsurgical coronary artery revascularization. J Am Coll Cardiol 1993; 21: 1087–93.

26. El-Said ES, Fioretti PM, Roelandt JR et al. Dobutamine stress-Doppler echocardiography before and after coronary angioplasty. Eur Heart J 1993; 14: 1011–21.

27. Pirelli S, Danzi GB, Massa D et al. Exercise thallium scintigraphy versus high dose dipyrida-mole echocardiography testing for detection of asymptomatic restenosis in patients with positive exercise test after coronary angioplasty. Am J Cardiol 1993; 71: 1052–6.

28. Hecht HS, DeBord L, Shaw R et al. Usefulness of supine bicycle stress echocardiography for detection of restenosis after percutaneous transluminal coronary angioplasty. Am J Cardiol 1993; 71: 293–6.

29. Heinle SK, Lieberman EB, Ancukiewicz M et al. Usefulness of dobutamine echocardio-graphy for detecting restenosis after percutaneous transluminal coronary angioplasty. Am J Cardiol 1993; 72: 1220–5.

30. Severi S, Picano E, Michelassi C et al. Diagnostic and prognostic value of dipyridamole echocardiography in patients with suspected coronary artery disease: Comparison with exercise electrocardiography. Circulation 1994; 89: 1160–73.

31. Picano E, Parodi O, Lattanzi F et al. Assessment of anatomic and physiological severity of single-vessel coronary artery lesions by dipyridamole echocardiography: Comparison with positron emission tomography and quantitative arteriography. Circulation 1994; 89: 753–61.

32. Lu C, Picano E, Pingitore A et al. Complex artery coronary lesion morphology influences results of stress echocardiography. Circulation 1995; 91: 1669–75.
33. Picano E, Landi P, Bolognese L et al. Prognostic value of dipyridamole echocardiography early after uncomplicated myocardial infarction: A large-scale, multicenter trial. Am J Med 1993; 95: 608–17.
34. Pingitore A, Bigi R, Mathias W et al. on behalf of the EDIC (Echo Dobutamine International Cooperative) study group. The prognostic value of dobutamine-atropine stress echocardiography: Early after acute myocardial infarction. Circulation 1994; 90 (4, part 2): I–452.
35. Pierard LA, De Landsheere CM, Berthe C et al. Identification of viable myocardium by echocardiography during dobutamine infusion in patients with myocardial infarction after thrombolytic therapy: Comparison with positron emission tomography. J Am Coll Cardiol 1990; 15: 1021–31.
36. Picano E, Marzullo P, Gigli G et al. Identification of viable myocardium by dipyridamole-induced improvement in regional left ventricular function assessed by echocardiography in myocardial infarction and comparison with thallium scintigraphy test. Am J Cardiol 1992; 70: 1703–10.
37. Pierard L. Assessment of viability in severely hypokinetic myocardium before revascularization and prediction of functional recovery: The role of echocardiography. In: Nienaber CA, Sechtem U, editors. Imaging and intervention in cardiology. Dordrecht: Kluwer Academic Publishers, 1995.
38. Miller DD, Verani M. Current status of myocardial perfusion imaging after percutaneous transluminal coronary angioplasty. J Am Coll Cardiol 1994; 24: 260–6.
39. Beleslin BD, Ostojic M, Stepanovic J et al. Stress echocardiography in the diagnosis of detection of ischemic heart disease: Head-to-head comparison between exercise, dobutamine and dipyridamole tests. Circulation 1994; 90: 1168–76.
40. Ostojic M, Babic R, Beleslin B et al. Comparative evaluation of exercise, dobutamine and dipyridamole echocardiography in the setting of interventional coronary revascularization. Circulation 1994; 90 (4, part 2): I–660 (Abstr).
41. Ostojic M, Djordjevic-Dikic A, Beleslin B et al. Detection of coronary restenosis upon performed transluminal coronary angioplasty and/or directional coronary atherectomy. Proceedings of the 10th meeting of invasive cardiology, Alghero, Italy, 26–29 June, 1994.
42. Sechtem U, Bachmann R, Voth E et al. Myocardial ischemia after successful coronary revascularization: Does intravascular ultrasound provide an explanation? Circulation 1994; 90 (4, part 2): I–448 (Abstr).
43. Picano E, Lattanzi F, Orlandini A et al. Stress echocardiography and the human factor: The importance of being expert. J Am Coll Cardiol 1991; 17: 666–9.

Corresponding Author: Dr Eugenio Picano, CNR, Institute of Clinical Physiology, Via Paolo Savi 8, 56100 Pisa, Italy

25. Predictors of restenosis after angioplasty: Morphologic and quantitative evaluation by intravascular ultrasound

UDO SECHTEM, HANS-WILHELM HÖPP and
DIRK RUDOLPH

Introduction

Restenosis remains the major limitation of angioplasty and restenosis rates vary from 30 to 60% [1, 2] The pathophysiologic mechanism of restenosis has been enigmatic so far, but accumulated evidence strongly suggests that intimal hyperplasia is a major mechanism [3]. The process of restenosis must be viewed as the vascular reaction to angioplasty-created injury and represents of form of wound healing. Vessel damage caused by the balloon is commonly observed in autopsy studies in patients dying early after angiographically successful angioplasty and intimal damage is often extensive and extends into the media in almost all specimens [4]. In addition to intimal hyperplasia, acute overstretching of the arterial wall and subsequent elastic recoil or fibrotic contraction is another important mechanism responsible restenosis formation [4, 5].

There have been numerous efforts to modify the restenosis process and reduce restenosis rates in order to improve the long term success after balloon angioplasty. However, neither modifications of the dilation protocol by varying inflation length, inflation pressure, or balloon size nor pharmacologic intervention led to significant reductions of the restenosis rate. Not unexpectedly, the vascular healing mechanism involved in the restenosis process is also activated by other interventional devices such as atherectomy [2], laser angioplasty [6], or high-speed coronary rotational angioplasty [7].

An impressive list of publications has defined the risk factors for restenosis [8, 9]. Knowledge of such risk factors would help to select patients for angioplasty or could lead to better understanding of the pathophysiology of the restenosis process. Three types of factors influencing restenosis rate have been described: patient-related factors, lesion-related factors, and procedure-related factors. Only very few patient-related factors have consistently been shown to be associated with an increased risk of restenosis such as diabetes mellitus and unstable angina [10, 11]. In contrast, a large number of lesion-related variables was found to be associated with a higher incidence of restenosis [8, 9].

C.A. Nienaber and U. Sechtem (eds.): Imaging and Intervention in Cardiology. 401–427.

Table 1. List of lesion-related factors associated with a higher incidence of restenosis.

Risk factors in preintervention angiogram	Risk factors in postintervention angiogram
Plaque eccentricity [11]	No visible dissections [1,11,15]
Calcification [65]	Residual stenosis [1, 11, 15, 56, 66]
Stenosis location [1, 15, 56, 66]	
Stenosis length [56, 67]	
Adjacent artery diameter [56]	
Baseline percentage diameter stenosis [11, 15, 55, 67, 68]	

All studies of the influence of lesion characteristics on the incidence of restenosis were conducted by using angiography to assess the coronary tree. There is growing evidence that intracoronary ultrasound has advantages over coronary angiography in assessing lesion severity and eccentricity [12], the composition of a plaque [13], and arterial responses to balloon coronary angioplasty [14]. Consequently, information obtained by intravascular ultrasound before and after coronary angioplasty may further elucidate whether lesion morphology influences the incidence of restenosis.

This chapter will review the currently available information on the relationship between ultrasound assessed lesion morphology and the inclination of the lesion to restenose after angiographically successful angioplasty.

Angiographic lesion-related factors associated with restenosis

Lesion related factors can be divided into two groups: Factors determined from preinterventional angiography and factors determined from postinterventional angiography. The former include a large variety of items, which are shown in Table 1. However, the factors found to influence the restenosis rate vary from study to study. This is not surprising because the odds ratio of each risk factor is relatively low (relative risk usually <1.5) and definitions and study designs differ in most reports. Another difficulty is that the relation between the variables examined and the underlying pathophysiologic process is hardly understood.

It is possible that lesion characteristics associated with an increased risk of restenosis simply reflect the propensity of the lesion to experience more injury during the intervention. Long lesions for instance, may be more commonly associated with dissection and re-endothelialization may occur later after the trauma. Calcified lesions which require higher balloon pressures may experience more barotrauma. Calcification is also common in ostial lesions resulting in a higher incidence of dissection. Deep medial dissections are also quite common in excentric stenoses where plaque disruption often occurs at the junction of the plaque and the disease-free wall. However,

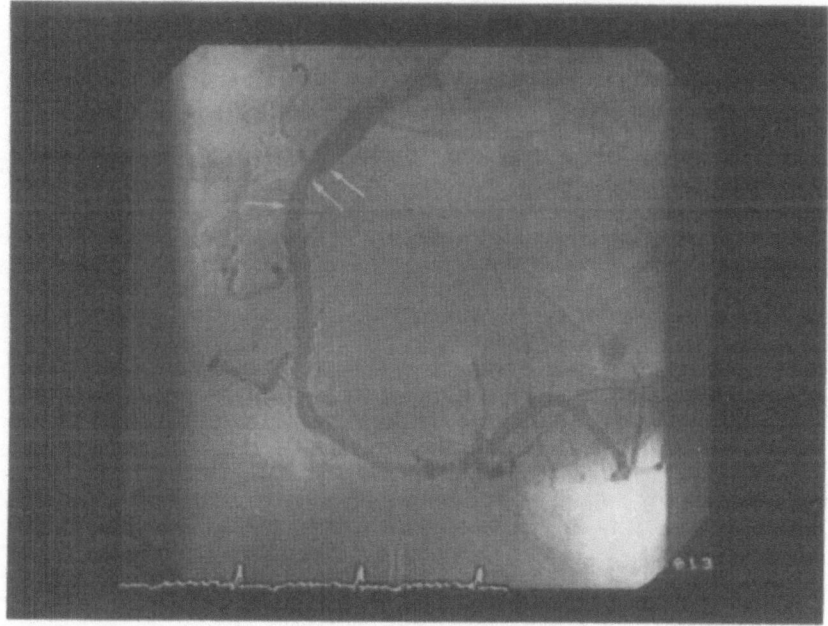

Figure 1a. The angiogram shows a right coronary artery with diffuse disease without high grade stenoses. Small white arrows mark the positions of the ultrasound cross sections.

there is an obvious contradiction between the postulation that larger injury, for instance dissection, causes restenosis and the repeated angiographic finding that restenosis rates are actually lower in lesions showing dissecting membranes [1, 11, 15].

Angiography versus intravascular ultrasound for assessment of lesion morphology and dimensions

Necropsy studies of coronary arteries performed soon after coronary angiography have demonstrated that the severity of coronary artery atherosclerosis in angiographically mildly diseased coronary arteries is often underestimated [16]. Comparative studies of angiography and intravascular ultrasound in patients with angiographically mildly diseased coronary arteries confirmed theses observations in vivo [17]. Intravascular ultrasound may detect substantial atheroma in patients with only slight changes in the coronary angiogram (Figure 1). In many patients, the proximal reference segment for determining percent narrowing on angiographic images exhibits substantial intimal thickening on intravascular ultrasound rendering angiographic stenosis calculations unreliable. Such significant atherosclerotic disease may go undetected

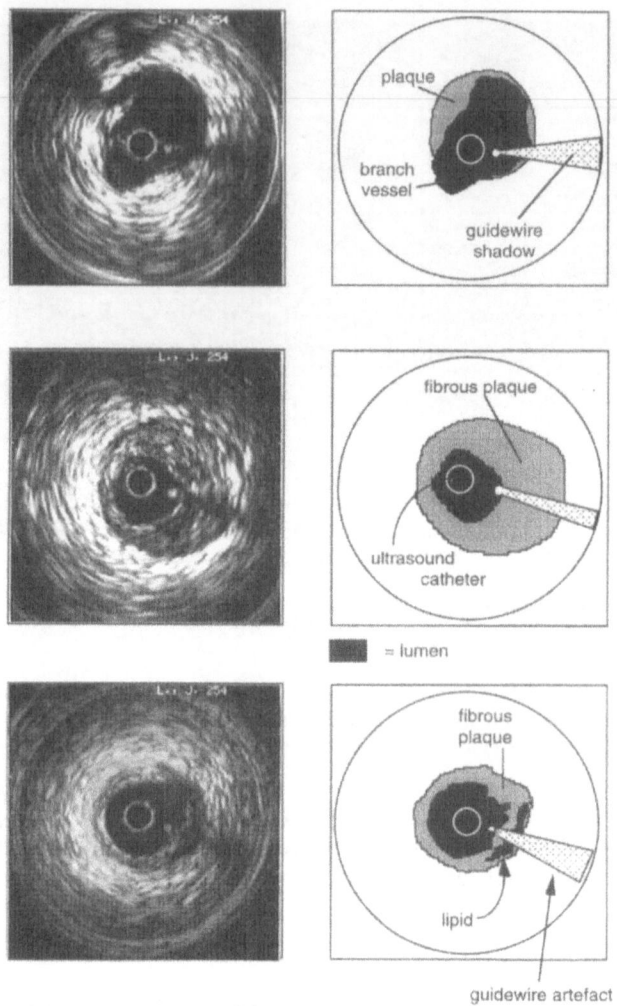

Figure 1b. In contrast to the angiogram, ultrasound images reveal marked focal plaque deposition. Upper panel: Proximal ultrasound position. At the take-off off the right ventricular branch there is mixed atherosclerotic plaque between 9.00 and 12.00 (see schematic drawing) containing some calcium. The lumen is widely patent. Middle panel: At the point of slight angiographic narrowing, there is substantial deposition of fibrous material with an area stenosis of >50%. Compensatory vessel remodeling with enlargement of the vessel cross sectional area encompassed by the media enables continued patency of the lumen despite the large plaque burden. Lower panel: Distal ultrasound position. Vessel cross sectional area is again much smaller and diffuse concentric thickening of the intima can be seen.

by angiography because diffuse atherosclerosis is often associated with compensatory arterial dilatation [18].

Despite the differences between angiographic and intravascular ultrasound findings, ultrasound measurements of diameters and cross sectional areas of normal or near-normal vessels correlate well with quantitative angiography although ultrasound measurements tend to be slightly larger [19, 20]. The correlation between the techniques is still acceptable in diseased concentric vessels (r = 0.93), but is much less close for eccentric sites (r = 0.77) [20] and even worse after coronary balloon angioplasty [21]. These data demonstrate the advantage of ultrasound, which provides a full circumferential image of the vessel, over contrast angiography, which shows the artery only in two projections. The fact that ultrasound must be regarded as the goldstandard for luminal quantifications is underscored by the accuracy of ultrasound lumen quantification as compared to histology [22].

Recent studies suggest that features of stenotic lesions such as true vessel and lumen size [23, 24] and lesion calcification are more accurately defined by intracoronary ultrasound [12, 25]. Although lesion calcification is extremely important for selecting the optimal interventional device, fluoroscopy is only able to detect long, circumferential calcifications whereas calcifications with a length of <6 mm [25], although they may involve more than half of the circumference of the vessel, may be overlooked. The GUIDE trial observed target lesion calcification in 62% of cases by ultrasound but in only 35% of cases on the angiogram [13].

Plaque characterization by intravascular ultrasound

Quantification of the "true" vessel lumen and the plaque burden within a vessel requires identification of the media to distinguish between the vessel wall and the surrounding soft tissues. In normal coronary arteries, the media appears relatively echolucent as compared to the more echogenic intima and adventitia. However, some degree of intimal thickening is required to show the typical three-layered appearance of a "normal" coronary artery (Figure 2). Ultrasound usually fails to demonstrate this three-layered appearance in young patients with truly normal arteries [26] because the very thin intima and the internal lamina do not produce enough echogenic reflections. Definition of the media on ultrasound images may also be difficult in patients with large plaques resulting in atrophy of the underlying media [27]. However, movement of the ultrasound catheter to a neighbouring location will usually result in better definition of a medial layer and thus enable quantification of plaque and vessel areas.

The ability of intravascular ultrasound to identify the different components of a plaque has been documented in a number of in vitro studies [22, 28–31]. Calcification is probably the plaque component which is most consistently identified by intravascular ultrasound (Figure 3). Ultrasound is also able to

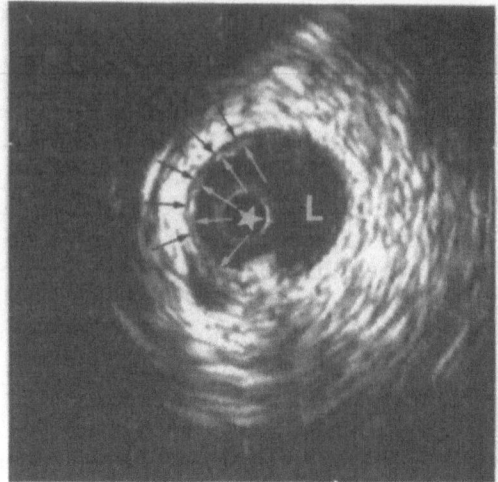

Figure 2. Three-layered appearance of "normal" coronary artery. Small black arrows point to the dark media from the outside soft tissue surrounding the left anterior descending artery. Small white arrows point to the slightly thickened intima, which is echogenic. L = free lumen; ☆ = central artefact caused by ultrasound catheter.

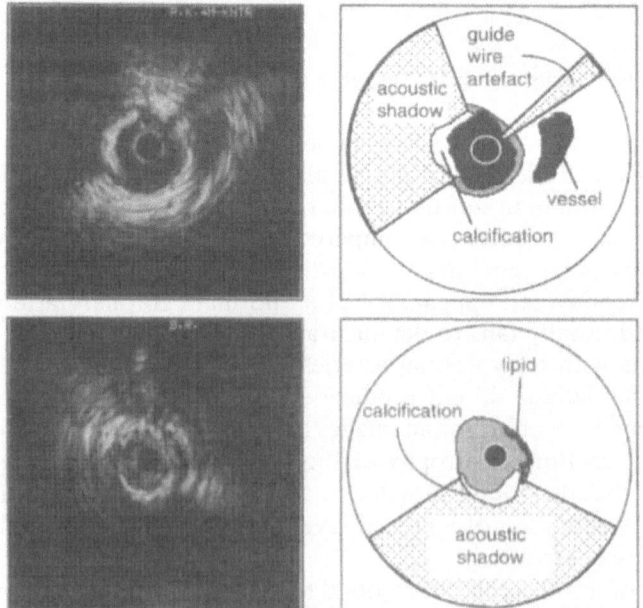

Figure 3. Upper panel: Calcification immediately adjacent to the lumen. "Normal" intima between 12.00 and 7.00. Lower panel: Calcification deeply embedded in soft plaque.

differentiate between calcifications which lie close to the lumen and those adjacent to the media. Typically, calcifications are recognized by their high echo reflectivity associated with a dark shadow more distal from the catheter. This shadowing precludes measurement of wall thickness, thickness of the calcification and vessel size at the site of intense calcifications. In order to make a reasonable judgement about vessel anatomy in such an area, it is necessary to look for a closely neighbouring site without calcification or with a different calcification pattern. Since calcification burden changes rapidly within a plaque, this can usually be accomplished without problems [25].

Fibrotic plaque is characterized by medium to high intensity echoes. A higher cellularity of the plaque is associated with decreased echo density whereas dense fibrosis with a high content of collagen causes bright echoes [22, 30]. Therefore, restenotic lesions, which are mainly composed of smooth muscle cells [32], have a typical appearance on ultrasound images (Figure 4). Differentiation between dense, collagen-rich fibrosis and calcification is possible on the basis of acoustic shadowing in the latter [30].

The detection of lipid and necrosis within a plaque is the most difficult part of plaque characterization by intravascular ultrasound [31, 33]. Large accumulations of extracellular lipids are relatively echolucent whereas the fibrous cap covering the lipid lake shows dense echoes [33]. However, in a systematic comparison of ultrasound images with histology, only 13 of 43 (30%) lipid lakes showed the expected circumscript zone of low signal intensity (Figure 5). Lipid detection was possible in 32 of 43 (74%) lipid lakes if a reduced echo density of more than a quarter of the plaque area was used as the criterion [31]. However, specificity declined to the unacceptably low value of 30%. The difficulty in detecting small areas of echolucency within a plaque is likely related to the presence of speckle noise. The ultrasound image may not reveal a low-contrast target due to interference noise from the surrounding multiscattering medium [34]. As speckle size decreases with increasing ultrasound frequency, 30 MHz and 40 MHz transducers may have advantages over 20 MHz transducers in the detection of lipids by intravascular ultrasound [29].

Mechanism of lumen enlargement by balloon angioplasty

The development of ultrasound catheters with diameters of 3.5 F and less made it possible to cross even tight coronary lesions before angioplasty. Consequently, one can measure the total vessel area surrounded by the media as defined by the outer bright boundary between the media and the adventitia, plaque area defined as total vessel area minus plaque area (see Figure 2), plaque eccentricity, and plaque morphology before altering vessel morphology by inflation of the balloon. By examining the vessel again after angioplasty, it is then possible to determine the relative contributions of the proposed mechanisms of vessel stretching, measured as the difference in total

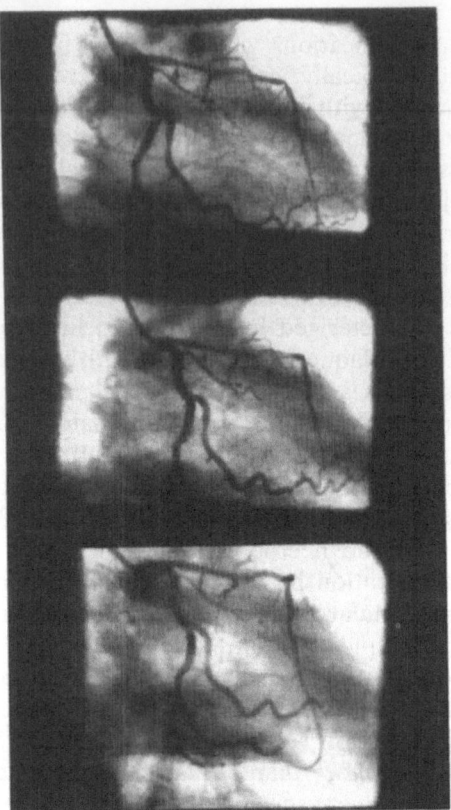

Figure 4a. Upper panel: Angiogram of successfully dilated LAD lesion (arrow). Middle panel: Transducer at the level of a septal branch at the site of previous maximal narrowing. Lower panel: At repeated catheterization 4 months later a 50% restenosis has developed at the level of the septal branch.

vessel area at baseline and after balloon angioplasty, and plaque reduction, measured as the difference in plaque area before and after the intervention. The challenge to the investigator is to exactly reposition the ultrasound catheter after angioplasty at the site of the previously tightest stenosis. However, ultrasound landmarks such as unique plaque calcifications and branching vessels as well as repeated contrast injections during fluoroscopy permit a highly reliable identification of identical measurement sites.

Braden and coworkers [35] published their results of such paired ultrasound measurements before and after balloon dilatation. They found that 81% of the mean total luminal gain in their group of 30 lesions could be accounted for by vessel stretching whereas plaque reduction was responsible for 19%. In 20 of the 30 lesions, lumen gain was solely due to vessel stretching and in 4 it was due to a reduction in plaque area, consistent with compression of soft, lipid rich plaque or redistribution along the long axis of the vessel.

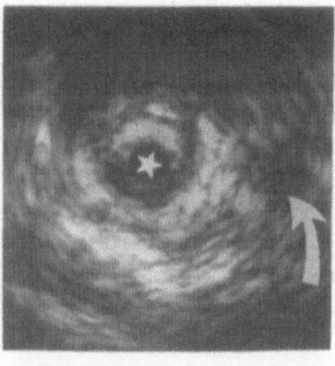

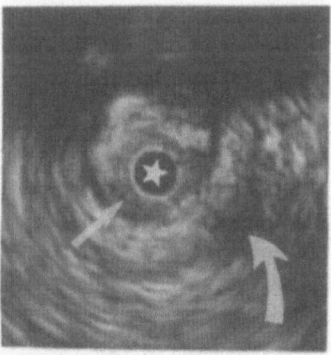

Figure 4b. Upper panel: The ultrasound image immediately after balloon dilatation shows the successfully dilated lumen and calcification between 6.00 and 12.00. ☆ = central catheter arte-fact. Lower panel: At repeated catheterization, ultrasound shows soft plaque, which fills the former lumen and abuts the catheter. Curved arrows point to small diagonal branch, which was used together with the calcification pattern and angiographic documentation to identify the same position of the transducer in the vessel.

In the remaining 20% of lesions, both mechanisms were involved. There was no influence of plaque eccentricity or lesion calcification on the mechanism of lumen enlargement.

Ultrasound examinations in 37 patients with 41 stenoses by other authors before and after balloon angioplasty showed [35a] different results. Vessel stretching accounted only for 34% of luminal gain, whereas plaque reduction was responsible for 66%. Lesion morphology after the intervention corre-lated with the predominant mechanism of luminal gain. Lesions with tears or dissections showed mainly vessel stretching (Figure 6) whereas lesions without major plaque deformation were characterized by predominant plaque reductions (Figure 7). Vessel stretch only was responsible for lumen gain in 5 lesions, whereas plaque reduction only was responsible in 12. In most

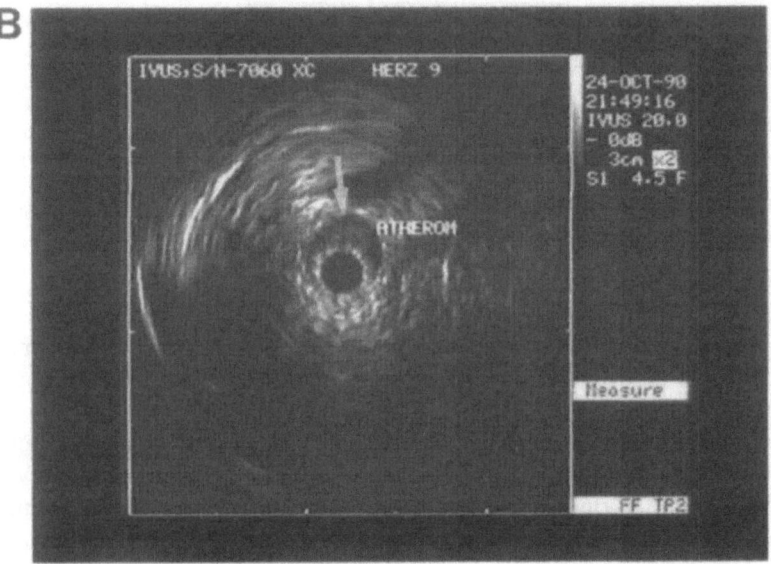

Figure 5. Histology of coronary artery from necropsy heart shows eccentric plaque with ather-oma embedded in fibrous material (HE-staining, ×25). Black line in the upper right corner indicates 1 mm. (B) The corresponding ultrasound image displays the lipid lake (white arrow, Atherom) as a low signal intensity structure lying deep in the plaque. (Reprinted from Sechtem et al. Z Kardiol 1993; 82: 618–27 with permission from the publisher.)

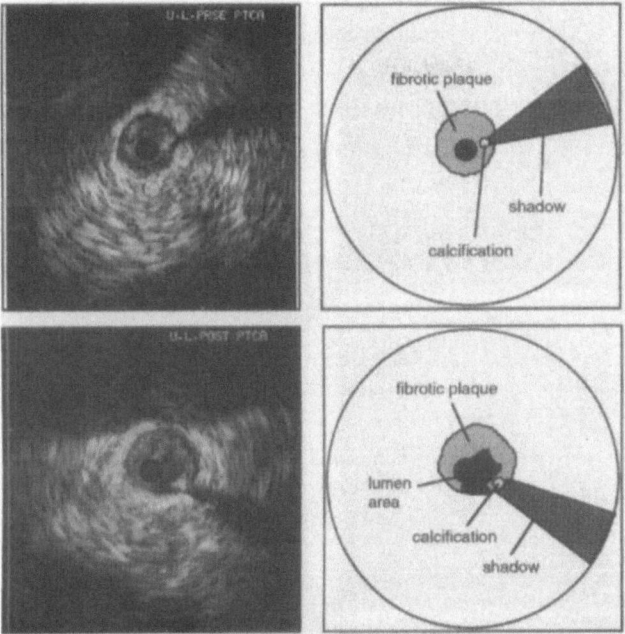

Figure 6. Upper panel: Intravascular ultrasound image of lesion before balloon dilatation. Total vessel area (determined as the area within the intima/adventitia interface = within thin dark line in schematic drawing around fibrous/lipid plaque) is 6.6 mm². and plaque area (determined as total vessel area–lumen area = area of catheter artefact) is 5.2 mm². Lower panel: After dilatation, total vessel area increases to 9.3 mm² and plaque area is reduced to 4.8 mm², resulting in a total luminal gain of 3.1 mm² (from 1.4 to 4.5 mm²). In this stenosis, the main mechanism responsible for enlargement of the perfused lumen is stretching of the vessel borders.

lesions, however, both mechanisms could be observed. The predominant role of plaque reduction for enlarging the free lumen after balloon angioplasty was also noted by Losordo and coworkers [36] in the iliac arteries. These conflicting results point to the need of further refining ultrasound measurements and finding universally applicable definitions before we will be able to tell how angioplasty really works in vivo.

Predictors of restenosis

Balloon angioplasty

Intracoronary ultrasound after balloon angioplasty has been performed by many groups in order to elucidate the mechanical effects on the arterial wall in vivo [35, 37–41] or to assess the impact of the ultrasound defined postinterventional appearance of the vessel wall on subsequent outcome [42,

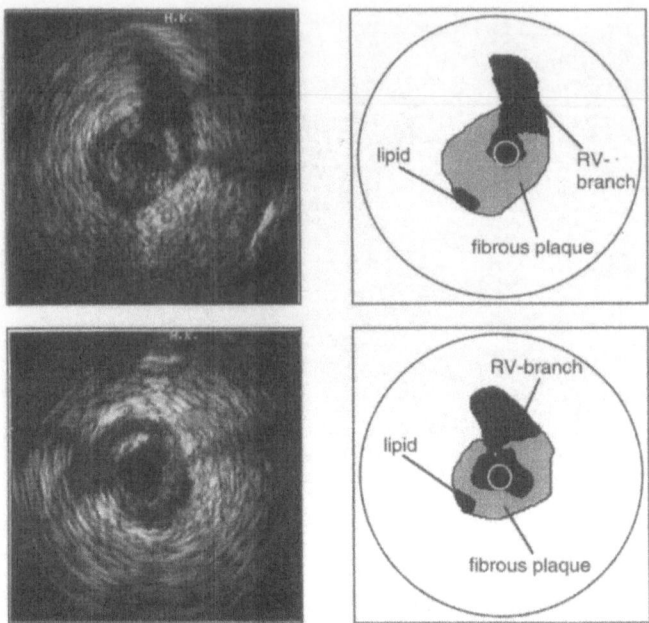

Figure 7. Upper panel: Eccentric plaque in the right coronary artery before balloon dilatation. Total vessel lumen is 18.4 mm^2 and plaque area is 15.8 mm^2. Lower panel: The ultrasound image shows predominant plaque reduction to 13.8 mm^2 as the main mechanism responsible for lumen enlargement from 2.6 to 5.2 mm^2. Total vessel area after balloon dilatation has only increased to 19.0 mm^2.

43]. As shown above, lumen expansion after balloon dilatation is achieved by a combination of plaque fracture [38, 44, 45], vessel stretch [36, 41, 46], and plaque compression [36]. There is substantial evidence from ultrasound studies that plaque fractures and dissections which have been commonly observed in animal [47] and autopsy studies [32, 44] after balloon dilatation are often missed by coronary angiography [13, 38]. However, some dissections, which are evident on angiographic images, may be missed by intravascular ultrasound because of a "stenting effect" of the intravascular ultrasound catheter itself. This effect was more likely in studies performed with catheter with diameters of 1.6 mm [38] than with the smaller catheters (<1 mm diameter) available today.

The terms dissection and tear have been used interchangeably by researchers to describe both the typical ultrasound finding of detachment of the plaque from the underlying media (Figure 8) or the more unusual observation of deep splitting of plaque substance, which runs parallel to linear deposits of calcification [48] but remains within the plaque and does not reach the media. Other commonly observed alterations of the plaque include fissuring perpendicular to the plaque surface with or without reaching the media

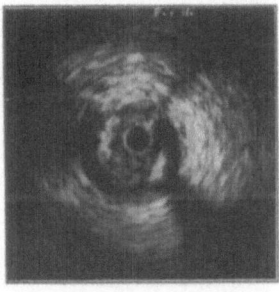 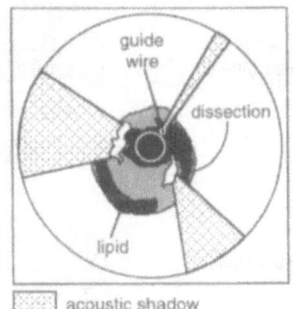 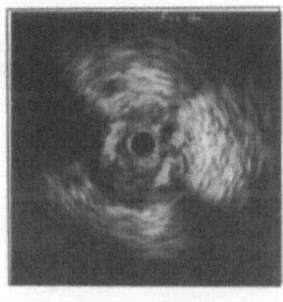

Figure 8. Left: Deep dissection after balloon dilatation detaching the calcified plaque from the underlying media. Middle: Schematic drawing of vessel structures. Right: After injection of contrast material through the guiding catheter, echogenic microbubbles fill the space created by the dissection. Note that no bubbles reach the echolucent space between 6.00 and 9.00 corresponding to lipid accumulation.

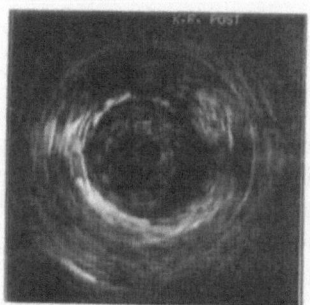 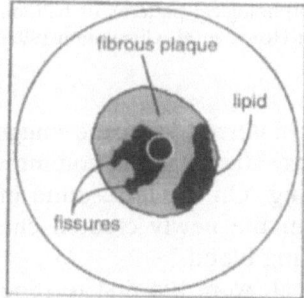

Figure 9. Fissures perpendicular to surface of plaque without reaching the media.

(Figure 9). Finally, the plaque may not show any sign of balloon created injury.

It is important to remember that dissections can easily be confused with linear deposits of lipid or necrosis which also appear dark on the ultrasound image. This lipid or necrosis space may appear directly connected to the vessel lumen suggesting an entry simply due to an unfavourable angle between the ultrasound beam and the surface of the plaque [49]. Therefore, to confirm the presence of dissection it is mandatory to inject contrast material through the guiding catheter during ultrasound imaging and observe the appearance of echogenic material in the suspected neolumen (Figure 8).

Several complex schemes have been proposed to classify balloon induced injury to the vessel wall [38, 40] based on the extent of the laceration (involvement of the media or not) and the eccentricity of the plaque (Figure 9). It must be pointed out, however, that involvement of the media can only

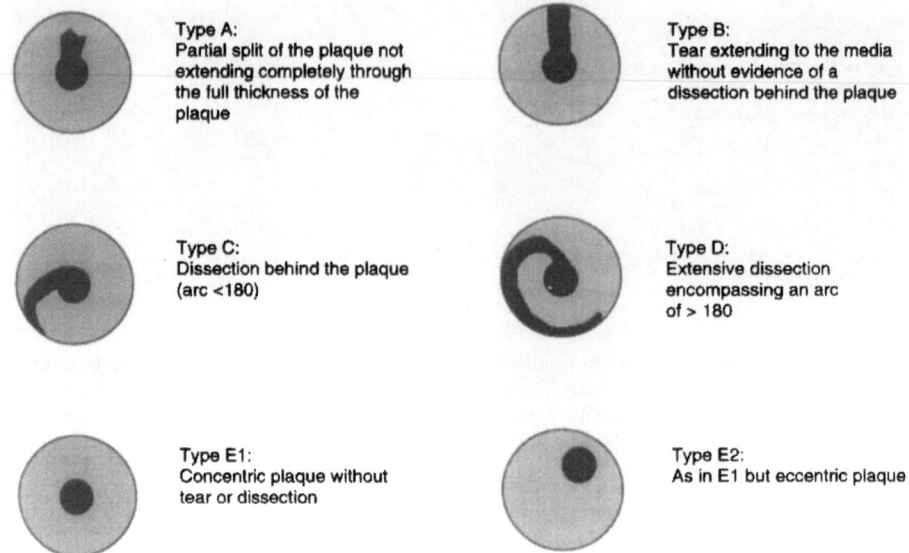

Type A:
Partial split of the plaque not extending completely through the full thickness of the plaque

Type B:
Tear extending to the media without evidence of a dissection behind the plaque

Type C:
Dissection behind the plaque (arc <180)

Type D:
Extensive dissection encompassing an arc of > 180

Type E1:
Concentric plaque without tear or dissection

Type E2:
As in E1 but eccentric plaque

Figure 10. Morphological patterns of balloon dilatation by intravascular ultrasound imaging. (Adapted from Honye et al. Circulation 1992; 85: 1012–1025 with permission.)

indirectly be inferred from the images on the basis of previous descriptions from necropsy studies about common disruption of the media with extensive plaque tearing. On the ultrasound image, the media itself cannot be distinguished from the newly created channel which also appears black due to rapidly flowing blood.

Honye et al. were the first to report an association between the morphological effects of balloon angioplasty assessed by intracoronary ultrasound imaging and restenosis [38]. Restenosis occurred in 50% of concentric plaques without a fracture or a dissection after angioplasty (type E1, Figure 10), whereas the mean rate of restenosis was only 12% in the remaining morphological groups (p = 0.053). There was no significant difference between lesions with and without restenosis with respect to mean percent diameter stenosis by angiography, and the ultrasound parameters mean percent area stenosis and residual plaque cross-sectional area.

Why should concentric plaques be more likely to restenose? The most likely explanation is that concentric stenoses are less likely to dissect than eccentric stenoses (4/18 = 22% vs 37/48 = 77% in the study of Honye et al. [38]). There are two reasons for this observation: first, concentric plaques have a similar thickness around their circumference and do not show a thin portion, which presumably represents the point of lowest resistance against the radial forces exerted by the inflated balloon (Figure 11). This thinnest portion of the plaque is the likely point of plaque splitting as could be shown in several autopsy studies [44, 50]. Second, concentric plaques often show

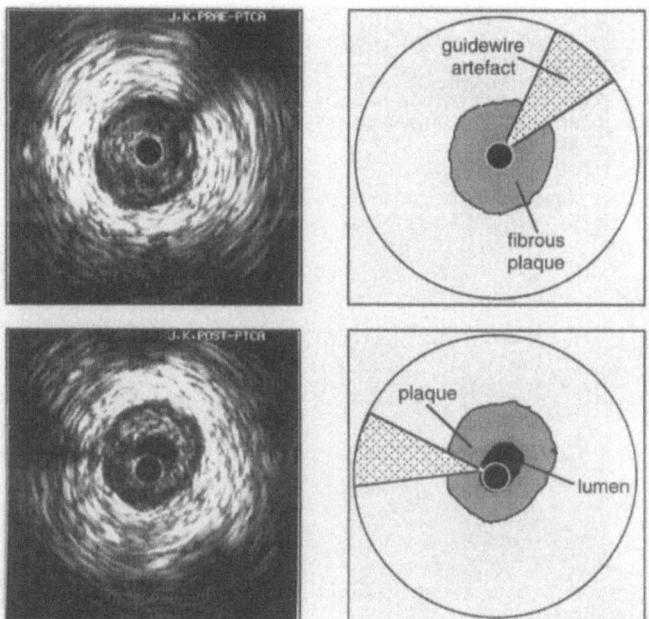

Figure 11a. Upper panel: Concentric stenosis consisting of soft plaque before balloon angioplasty. Lower panel: After PTCA there are no tears or dissections created within the plaque and luminal gain is mainly achieved by plaque reduction.

little or no calcification and calcifications are more likely to fracture [25, 38] because they cannot stretch as may do softer, noncalcified atheromas. As noted above, the absence of dissections after balloon angioplasty has been repeatedly linked to a higher restenosis rate in angiographic studies [1, 11, 15] which would support the ultrasound observations by Honye et al. [38].

Another mechanism possibly explaining the higher restenosis rate in concentric plaque without plaque splitting is elastic recoil after deflation of the balloon which may be larger in this type of stenosis. However, a study of angiographic recoil in stenoses defined as concentric, eccentric, or eccentric with a partially normal vessel wall by intravascular ultrasound found no significant difference between the first two entities [51] whereas recoil was significantly larger in eccentric stenoses with a segment of a "normal" appearing vessel wall (Figures 12 and 13), which argues against the recoil theory in concentric plaques. The important limitation is that only 20% of their patients, all of whom had symptoms or other evidence of restenosis underwent repeated angiography, which may have resulted in underestimating true restenosis rate [52].

Tenaglia et al. [42] used a more simple classification of postangioplasty results seen by intravascular ultrasound than Honye and coworkers. They

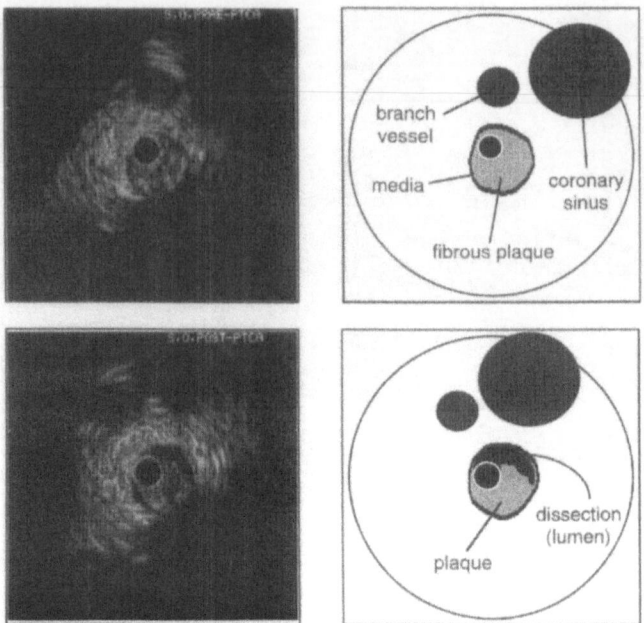

Figure 11b. Upper panel: Eccentric stenosis, which shows area of thinning between 11.00 and 12.00 before PTCA. Lower panel: After PTCA, plaque rupture with dissection behind the plaque has occurred at this point of lowest resistance.

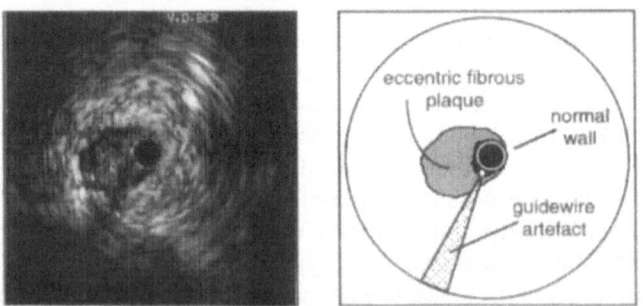

Figure 12. Eccentric stenosis with normal wall.

distinguished between lesions showing a dissection (= separation of the plaque from the media) and those showing no dissections. The presence of a dissection was found to be the only ultrasound variable associated with subsequent adverse events (25 of 30 events were restenosis) after angioplasty (63% dissections in adverse outcome group as compared to 35% in no adverse outcome group; $p < 0.05$) Major dissections encompassing >33% of

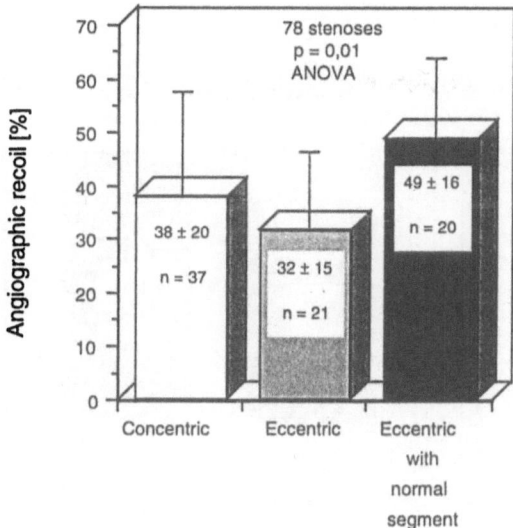

Plaque morphology by IVUS

Figure 13. Percent recoil as measured by quantitative angiography (measured as: [1-minimal balloon diameter at maximal inflation pressure/minimal lumen diameter after PTCA] (×100) for stenoses defined as concentric, eccentric, or eccentric with segment of normal wall by intravascular ultrasound.

the circumference occurred four times more frequently in patients with than in those without an adverse event, whereas minor dissections occurred 50% more frequently in this group. Variables such as plaque composition, plaque eccentricity, lumen area, plaque area and percent area stenosis after the intervention were not different between those with or without a later adverse outcome.

These results are in obvious contradiction to those found by Honye et al. [38] and several angiographic studies, which demonstrated that dissections portend a *better* long term result with lower restenosis rates. However, some authors reported that major dissections were followed by higher restenosis rates [53] and others believed that restenosis was not related to the presence or absence of dissection [54–56]. It must therefore be concluded that it is presently not clear whether dissection initiates the restenosis process by inducing smooth muscle cell proliferation due to deep injury or whether it prevents it by creating a better initial result, which prevents restenosis as defined on a binary scale.

Based on their classification scheme [40], preliminary data on restenosis rates were reported by the Mainz group [57]. They confirmed the observation of Tenaglia et al. that extensive dissections were frequently followed by adverse outcomes including restenosis, whereas concentric stenoses without

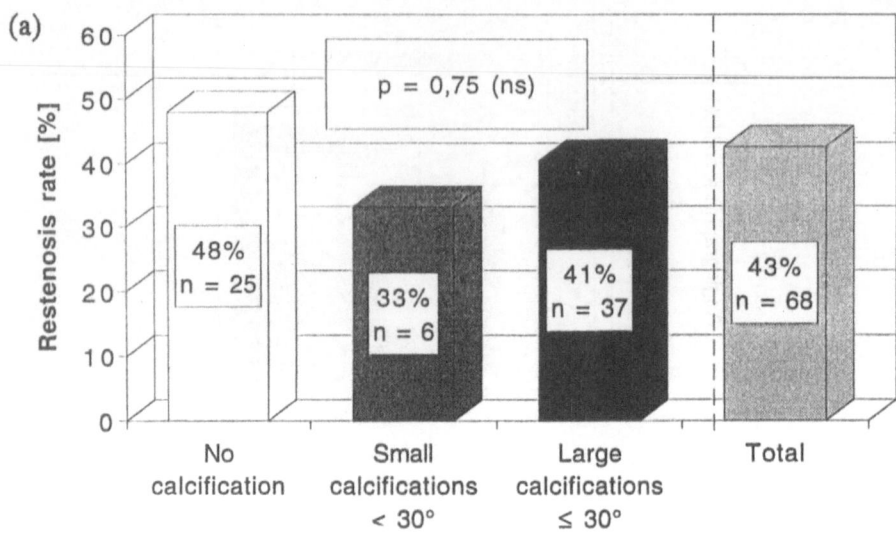

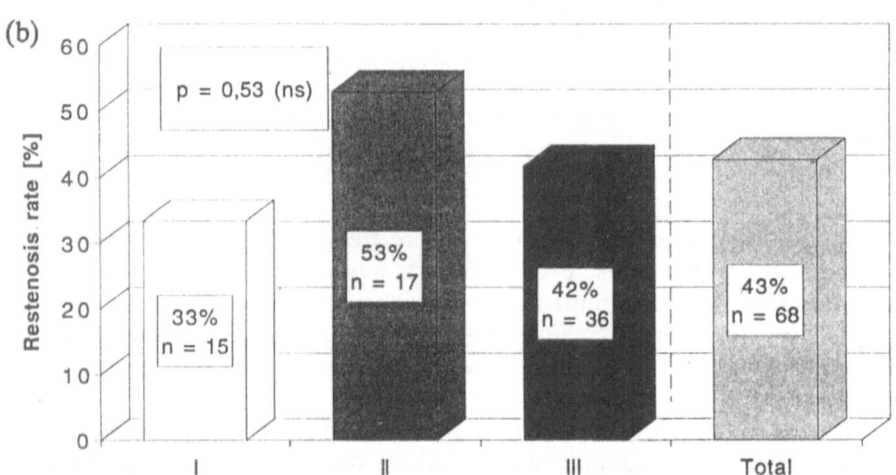

Figure 14. Angiographic restenosis rates (diameter stenosis ≧50%) in 68 lesions treated by balloon angioplasty depending on lesion characteristics as assessed by postinterventional intravascular ultrasound. (a) Extent of plaque calcification. (b) Extent of plaque disruption caused by balloon inflation. I = no tear, no dissection; II = tears not reaching media; III = tear or dissection with media involvement. (c) Influence of balloon/vessel ratio (BVR). Balloon size was determined as balloon area in stenosis from biplane angiographic documentation of maximally inflated balloon. Vessel size was determined as total vessel area within intima/adventitia interface from ultrasound images. BVR = Balloon size/vessel size. (d) Influence of residual plaque burden (area stenosis) as measured from ultrasound images as ratio (plaque area/total vessel area) after intervention. ns = not significant at level p < 0.05.

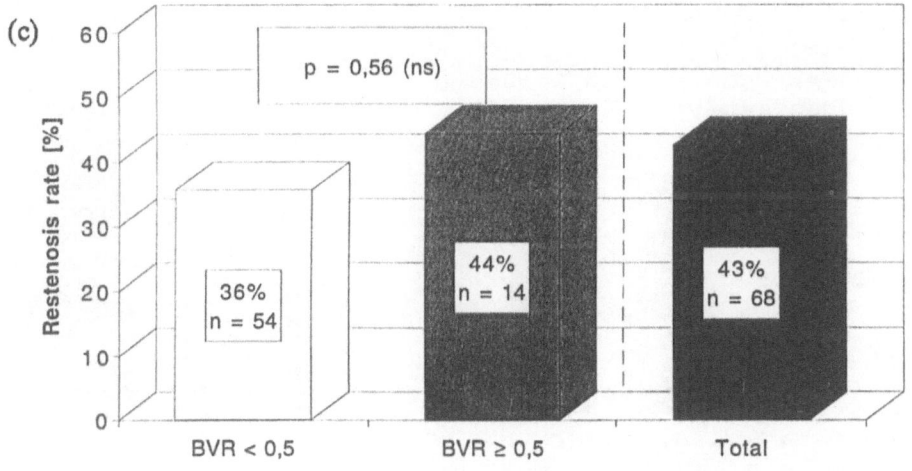

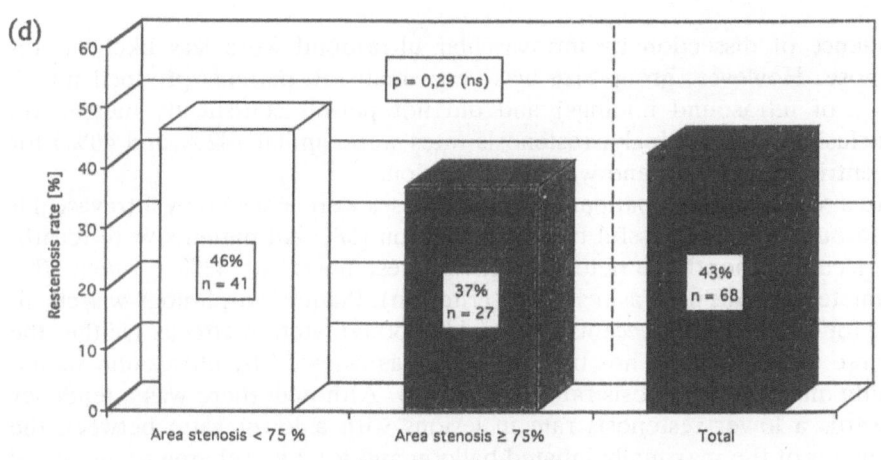

Figure 14. Continued.

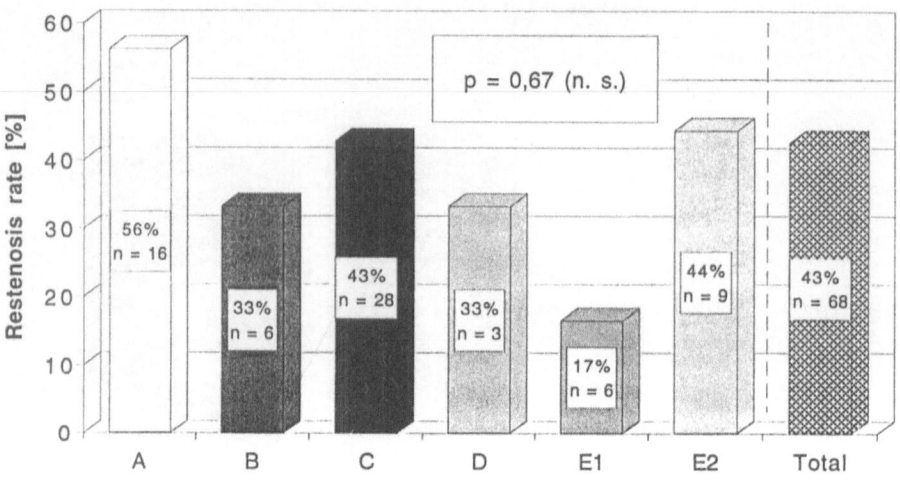

Figure 15. Restenosis rates in 68 lesions depending on plaque classification (see Figure 10) described by Honye et al. [38]. ns = not significant at level p < 0.05.

evidence of dissection by intravascular ultrasound were less likely to restenose. However, group size was very small (56 patients grouped into 7 types of ultrasound findings) and did not permit statistically meaningful conclusions. Interestingly, restenosis rates were similar (42% and 40%) for eccentric lesions with and without dissections.

In a recent study 61 patients with 68 stenoses were assessed by intravascular ultrasound after successful balloon dilatation [58]. All patients were recatheterized at 4 months to detect restenosis (restenosis rate 43% = 29/68; 50% diameter stenosis used as restenosis criterion). Plaque morphology was classified for calcifications, eccentricity, and balloon dilatation effects. Neither the degree of calcification nor balloon effects as assessed by ultrasound significantly influence restenosis rates (Figure 14). Although there was a tendency towards a lower restenosis rate in lesions with a lower ratio between the diameter of the maximally inflated balloon and total vessel area as measured form ultrasound images, this trend was not statistically significant. Interestingly, there was a trend towards lower restenosis rates for lesions with a higher residual plaque burden after balloon dilatation as compared with those with a lower plaque burden. When we used the Honye classification in our population to classify postdilatation plaques, we found that type E1 (concentric plaque without tears) had the *lowest* restenosis rate (Figure 15). The difference in restenosis rates between groups classified for plaque eccentricity approached significance and eccentric lesions featuring some normal appearing part of the vessel's circumference had the lowest tendency to restenose (Figure 16).

There are some limitations of the ultrasound technique for assessing

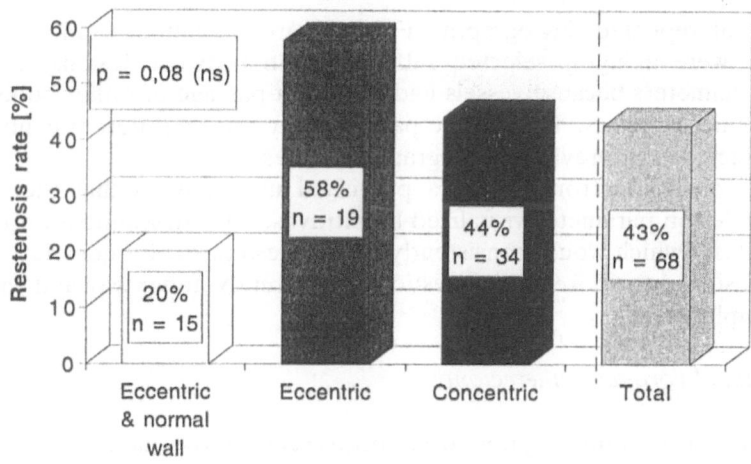

Figure 16. Restenosis rate based on postinterventional ultrasound classification of plaque eccentricity in 68 stenoses. Concentric = maximal plaque diameter/minimal plaque diameter <2. Eccentric & normal wall = eccentric stenoses with segment of "normal" appearing wall. ns = not significant at level $p < 0.05$.

stenosis morphology after balloon dilatation. First, selection of one particular cross-section for classifying stenosis morphology does not take into account that this morphology may change along the length of a lesion. Therefore, slightly different mechanisms of plaque disruption may occur at different positions of the ultrasound catheter along the vessel segment which was in contact with the balloon. Second, dissections must be carefully confirmed by injecting contrast material through the guiding catheter, which may be difficult in the presence of additional proximal lesions or guiding catheters with sideholes. Third, the acoustic shadow of calcification sometimes prevents an unequivocal diagnosis of the presence or absence of a dissection. Fourth, in smaller vessels and suboptimal luminal enlargement after balloon dilatation, near field artifacts may obscure the free lumen, leading to erroneously low measurements of lumen size. Moreover, similar to angiography, various definitions exist of what constitutes an eccentric plaque, what is a severe calcification and how the extent of a dissection should be classified. Finally, most studies obtained ultrasound images only after angioplasty, which did not allow to study other mechanisms likely involved in the creation of a larger coronary lumen such as plaque reduction and vessel stretch [35]. All of these limitations may contribute to the present failure of intravascular ultrasound examinations to predict restenosis following balloon angioplasty.

The differences between studies discussed above are in part explained by the different ultrasound definitions used for plaque eccentricity in ultrasound images, calcification gradings, and especially of dilatation effects. Another difficulty in comparing the results of these studies is the different extent and timing of repeated angiography. Furthermore, patients included in these studies were a highly selected subgroup with proximal lesions and large vessel diameters because vessels had to permit passage of rather bulky 4.8 F ultrasound catheters. Thus, these patients may form a different cohort than those included in previous angiographic studies.

The conclusion from the data published until now is that there is no specific lesion parameter visualized by intravascular ultrasound after balloon angioplasty which would consistently predict restenosis. Larger trials specifically designed to address this question are currently under way and will soon be completed.

Directional coronary atherectomy

Although several investigators used intravascular ultrasound to examine the effect of atherectomy on coronary lesions [13, 35, 41, 59–62], there are only few data regarding the occurrence of restenosis in lesions treated by atherectomy [59, 63]. Suarez de Lezo and coworkers used a phased-array type of ultrasound catheter to study 52 patients after successful atherectomy without adjunct balloon angioplasty. They classified plaque into two groups: predominantly echogenic and predominantly echolucent. Echogenic plaque had a greater collagen and calcium content, whereas echolucent plaques had a higher content of thrombotic material, nuclei and lipids [59]. Angiographic restudy was performed in 22 patients and showed restenosis in 13. Although there were no angiographic predictors of restenosis identified in this group of patients, the incidence of restenosis in primary lesions (n = 19) was influenced by the echogenicity of the plaque. All 7 echolucent lesion were restenosed as compared to only 4 of 12 echogenic lesions (p < 0.07). Pathology confirmed that patients with restenosis had a higher cellular content than patients who did not develop restenosis (p < 0.05). Interestingly, the percent plaque reduction after atherectomy was higher in echolucent than in echogenic plaques, suggesting that the primary result is less important than plaque composition for predicting restenosis. However, a large subgroup of patients in this study had unstable angina or was studied shortly after thrombolysis. Therefore, thrombotic material may have caused the plaques to appear more echolucent and the higher restenosis rate in this subgroup may have only reflected the well known propensity of unstable lesions to restenose [9].

The influence of ultrasound appearance of plaque material on restenosis rate found by Suarez de Leso must be also viewed in the light of another large ultrasound study, which included patients treated with various forms of transcatheter therapy (one third directional atherectomy) [63]. This study suggested that 1) less intralesional calcium (soft plaque) was associated with less restenosis, 2) a better acute result (larger lumen, fewer dissections) showed fewer restenoses, 3) the magnitude of luminal gain was related to freedom of restenosis. Consequently, no clear answer has yet emerged as to whether intravascular ultrasound may have a role in preventing restenosis after directional atherectomy by assessing pre- and/or postinterventional plaque morphology. However, identification of soft and eccentric plaque morphology before intervention may be useful for selecting directional atherectomy as the ideal interventional device for achieving an optimal initial result [12].

Rotational atherectomy

No data are yet available addressing the relationship between the ultrasound appearance of a lesion and the occurrence of a restenosis after rotational atherectomy.

Conclusions

As of now, there are conflicting data as to what constitutes a postangioplasty vessel morphology on intracoronary ultrasound examination with a high likelihood for restenosis. Consequently, larger studies using commonly accepted ultrasound definitions have to further clarify whether the ultrasound image can be used to predict restenosis. Interesting data can be expected from serial ultrasound studies before and immediately after angioplasty and at the time of recatheterization between 4 and 6 months after the initial procedure. These studies may be able to demonstrate the localization of extracellular matrix and smooth muscle cells with respect to the remaining plaque after intervention. Although is has yet to be proven that the use of ultrasound catheters in conjunction with coronary interventions improves outcome and is cost effective, some clinically relevant applications beyond scientific interest have emerged lately. Preprocedural ultrasound is now feasible in many lesions and the choice of the interventional tool can be much better targeted if lesion morphology is precisely known. Postinterventional ultrasound may demonstrate a larger extent of atherosclerosis at reference sites which seems to predict an unfavourable clinical outcome [64]. Moreover, examining the lesion by ultrasound after balloon dilatation may reveal suboptimal lumen enlargement despite a satisfactory angiographic result. This finding will prompt another attempt to improve lumen size ("bigger is better") which may ultimately result in lower restenosis rates without increasing acute complication rates [65].

Acknowledgements

We thank the staff in the catheterization laboratory, Gertrud Sogorski, Ida Steinhoff, Dagmar Clauß, and Jurgen Korsten, who were supportive and helpful for performing intravascular ultrasound research at our institution. Invaluable support was also provided by Rosemarie Floridia, Thomas Keweloh, Antje Struck, Oliver Klass, Rolf Fussl, Stefan Kaspers, Jorg Schroder and Martin Weihrauch, who assisted during the procedure and handled the ultrasound machine with expertise. We also thank Hans Deutsch, M.D. who performed several of the intracoronary ultrasound examinations shown as figures in this chapter.

References

1. Leimgruber PD, Roubin GS, Hollman J et al. Restenosis after successful coronary angioplasty in patients with single vessel disease. Circulation 1986; 73: 710–7.
2. Topol EJ, Leya F, Pinkerton CA et al. A comparison of directional atherectomy with coronary angioplasty in patients with coronary artery disease. The CAVEAT Study Group. N Engl J Med 1993; 329: 221–7.
3. Liu MW, Roubin GS, King SB. Restenosis after coronary angioplasty. Potential biologic determinants and role of intimal hyperplasia. Circulation 1989; 79: 1374–87.
4. Potkin BN, Roberts WC. Effects of percutaneous transluminal coronary angioplasty on atherosclerotic plaques and relation of plaque composition and arterial size to outcome. Am J Cardiol 1988; 62: 41–50.
5. Rensing BJ, Hermans WR, Beatt KJ et al. Quantitative angiographic assessment of elastic recoil after percutaneous transluminal coronary angioplasty. Am J Cardiol 1990; 66: 1039–44.
6. de Marchena EJ, Mallon SM, Knopf WD et al. Effectiveness of holmium laser-assisted coronary angioplasty. The Holmium Laser Coronary Registry. Am J Cardiol 1994; 73: 117–21.
7. Safian RD, Niazi KA, Strzelecki M et al. Detailed angiographic analysis of high-speed mechanical rotational atherectomy in human coronary arteries. Circulation 1993; 88: 961–8.
8. Hermans WR, Rensing BJ, Strauss BH, Serruys PW. Prevention of restenosis after percutaneous transluminal coronary angioplasty: The search for a "magic bullet". Am Heart J 1991; 122: 171–87.
9. Califf RM, Fortin DF, Frid DJ et al. Restenosis after coronary angioplasty: An overview. J Am Coll Cardiol 1991; 17 (Suppl B): 2B-13B.
10. Carrozza JJ, Kuntz RE, Fishman RF, Baim DS. Restenosis after arterial injury caused by coronary stenting in patients with diabetes mellitus. Ann Intern Med 1993; 118: 344–9.
11. Weintraub WS, Kosinski AS, Brown CL, King SB. Can restenosis after coronary angioplasty be predicted from clinical variables? J Am Coll Cardiol 1993; 21: 6–14.
12. Mintz GS, Pichard AD, Kovach JA et al. Impact of preintervention intravascular ultrasound imaging on transcatheter treatment strategies in coronary artery disease. Am J Cardiol 1994; 73: 423–30.
13. Fitzgerald PJ, Yock PG. Mechanisms and outcomes of angioplasty and atherectomy assessed by intravascular ultrasound imaging. J Clin Ultrasound 1993; 21: 579–88.
14. Potkin BN, Keren G, Mintz GS et al. Arterial responses to balloon coronary angioplasty: an intravascular ultrasound study. J Am Coll Cardiol 1992; 20: 942–51.
15. Ellis SG, Roubin GS, King SB et al. Importance of stenosis morphology in the estimation of restenosis risk after elective percutaneous transluminal coronary angioplasty. Am J Cardiol 1989; 63: 30–4.
16. Arnett EN, Isner JM, Redwood DR et al. Coronary artery narrowing in coronary artery disease: comparison of cineangiographic and necropsy findings. Ann Intern Med 1979; 91: 350–6.
17. Porter TR, Sears T, Xie F et al. Intravascular ultrasound study of angiographically mildly diseased coronary arteries. J Am Coll Cardiol 1993; 22: 1858–65.

18. Glagov S, Weisenberg E, Zarins CK et al. Compensatory enlargement of human atherosclerotic coronary arteries. N Engl J Med 1987; 316: 1371–5.
19. St Goar FG, Pinto FJ, Alderman EL et al. Intravascular ultrasound imaging of angiographically normal coronary arteries: An in vivo comparison with quantitative angiography. J Am Coll Cardiol 1991; 18: 952–8.
20. Nissen SE, Gurley JC, Grines CL et al. Intravascular ultrasound assessment of lumen size and wall morphology in normal subjects and patients with coronary artery disease. Circulation 1991; 84: 1087–99.
21. De Scheerder I, De Man F, Herregods MC et al. Intravascular ultrasound versus angiography for measurement of luminal diameters in normal and diseased coronary arteries. Am Heart J 1994; 127: 243–51.
22. Nishimura RA, Edwards WD, Warnes CA et al. Intravascular ultrasound imaging: in vitro validation and pathologic correlation. J Am Coll Cardiol 1990; 16: 145–54.
23. Dietz WA, Tobis JM, Isner JM. Failure of angiography to accurately depict the extent of coronary artery narrowing in three fatal cases of percutaneous transluminal coronary angioplasty. J Am Coll Cardiol 1992; 19: 1261–70.
24. Ehrlich S, Honye J, Mahon D et al. Unrecognized stenosis by angiography documented by intravascular ultrasound imaging. Cathet Cardiovasc Diagn 1991; 23: 198–201.
25. Mintz GS, Douek P, Pichard AD et al. Target lesion calcification in coronary artery disease: an intravascular ultrasound study. J Am Coll Cardiol 1992; 20: 1149–55.
26. Fitzgerald PJ, St Goar FG, Connolly AJ et al. Intravascular ultrasound imaging of coronary arteries. Is three layers the norm? Circulation 1992; 86: 154–8.
27. Gussenhoven EJ, Frietman PA, The SH et al. Assessment of medial thinning in atherosclerosis by intravascular ultrasound. Am J Cardiol 1991; 68: 1625–32.
28. Tobis JM, Mallery J, Mahon D et al. Intravascular ultrasound imaging of human coronary arteries in vivo: Analysis of tissue characterizations with comparison to in vitro histological specimens. Circulation 1991; 83: 913–26.
29. Di Mario C, The SH, Madretsma S et al. Detection and characterization of vascular lesions by intravascular ultrasound: An in vitro study correlated with histology. J Am Soc Echocardiogr 1992; 5: 135–46.
30. Gussenhoven EJ, Essed CE, Lancée CT et al. Arterial wall characteristics determined by intravascular ultrasound imaging: An in vitro study. J Am Coll Cardiol 1989; 14: 947–52.
31. Sechtem U, Arnold G, Keweloh T et al. In-vitro-Diagnose der koronaren Plaquemorphologie mit intravaskularem Ultraschall: Vergleich mit histopathologischen Befunden. Z Kardiol 1993; 82: 618–27.
32. Waller BF, Pinkerton CA, Orr CM et al. Morphological observations late (greater than 30 days) after clinically successful coronary balloon angioplasty: An analysis of 20 necropsy patients and literature review of 41 necropsy patients with coronary angioplasty restenosis. Circulation 1991; 83 (Suppl I): I-28-I-41.
33. Potkin BN, Bartorelli AL, Gessert JM et al. Coronary artery imaging with intravascular high-frequency ultrasound. Circulation 1990; 81: 1575–85.
34. Finet G, Maurincomme E, Tabib A et al. Artifacts in intravascular ultrasound imaging: Analyses and implications. Ultrasound Med Biol 1993; 19: 533–47.
35. Braden GA, Herrington DM, Downes TR et al. Qualitative and quantitative contrasts in the mechanisms of lumen enlargement by coronary balloon angioplasty and directional coronary atherectomy. J Am Coll Cardiol 1994; 23: 40–8.
35a. Füessl R, Burkhard-Meier C, Kaspers S et al. Dissektion nach Ballonangioplastie: Vorhersagemöglichkeit mit präinterventionellem intra-vaskulärem Ultraschall. Z Kardiol 1995; 84: 205–15.
36. Losordo DW, Rosenfield K, Pieczek A et al. How does angioplasty work? Serial analys' of human iliac arteries using intravascular ultrasound. Circulation 1992; 86: 1845–58.
37. Werner GS, Sold G, Buchwald A et al. Intravascular ultrasound imaging of human coronary arteries after percutaneous transluminal angioplasty: Morphologic and quantitative assessment. Am Heart J 1991; 122: 212–20.

38. Honye J, Mahon DJ, Jain A et al. Morphological effects of coronary balloon angioplasty in vivo assessed by intravascular ultrasound imaging. Circulation 1992; 85: 1012–25.
39. Tobis JM, Mallery J, Mahon D et al. Intravascular ultrasound imaging of human coronary arteries in vivo. Analysis of tissue characterizations with comparison to in vitro histological specimens. Circulation 1991; 83: 913–26.
40. Gerber TC, Erbel R, Gorge G et al. Classification of morphologic effects of percutaneous transluminal coronary angioplasty assessed by intravascular ultrasound. Am J Cardiol 1992; 70: 1546–54.
41. Tenaglia AN, Buller CE, Kisslo KB et al. Mechanisms of balloon angioplasty and directional coronary atherectomy as assessed by intracoronary ultrasound. J Am Coll Cardiol 1992; 20: 685–91.
42. Tenaglia AN, Buller CE, Kisslo KB et al. Intracoronary ultrasound predictors of adverse outcomes after coronary artery interventions. J Am Coll Cardiol 1992; 20: 1385–90.
43. Hodgson JM, Reddy KG, Suneja R et al. Intracoronary ultrasound imaging: Correlation of plaque morphology with angiography, clinical syndrome and procedural results in patients undergoing coronary angioplasty. J Am Coll Cardiol 1993; 21: 35–44.
44. Block PC, Myler RK, Stertzer S, Fallon JT. Morphology after transluminal angioplasty in human beings. N Engl J Med 1981; 305: 382–6. 45.
45. Tobis JM, Mallery JA, Gessert J et al. Intravascular ultrasound cross-sectional arterial imaging before and after balloon angioplasty in vitro. Circulation 1989; 80: 873–82.
46. Farb A, Virmani R, Atkinson JB, Kolodgie FD. Plaque morphology and pathologic changes in arteries from patients dying after coronary balloon angioplasty. J Am Coll Cardiol 1990; 16: 1421–9.
47. Block PC, Baughman KL, Pasternak RC, Fallon JT. Transluminal angioplasty: Correlation of morphologic and angiographic findings in an experimental model. Circulation 1980; 61: 778–85.
48. Fitzgerald PJ, Ports TA, Yock PG. Contribution of localized calcium deposits to dissection after angioplasty. An observational study using intravascular ultrasound. Circulation 1992; 86: 64–70.
49. Di Mario C, Madretsma S, Linker DL et al. The angle of incidence of the ultrasonic beam: a critical factor for the image quality in intravascular ultrasonography. Am Heart J 1993; 125: 442–8.
50. Lyon RT, Zarins CK, Lu CT et al. Vessel, plaque, and lumen morphology after transluminal balloon angioplasty: Quantitative study in distended human arteries. Atherosclerosis 1987; 7: 306–14.
51. Sechtem U, Hopp HW, Rudolph D et al. Recoil after percutaneous transluminal coronary angioplasty depends on stenosis morphology: Assessment by intravascular ultrasound (Abstr). Eur Heart J 1993; 14 (Suppl B): 128.
52. Kuntz RE, Keaney KM, Senerchia C, Baim DS. A predictive method for estimating the late angiographic results of coronary intervention despite incomplete ascertainment. Circulation 1993; 87: 815–30.
53. Matthews BJ, Ewels CJ, Kent KM. Coronary dissection: A predictor of restenosis? Am Heart J 1988; 115: 547–54.
54. Bourassa MG, Lesperance J, Eastwood C et al. Clinical, physiologic, anatomic and procedural factors predictive of restenosis after percutaneous transluminal coronary angioplasty. J Am Coll Cardiol 1991; 18: 368–76.
55. Lambert M, Bonan R, Cote G et al. Multiple coronary angioplasty: A model to discriminate systemic and procedural factors related to restenosis. J Am Coll Cardiol 1988; 12: 310–4.
56. Hirshfeld JJ, Schwartz JS, Jugo R et al. Restenosis after coronary angioplasty: A multivariate statistical model to relate lesion and procedure variables to restenosis. The M-HEART Investigators. J Am Coll Cardiol 1991; 18: 647–56.
57. Gorge G, Erbel R, Gerber T et al. Morphologie im intravasalen Ultraschall nach PTCA und klinischer Verlauf (Abstr). Z Kardiol 1993; 82 (Suppl 1): 567.
58. Sechtem U, Rudolph D, Klass O et al. Restenosis after balloon angioplasty: Influence of

postinterventional vessel morphology as assessed by intracoronary ultrasound (Abstr). Eur Heart J 1994; 16 (Suppl).

59. Suarez de Lezo J, Romero M, Medina A et al. Intracoronary ultrasound assessment of directional coronary atherectomy: Immediate and follow-up findings. J Am Coll Cardiol 1993; 21: 298–307.
60. Kimura BJ, Fitzgerald PJ, Sudhir K et al. Guidance of directed coronary atherectomy by intracoronary ultrasound imaging. Am Heart J 1992; 124: 1365–9.
61. Keren G, Pichard AD, Kent KM et al. Failure or success of complex catheter-based interventional procedures assessed by intravascular ultrasound. Am Heart J 1992; 123: 200–8.
62. Suneja R, Nair RN, Reddy KG et al. Mechanisms of angiographically successful directional coronary atherectomy: Evaluation by intracoronary ultrasound and comparison with transluminal coronary angioplasty. Am Heart J 1993; 126: 507–14.
63. Mintz GS, Pichard AD, Ditrano CJ et al. Intravascular ultrasound predictors of angiographic restenosis (Abstr). Circulation 1993; 88 (Suppl): I-598.
64. Nissen SE, Tuzcu EM, de Franco AC et al. Intravascular evidence of atherosclerosis at "normal", reference sites predicts adverse clinical outcomes following percutaneous coronary interventions (Abstr). J Am Coll Cardiol 1994; 271A.
65. Mudra H, Blasini R, Klauss V et al. Verbesserung des Akut- und Langzeitresultats durch Ultraschall-gesteuerte Ballonangioplastie (Abstr). Z Kardiol 1994; 83 (Suppl 1): 12.
66. Mata LA, Bosch X, David PR et al. Clinical and angiographic assessment 6 months after double vessel percutaneous coronary angioplasty. J Am Coll Cardiol 1985; 6: 1239–44.
67. Vandormael MG, Deligonul U, Kern MJ et al. Multilesion coronary angioplasty: Clinical and angiographic follow-up. J Am Coll Cardiol 1987; 10: 246–52.

Corresponding Author: Prof. Dr Udo Sechtem, Klinik für Innere Medizin, University of Cologne, Joseph-Stelzmannstrasse 9, D-50924, Cologne, Germany

26. How to evaluate and to avoid vascular complications at the puncture site

FRANZ FOBBE

Introduction

The technique for transfemoral vascular puncture described by Seldinger in 1953 [1] is basically still used today. The procedure can also be used for puncturing the axillary artery or brachial artery. Although it is regarded as the method of choice, the Seldinger technique can lead to various complications at the puncture site. This chapter deals with possible causes and the diagnostic evaluation of such complications and their therapeutic management.

Types of local complications and possible causes

The most frequent complications are hematomas at the puncture site, though the precise incidence of such hematomas is difficult to estimate reliably. Basically, every arterial puncture will result in a hematoma, although it may be a very small one. There is no generally accepted definition of a clinically relevant hematoma, i.e., one that impairs the patient's condition and/or requires surgical management. Most studies address only those hematomas that have to be treated surgically or prolong the patient's hospitalization period. The frequencies given range from 0.26 to 2.0% [2–4] depending on the type of procedure (diagnostic or therapeutic) and the artery chosen for puncture (femoral, axillary or brachial).

If there is insufficient coagulation of the escaping blood, a false aneurysm may form. In a prospective study by Kresowik et al. [5], 9 (6.35%) of 144 patients developed a false aneurysm after percutaneous coronary angioplasty. Seven of these pseudoaneurysms thrombosed spontaneously. Although this observation of an 80% rate of spontaneous healing is consistent with the clinical impression of the author, this percentage is markedly above the frequencies reported by other authors. However, most studies reporting a lower incidence of spontaneous closure of pseudoaneurisms were performed

C.A. Nienaber and U. Sechtem (eds): Imaging and Intervention in Cardiology, 429–441.
© 1996 Kluwer Academic Publishers. Printed in the Netherlands.

retrospectively and included only patients who had clinically manifest symptoms or required surgical treatment [3, 5].

If the puncture needle pierces not only the artery but also the accompanying vein, an ateriovenous fistula may develop. There are again no generally accepted data on the frequency of such fistulas. In the above-mentioned prospective study by Kresowik et al. [5], arteriovenous fistulas were observed in 2% of the patients. Another local complication is the occlusion of the vessel at the puncture site. Such occlusions may be caused by dissection of the vessel wall or the separation of an arteriosclerotic wall plaque from the wall due to the manipulations of the intima with the puncture needle or the guiding wire. The clinical effects of such an occlusion depend on the condition of the vascular system: In a patient with hemodynamically relevant stenoses which have been present for some time, such an occlusion may cause only minor or no clinical changes. If, however, the punctured vessel is normal, there is a high risk of acute ischemia with jeopardy of the leg. Ischemia occurring after an uncomplicated puncture with proper positioning of the needle tip in the vessel lumen and unproblematic advancement of the guide wire may also be due to an occlusion caused by the properly positioned vessel sheath itself. The latter primarily occurs when a sheath with a large lumen is used or in patients with diffuse arteriosclerotic plaques affecting a segment of the distal external iliac artery.

The frequency of local complications is determined by various factors. The most important one is the puncture site. Arterial puncture should only be performed in those areas where a large artery takes a superficial course and the vessel can be compressed against an underlying bony structure. For examinations of the heart, only three sites fulfill this criterion: the groin, the axilla, and the elbow. Diagnostic or therapeutic interventions in the heart are easiest to perform by puncturing the common femoral artery, which has a rather large lumen. This site is associated with the lowest complication rate and the procedure can be performed with the patient in a normal and comfortable supine position. In the vicinity of the femoral artery, there is the femoral vein in a medial direction and the femoral nerve in a lateral direction. In case of a hemorrhage into the surrounding tissue, the blood can disperse in all directions without the risk of pressure damage to the nerve. However, a hematoma may result in compression of the lumen of the femoral vein. Access via the axillary artery is more difficult: 1) the patient must be positioned with the arm abducted (stretching of the vessel by positioning the upper arm at an angle of 90° to the trunk), 2) the vessel has a smaller diameter than the femoral artery, 3) the required position and the structure of the surrounding soft tissue (e.g., due to muscular tension required for elevating the arm) make it more difficult to palpate the vessel, and 4) the examination of the heart via this access is more complicated (because the examiner is impeded by the X-ray tube). In addition, the distal third of the axillary artery is surrounded on all sides by branches of the brachial plexus, which results in a higher incidence of pressure damage to individual nerve fibers if there is bleeding from the puncture site. The brachial artery is typically punctured in the proximal bend of the elbow, where the vessel has a relatively thin lumen. The most frequent complication is an occlusion of the artery resulting from the manipulation. All large studies demonstrate that the complication rate is lowest after puncture of the femoral artery and much higher (2–8 times) after access via the axillary or brachial artery. This holds for both diagnostic examinations and therapeutic interventions [3, 4, 7–9].

Most patients with coronary heart disease also suffer from peripheral arterial occlusive disease. Many patients with occlusion or extensive arteriosclerotic changes at the level of the abdominal aorta or iliac arteries underwent implantation of a vascular prosthesis before being referred for coronary angiography and catheter intervention at a later stage. Some centers prefer the access via the axillary artery or the brachial artery in these patients and do not puncture the graft – even if there is complete patency of the prosthesis. Puncture or dilation of the puncture site by the catheter can theoretically produce a leak in the prosthesis wall which may not close spontaneously after removal of the catheter. An even more severe complication could be the development of an infection resulting from manipulation of the prosthesis. However, a number of studies has shown that the prosthesis can be punctured directly in the same way as the normal vessel without a higher risk of complications [10–12]. Therefore, facing the higher complication rates associated with using the brachial or axillary artery approach, it is recommended to access the arterial system in patients with previous graft surgery through the graft.

The artery should always be punctured at a site where a bony structure can be used as an abutment to ensure sufficient compression after removal of the catheter. If the femoral artery is punctured immediately below the inguinal ligament, the vessel can be compressed against the femoral head. The inguinal ligament may be difficult to localize in obese patients, since the fold that becomes visible between the proximal thigh and the ventral abdominal wall in the recumbent position corresponds to the inguinal ligament only in slender individuals. In obese patients, this fold is shifted in a caudal direction and does not indicate the position of the inguinal ligament. If this fold is used for orientation, the examiner will puncture the superficial femoral artery or the deep femoral artery rather than the common femoral artery. In these vessel segments, however, there is no underlying bony structure and the accompanying vein runs dorsal and not medial to the artery. Several authors have demonstrated that most false aneurysms and arteriovenous fistulas occur after puncture of the superficial or deep femoral artery [4, 5, 13–17]. It is therefore important to avoid puncture of the artery at a site too far down from the inguinal ligament. If palpation of the bony landmarks (anterior superior iliac spine, symphysis) does not reliably indicate the course of the inguinal ligament, the femoral head should be focussed in the center of the monitor under fluoroscopic control and the center of the femur head

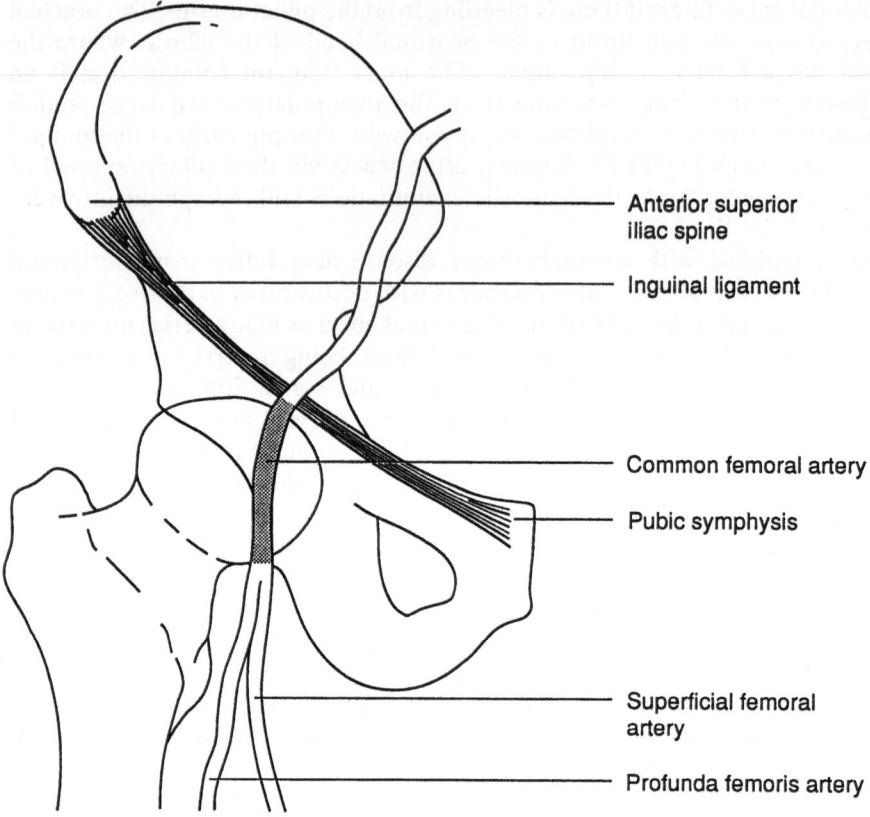

Anterior superior
iliac spine

Inguinal ligament

Common femoral artery

Pubic symphysis

Superficial femoral
artery

Profunda femoris artery

Figure 1. Schematic drawing of the anatomy of the groin: The needle should puncture the arterial wall only in that area where the vessel courses ventral of the femoral head (shaded area).

should then be indicated by skin marks (Figure 1). If the vessel is punctured in this segment, there will be a markedly lower complication rate. The vessels in this area are rather close to the surface even in very obese patients, the artery is easier to palpate and puncture is easier to perform.

The complication rate can additionally be influenced by the puncture needle and technique used for the intervention. Two types of puncture needles are available: a sharpened hollow needle or a blunt hollow cannula with a sharp-pointed trocar. The sharp hollow cannula has the advantage that, theoretically, only the ventral wall of the vessel has to be punctured. However, the lumen of the cannula might get obstructed (e.g., by a punched-out fatty-tissue segment) while the cannula is advanced through the subcutaneous soft-tissue structures. In addition, the sharp needle tip might damage the intima of the vessel. When the trocar needle is used, the examiner should perforate both the ventral and the dorsal vessel wall and advance the needle tip to the underlying bone. The mandrin is then removed and the needle slowly drawn back until a strongly pulsating stream of blood flows from the needle. This indicates that the (blunt!) needle tip is completely within the lumen and that the guide wire can be inserted safely. The latter technique has reduced the frequency of intimal dissections [4]. Theoretically, there might be formation of a relevant hematoma as a result of bleeding from the puncture site in the dorsal vessel wall, but this complication does not seem to occur in clinical practice. Frooed et al. [18] used these two needle types to puncture the iliac arteries of fresh corpses and did not find any difference in the extent of wall damage. However, the application of these experiments to the actual clinical setting is very limited. There are no prospective studies comparing the rate of complications in relation to the puncture technique or type of needle. Nevertheless, the results appear to be more favorable when the trocar needle is used.

As a rule, the puncture site should be compressed manually for 5–10 min after removal of the catheter from the vessel. Subsequent application of a pressure bandage can further reduce the risk of hematoma formation, but there is no agreement on the optimal type of pressure bandage. One possibility is to exert a constant pressure on the puncture site by wrapping elastic bandages around the trunk and the affected leg. However, the pressure thus achieved is low, application of this type of bandage is difficult, and the puncture site and the area around it can no longer be inspected because they are covered by the bandages. A very simple, inexpensive and effective method appears to be the application of a bridle strapping: with the affected leg maximally flexed and abducted in the hip, a firm roll of bandaging material is placed on the puncture site and secured by several wide strips of adhesive silk tape attached to the inner thigh and lateral cranial thoracic wall. When the patient then stretches his leg, the roll exerts a high pressure on the puncture site. This bandage covers the puncture area only minimally and it can be removed rapidly. To prevent skin damage, the tape should be removed or (in case of rebleeding) changed after 4 to 6 hours. In most cases, this period is sufficient to prevent further bleeding from the puncture site [19]. Commercially available devices for compression of the puncture site [20] offer no major advantage.

Diagnostic assessment

The most frequent complication occurring after arterial angiography is the formation of a hematoma. The assessment of the size of such a hematoma is limited by the induration resulting from the effusion of blood into the tissue. In the setting where a diffuse hematoma has already developed, it is especially difficult to clinically identify any additional pathologic changes such as a pseudoaneurysm or an arteriovenous fistula. Until recently, such changes could only be diagnosed by angiography, but this procedure is no longer required, as sonography, and especially color-coded duplex sonography (CCDS), have been shown to be reliable procedures for diagnosing all local complications occurring at the puncture site. CCDS yields a good survey of both the anatomy of soft-tissue structures and blood flow in a single image. The groin and the axilla can best be examined with a linear 5 MHz transducer. A transducer with a lower frequency is only required in very obese patients and/or in the presence of a large hematoma. A curved-array transducer is more suitable only in the treatment of a false aneurysm (see below). The examiner should first obtain a grey-scale image to identify any morphological changes and then visualize the blood flow in a color-coded image. To reduce artifacts in the color-coded mode, only frequency shifts higher than 50 Hz should be encoded (="wall filter"). In the presence of an arteriovenous fistula with a high flow rate, a considerable reduction of artifacts can be achieved with encoding starting at 100 Hz (using a 5 MHz transducer). When the vessel is examined in a transverse plane, it is important to always keep the transducer in a slightly oblique position (to avoid a 90° angle between the course of the vessel and the direction of sound wave propagation) [21].

A perivascular hematoma is visualized in the grey-scale image as an inhomogeneous and hypoechoic structure, which is often difficult to distinguish from muscle tissue. A perfused area within a hematoma is likewise not seen on the grey-scale scan. A clear-cut differentiation can only be achieved with CCDS: perfused areas are immediately identified by the assignment of red and blue color encoding of the flowing blood (Figures 2a–c). In addition to the differentiation of thrombosed from perfused areas, CCDS can also identify the leak in the vessel wall (the "neck of the aneurysms") where the blood leaves the vessel (Figure 2b) [21–23]: the connection between the vessel and the aneurism is frequently fromed by a thin canal presumably created by the needle with a relatively high flow rate (indicated by light red or light blue), from which the blood spreads out into a more or less wide area. The pseudoaneurism often shows circular blood flow, which can be identified by the regular distribution of the color-coded flow signals, e.g., blood flow towards the transducer (red color) in the right half of the aneurysm and away from the transducer (blue color) in the left half (Figure 2a).

An additional frequency analysis is not required for the diagnosis of a pseudoaneurysm.

In the presence of an arteriovenous fistula, the high pressure gradient between the artery and the vein will considerably increase the flow velocity in the fistula, which in turn leads to vibrations in the perivascular tissue. These vibrations have a much higher velocity than those which are caused by the normal motion of the vessel wall and which are cut off by the so-called wall-filter and therefore not visualized on the scan. This phenomenon has a typical appearance in CCDS: A circumscribed area around the fistula with a mosaic-like accumulation of red and blue dots. The "color fog" corresponds to the diffuse vibrations of the perivascular soft-tissue structures.

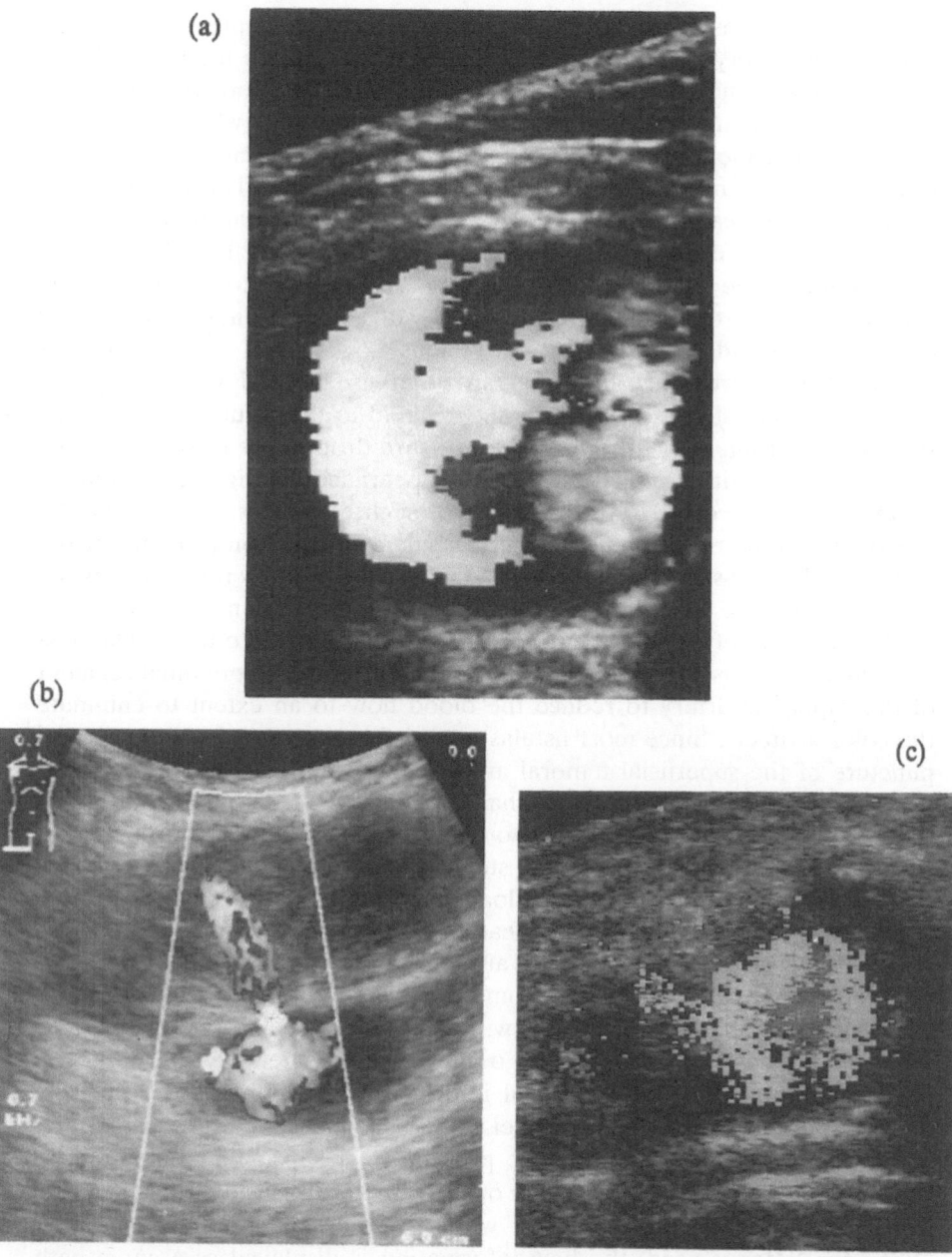

Figure 2. CCDS images of pseudoaneurysms of the femoral artery (three different patients).
(a) Transverse scan of the right proximal thigh: almost circular flow pattern inside the pseudoaneurysm with red encoding (flow towards the transducer) on the lateral and blue encoding (flow away from the transducer) on the medial site. The feeding artery is displaced medially and not visualized. (b) Almost completely thrombosed large pseudoaneurysm with the feeding artery (dorsal) and the neck of the aneurysm with the defect in the arterial wall (encoding in bright blue). Perfusion is displayed only in the center of the the lesion. (c) Transverse scan of the left proximal thigh: diffuse fresh parially thrombosed pseudoaneurysm lateral to the femoral artery, femoral vein with blue encoding. (For colour plate of this figure see **page 539.**)

In the presence of an arteriovenous fistula, the high pressure gradient between the artery and the vein will considerably increase the flow velocity in the fistula, which in turn leads to vibrations in the perivascular tissue. These vibrations have a much higher velocity than those which are caused by the normal motion of the vessel wall and which are cut off by the so-called wall-filter and therefore not visualized on the scan. This phenomenon has a typical appearance in CCDS: A circumscribed area around the fistula with a mosaic-like accumulation of red and blue dots. The "color fog" corresponds to the diffuse vibrations of the perivascular soft-tissue structures. Because of this artifact, the arteriovenous fistula itself cannot be delineated on the ultrasound scan (Figure 3). Venous flow cranial to the fistula is increased and turbulent, and – in an otherwise normal vascular system without relevant stenoses – arterial flow caudal to the fistula loses its usual three-phase profile [22, 24] due to the pressure drop in the fistula. The only other condition with a similar ultrasound appearance is a high-grade stenosis in an artery. However, in the presence of such a stenosis, there would be loss of the laminar flow and extensive turbulence formation (mixture of red and blue dots) distal of the stenosis. In contrast, an arteriovenous fistula does not affect the laminar flow in the artery. If this criterion does not permit a differentiation of these two entities, the arterial influx into the fistula must be reduced. This is achieved by manually compressing the proximal segment of the supplying artery to reduce the blood flow to an extent to eliminate the color artifacts. Since most fistulas occur after too caudal puncture (i.e., puncture of the superficial femoral artery), the examiner can compress the distal external iliac artery and thus has enough space left to apply the transducer. With this maneuver, it is also possible to register the morphological features of a fistula or to exclude a stenosis. Arteriovenous fistulas can also occur in combination with a pseudoaneurysm. In the presence of a large hematoma, the examiner should bear in mind that there might be an increased flow velocity and possibly also turbulence formation due to compression of the vein by the hematoma. However, the mosaic-like accumulation of colours typical of a fistula will be absent in such cases.

In most cases, an acute arterial occlusion can be reliably diagnosed on clinical grounds alone. If additional information is required, CCDS shows an hypoechoic lumen of the vessel with an absence of flow signals. If symptoms already occur during the procedure, the examination should be repeated after removal of the sheath or the catheter. Basically, the diagnostic assessment can also be performed with conventional duplex sonography. When the latter is used, the flow information is displayed as a curve path and not superimposed on the grey-scale image. A major drawback of this technique is the fact that flow information can only be obtained from one small circumscribed area at a time. The examiner therefore has to move the cursor over the entire image to assess blood flow. This is a very time-consuming procedure, and the interpretation of the findings is more difficult.

(a)

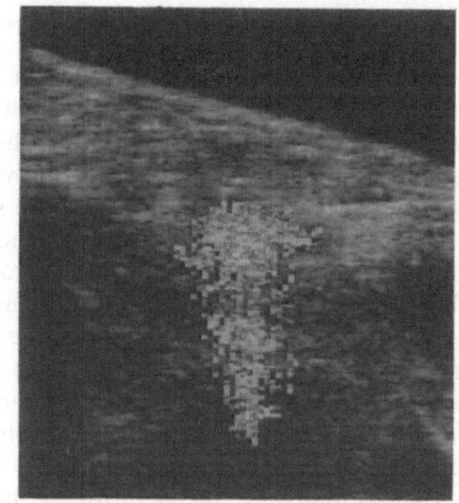

(b)

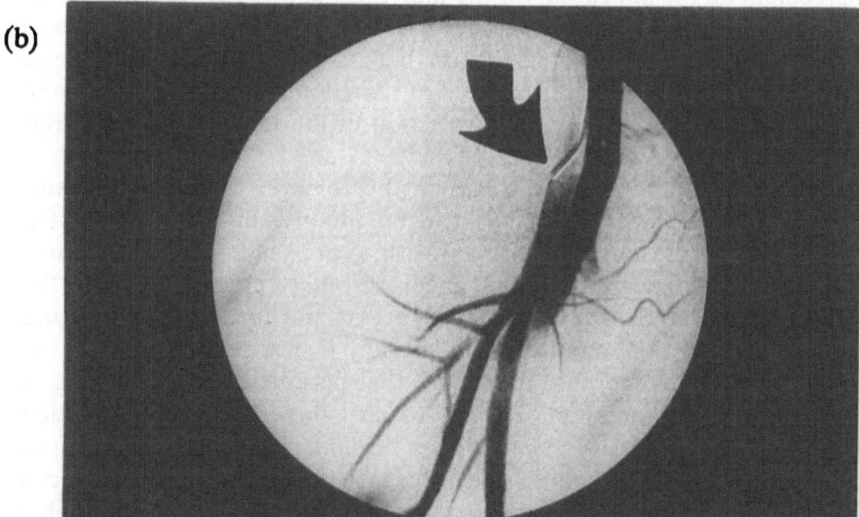

Figure 3. Arteriovenous fistula of superficial femoral artery: (a) Transverse CCDS images shows typically a fog like mixture of red and blue dots (due to the high blood velocity in the fistula which causes high speed vibration of the soft tissue) which superimpose the artery and vein. (b) Corresponding selective angiogramm: immediate visualization of the femoral vein after contrast application in the commo n femoral artery (arrow = tip of the catheter). The lesion is localized in the proximal superficial artery. (For colour plate of Figure 3a see **page 540**.)

Treatment

Most complications occurring at the puncture site do not need any specific treatment. Only acute vascular occlusion requires immediate surgical management. Hematomas are removed by surgery only if they are very large and/or impair the mobilization of the patient. Prospective studies (which, however, included only rather small numbers of patients) show that at least 60% of all false aneurysms thrombose spontaneously. The smaller the perfused false lumen, the greater the probability of spontaneous healing [5, 25, 26]. There is a relatively great difference between the number of surgically treated aneurysms reported in retrospective studies and the number of aneurysms diagnosed in prospective studies (see section "Types of local complications and possible causes"). This difference can be explained by the fact that most pseudoaneurysms escape clinical detection and resolve spontaneously. The same probably also holds for arteriovenous fistulas.

Three basic therapeutic options are available for the management of an arteriovenous fistula or a false aneurysm: conservative treat ment (e.g., bed rest, pressure bandage), surgery, and compression with the transducer. There is no agreement on the indication for the individual approaches or the optimal technique, while it is generally accepted that very large aneurysms (perfused lumen > 4 cm) and arteriovenous fistulas that affect cardiac function require surgical management. The latter consists of resection of the false lumen and patching of the arterial leak or reconstruction of the lumen by a vein graft or a vascular prosthesis [6, 27].

A fairly new procedure is the treatment by compression with the transducer. This is done under CCDS control by compressing the neck of the aneurysm with the transducer in such a way as to preserve arterial flow while preventing blood from entering the aneurysm. It is crucial to apply the pressure exactly over the neck of the aneurysm and to keep the pressure constant for about 10–20 minutes. This therapy is best performed with the aid of CCDS, which is the only procedure that permits close monitoring of blood flow during compression. The approach is based on the assumption that the blood in the aneurysm undergoes thrombosis during compression. If there is only partial thrombosis after the first session, the procedure can be repeated with promising results. There are also commercially available compression devices which can be used instead of the transducer. When such a device is used, however, the clamp, which exerts the pressure, is difficult to keep in place. Blood flow during compression can be monitored by placing the transducer directly next to the clamp. Since compression with such a device may be very painful, most patients require analgetics [28–31].

Reports in the literature indicate that the success rate of this procedure varies between 30 and 90%. The patient groups investigated in each study are very small [28–31] and the authors did not investigate to what extent the therapeutic effect was influenced by the size, age and configuration of an aneurysm. The experience available so far suggests that the therapeutic success decreases with size and the age of the aneurysm. No major complications of compression have been reported so far. A rupture of the aneurysm induced by the external pressure, which some authors suggested as a possible complication, has not been reported in the literature. However, one group reported a thrombosis of the accompanying vein after compression [32]. It is therefore emphasized again that the pressure exerted on the tissue should just be sufficient to interrupt the blood flow into the aneurysm without affecting flow in the other vessels. The same technique can also be used to treat arteriovenous fistulas, but there are as yet no data on the success rate. Our experience suggests that it is much more difficult to sufficiently compress the often very short communication between the artery and the vein to induce thrombosis.

Conclusion

The frequency and severity of complications at the puncture site can be reduced by using an appropriate technique. Color-coded duplex sonography is the method of choice for diagnosing such complications. This procedure can additionally be used to treat false aneurysms and arteriovenous fistulas.

References

1. Seldinger SI. Catheter replacement of the needle in percutaneous arteriography. A new technique. Acta Radiol 1953; 39: 368–76.
2. Cumberland DC. Percutaneous angioplasty. In: Ansel G, Wilkins RA, editors. Complications in diagnostic radiology. Oxford: Blackwell, 1987.
3. Hessel SJ, Adams DF, Abrams HL. Complications of angiography. Radiology 1981; 138: 273–81.
4. Wilkins RA, Garvey CJ. Diagnostic arteriography. In: Ansel G, Wilkins RA, editors. Complications in diagnostic radiology. Oxford: Blackwell, 1987.
5. Kresowik TF, Khoury MD, Miller BV et al. A prospective study of the incidence and natural history of femoral vascular complications after percutaneous transluminal coronary angioplasty. J Vasc Surg 1991; 13: 328–36.
6. Skillman JJ, Kim D, Baim DS. Vascular complications of percutaneous femoral cardiac interventions. Arch Surg 1988; 123: 1207–12.
7. Babu SC, Piccorelli GO, Shah PM et al. Incidence and result of arterial complications among 16350 patients undergoing cardiac catheterization. J Vasc Surg 1989; 10: 113–6.
8. Davis K, Kennedy JW, Kemp HG et al. Complications of coronary arteriography from the collaborative study of coronary artery surgery (CASS). Circulation 1979; 59: 1105–12.
9. McCollum CH, Mavor E. Brachial artery injury after cardiac catheterization. J Vasc Surg 1986; 4: 355–9.
10. AbuRahma AF, Robinson PA, Boland JP. Safety of arteriography by direct puncture of a vascular prosthesis. Am J Surg 1992; 164: 233–6.

440   F. Fobbe

11. Mohr LL, Smith DC, Schaner GJ. Catheterization of synthetic vascular grafts. J Vasc Surg 1986; 3: 854–6.
12. Smith, DC. Catherization of prosthetic vascular grafts. Acceptable technique. Am J Radiol 1984; 143: 1117–1118.
13. Almgren B, Karacagil S, Nybacka O. Arteriovenous fistula following transfemoral angiography. Aust N Z J Surg 1990; 60: 549–50.
14. Altin RS, Flicker S, Naidech HJ. Pseudoaneurysm and arteriovenous fistula after femoral artery catheterization: Association with low femoral punctures. Am J Radiol 1989; 152: 629–31.
15. Grier D, Hartnell G. Percutaneous femoral artery puncture: Practice and anatomy. Br J Radiol 1990; 63: 602–4.
16. Rapoport S, Sniderman KW, Morse SS et al. Pseudoaneurysm: A complication of faulty technique in femoral arterial puncture. Radiology 1985; 154: 529–30.
17. Spijkerboer AM, Scholten FG, Mali PTM, van Schaik JPJ. Antegrade puncture of the femoral artery: Morphologic study. Radiology 1990; 176: 57–60.
18. Frood LR, Smith DC, Pappas JM et al. Use of angiographic needles with or without stylets: Pathologic assessment of vessel walls after puncture. J Vasc Intervent Radiol 1991; 2: 269–72.
19. Haygood TM, Spar J, Orrison WW, Eldevik OP. A simple and effective postangiographic femoral artery pressure dressing. Cardiovasc Intervent Radiol 1993; 16: 262–3.
20. Wolf KJ, Fobbe F. Color duplex sonography. Stuttgart, New York: Thieme, 1995.
21. Colapinto RF, Harty PW. Femoral artery compression device for outpatient angiography. Radiology 1988; 166: 890–1.
22. Foshager MC, Finlay DE, Longley DG, Letourneau JG. Duplex and color Doppler sonography of complications after percutaneous interventional procedures. Radio Graphics 1994; 14: 239–53.
23. Mitchell DG, Needleman L, Bezzi M et al. Femoral artery pseudoaneurysm: Diagnosis with conventional duplex and color Doppler US. Radiology 1987; 165: 687–90.
24. Igidbashian VN, Mitchell DG, Middleton WD et al. Iatrogenic femoral arteriovenous fistula: Diagnosis with color Doppler imaging. Radiology 1989; 170: 749–52.
25. Johns JP, Pupa LE, Bailey SR. Spontaneous thrombosis of iatrogenic femoral artery pseudoaneuryms: Documentation with color Doppler and two dimensional ultrasonography. J Vasc Surg 1991; 14: 24–2.
26. Paulson EK, Hertzberg BS, Paine SS, Caroll BA. Femoral artery pseudoaneuryms: Value of color Doppler sonography in predicting which ones will thrombose without treatment. Am J Radiol 1992; 159: 1077–81.
27. Roberts SR, Main D, Pinkerton J. Surgical therapy of femoral artery pseudoaneurysm after angiography. Am J Surg 1987; 154: 676–80.
28. Agrawal SK, Pinheiro L, Roubin GS et al. Nonsurgical closure of femoral pseudoaneurysms complicating cardiac catheterization and percutaneous transluminal coronary angiography. JACC 1992; 20: 610–5.
29. Feld R, Patton GM, Carabasi RA et al. Treatment of iatrogenic femoral artery injuries with ultrasound-guided compression. J Vasc Surg 1992; 16: 832–40.
30. Fellmeth BD, Roberts AC, Bookstein JJ et al. Postangiographic femoral artery injuries: Nonsurgical repair with US-guided compression. Radiology 1991; 178: 671–5.
31. Sorrell KA, Feinberg RL, Wheeler JR et al. Color-flow duplex-directed manual occlusion of femoral false aneurysms. J Vasc Surg 1993; 17: 571–7.

32. Hilborn M, Downey D. Deep venous thrombosis complicating sonographically guided compression repair of a pseudoaneurysma of the common femoral artery. Am J Radiol 1993; 161: 1334–5.

Corresponding Author: Dr F. Fobbe, Department of Diagnostic Radiology, Freie Universität Berlin, Universitätsklinikum Benjamin Franklin, Hindenburgdamm 30, D-12200 Berlin 45, Germany

27. Selection of patients and transesophageal echocardiography guidance during balloon mitral valvuloplasty

STEVEN A. GOLDSTEIN

Introduction

Cardiac ultrasound has evolved rapidly over the past 20 years. In addition to its powerful diagnostic role, echocardiography has expanded into what has been termed *interventional echocardiography*, that is, the use of echocardiography to guide and monitor more invasive techniques, such as pericardiocentesis, cardiac surgery, endomyocardial biopsy, transseptal puncture, transcatheter closure of atrial septal defects, balloon and blade atrial septostomy, positioning of radio frequency ablation catheters, implantation of ventricular assist devices, and guidance of percutaneous balloon mitral valvuloplasty (PBMV).

PBMV has become an established and effective method of treating symptomatic patients with rheumatic mitral stenosis [1–5]. This procedure can be performed with low risk and excellent, immediate and long-term results [6–12] in properly selected patients. Symptomatic and hemodynamic improvement are comparable to that with closed surgical commissurotomy [13, 14]. This report reviews the role of echocardiography in the preprocedure selection of patients and of transesophageal echocardiography (TEE) to assist PBMV on awake patients in the cardiac catheterization laboratory (Table 1). It is based on the experience with more than 100 patients with symptomatic mitral stenosis [15–18].

Patient selection

Echocardiographic assessment of the morphology of the mitral apparatus has been found to be useful for patient selection and prediction of optimal hemodynamic outcome. A transthoracic echocardiographic (TTE) scoring system or "splittability score" based on severity of leaflet mobility, leaflet thickness, leaflet calcification, and subvalvular disease has become a standard

C.A. Nienaber and U. Sechtem (eds): Imaging and Intervention in Cardiology, 443–458.
© 1996 *Kluwer Academic Publishers. Printed in the Netherlands.*

Table 1. Role of transesophageal echocardiography before and during balloon mitral valvuloplasty.

1. Patient selection
2. Guidance of transseptal puncture
3. Guidance of balloon positioning and dilatation
4. Immediate assessment of results
5. Early detection of complications

part of the preprocedural assessment [19, 20]. Several studies have attempted to address whether or not TEE provides important additional information or a more comprehensive assessment of mitral apparatus morphology compared to TTE [21–26]. Most agree that these two modalities are of equal value and that TEE does not provide greater accuracy than TTE. In fact, TEE may underestimate subvalvular disease and calcification since subvalve structures are in the far field as the echocardiographic beam traverses the enlarged left atrium. Moreover, the echocardiographic beam may be partly attenuated by the thickened and often calcified mitral valve and annulus. Nevertheless, in some patients, the longitudinal transgastric view of the left ventricle provides excellent visualization of the chordae and papillary muscles. Therefore assessment of mitral valve morphology by TEE may be complementary but not superior to assessment by TTE.

TEE is, however, clearly superior to TTE for the detection of thrombi in the left atrium (LA) or left atrial appendage (LAA) [21, 27, 28]. The presence of a left atrial thrombus is generally considered to be a contraindication for PBMV because of the potential for systemic embolization when catheters and wires are manipulated in the left atrium. As opposed to TTE, TEE provides optimal imaging of the entire LA, LAA, and atrial septum which are common sites for thrombus formation (Figure 1).

For this reason several investigators have recommended that TEE be performed in all patients before PBMV [29–31]. However, it is not clear whether patients with small, non-mobile thrombi confined to the apex of the LAA should be excluded for consideration for PBMV. Several groups have performed PBMV without incident in such patients [18, 21, 30] (Figure 2). Clearly, such experiences are still anecdotal and the optimal management and risk of PBMV in patients with small thrombi in the LAA are unclear. However, TEE guidance seems to minimize the inadvertent placement of catheters and wires in the LAA, and, thus, avoids dislodgement of clots.

A second widely accepted contraindication to PBMV (in addition to left atrial thrombi) is greater than moderate (2 + /4) mitral regurgitation. The majority of patients can be satisfactorily screened for moderate mitral regurgitation by TTE, but TEE may be necessary for this purpose in the occasional patient with poor precordial image quality or acoustic masking of the LA by heavy calcium deposits in the mitral valve or annulus.

A few additional anatomic features detectable by TEE have relevance for

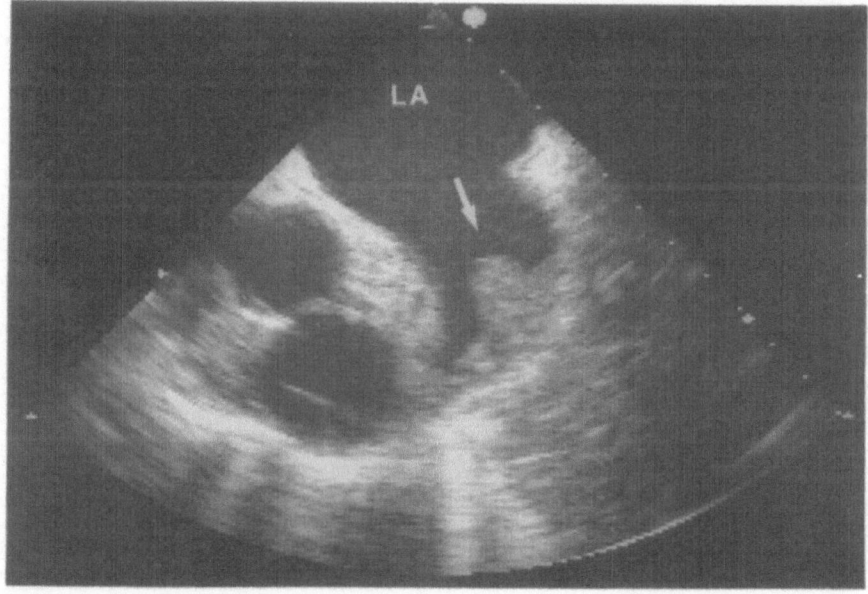

Figure 1. Relatively large thrombus (arrow) which was slightly mobile and projected toward the "mouth" of the left atrial appendage. PBMV was aborted in this patient. LA = left atrium. (With permission from Goldstein et al. J Heart Valve Dis 1994; 3: 138.)

the operators performing PBMV. First, small left ventricles can present a problem during PBMV when using the double-balloon technique. These Mansfield (Mansfield, MA) balloons are long (5.5 cm), cylindrical, and non-compliant, and have a pointed tip. These characteristics increase the risk of perforation of the left ventricle beyond that encountered with the round, shorter (3 cm) Inoue balloon [32, 33]. Second, the shape and orientation of the mitral stenotic orifice may influence the approach and manipulation of the dilating catheter [17]. Lastly, variability in the anatomy of the atrial septum can influence transseptal puncture [17]. These features and the anatomy of the mitral apparatus are reviewed with the operators at the beginning of the procedure, because these features may influence the approach taken.

Guidance of transseptal puncture

Although transseptal puncture is standardly performed with fluoroscopic guidance, even experienced operators can be misled by X-ray anatomic landmarks. By providing excellent visualization of the atrial septum, the transseptal needle, and the relationship of the tip of the needle to other intracardiac structures, TEE guidance facilitates safe crossing of the atrial

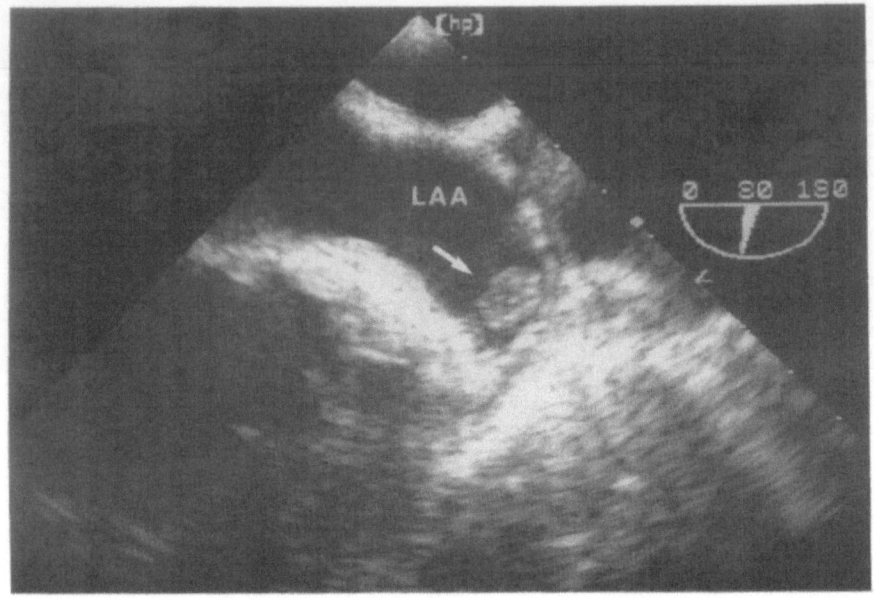

Figure 2. Small thrombus (arrow) near the apex of the left atrial appendage (LAA). Uneventful PBMV was performed in this patient using TEE-guidance. (With permission from Goldstein, et al. J Heart Valve Dis 1994; 3: 139.)

septum by the transseptal needle. In the catheterization laboratory, echocardiographic images can be displayed on a monitor adjacent to the fluoroscopic image so that both can be viewed simultaneously by the operators. With increasing experience, operators rely more and more upon the echocardiographic images. This approach has been particularly useful in patients with chamber enlargement (especially right atrial enlargement), aortic root dilatation, or cardiothoracic deformity. In these circumstances, it may be more difficult to identify the safe region for atrial septal puncture using only fluoroscopy and the risk of puncture of the aorta, right ventricular wall, right atrial wall, left atrial wall, or coronary sinus is increased [34]. When TEE is employed in the laboratory, a routine prepuncture right atriogram to help delineate the atrial septum is no longer necessary, reducing the contrast load to the patient.

The excellent image quality of TEE allows the operators to confirm correct needle position prior to advancing the needle or to redirect the location of the transseptal needle as necessary. In almost all instances, as the advancing transseptal needle contacts the atrial septum, it bulges or "tents" toward the LA before the actual puncture (Figure 3). If this position is satisfactory, the needle is then advanced further into the LA, and the atrial septum can be seen to snap partially or wholly back to its original position.

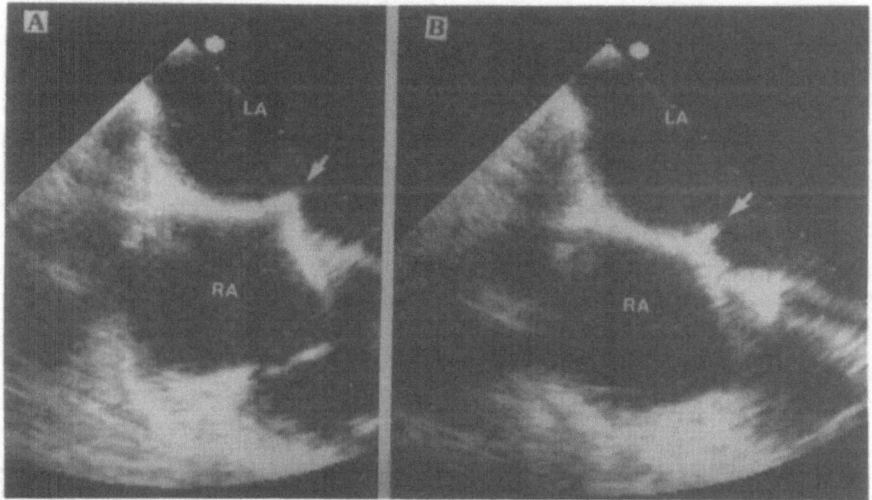

Figure 3. Left panel (A), illustrates "tenting" of the mid-portion of the atrial septum (arrow) due to the advancing transseptal needle. Right panel (B), illustrates partial return of the atrial septum toward its original position as the needle tip (arrow) punctures the atrial septum and enters the left atrium (LA). RA = right atrium. (With permission from Goldstein and Campbell. Cardiology Clinics 1993; 11: 415.)

TEE-guidance of transseptal puncture helps avoid several problems. Such guidance has prevented transseptal puncture that is either too high or too low (Figure 4). Occasionally, a thick or even calcified atrial septum can hinder puncture into the LA [35]. In the experience of the author, operators would have abandoned the procedure in several patients had TEE not detected marked tenting of the atrial septum in the correct position. In three other instances the transseptal needle punctured the septum primum but not the septum secundum and was wedged in the intervening space. Appreciation and correction of the problem was possible only by TEE. In a single imaging plane, correct identification of the needle tip can be difficult. Accurate identification of the tip of the transseptal needle requires experience and frequent manipulations of the TEE probe. Biplane and multiplane TEE probes are helpful.

After transseptal puncture, contrast material can be injected to confirm that the catheter is free within the LA (Figure 5).

Guidance of balloon positioning and dilatation

Once the balloon dilating catheter is in the left atrium, TEE can facilitate manipulation of the balloon catheter through the mitral orifice. Although

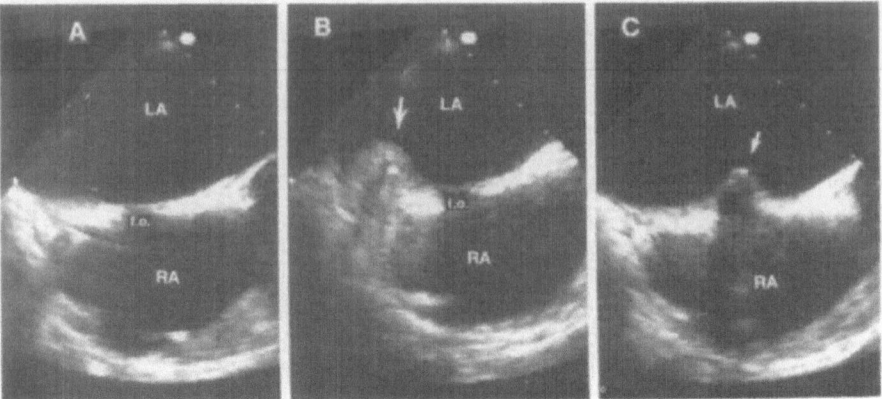

Figure 4. TEE view showing the atrial septum separating the left atrium (LA) from the right atrium (RA). Left panel (A) illustrates the thin fossa ovalis (f.o.) region of the atrial septum. Center panel (B) shows improper position of the advancing transseptal needle indicated by "bowing" of the atrial septum (arrow) above the fossa ovalis. Right panel (C) shows the corrected placement of the transseptal needle by "tenting" of the thin fossa ovalis region (arrow) toward the left atrium.

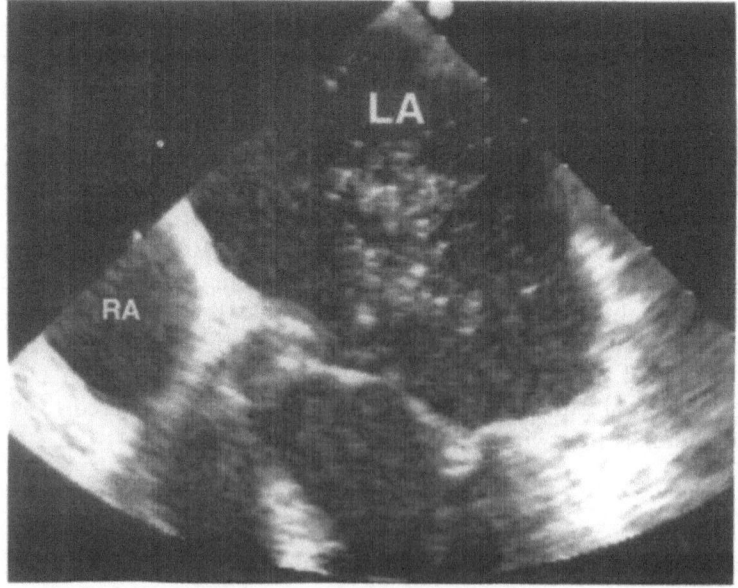

Figure 5. Contrast effect from injection of 3 ml of normal saline confirms the presence of the catheter in the mid left atrium (LA). RA = right atrium. (With permission from Goldstein, et al. J Heart Valve Dis 1994; 3: 137.)

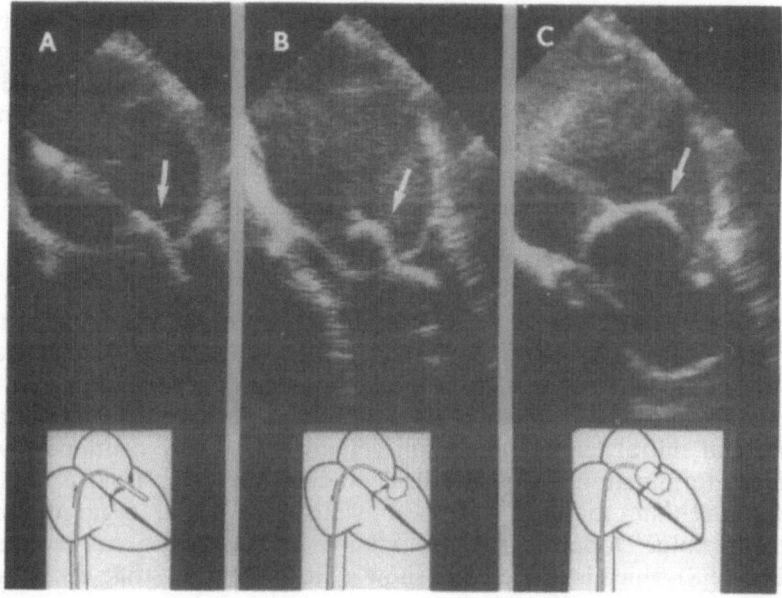

Figure 6. Arrows point to the Inoue balloon during three stages of inflation, corresponding to the diagrams inserted below the figures: Uninflated (A); partly inflated (B); and fully inflated (C). (With permission from Goldstein and Campbell, Cardiology Clinics 1993; 11: 417.)

the stenotic mitral orifice is usually crossed relatively easily, in some instances the shape and orientation of the mitral annulus and orifice requires that the catheter be advanced at an angle from either the medial or lateral side. TEE can be helpful in properly orienting the catheter in situations in which crossing the stenotic orifice is difficult.

TEE can also assist the optimal orientation of the balloon catheter in the mitral orifice before and during dilatation (Figure 6). The unique "self-seating" design of the Inoue balloon generally reduces the need for TEE [1]. However, because of the 5.5 cm length of the double balloons, care must be taken to avoid positioning the proximal end of the dilating balloon in the atrial septum at the time of inflation. Inadvertent dilatation of the atrial septum may result [4, 36, 37]. This problem can be recognized by TEE and corrected by slight advancement of the catheter. In addition, TEE monitoring can detect failure to deflate the balloon fully before withdrawal, which can result in the creation of a large defect in the atrial septum [38].

The ability of TEE-guidance to detect and minimize the presence of catheters and wires in the LAA and the pulmonary veins may be even more important. Guide-wires and catheters often enter the LAA during their manipulation. This is usually not appreciated by fluoroscopy, but is readily detected by TEE. Therefore, TEE imaging can potentially prevent dislodgement of a thrombus or perforation of the atrial wall. In addition, entry of catheters and guide-wires into one of the left pulmonary veins may appear on fluoroscopy to lie across the mitral orifice in a position suitable for dilatation, when, in fact, TEE demonstrates the catheter to be located in the left upper pulmonary vein.

Immediate assessment of results

During PBMV, one or multiple balloon inflations are performed until satisfactory results are obtained. On-line TEE during the procedure is ideally suited for immediate assessment of the hemodynamic results after each balloon inflation. Adequacy of the dilatation can be determined by evaluating the maximal mitral leaflet separation (Figure 7) and by continuous-wave Doppler determination of mean mitral gradient and mitral valve area (by pressure half-time method). New or worsening mitral regurgitation is dectable by color Doppler. It is also possible to reassess pulmonary venous flow (Figure 8) which is expected to show a more rapid diastolic deceleration after successful PBMV [39, 40].

Several investigators have pointed out that immediately after PBMV,

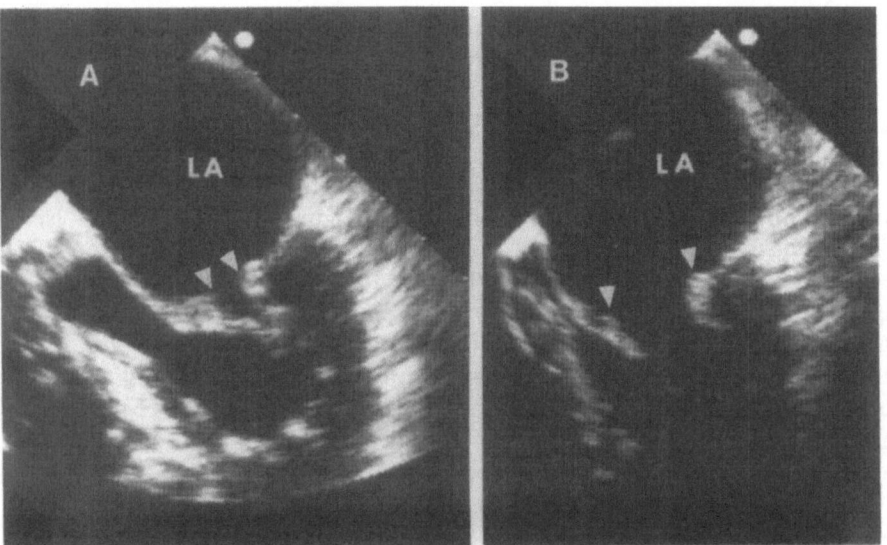

Figure 7. Left panel (A): Pre-percutaneous mitral valvuloplasty (PRE-PTMV) image illustrates fused mitral leaflet tips and narrow orifice (arrows) prior to balloon dilatation. Right panel (B): POST-PTMV illustrates increased leaflet separation after successful balloon valvuloplasty.

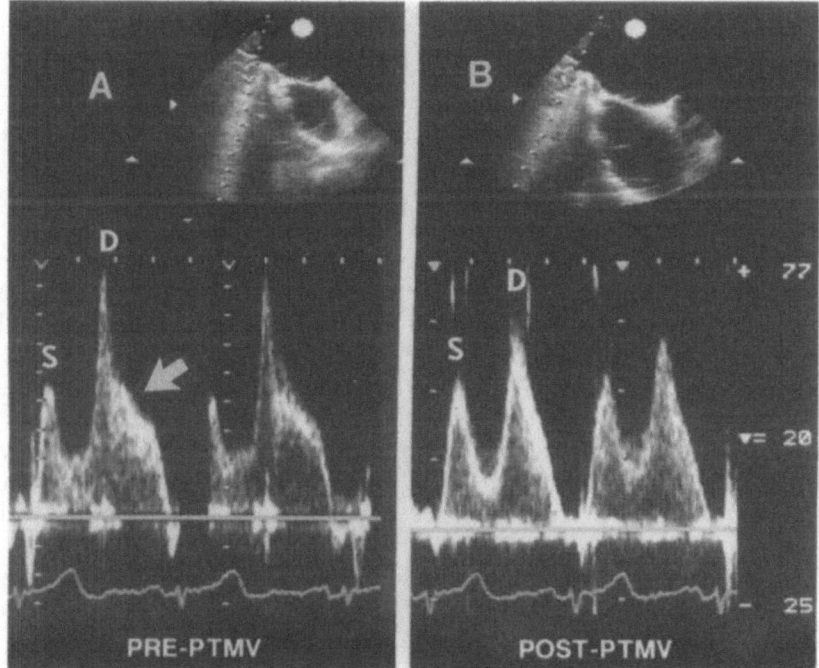

Figure 8. Left panel (A): PRE-PTMV illustrates the typical pulmonary venous flow pattern of mitral stenosis with delayed diastolic deceleration (arrow). Right panel (B): POST-PTMV shows a more rapid deceleration consistent with successful balloon valvuloplasty. S = systole; D = diastole.

evaluation of these results should be interpreted with caution, because their correlation with catheter-derived measurements of mean gradient and valve area is reduced [41–44]. This discrepancy may be related in part to acute alterations in left atrial and left ventricular compliance. It may also be related to mitral valve "recoil" [14, 45, 46], but the role of this phenomenon is unclear. Despite these limitations, decisions about the adequacy of the procedure versus the need for further dilatations can be aided by this data.

When the procedure is deemed satisfactory, all wires and catheters are removed, and several final aspects are examined. Trivial atrial septal defects due to the atrial septostomy are almost always present. Because the hole is usually small and because left atrial pressure in these patients is high, these small left-to-right shunting jets are easily detected by TEE color Doppler. It is well-recognized that the majority of these small defects close over time [6, 11, 21]. Lastly, one looks for a pericardial effusion before removing the probe.

Early detection of complications

Although uncommon, serious complications do occur with PBMV. The majority of these (e.g., severe mitral regurgitation, cardiac perforation and tamponade, and significant atrial septal defect) can be accurately and quickly detected by on-line TEE during the procedure. The rapid identification of these complications facilitates proper management and can help prevent unnecessary clinical deterioration due to delays in appropriate therapy.

Listed in Table 2 are complications from several large series (each with at least 100 patients). An increase in the degree of mitral regurgitation (MR) occurs in approximately half of patients after PBMV [1, 3, 6, 8, 41, 56]. In most, this increase is mild, but the reported incidence of severe MR is 1% to 7% [5, 7–9, 30, 47–55]. At the institution of the author more than 3 + /4 MR was detected in 4/105 (4%). Acute, severe MR may be caused by tear or rupture of the mitral leaflets, by ruptured chordae tendinae, or rarely, by avulsion of a papillary muscle [52, 57]. Each of these can be detected by TEE. Moreover, the presence and severity of MR can be determined without the need for left ventriculography.

The incidence of cardiac tamponade during PBMV has been reported to be between 0 and 9% [7, 9, 47–55, 58–61]. Perforation of the atrial wall at the time of transseptal puncture is the most common cause of bleeding into the pericardial space [11, 61]. On-line TEE can lead to rapid detection and treatment of this potentially life-threatening complication (Figure 9).

The reported incidence of atrial septal defect resulting from PBMV is

Table 2. Serious complications after percutaneous balloon mitral valvuloplasty.

Study group	No.	Mortality (%)	Embolism (%)	Severe MR (%)	Tamponade (%)	Reference
Hopital Tenon, Paris	200	0	4.0	4.0	3.0	8
Kochi, Japan	106	0	0	4.7	1.9	7
Loma Linda, California	407	1.2	1.0	7.2	0.75	47
Massachusetts General Hospital, Boston	250	1.0	1.0	1.0	1.0	48
Beth Israel Hospital Boston	146	0.7	2.0	1.5	4.1	49
Inoue	527	0	0.6	1.9	1.5	50
Cordoba, Spain	288	2.8	1.1	6.3	2.8	51
Besancon, France	232	NR	6.5	4.7	1.4	52
Taiwan, Republic of China	219	0.5	1.4	6.0	0	9
NHLBI Registry	738	1.1	2.2	3.3	3.6	53
Belgrade, Yugoslavia	294	0.7	2.4	2.3	1.7	54
Athens, Greece	200	0.5	0	3.5	0	55

MR = mitral regurgitation; NR = not reported; NHLBI = National Heart, Lung and Blood Institute.

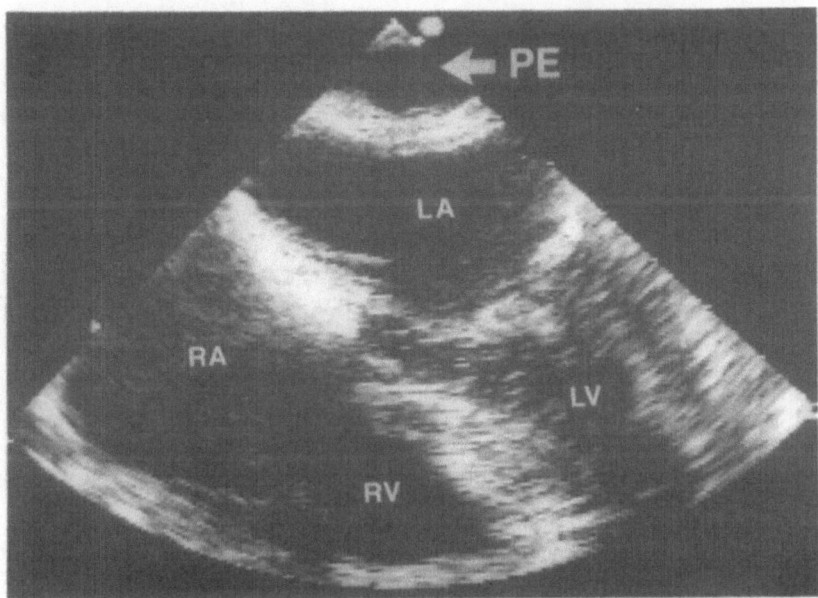

Figure 9. Pericardial effusion (PE, arrow) complicating PBMV invaginates the left atrial (LA) wall in this patient with mitral stenosis. The effusion was recognized immediately by TEE, evacuated successfully and safely in the cath lab, and the patient underwent successful PBMV several weeks later. RA = right atrium; RV = right ventricle; LV = left ventricle.

highly variable depending on the technique used for its detection [8, 13, 14, 47, 48, 51–55, 62]. Using on line TEE immediately after PBMV, an atrial septal defect was detected in 88% of patients [18]. The creation of a small atrial septal defect (ASD) should be considered an expected consequence rather than a true complication in the majority of patients. Most result in a QP/QS ratio of less than 1.5/1 [1, 3, 6, 8] and are clinically well-tolerated. Moreover, hemodynamic and echocardiographic studies have demonstrated that 50 to 95% of the atrial septal defects created by PBMV close spontaneously within 6 to 12 months [1, 9, 10, 12–14, 63]. We found a jet width greater than 5 mm in only 3/93 (3%) and these defects are considered to be large [18].

The incidence of clinically detected systemic embolism is approximately 1 to 6% (Table 2). The role of TEE in screening patients before PBMV to detect left atrial thrombi has already been discussed. However, the potential mechanisms for systemic embolization include not only dislodgement of preformed thrombi in the LA/left atrial appendage, but also embolism of valve material/debris, disruption of atheromatous debris in the aorta, thrombus formation on intravascular devices (catheters and wires) during the procedure, and air embolism [8, 52]. Using continuous on-line TEE, a surprisingly

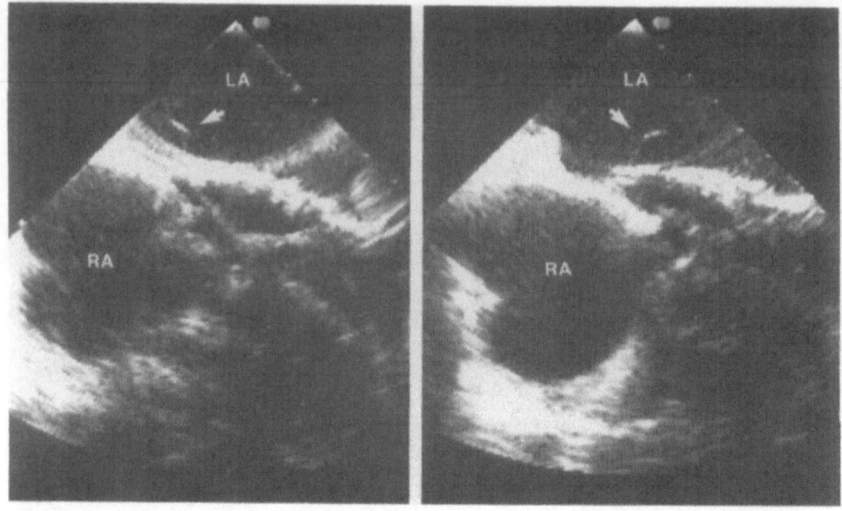

Figure 10. Arrows point to a small, mobile, filamentous thrombus attached to a catheter in the left atrium (LA). RA = right atrium. (With permission from Goldstein and Campbell, Cardiology Clinics 1993; 11: 415.)

high prevalence (59%) of catheter-related thrombi can be detected during PBMV [16, 64] (Figure 10). Despite the presence of thrombi on catheters in the left atrium, no clinical embolic events occurred. However, when thrombi are detected in the LA, supplemental heparin should be given.

Summary

Percutaneous transvenous balloon mitral valvuloplasty is normally performed with fluoroscopic guidance. However, even the experienced operator can be misled by radiographic landmarks. TEE has a number of unique advantages that make it a useful adjunct to fluoroscopic guidance and monitoring of patients during PBMV, including a) high quality images (especially of the atrial septum and surrounding structures which can facilitate transseptal catheterization), b) ability to image continuously without interfering with or interrupting the procedure, c) reduction in X-ray radiation time, d) immediate assessment of results, and e) immediate detection of complications. Finally, TEE during PBMV is feasible, safe, and well-tolerated by awake patients.

Acknowledgements

The author wishes to thank Drs Joseph Lindsay Jr and Gary S. Mintz for their helpful review of this manuscript. The author also wishes to thank Pushpa Gulati for her expert assistance in preparing this manuscript.

References

1. Inoue K, Owaki T, Nakamuara T et al. Clinical application of transvenous mitral commissurotomy by a new balloon catheter. J Thorac Cardiovasc Surg 1984; 87: 394–402.
2. Zaibag MA, Kasab SA, Ribeiro PA, Fagih MRA. Percutaneous double balloon mitral valvotomy for rheumatic mitral valve stenosis. Lancet 1986; 1: 757–61.
3. Palacios I, Block PC, Brandi S et al. Percutaneous balloon mitral valvotomy for patients with severe mitral stenosis. Circulation 1987; 75: 778–84.
4. McKay CR, Kawanishi DT, Rahimtoola SH. Catheter balloon valvuloplasty of the mitral valve in adults using a double-balloon technique. Early hemodynamic results. JAMA 1987; 257: 1753–61.
5. Ruiz CE, Allen JW, Lau FYK. Percutaneous double balloon valvotomy for severe rheumatic mitral stenosis. Am J Cardiol 1990; 65: 473–7.
6. Palacios IF, Block P, Wilkins GT, Weyman AE. Follow-up of patients undergoing percutaneous mitral balloon valvotomy. Analysis of factors determining restenosis. Circulation 1989; 79: 573–9.
7. Nobuyoshi M, Hamasaki, N, Kimura T et al. Indications, complications, and short-term clinical outcome of percutaneous transvenous mitral commissurotomy. Circulation 1989; 80: 782–92.
8. Vahanian A, Michel PL, Cormier B et al. Results of percutaneous mitral commissurotomy in 200 patients. Am J Cardiol 1989; 63: 847–52.
9. Hung JS, Chern MS, Wu JJ et al. Short and long-term results of catheter balloon percutaneous transvenous mitral commissurotomy. Am J Cardiol 1991; 67: 854–62.
10. Block PC, Palacios IF, Block EH et al. Late (two-year) follow-up after percutaneous balloon mitral valvotomy. Am J Cardiol 1992; 69: 537–41.
11. Desideri A, Vanderperren O, Serra A et al. Long-term (9 to 33 months) echocardiographic follow-up after successful percutaneous mitral commissurotomy. Am J Cardiol 1992; 69: 1602–6.
12. Tuzcu EM, Block PC, Griffin BP et al. Immediate and long-term outcome of percutaneous mitral valvotomy in patients 65 years and older. Circulation 1992; 85: 963–71.
13. Patel JJ, Sharma D, Mithu AS et al. Balloon valvuloplasty versus closed commissurotomy for pliable mitral stenosis: A prospective hemodynamic study. J Am Coll Cardiol 1991; 18: 1318–22.
14. Turi ZG, Reyes VP, Raju BS et al. Percutaneous balloon versus surgical closed commissurotomy for mitral stenosis. A prospective, randomized trial. Circulation 1991; 83: 1179–85.
15. Milner MR, Goldstein SA, Lindsay J et al. Transesophageal echocardiographic guidance for percutaneous balloon mitral valvuloplasty (Abstr). Circulation 1990; 82 (Suppl III): 81.
16. Campbell AN, Hong MK, Pichard AD et al. Routine transesophageal echocardiographic guidance is useful during percutaneous transvenous mitral valvuloplasty (Abstr). J Am Soc Echocadiogr 1992; 5: 330.
17. Goldstein SA, Campbell AN. Mitral stenosis: Evaluation and guidance of valvuloplasty by transesophageal echocardigoraphy. Cardiol Clinics 1993; 11: 409–25.
18. Goldstein SA, Campbell AC, Mintz GS et al. Feasibility of on-line transesophageal echocardiography during balloon mitral valvulotomy: Experience with 93 patients. J Heart Valve Dis 1994; 3: 136–48.

19. Wilkins GT, Weyman AE, Abascal VM et al. Percutaneous balloon dilation of the mitral valve: An analysis of echocardiographic variables related to outcome and the mechanism of dilatation. Br Heart J 1988; 60: 299–308.

20. Abascal VM, Wilkins GT, O'Shea JP et al. Prediction of successful outcome in 130 patients undergoing percutaneous balloon mitral valvotomy. Circulation 1990; 82: 448–56.

21. Cormier B, Vahanian A, Michel Pl et al. Transesophageal echocardiography in the assessment of percutaneous mitral commissurotomy. Eur Heart J 1991; 12 (Suppl B): 61–5.

22. Marwick TH, Torelli J, Obarski T et al. Assessment of the mitral valve splitability score by transthoracic and transesophageal echocardiography. Am J Cardiol 1991; 68: 1106–7.

23. Levin TN, Feldman T, Bednarz J et al. Transesophageal echocardiographic evaluation of mitral valve morphology to predict outcome after balloon mitral valvotomy. Am J Cardiol 1994; 73: 707–10.

24. Hutchinson SJ, Smalling RG, Ma A et al. Transthoracic and transesophageal echocardiography pre and post percutaneous mitral catheter balloon valvotomy. J Heart Valve Dis 1994; 3: 149–54.

25. Thomas MR, Monaghan MJ, Smyth DW et al. Comparative value of transthoracic and transesophageal echocardiography before balloon dilatation of the mitral valve. Br Heart J 1992; 68: 493–7.

26. Rittoo D, Sutherland GR, Currie P et al. The comparative value of transesophageal and transthoracic echocardiography before and after percutaneous mitral balloon valvotomy: A prospective study. Am Heart J 1993; 125: 1094–105.

27. Aschenberg W, Schluter M, Kremer P et al. Transesophageal two-dimensional echocardiography for the detection of left atrial appendage thrombus. J Am Coll Cardiol 1986; 7: 163–6.

28. Kronzon I, Tunick PA, Glassman E et al. Transesophageal echocardiography to detect atrial clots in candidates for percutaneous transseptal mitral balloon valvuloplasty. J Am Coll Cardiol 1990; 16: 1320–2.

29. Casale PN, Whitlow P, Currie PJ, Stewart WJ. Transesophageal echocardiography in percutaneous balloon valvuloplasty for mitral stenosis. Cleve Clin J Med 1989; 56: 597–600.

30. Chan KL, Marquis JF, Ascah C et al. Role of transesophageal echocardiography in percutaneous balloon mitral valvuloplasty. Echocardiography 1990; 7: 115–23.

31. Manning WJ, Reis GJ, Douglas PS. Use of transesophageal echocardiography to detect left atrial thrombi before percutaneous balloon dilatation of the mitral valve: A prospective study. Br Heart J 1992; 67: 170–3.

32. Robertson JM, de Virgilio C, French W et al. Fatal left ventricular perforation using mitral balloon valvuloplasty. Ann Thorac Surg 1990; 49: 819–21.

33. Shawl FA, Domanski MJ, Yackee JM et al. Left ventricular rupture complicating percutaneous mitral commissurotomy: Salvage using percutaneous cardiopulmonary bypass support. Cathet Cardiovasc Diagn 1990; 21: 26–7.

34. Baim DS, Grossman W. Percutaneous approach and transseptal catheterization. In: Grossman W, editor. Cardiac catheterization and angiography, 3rd ed. Philadelphia: Lea and Febiger, 1974: 59–75.

35. Sheikh KH, Davidson CJ, Skelton TN et al. Interatrial thickening preventing percutaneous mitral valve balloon valvuloplasty. Am Heart J 1989; 117: 206–10.

36. Palacios IF, Lock JE, Keane JF, Block PC. Percutaneous transvenous balloon valvotomy in a patient with severe calcific mitral stenosis. J Am Coll Cardiol 1986; 7: 1416–9.

37. Nishimura RA, Holmes DR, Reeder GS. Efficacy of percutaneous mitral balloon valvuloplasty with the Inoue balloon. Mayo Clin Proc 1991; 66: 276–82.

38. Fields CD, Isner JM. Size of atrial septostomy resulting from transseptal delivery of balloon catheters used for mitral valvuloplasty (Abstr). Circulation 1988; 78 (Suppl II): 488.

39. Keren A, Pardes A, Miller HI et al. Pulmonary venous flow determined by Doppler echocardiography in mitral stenosis. Am J Cardiol 1990; 65: 246–9.

40. Klein Al, Bailey AS, Cohen GI et al. Effects of mitral stenosis on pulmonary venous flow

as measured by Doppler transesophageal echocardiography. Am J Cardiol 1993; 72: 66–72.

41. Abascal VM, Wilkins GI, Choong CY et al. Echocardiographic evaluation of mitral valve structure and function in patients followed for at least 6 months after percutaneous balloon mitral valvuloplasty. J Am Coll Cardiol 1988; 12: 606–15.

42. Come PC, Riley MF, Diver DJ et al. Noninvasive assessment of mitral stenosis before and after percutaneous balloon mitral valvuloplasty. Am J Cardiol 1988; 61: 817–25.

43. Reid CL, McKay CR, Chandraratna PAN et al. Mechanisms of increase in mitral valve area and influence of anatomic features in double-balloon, catheter balloon valvuloplasty in adults with rheumatic mitral stenosis: A Doppler and two-dimensional echocardiographic study. Circulation 1987; 76: 628–36.

44. Thomas JD, Wilkins GT, Choong CYP et al. Inaccuracy of mitral pressure half-time immediately after percutaneous mitral valvotomy. Circulation 1988; 78: 980–93.

45. Nabel E, Bergin PJ, Kirsh MM. Morphologic analysis of balloon mitral valvuloplasty: Intraoperative results (Abstr). J Am Coll Cardiol 1990; 15: 97A.

46. Nakatani S, Nagata S, Beppu S et al. Acute reduction of mitral valve area after percutaneous balloon mitral valvuloplasty. Assessment with Doppler continuity equation. Am Heart J 1991; 121: 770–5.

47. Ruiz, CE, Zhang HP, Macaya C et al. Comparison of Inoue single-balloon versus double-balloon technique for percutaneous mitral valvotomy. Am Heart J 1992; 123: 942–7.

48. Block PC, Palacios IF. Aortic and mitral balloon valvuloplasty: The United States experience. In: Topol EJ, editor. Textbook of international cardiology. Philadelphia: WB Saunders, 1990: 845.

49. Cohen DJ, Kuntz RE, Gordon SPF et al. Predictors of long-term outcome after percutaneous balloon mitral valvuloplasty. N Engl J Med 1992; 327: 1329–35.

50. Inoue K, Hung JS. Percutaneous transvenous mitral commissurotomy (PTMC): The Far East experience. In: Topol EJ, editor. Textbook of international cardiology. Philadelphia: WB Saunders, 1990: 897.

51. Cequier A, Nonan R, Serra A et al. Left-to-right atrial shunting after percutaneous mitral valvuloplasty: Incidence and long-term hemodynamic follow-up. Circulation 1990; 81: 1190–7.

52. Bassand JP, Schiele F, Bernard Y et al. The double balloon and Inoue techniques in percutaneous mitral valvuloplasty: Comparative results in a series of 232 cases. J Am Coll Cardiol 1991; 18: 982–9.

53. Report from the NHLBI Balloon Valvuloplasty Registry. Complications and mortality of percutaneous balloon mitral commissurotomy. Circulation 1992; 85: 2014–24.

54. Babic UU, Grujicic S, Popovic Z et al. Percutaneous transarterial balloon dilatation of the mitral valve: Five year experience. Br Heart J 1992; 67: 185–9.

55. Stefanadis C, Toutouzas P. Balloon mitral valvuloplasty: Where are we now? J Invasc Cardiol 1993; 5: 203–11.

56. Abascal VM, Wilkins GT, Choong CY et al. Mitral regurgitation after percutaneous mitral valvuloplasty in adults: Evaluation by pulsed Doppler echocardiography. J Am Coll Cardiol 1987; 11: 257–63.

57. Waksmonski CA, McKay RG. Echocardiographic diagnosis of valve disruption following percutaneous balloon valvuloplasty. Echocardiography 1989; 6: 277–81.

58. Block PC. Early results of mitral balloon valvuloplasty for mitral stenosis: Report from the NHLBI registry. Circulation 1988; 78 (Suppl II): 489.

59. Hermann HC, Kleaveland P, Hill JA et al. The M-Heart percutaneous balloon mitral valvuloplasty registry: Initial results and early follow-up. J Am Coll Cardiol 1990; 15: 1221–6.

60. Pan M, Medina A, de Lezo JS et al. Balloon mitral valvuloplasty for mild mitral stenosis. Cathet Cardiovasc Diagn 1991; 24: 1–5.

61. Pan M, Medina A, de Lezo JS et al. Cardiac tamponade complicating mitral balloon valvuloplasty. Am J Cardiol 1991; 68: 802–5.

62. Rittoo D, Sutherland GR, Shaw TRD. Quantification of left-to-right atrial shunting and defect size after balloon mitral commissurotomy using biplane transesophageal echocardiography, color flow Doppler mapping, and the principle of proximal flow convergence. Circulation 1993; 87: 1591–1603.
63. Nigri A, Alessandri N, Martuscelli E et al. Clinical significance of small left-to-right shunts after percutaneous mitral valvuloplasty. Am Heart J 1993; 125: 783–6.
64. Milner MR, Goldstein SA, Pichard AD et al. Transesophageal echocardiographic detection of transseptal catheter-related thrombi in patients with mitral stenosis (Abstr). J Am Coll Cardiol 1991; 17: 261A.

Corresponding Author: Dr Steven A. Goldstein, Washington Hospital Center, 110 Irving St, NW, Washington, DC 20010, USA

28. Echocardiography for intraprocedural monitoring and postinterventional follow-up of mitral balloon valvuloplasty

LIANGLONG CHEN, LINDA GILLAM, RAYMOND MCKAY
and CHUNGUANG CHEN

Introduction

Since first introduced in 1982 [1], percutaneous balloon mitral valvuloplasty (PMV) has been widely performed to relieve mitral stenosis, and in many instances, as an alternative to cardiac surgery [2–4]. Two-dimensional and Doppler echocardiography with the ability to assess mitral valvular and subvalvular structures and their function is routinely used to help select candidates for mitral balloon valvuloplasty, to evaluate immediate results and to follow up mid- and long-term results of this procedure [5–7]. In this chapter, we will briefly review current applications of conventional transthoracic echocardiography and transesophageal echocardiography for intraprocedural monitoring and postinterventional follow-up of mitral balloon valvuloplasty.

Intraprocedural monitoring by echocardiography

Currently, percutaneous mitral balloon valvuloplasty is performed at the cardiac catheterization laboratory with X-ray fluoroscopy guidance and hemodynamic monitoring [2–4]. Neither transthoracic echocardiography (TTE) nor transesophageal echocardiography (TEE) is routinely used at the cardiac catheterization laboratory to monitor patients. However, if there is any suspicion of severe complications of the procedure, such as cardiac perforation and severe mitral regurgitation, transthoracic echocardiography is very sensitive for detecting such complications and can be performed to confirm clinical suspicions during valvuloplasty procedure.

The lack of the routine use of conventional echocardiography during valvuloplasty procedure is probably due to additional cost imposed on the procedure and technical inconvenience. However, if the valvuloplasty procedure can be performed in a safer, and more effective manner with improved short-term and long-term results with the addition of echocardiographic monitoring, which could reduce later repeated interventional procedures

C.A. Nienaber and U. Sechtem (eds): Imaging and Intervention in Cardiology. 459–469.

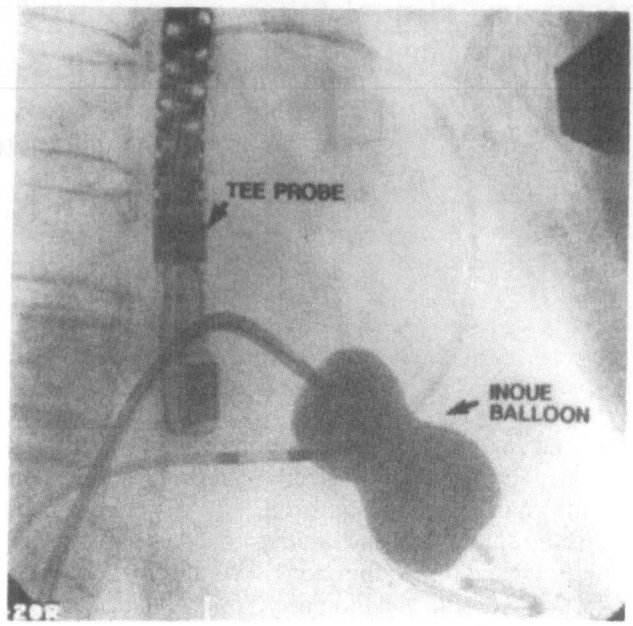

Figure 1. This fluoroscopic image shows an example of intraprocedural transesophageal echocardiography (TEE) for monitoring mitral valvuloplasty procedure. Note that the TEE probe is in the mid esophagus to monitor the balloon inflation (Inoue Balloon). (Adopted from: Goldstein, Campbell. Cardiology Clinics 1993; 11: 409–25 [8].)

and/or surgical valve replacement, the overall long-term cost may be reduced with improvement in the quality of care. Conventional echocardiography is technically limited in the cardiac catheterization laboratory due to restrained supine position of the patient and limited access of echocardiographic windows with possible interference of the sterile catheterization field.

Transesophageal echocardiography introduces the ultrasound imaging transducer with a flexible endoscopic tube in the esophagus/stomach (Figure 1) and is able to continuously monitor cardiac and great vessel structures and function with better imaging resolution and quality without interfering or interrupting the catheterization procedure during the valvuloplasty procedure. Therefore, transesophageal echocardiography has theoretical advantages over conventional transthoracic echocardiography for intraprocedural monitoring in the cardiac catheterization laboratory.

Several centers have investigated feasibility and clinical value of transesophageal echocardiography and intracardiac echocardiography for the intraoperative monitoring of the valvuloplasty procedure [8–11]. Goldstein et al. [8] reported experience of TEE monitoring of 80 consecutive awake patients during mitral balloon valvuloplasty (Figure 1). With mild sedation by intravenous meperidine (20–50 mg) and diazepam (1–5 mg), all patients tolerated TEE monitoring well without major complications. Other authors reported similar experiences both in awake and anesthetized patients [9–11]. Therefore, it appears that TEE is feasible and safe in intraprocedural monitoring of the valvuloplasty procedure.

However, the clinical value of TEE in intraoperative monitoring is not well established. More detailed and accurate assessment of mitral valve and subvalvular structures may help to select patients for successful valvuloplasty and avoid major complications such as severe mitral regurgitation. At the current stage, transesophageal echocardiography does not appear to provide additional information on morphological characteristics of the mitral valve and the subvalvular structures that lead to improved results of valvuloplasty and reduced complications if an adequate quality of transthoracic echocardiogram is already available. Cormier et al. [12] compared TTE and TEE for selecting candidates for mitral valvuloplasty in 110 patients and found that the two modalities were of equal value in assessing leaflet mobility, calcification, and subvalvular disease. Their results suggested that TEE is not more accurate than TTE in assessing anatomy of the mitral valvular and subvalvular apparatus. In their study, Marwick et al. [13] reported that there is no significant difference between TTE and TEE for evaluating valve thickness and mobility but that TEE may underestimate subvalvular disease and calcification due to shielding of the subvalvular structure by the thickened and calcified mitral valve leaflets. Neither the valve orifice nor the degree of commissural fusion appears to be adequately assessed by TEE using a monoplane probe [14]. Furthermore, detailed assessment of subvalvular thickening, shortening, and fusion is usually best achieved with TTE and often requires a modified parasternal long axis view [8, 14]. With TEE, the subvalvular structures are in the far field as the ultrasound beam transverses the enlarged LA. Moreover, the echocardiographic beam is attenuated in part by the thickened and often calcified mitral valve and annulus. Nevertheless, in patients with inadequate quality of conventional transthoracic echocardiography, the transesophageal technique is certainly an alternative complementary approach for assessment of mitral morphology.

Using biplane transesophageal echocardiography, an improved assessment of mitral valve and subvalvular structure may be achieved. Fraser et al. [15] examined 8 hearts from patients who died of noncardiac disease with biplane transesophageal two-dimensional echocardiography in transverse and longitudinal transesophageal equivalent planes. They observed that the transverse plane of the esophageal approach could image the anterolateral commissure and the adjacent leaflets and the longitudinal plane was ideally aligned for studying the posteromedial commissure and medial thirds of the leaflets. Since the commissures of the mitral valve are not linear, transthoracic imaging may be limited by the restricted windows. Thus, the transesophageal biplane approach appears to have advantages in detailed noninvasive assessment of mitral commissure and valve morphology [14, 15]. With careful manipulation, the longitudinal plane of the TEE can sometimes provide excellent visualization of mitral subvalvular apparatus. With technical development, multi-plane transesophageal echocardiography may have advantages over TTE. This awaits further investigation.

It is well established that transesophageal echocardiography is more sensitive than conventional echocardiography in detecting left atrial thrombus, especially in the atrial appendage [16]. Conventionally, presence of atrial thrombus is considered a contraindication for balloon mitral valvuloplasty. However, mitral balloon valvuloplasty has been performed safely in patients with thrombus in left atrial appendage when catheters were carefully manipulated to avoid entering the atrial appendage [17]. In some large centers, mitral balloon valvuloplasty has been performed safely with careful TTE examination without routine TEE for pre- or intraoperative assessment to rule out atrial appendage thrombus [2, 7]. Therefore, large series of patients should be investigated to determine whether TEE should be performed preoperatively or intraoperatively to rule out thrombus in the atrial appendage.

The use of transesophageal echocardiography has been reported to guide the transeptal catheterization procedure [8–11, 18]. The interatrial septum, particularly that of the oval fossa, commonly presents a thin, clear-cut, well-defined area and can be visualized by transesophageal echocardiography. When the tip of the transseptal needle reaches the atrial septum and some pressure is applied, the atrial septum changes its shape to a triangular configuration and tents or bulges toward the left atrium (see Figure 3 in the previous chapter) [8, 11, 18]. In a study of 15 patients undergoing mitral balloon valvuloplasty with general anesthesia, Visser et al. [18] showed that in 2 cases this monitoring was necessary to guide appropriate positioning of the transseptal puncture device. More recently, Goldstein et al. [8] reported that TEE guided transseptal punctures in 80 consecutive patients undergoing balloon mitral valvuloplasty. They confirmed that recognition of the tenting sign (Figure 2) of the atrial septum as advancing the transseptal needle contacted the atrial septum was extremely important. They also found that accurately locating the tip of the transseptal needle requires operator's experience with careful manipulation of the TEE probe. The longitudinal plane appears an important complimentary plane for visualizing the transseptal needle. However, in most centers, experienced operators usually have no difficulty with the transseptal puncture under X-ray fluoroscopy. Nevertheless, significant dilatation of the right atrium may change radiographic anatomic landmarks and make the transseptal puncture complicated [8]. In these cases, TEE monitoring may be helpful.

Another potential use of TEE may be to guide the positioning of the balloon catheter through the mitral valve to avoid unsuccessful inflation of the balloon catheters (see Figure 6 in the previous chapter) [8, 14]. It has also been demonstrated that transesophageal monitoring shortens the X-ray exposure time during valvuloplasty [10]. Transesophageal echocardiography provides an on-table (catheterization table) assessment of commissural separation and complications including pericardial effusion by cardiac perforation, severe mitral regurgitation with mitral leaflet tear or rupture of chordae tendinae [8–14, 19, 20]. TEE is also more sensitive for detecting atrial septal defects (ASD) created by transseptal catheterization although this type of small ASD usually closes spontaneously (see the follow-up section).

The incidence of cardiac tamponade during percutaneous balloon mitral valvuloplasty has been reported to be 4% in large series [20]. Intraprocedural cardiac tamponade is often due to cardiac perforation by the transseptal needle entering the aortic root, atrial free wall or by guide wire or tip of the balloon catheter perforating the left ventricle. TEE monitoring can rapidly detect this life-threatening complication.

TEE can provide immediate assessment of the increase in mitral valve area by balloon valvuloplasty. Although the increase in mitral valve area can be assessed by hemodynamic data, in the presence of severe tricuspid regurgitation or significant iatrogenic atrial septal defect, the thermodilution technique of measurement of cardiac output may be misleading and may result in an error of calculation of the mitral valve area. In this case, two-dimensional echocardiographic planimetery of mitral valve area in the parasternal short-axis view may be helpful [5–7]. Recently, color Doppler jet widths from two orthogonal planes intersecting the major and minor axis of the oval mitral orifice have been shown to accurately predict mitral valve area [21]. Biplane TEE can provide two such orthogonal planes for calculating mitral valve area and may be useful in intraprocedural assessment of adequacy of mitral orifice size (Figure 2).

Therefore, transesophageal echocardiography is certainly a complimentary to fluoroscopy and hemodynamic monitoring, providing important additional information during valvuloplasty. However, whether these additional data provided by intraoperative TEE monitoring can translate into improvement of immediate and long-term results, and reduction in procedural complications has not been documented and requires further investigation.

Echocardiography in follow-up of patients after valvuloplasty

Being noninvasive, convenient and readily available, conventional transthoracic echocardiography is an ideal tool for repeat assessment of results and complications of valvuloplasty including mitral valve area, presence and severity of mitral regurgitation, and iatrogenic atrial septal defect after mitral balloon valvuloplasty.

Mitral valve area

Immediately after successful valvuloplasty, the morphology of the mitral valve, as seen using two-dimensional echocardiography, frequently changes with great improvement of motion of mitral valve with some degree of

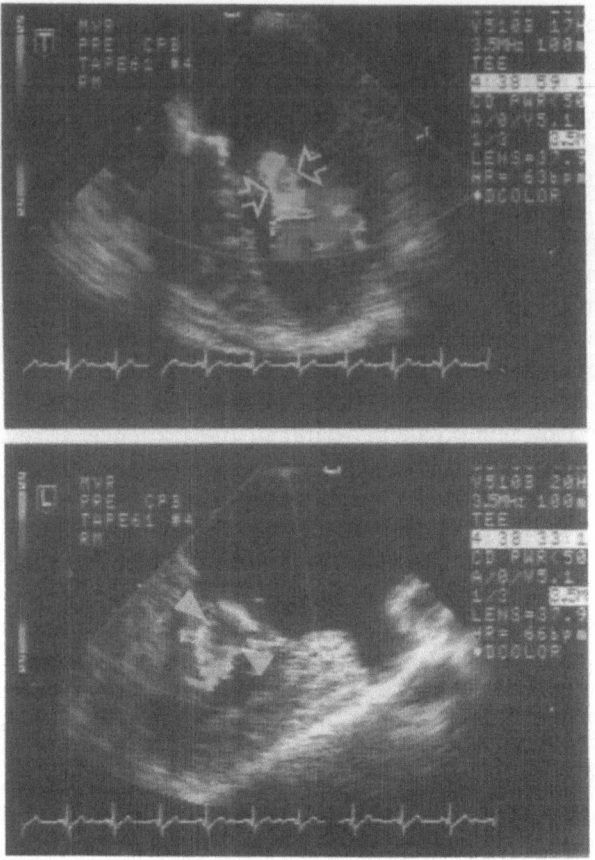

Figure 2. An example of biplane color Doppler transesophageal echocardiographic (TEE) assessment of severity of mitral stenosis with the use of stenotic jet widths from two orthogonal planes. Note that the stenotic jet width (JW_1, indicated by open arrows) from a TEE horizontal plane at the top is smaller than the jet width (JW_2, indicated by arrow heads) from a vertical TEE plane at the bottom. The mitral valve area is calculated by assuming an oval mitral orifice: $\pi \times JW_1/2 \times JW_2/2$. (For colour plate of this figure see **page 540.**)

residual doming and restriction. Obvious increase of mitral valve area can be appreciated by planimetry of the mitral valve orifice from the two-dimensional parasternal short-axis view [6, 7]. With continuous wave Doppler, mitral inflow velocity profile can be recorded and used to calculate peak and mean pressure gradient across mitral valve. The descending slope of mitral inflow velocity profile can be used to determine pressure half-time ($T_{1/2}$, time required for mitral gradient to fall to its half value). Pressure half-time has been used to estimate mitral valve area with convenience and accuracy both in native and prosthetic valves. However, pressure half-time has been reported to be less reliable and accurate for estimation of mitral valve area immediately (within 24 hours) after mitral valvuloplasty [22] because pressure half-time is not only related to mitral valve area but also critically dependent on net atrioventricular compliance and peak transmitral pressure gradient:

$$T_{1/2} = 11.6 \, C_n \, \Delta p_0^{1/2} / (C_c MVA)$$

where $T_{1/2}$ is pressure half-time, C_n is net atrio-ventricular compliance, Δp_0 is the initial peak gradient, C_c is coefficient of orifice and MVA is the mitral valve area [21]. Dramatic changes in left atrial and ventricular compliance and decrease in initial peak mitral valve gradient render $T_{1/2}$ an unreliable measure of mitral valve area in the setting of acute mitral valvotomy. However, 24–48 hours after valvuloplasty, an accurate estimation of mitral valve area can be obtained by $T_{1/2}$ again [23]. Therefore, pressure half-time is recommended to be used for assessment of mitral valve area 24 hours after mitral valvuloplasty procedure.

Long-term results of mitral valvuloplasty are related to mitral valvular and subvalvular morphology assessed by two-dimensional echocardiography [5–7, 24, 25]. The echocardiography score for evaluating valvular and subvalvular structures and functions has been proposed for evaluating mitral valve pre-valvuloplasty [24]. Using this echocardiography score system, Palacios et al. [26] demonstrated that only 2 of 45 (4.4%) patients with echo score <8 had restenosis, whereas 7 of 10 (70%) patients with the echo score > 8 experienced restenosis at an average of 13 months follow-up. The patients with echocardiographic evidence of high echo score also had severe symptoms of New York Heart Association function class III–IV (42% of patients in NYHA classes III and IV) at follow-up. Nobuyoshi et al. [27] found a similar relationship between echocardiographic morphological features and results of mitral balloon valvuloplasty in 97 patients at short-term (9 ± 4 months) follow-up after valvuloplasty. In patients with pliable and semipliable mitral valves, both immediate and follow up results including symptomatic improvement, mitral valve area and incidence of mitral regurgitation were significantly better than those in patients with rigid valves [27]. In a preliminary report of 2–4 year clinical follow-up (mean 20 ± 1 months) in 320 patients after valvuloplasty, Palacios et al. [28] demonstrated that 80% of patients with echo score < 8 were free from total clinical events (death, mitral valve replacement and NYHA class III or IV). In contrast, 40% of patients with echo score more than 8 had at least one of these clinical events. The survival at follow-up period was 99% in patients with the echo score of less than 8 and 75% in patients with an echo score of greater than 8. Similar results were reported by other investigators [24, 25]. Cohen et al. [25] followed 146 patients up to 6 years and found that risk factors for early restenosis were echocardiographic score of > 8, left ventricular enddiastolic pressure > 10 mm Hg or NYHA functional class IV. Patients without any of these risk factors had a predicted five-year event free survival rate of 60–84%, whereas patients with two or three risk factors had a predicted five-year event free survival rate of only 13 to 41%.

Mitral regurgitation

Mild mitral regurgitation is often seen at the site of commissural split during post mitral valvuloplasty [19, 20, 24, 25, 29]. Severe mitral regurgitation occurred in 3% of 738 patients who underwent balloon mitral valvuloplasty according to the National Heart, Lung and Blood Institute Balloon Valvuloplasty Registry [20]. Acute severe mitral regurgitation is often due to tearing of a mitral leaflet or rupture of the chords and often requires surgical repair or replacement of the valve [20, 29]. Herrmann et al. [29] reported that during 9–66 month follow-up 71% of patients with severe mitral regurgitation were treated surgically. It is clear that severe mitral regurgitation increases mortality and morbidity after mitral valvuloplasty. Echocardiography with color Doppler technique is highly sensitive and specific for the detection of mitral regurgitation. Severity of mitral regurgitation after valvuloplasty can be estimated semi-quantitatively by pulsed wave Doppler and color Doppler methods. Two-dimensional echocardiography also provides information about mechanisms of mitral regurgitation after balloon mitral valvuloplasty and can be used to guide selection of a therapeutic options such as valve repair or replacement [19, 20, 24–29]. On echocardiogram, rupture of chordal apparatus is characterized by random movements of interrupted chords with loss of coaptation of the interrupted leaflet.

Mild to moderate mitral regurgitation developed in 25–40% of patients after mitral balloon valvuloplasty. Abascal et al. [30] showed that mitral regurgitation remained unchanged in 35% of patients, decreased at least by 1 degree in 55% of patients, and increased in 10% of patients in mitral regurgitation at 6-month follow-up. Pan et al. [31] followed 59 patients for one year after mitral valvuloplasty and found similar results. However, long-term effects of moderate mitral regurgitation on survival and event free survival of patients post valvuloplasty is still unknown.

Atrial septal defect

During mitral balloon valvuloplasty most operators use the transseptal approach to introduce balloon catheters through the stenotic mitral valve. It has been demonstrated in a canine study that persistence of a small (<5 mm) atrial septal defect was found after a transseptal puncture with a 7 mm catheter [1]. An iatrogenic atrial septal defect after mitral balloon valvuloplasty was reported to occur in about 87–98% of patients detected by TEE [8]. Although the interatrial shunt was often small (<1/1.5 of Qs/Qp), acute creation of an interatrial communication could theoretically be deleterious in patients with longstanding pulmonary hypertension secondary to mitral stenosis because the added volume overload in the right ventricle could theoretically lead to worsening hemodynamic consequences. An interatrial shunt may also hinder the accurate calculation of the mitral valve area using thermodilution cardiac output. Although an oxygen step-up of >7% of saturation or >2% of volume in the right atrium at cardiac catheterization is conventionally used to define an interatrial shunt, this technique is insensitive for small shunts, costly for follow-up of patients, and carries some risk of the common complications of an invasive technique. Two-dimensional echocardiography with color Doppler technique is very sensitive for detecting small ASDs and the consequences of a left-to-right shunt (right ventricular dilatation and paradoxical motion of interventricular septum) [32]. A moderate size (>1.0 cm) defect of the interatrial septum may be directly identified by two-dimensional echocardiography. However, a small atrial septal defect (<5 mm) after balloon mitral valvuloplasty may not be recognized by two-dimensional technique. Doppler techniques permit noninvasive evaluation of intracardiac blood flow velocity and direction and have a widely established record of accuracy in the detection and quantification of atrial septal defects. Come et al. [33] reported that an interatrial shunt was detected in 12/37 (32%) of patients after mitral valvuloplasty by contrast or pulse wave Doppler echocardiography or both and in 9/37 (24%) of patients by oximetry. Echocardiographic and oximetric diagnoses of the presence or absence of an atrial septal defect were concurrent in 30 patients. One patient with a shunt of Qp/Qs = 1.2 was not detected by echocardiography. Five patients with echocardiographic findings of a left-to-right shunt had no diagnostic oxygen step-up in the right heart. Thus, pulse wave Doppler and contrast echocardiography appear to be more sensitive for detecting small interatrial shunting [34]. Transesophageal color Doppler flow mapping has considerably enhanced detection of small interatrial left-to-right shunts. Using transesophageal color Doppler, Yoshida et al. [35] detected an atrial left-to-right shunting flow in 13/15 (87%) of patients, in 73% of patients and in 47% of patients at intervals of one day, one week and one month after balloon mitral valvuloplasty, respectively. Only 2/15 patients with a shunt detected by transesophageal echocardiography could be identified by transthoracic echocardiography at one day. However, the correlation between transesophageal color Doppler technique and other more sensitive techniques (such as indicator dilution curve technique) for detecting shunts has not been tested. From available data, it appears that a small shunt has no significant hemodynamic impact during long-term follow-up and most of the atrial septal defects (about two thirds) created intraprocedurally close spontaneously within 6 to 12 months [8, 34–36].

References

1. Inoue K, Owani T, Nakamura F, Miyamoto N. Clinical application of transvenous mitral commissurotomy by a new balloon catheter. J Thorac Cardiovasc Surg 1984; 87: 394–9.
2. Palacios I, Block PC, Brandi S et al. Percutaneous balloon valvotomy for patients with severe mitral stenosis. Circulation 1987; 75: 778–84.
3. Chen C, Wang Y, Qing D et al. Percutaneous mitral balloon dilatation by a new sequential single- and double-balloon technique. Am Heart J 1988; 116: 1161–7.

4. Lock JE, Khalilullah M, Shrivastava S et al. Percutaneous catheter commissurotomy in rheumatic mitral stenosis. N Engl J Med 1985; 313: 1515–8.
5. Abascal VM, Wilkins GT, Choong CY et al. Echocardiographic evaluation of mitral valve structure and function in patients followed for at least 6 months after percutaneous balloon mitral valvuloplasty. J Am Coll Cardiol 1988; 12: 606–15.
6. Chen C, Wang X, Wang Y, Lan Y. Value of two-dimensional echocardiography in selecting patients and balloon sizes for percutaneous balloon mitral valvuloplasty. J Am Coll Cardiol 1989; 14: 1651–8.
7. Reid CL, Chandraratna AN, Kawanishi DT et al. Influence of mitral valve morphology on double-balloon catheter balloon valvuloplasty in patients with mitral stenosis: Analysis of factors predicting immediate and 3-month results. Circulation 1989; 80: 515–24.
8. Goldstein SA, Campbell AN. Mitral stenosis: Evaluation and guidance of valvuloplasty by transesophageal echocardiography. Cardiol Clinics 1993; 11(3): 409–25.
9. Kronzon I, Tunick PA, Schwinger ME et al. Transesophageal echocardiography during percutaneous mitral valvuloplasty. J Am Soc Echo 1989; 2: 380–5.
10. Vilacosta I, Iturralde E, San Roman JA et al. Transesophageal echocardiographic monitoring of percutaneous mitral balloon valvuloplasty. Am J Cardiol 1992; 70: 1040–4.
11. Ballal RS, Mahan EF, Nanda NC, Dean LS. Utility of transesophageal echocardiography in interatrial septal puncture during percutaneous mitral balloon commissurotomy. Am J Cardiol 1990; 66: 230–2.
12. Corminer B. Transesophageal echocardiography in the assessment of percutaneous mitral commissurotomy. Eur Heart J 1991; 12 (Suppl B): 61–5.
13. Marwick TH. Assessment of mitral valve splitality score by transthoracic and transesophageal echocardiography. Am J Cardiol 1991; 68: 1106–7.
14. Rittoo D, Sutherland GR, Currie P, Starkey IR, Show TR. The comparative value of transthoracic and transesophageal echocardiography before and after percutaneous mitral balloon valvotomy: A prospective study. Am Heart J 1993; 125: 1094–1105.
15. Fraser AG, Stumper OFW, van Herwerden LA et al. Anatomy of imaging planes used to study the mitral valve: Advantages of biplane transesophageal echocardiography. Circulation 1990 (Suppl): III–668 (Abstr).
16. Hwang JJ, Chen JJ, Lin SC et al. Diagnostic accuracy of transesophageal echocardiography for detecting left atrial thrombi in patients with rheumatic heart disease undergoing mitral valve operation. Am J Cardiol 1993; 72: 677–81.
17. Chen WJ, Chen MF, Liau CS, Lee YT. Safety of percutaneous transvenous balloon mitral commissurotomy in patients with mitral stenosis and thrombus in the left appendage. Am J Cardiol 1992; 70: 117–25.
18. Visser CA, Jaarsma W et al. Transesophageal echocardiographic observations during percutaneous balloon mitral valvuloplasty. In: Erbel R, Khandheria BK, Brennecke R et al. editors. Transesophageal echocardiography. Berlin: Springer-Verlag, 1989: 244–52.
19. Essop MR, Wisenbaugh T, Skoulariigis S et al. Mitral regurgitation following mitral balloon valvotomy: Differing mechanism for severe vs mild-to-moderate lesions. Circulation 1991; 84: 1669–79.
20. National Heart, Lung and Blood Institute Balloon Valvuloplasty Registry. Complications and mortality of percutaneous balloon mitral commissurotomy. Circulation. 1992; 85: 2014–24.
21. Chen C, Schneider B, Sievers B et al. Estimation of mitral valve area using biplane transesophageal color Doppler echocardiography. Circulation 1991; 84: II–129.
22. Thomas JD, Wilkins GT, Choong CYP et al. Inaccuracy of mitral presure half-time immediately after percutaneous mitral valvotomy: Dependence on transmitral gradient and left atrial and ventricular compliance. Circulation 1988; 78: 980–93.
23. Chen C, Wang X, Gou B, Lin Y. Reliability of the Doppler presure half-time method for assessing effects of percutaneous mitral balloon valvuloplasty. J Am Coll Cardiol 1989; 13: 1309–13.

24. Abascal VM, Wilkins GT, O'Shea JP et al. Prediction of successful outcome in 130 patients undergoing percutaneous balloon mitral valvotomy. Circulation 1990; 82: 448–56.
25. Cohen DJ, Kunz RE, Gordon SPF et al. Predictors of long-term outcome after percutaneous balloon mitral valvuloplasty. N Engl J Med 1992; 327: 1329–35.
26. Palacios IF, Block PC, Wilkins GT, Weyman AE. Follow-up of patients undergoing percutaneous mitral balloon valvotomy. Circulation 1989; 79: 573–9.
27. Nobuyoshi M, Hamasaki N, Kimura T et al. Indications, complications, and short-term clinical outcome of percutaneous transvenous mitral commissurotomy. Circulation 1989; 80: 782–92.
28. Palacios IF, Tuzcu EM, Newell JB, Block PC. Four year clinical follow-up of patients undergoing percutaneous mitral balloon valvotomy. Circulation 1990 (Suppl): III–545 (Abstr).
29. Herrmann HC, Lima JAC, Feldman T et al. Mechanisms and outcome of severe mitral regurgitation after Inoue balloon valvuloplasty. J Am Coll Cardiol 1993; 22: 783–9.
30. Abascal VM, Wilkins GT, Choong XY et al. Mitral regurgitation after percutaneous mitral valvuloplasty in adults: Evaluation by pulsed Doppler echocardiography. J Am Coll Cardiol 1988; 11: 257–63.
31. Pan JP, Lin SL, Go JU et al. Frequency and severity of mitral regurgitation one year after balloon mitral valvuloplasty. Am J Cardiol. 1991; 67: 264–8.
32. Chen C, Kremer P, Shroeder E et al. Usefulness of anatomic parameters derived from two-dimensional echocardiography for estimating magnitude of left to right shunt in patients with atrial septal defect. Clin Cardiol 1987; 10: 316.
33. Come PC, Riley MF, Diver DJ et al. Noninvasive assessment of mitral stenosis before and after percutaneous balloon mitral valvuloplasty. Am J Cardiol 1988; 61: 817–25.
34. Nigri A, Alessaandri N, Martuscelli E et al. Clinical significance of small left-to-right shunts after percutaneous mitral valvuloplasty. Am J Cardiol. 1993; 125: 783–5.
35. Yoshida K, Yoshikawa J, Akasaka T et al. Assessment of left-to-right atrial shunting after percutaneous mitral valvuloplasty by transesophageal color Doppler flow-mapping. Circulation 1989; 80: 1521–6.
36. Reid C, Kawanishi DT, Stellar W et al. Long-term incidence of atrial septal defects after catheter balloon commissurotomy for mitral stenosis. J Am Coll Cardiol 1991; 17: 339A.

Corresponding Author: Chunguang Chen, Echocardiography Laboratory, Hartford Hospital, 80 Seymour Street, Hartford, CT 06102, USA

29. Preinterventional imaging in paediatric cardiology

GERD HAUSDORF

Introduction

Compared to the surgical therapy of children with congenital heart disease interventional techniques have been of minor importance for years. This has changed dramatically since the development of new and refined transcatheter techniques. Today, the number of interventional procedures is higher than that of diagnostic cardiac catheterizations in many centres. Adequate preinterventional imaging is crucial for patient-selection, in order to accurately plan the specific interventional procedure and to calculate its risk and complexity. Another reason for establishing the diagnosis noninvasively before catheterization is to gain time to adequately inform the patient and the parents about the therapeutic choices and the potential side effects and outcome of the intervention. Informed consent cannot usually be obtained between diagnostic catheterization and intervention because both steps should be performed in children as a single procedure to minimize traumatic laceration of the vessels and reduce the risk of later vessel occlusion [1–3]. The main value of catheterization is to confirm the noninvasive findings and, based on these findings, the diagnostic part of the catheterization procedure can be made as short as possible to save contrast material and fluoroscopy time.

Preinterventional imaging in children is complicated by the minute anatomic details that have to be delineated particularly in newborns, the accelerated heart rate and respiration rate within this group of patients. Thus, spatial and temporal resolution have to be extremely high. Since these patients are usually not able to cooperate, sedation or general anesthesia is frequently required to eliminate motoric activity during image acquisition. This limits the applicability of imaging techniques with long acquisition times, as well as those with the need of ECG-triggered data sampling and suspended respiration.

Thus, the most important and widespread used technique for preinterventional imaging in paediatric cardiology is echocardiography. Transthoracic echocardiography is non-invasive and has adequate spatial and temporal

C.A. Nienaber and U. Sechtem (eds): *Imaging and Intervention in Cardiology*, 471–504.
© 1996 Kluwer Academic Publishers. Printed in the Netherlands.

resolution for this particular age-group [4–5]. Usually there is no need for sedation and echocardiography can be repeated as often as necessary before and even during interventional procedures [6]. In paediatric patients transthoracic echocardiography is usually sufficient for diagnostic imaging alone. In contrast, transesopageal echocardiography has superior imaging-quality in older children and adult patients, particularly if the interatrial septum, pulmonary veins, atrioventricular valves and the relation between ventricular septal defects, atrioventricular valves and semilunar valves have to be evaluated [7–14]. However, consequent sedation using ketamine or ethomidate is generally required for transesophageal echocardiography in children. An additional disadvantage is near field distortion, which limits the use of transesophageal echocardiography in small infants, so that accurate delineation of the interatrial septum and the atrioventricular valves can be impossible due to the small distance between these structures and the transducer. However, this problem may be solved within the near future with the development of transducers with negligible near field distortion. Although 3D-echocardiography is an interesting new concept, it cannot yet be decided if this method will provide crucial additional information for the intervention. Currently, spatial resolution and time needed for the generation of 3D-reconstructions are not adequate for a routine use in children [15–19].

Echocardiographic techniques are limited by the physics of ultrasound, which cannot penetrate bone, calcifications and air. Therefore, intrapulmonary structures or those covered by lung tissue cannot be delineated adequately. These technical limitations are not inherent to computerized tomography and magnetic resonance imaging [20–30]. However, even with ultrafast CT imaging consequent sedation or even general aesthesia is required in paediatric patients to achieve adequate images. Both with MR and CT implantable devices as stents, coils or umbrellas may result in significant image distortion, thereby limiting the usefulness and accuracy of these techniques for some staged interventional procedures [31–33].

For preinterventional imaging the technical advantages of complex imaging techniques are less important than the requirements crucial for the specific interventional procedure. Thus, from the interventionalist's point of view the preinterventional imaging techniques are chosen according to the specific intervention. Preinterventional imaging has several purposes. First, the clinical diagnosis needs to be confirmed and refined in order to reduce the requirement for cardiac catheterization. Second, sufficient information has to be obtained to decide whether a patient should be selected for an interventional procedure or for surgery. Third, optimal preinterventional imaging should enable the interventionalist to plan the interventional procedure in detail, in order to make all preparations for specific interventional techniques preinterventionally, including the selection of specific balloon catheters, or the decision for stent-implantation [34–40]. Fourth, the imaging technique used for preinterventional imaging should be applicable during the intervention, a feature restricted to echocardiography today. However, "open" magnetic resonance machines may provide this option in the near future. Finally, preinterventional imaging should minimize the duration of the procedure and reduce the exposure to radiation as much as possible. In this chapter, the role of imaging techniques in preparing for all types of transcatheter interventions in congenital heart disease is discussed.

Interventional techniques in paediatric cardiology are of increasing complexity, however, some interventions can be summarized as "basic" interventional techniques. For these "basic" procedures preinterventional imaging has to confirm the exact diagnosis and to allow precise measurements of the anatomic details important for the interventional procedure, such as the valve ring of a stenotic valve or the critical diameter of a stenotic vessel. For most "basic" interventions echocardiography alone is sufficient for preinterventional imaging.

Atrial septostomy

Balloon atrial septostomy was first reported by Rashkind in 1967 [41]. This procedure is life-saving in patients with d-transposition of the great arteries without adequate mixing through a ventricular septal defect, in patients with univentricular circulation and restrictive interatrial communication (tricuspid atresia, mitral atresia) and rarely in double outlet ventricles with inadequate mixing. Preinterventional imaging has to confirm the diagnosis and has to demonstrate the interatrial septum, the size of the foramen ovale and finally the size of the left atrium. Originally, the diagnosis was made using angiography, but nowadays diagnosis is exclusively based on echocardiographic findings and even the septostomy is usually performed under echocardiographic guidance (Figure 1) [42–44]. The major advantage of echocardiography is the precise on-line visualization of the interatrial septum and the relation between balloon, pulmonary veins, mitral valve and interatrial septum during the septostomy. The same holds true for blade-septostomy as described by Park [45–47], which is also performed in most centres under echocardiographic guidance, as this is superior in showing the relation of the blade in relation to both atria and the interatrial septum.

Balloon valvuloplasty

Valvular pulmonic stenosis

The most widely accepted and established interventional procedure in paediatric cardiology is balloon valvuloplasty of valvular pulmonic stenosis [48–53]. For preinterventional imaging echocardiography is usually sufficient, because the diagnosis is made easily using echocardiography and most associated anomalies such as atrial septal defects, ventricular septal defects, patent

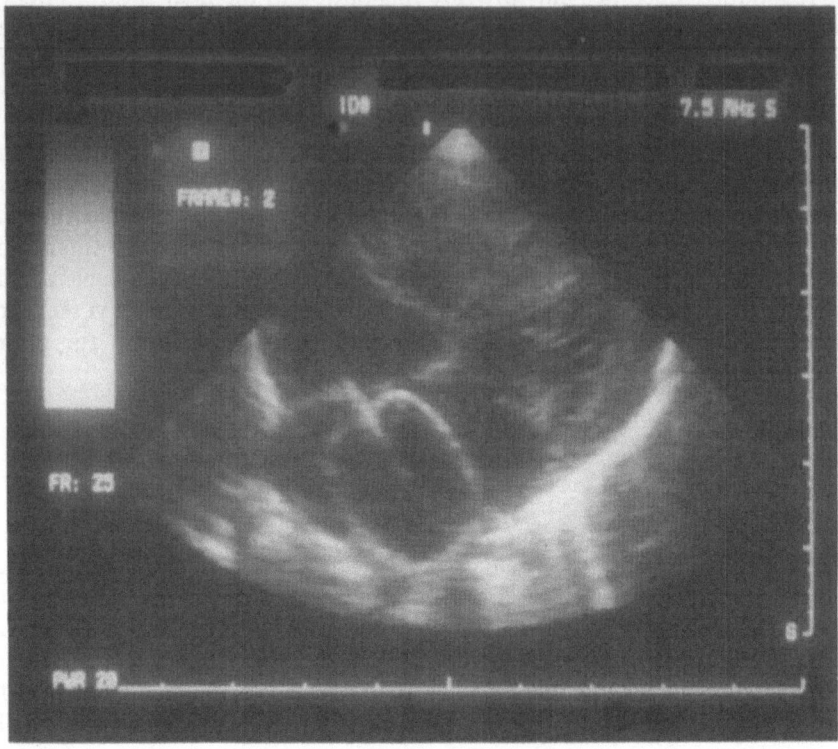

Figure 1. Balloon atrial septostomy is nowadays performed at the bedside under echocardio-graphic guidance. The figure shows a subxiphoidal 2D-echocardiographic view of the Rashkind-BAS-catheter inflated within the left atrium, immediately before it is pulled back into the right atrium.

ductus arteriosus, or Ebstein's malformation of the tricuspid valve can be detected or excluded. The precise differentiation between valvular and infundibular stenosis can also be achieved by using echocardiography. Even the pressure gradient and the diameter of the pulmonic valve ring can be accurately measured using echocardiography, which permits the appropriate choice of the balloon before intervention [7].

Echocardiography is sometimes limited in the diagnosis of dysplastic valves, which are best demonstrated using angiography. In dysplastic pulmonic valves balloon dilatation often fails, so that valvuloplasty is not attempted in some centres. However, pulmonary balloon valvuloplasty carries only a minute risk in experienced hands and the success of valvuloplasty cannot be predicted preinterventionally in dysplastic valves. Therefore, it is the opinion of the author that valvuloplasty should also be attempted in dysplastic valves. Consequently, a precise echocardiographic diagnosis of valve morphology is not of paramount importance.

Supravalvular pulmonic stenosis

Supravalvular pulmonic stenosis which occurs often after pulmonary debanding is usually well visualized by echocardiography. However, in contrast to valvular pulmonic stenosis delineation of the bifurcation and the proximal portion of the main branches is crucial, as a residual stenosis after pulmonary debanding is regularly associated with pulmonary branch stenosis and is sometimes even associated with complete occlusion of one main pulmonary branch [22, 25, 27]. If echocardiography does not visualize both pulmonary branches sufficiently, magnetic resonance imaging should be performed to demonstrate both pulmonary branches. This technique has been shown to visualize the peripheral pulmonary arteries more complete than echocardiography [25, 54–57].

Aortic stenosis

While balloon valvuloplasty of aortic stenosis is rarely performed in adult patients, it is widely practised in paediatric cardiology [7, 9, 58–64]. In contrast to the adult population calcification of the stenotic valve is extremely rare during childhood, so that the risk for cerebral embolization and early restenosis is minimal. For preinterventional imaging echocardiography is usually sufficient [59, 60]. The diagnosis is easily made using echocardiography and it is also possible to confirm or exclude associated malformations such as coarctation, persistent ductus, dysplastic mitral valve and subvalvular stenosis at the same time. As aortic valvuloplasty aggravates aortic regurgitation severe aortic regurgitation > grade 2 has to be excluded preinterventionally [58–62]. The pressure gradient and the diameter of the aortic valve ring can be measured precisely using echocardiography. Therefore, the size of the balloon catheter can be chosen accordingly. The exact determination of the diameter of the aortic valve ring is crucial, because a balloon diameter only 1 mm larger than the aortic ring may cause severe aortic regurgitation. Finally, assessment of the left ventricle is critical for decision making in neonates with aortic stenosis. If the left ventricle shows significant hypoplasia, neither interventional valvuloplasty nor surgical valvotomy should be performed, as the left ventricle will not be able to take over the systemic work load [65, 66]. Instead, univentricular repair with the right ventricle serving as the systemic ventricle should be performed.

Depiction of the anatomy of the mitral valve by echocardiography is also essential if antegrade balloon valvuloplasty of aortic stenosis is attempted. The anatomy of the mitral valve is critical when the retrograde venous approach is employed because tension may be exerted upon the anterior (aortic) leaflet by the balloon catheter during inflation [60, 63].

Supravalvular aortic stenosis

Although the anatomy and exact diameter of the stenotic segment in supravalvular aortic stenosis are easily assessed using echocardiographic imaging, the exact anatomy of the coronary ostia and their distance to the stenosis are usually not sufficiently delineated. The relation between the coronary arteries and the supravalvular stenosis is of critical importance, because an intimal tear caused by the intervention could extend into the coronary ostia leading to occlusion or stenosis of a coronary artery. Thus, aortography and selective coronary angiography are necessary before the decision for an interventional approach is made. Magnetic resonance imaging may be used as an alternative to angiography in the future but adequate data supporting such a strategy have not yet been presented.

Aortic coarctation

While echocardiography is sufficient for preinterventional imaging in most of the basic interventional procedures, this is not the case for balloon angioplasty of coarctation [67–70]. Although the diagnosis of coarctation is routinely made by echocardiography, exact visualization of the stenotic area is usually not possible in older children or adults using echocardiography alone. This is in part due to the fact that the descending aorta and the ultrasound beam parallel each other if the suprasternal approach is applied. Additionally echocardiographic images may be distorted by artefacts from air-filled structures such as the oesophagus, trachea and lung. Although intravascular ultrasound can be used to image the area of interest immediately before the intervention, it seems to have little advantages when compared with angiography [71].

In contrast to echocardiography, the exact anatomy of coarctation is clearly shown by magnetic resonance imaging in most patients, if care is taken to exclude "pseudocoarctation" [72–74]. Furthermore, aneurysms which can occur postinterventionally or postsurgically are detected by magnetic resonance imaging but may not be visualized by echocardiography. Thus, magnetic resonance imaging is the superior preinterventional imaging technique for coarctation, particularly in older children and in re-coarctation when aortic aneurysms have to be excluded (Figure 2) [24, 25, 37–39, 72–74]. Nevertheless, associated malformations such as a patent duct, aortic stenosis, dysplasia of the mitral valve or a ventricular septal defect, are easily detected by echocardiography. The measurement of the descending aorta at the diaphragm, which is necessary to select an adequately sized balloon catheter, is done either by magnetic resonance or by ultrasound. If an antegrade approach is attempted for balloon dilation of coarctation the size of the left

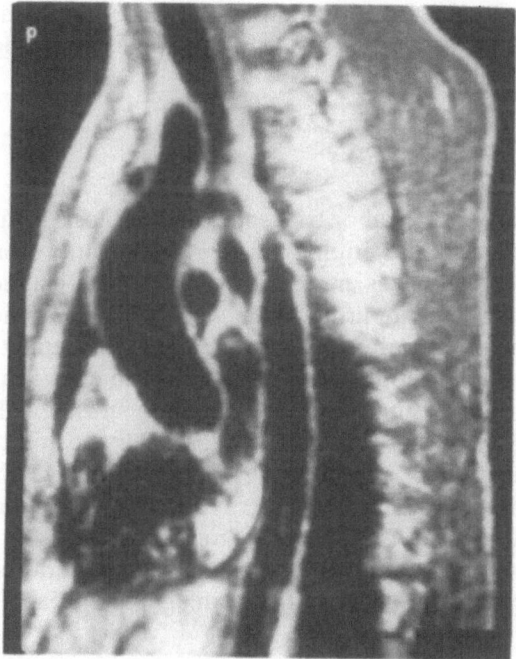

Figure 2. Magnetic resonance imaging of re-coarctation. Hypoplasia of the aortic arch is shown, the distal aortic arch is not visualized due to extreme narrowing.

ventricle and the exact anatomy of the mitral valve are essential, both being delineated by echocardiography as discussed above [60–63].

In newborns and small infants echocardiographic imaging of coarctation is often adequate for preinterventional imaging. In this age group visualization of a patent duct is of particular importance, as the descending aorta is usually perfused through a patent duct. Before balloon angioplasty is performed, the duct should be closed pharmacologically, which also results in contraction of the ductal tissue within the coarctation rendering balloon dilatation more effective. Another important feature of coarctation in newborns is a "tubular" hypoplasia of the aortic arch, which is clearly visualized using echocardiography.

Stent implantation into coarctation is a new technique in paediatric interventional cardiology [75]. Ineffective balloon angioplasty of re-coarctation seems to be an indication for stent implantation. Another indication for stent implantation is the newborn infant with coarctation and severe hypoplasia of the aortic arch. Criteria for stent implantation are inadequate balloon angioplasty and a diameter of the aortic arch below 3.5 mm with the aim to achieve adequate growth of the aortic arch. A normal sized arch would likely improve results when surgical correction is performed later. Angiography

(Figure 3) and intravascular ultrasound are probably the ideal imaging techniques to immediately assess the results of angioplasty in order to decide on whether a stent should be implanted.

Mitral and tricuspid valve stenosis

Balloon valvuloplasty of mitral or tricuspid valve stenosis is rarely performed in children [76], because the etiology differs significantly from that in adult patients. In children the valves are usually dysplastic with abnormal chordae. Most often the valve is hypoplastic, with short, thickened and rarified chordae. In addition the insertions of the chordae are often found to be abnormal, varying from a hypoplastic mitral valve to a parachute mitral valve with all chordae inserting into a single isolated papillary muscle. The decision for balloon valvuloplasty of these valvular stenoses depends on the exact preinterventional delineation of the chordae to avoid rupture of chordae with subsequent life-threatening mitral or tricuspid regurgitation. Echocardiography, in particular transesophageal echocardiography, is the method of choice to delineate the anatomy and mechanics of the chordae, and is therefore the most important preinterventional imaging approach.

Peripheral pulmonic stenosis

Preinterventional imaging of peripheral pulmonic stenosis is more complex. Imaging of peripheral stenosis is impossible using echocardiography (Figure 4). Magnetic resonance imaging or computerized tomography are clearly superior to echocardiography in detecting stenoses of the main pulmonary artery branches. However, both techniques are limited in depicting more peripheral stenoses [25, 34, 54–57, 77–80]. Thus, pulmonary angiography and selective angiography is still the gold standard for making the diagnosis of multiple peripheral stenoses and exactly evaluating vessel diameters. To discriminate tubular from circumscript peripheral pulmonic stenosis the inflation of a balloon catheter is required. Even when angiography demonstrates a typical tubular stenosis, an inflated balloon may show a circumscript waist during low-pressure inflation (Figure 5). Thus, for accurate "pre"-interventional imaging inflation of a balloon seems mandatory to delineate the exact anatomy, so that the intervention itself becomes an important "imaging" method in this particular entity. Even intravascular ultrasound is not sufficient to show the abnormalities within the vessel wall responsible for this phenomenon.

Balloon angioplasty of peripheral pulmonary stenosis and pulmonary branch stenosis is successful in about 50% of cases, independent of the etiology (native or postsurgical). No valid parameters predictive for the success or failure of balloon dilatation are known. Therefore, balloon dilatation should be performed in all patients and the result of the intervention

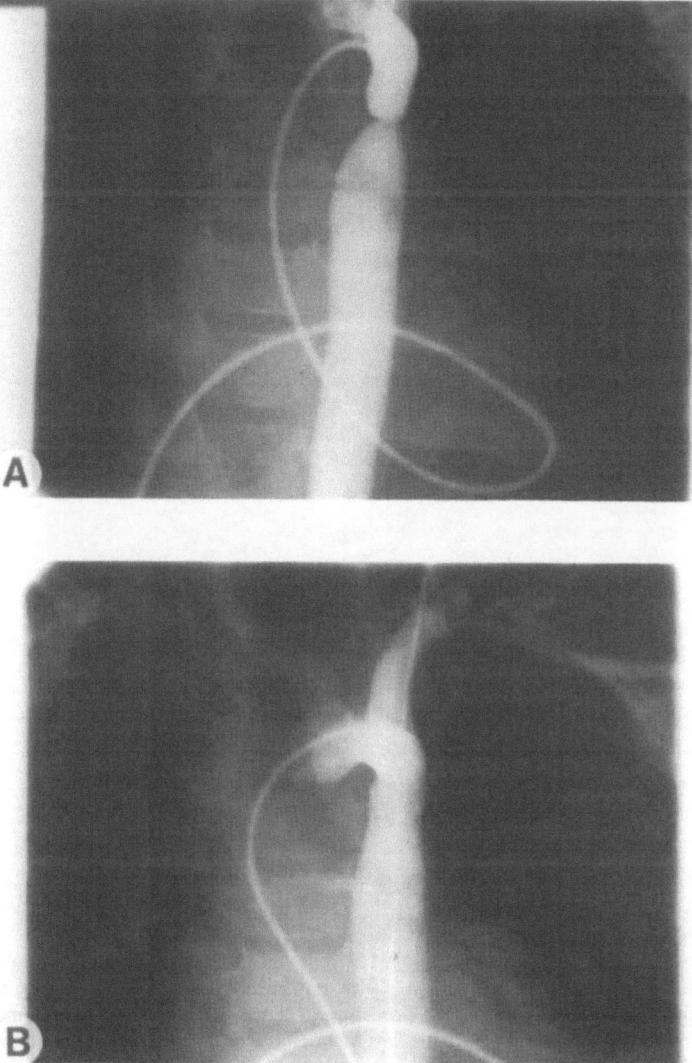

Figure 3. (A) A native coarctation after failed balloon angioplasty is shown (aortogram, posteroanterior view). Although the waist in the balloon disappeared during dilatation, the circumscript stenosis persisted after angioplasty, obviously due to elastic recoil. (B) After stent-implantation (12 mm diameter, palmaz iliac stent) into the coarctation, the stenosis completely disappeared (aortogram, posteroanterior view).

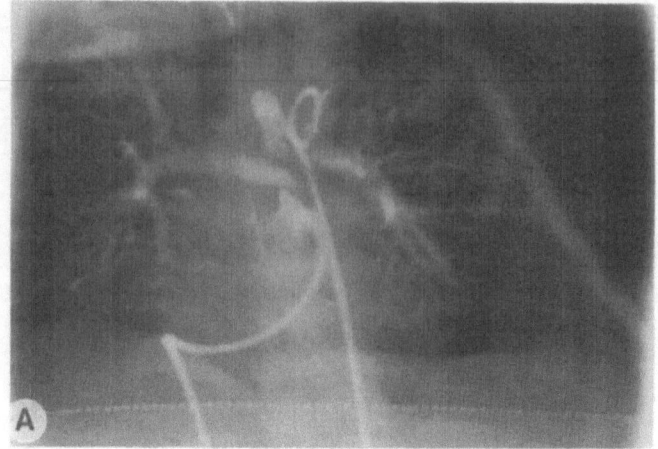

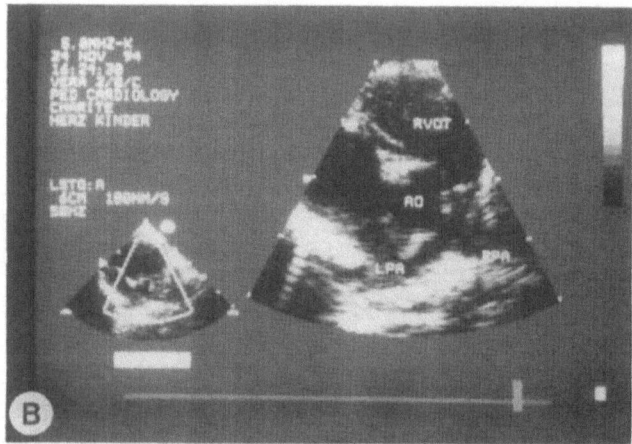

Figure 4. Imaging of pulmonary atresia in an newborn infant (2.8 kg). While angiography delineates the exact anatomy during the procedure, echocardiography does not demonstrate the narrowing of the infundibulum and the left pulmonary branch stenosis. (A) Simultaneously selective injections into the ductus arteriosus and the right ventricular infundibulum are performed immediately before perforation is performed, demonstrating left pulmonary branch stenosis and the atresia between infundibulum and main pulmonary artery. Due to the tension of the catheter within the infundibulum the anatomy is distorted so that the tip of the catheter (4F) points to the right of the main pulmonary artery. (B) Echocardiography (short axis view) reveals a membraneous atresia (RVOT – right ventricular outflow tract; Ao – ascending aorta; LPA – left pulmonary artery; RPA – right pulmonary artery). (C) Right ventricular angiogram after radiofrequency perforation of the atresia, balloon dilatation of the atresia and the left pulmonary branch stenosis.

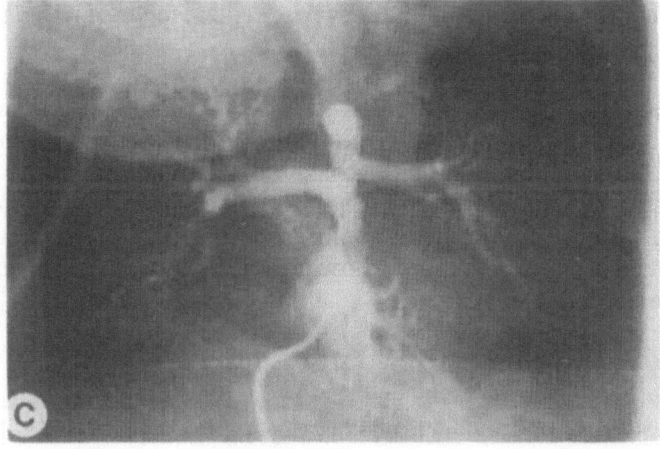

Figure 4. Continued.

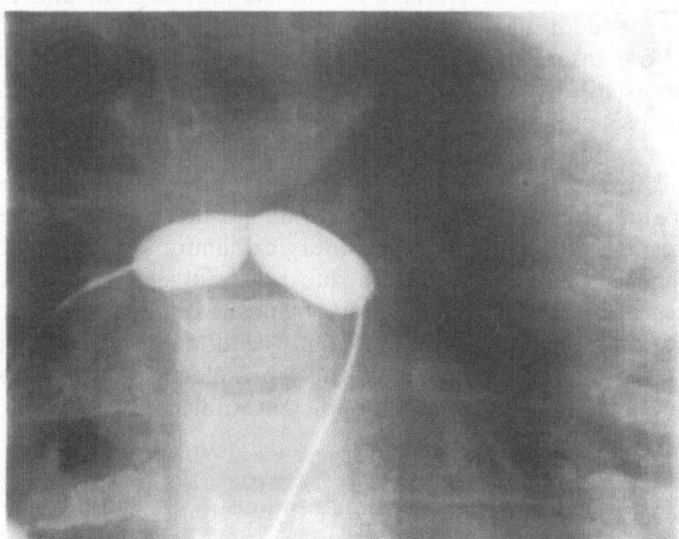

Figure 5. A circumscript stenosis of the right pulmonary branch is shown by inflating a balloon within the stenosis (posteroanterior view). During low-pressure inflation of the balloon the waist in the balloon demonstrates the diameter and length of the stenosis. Even when angiography shows a typical tubular stenosis, inflating the balloon reveals often a circumscript waist.

should be controlled after 3 months by magnetic resonance imaging or angiography.

In patients with primary failure of angioplasty or restenosis at 3 months, stent-implantation (Figure 6) is an established therapeutic approach [81–83]. Preinterventional imaging has to delineate the accurate anatomy of the stenotic site, including inflation of a balloon in tubular stenosis, because this often reveals circumscript stenosis, as discussed above. Therefore before implanting a stent into a tubular stenosis "diagnostic" pre-dilatation should be performed to demonstrate and localize a circumscript stenotic segment and to size its diameter (Figure 5).

Pulmonary veins

Stenotic lesions of pulmonary veins are observed in obstructed total anomalous pulmonary venous drainage and after surgical correction of this entity. They are rarely observed after atrial repair of transposition of the great arteries. Preinterventional imaging is usually performed by echocardiography which shows an increased flow velocity in the pulmonary veins or within the common vein, which drains the pulmonary venous blood. However, imaging is often technically difficult because the stenotic segment is covered by lung tissue and may therefore not be visualized by echocardiography. Chest X-ray often fails to show pulmonary congestion in those segments with impaired drainage. Alternative approaches to echocardiography are magnetic resonance imaging and cine- or spiral CT. The stenotic region, and congestion within the dependent lung segments can be depicted by these techniques and MRI can also measure the increased flow velocity within the vein. However, angiography is still the most valid imaging technique and the gold standard for the diagnosis of pulmonary venous stenosis. It is of particular importance that stenosis is often due to the constricting residual tissue of the common vein which drained the pulmonary venous blood before surgical correction and is not due to scar formation or shrinkage at the site of the surgical anastomoses [84, 85]. While a stenotic surgical anatomosis is usually susceptible to balloon dilatation, stenoses due to shrinkage of abnormal tissue require stent-implantation into pulmonary veins to obtain satisfactory results. Thus, in the opinion of the author, preinterventional imaging of pulmonary venous stenosis still requires selective and supraselective angiograms whereas non-invasive techniques do not give sufficient information.

Occlusion of abnormal vascular communications

Coil embolization or embolization using detachable balloons for the occlusion of abnormal vessels are established techniques. Coil embolization can be used to occlude aortopulmonary fistulae, coronary fistulae, intrapulmonary fistulae, aortopulmonary (surgical) shunts and patent ducts (Figure 7). For

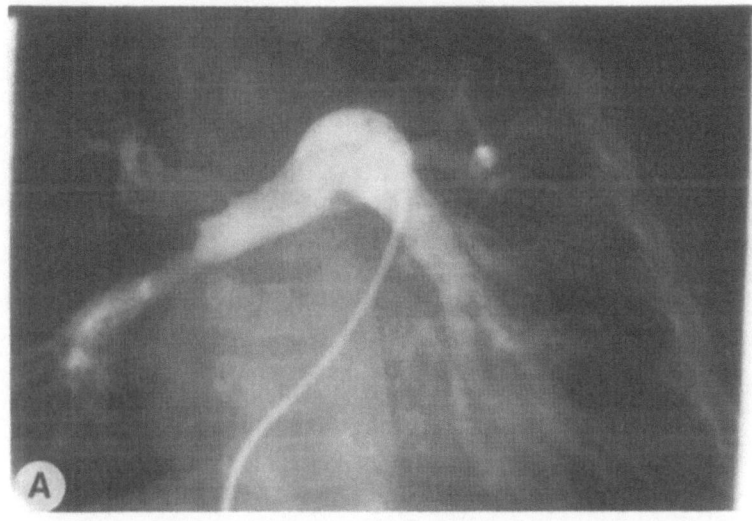

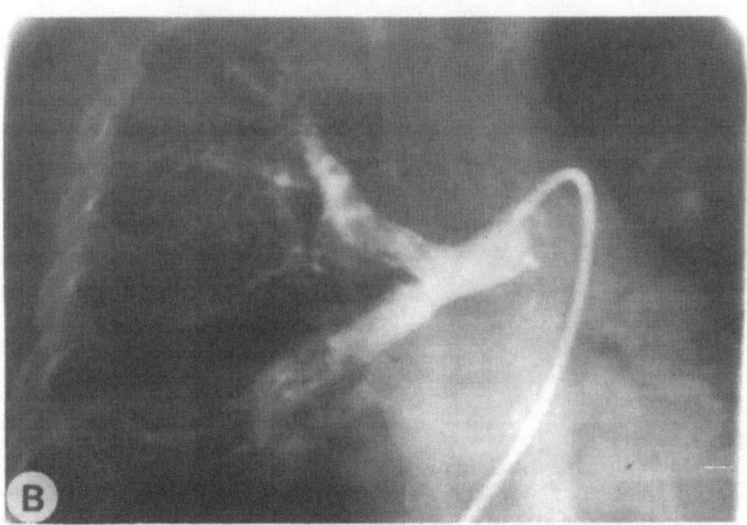

Figure 6. (A) A pulmonary angiogram in a 3-month-old infant shows severe stenosis of the branch of the pulmonary artery to the right upper lobe and right lower lobe. The branch to the right middle lobe is completely occluded and opacifies retrogradely from the right upper lobe (posteroanterior view). (B) After implanting two stents (palmaz iliac stents, 8 mm diameter) into the stenotic segments the right sided perfusion is significantly improved (angiogram of the right pulmonary artery, posteroanterior view).

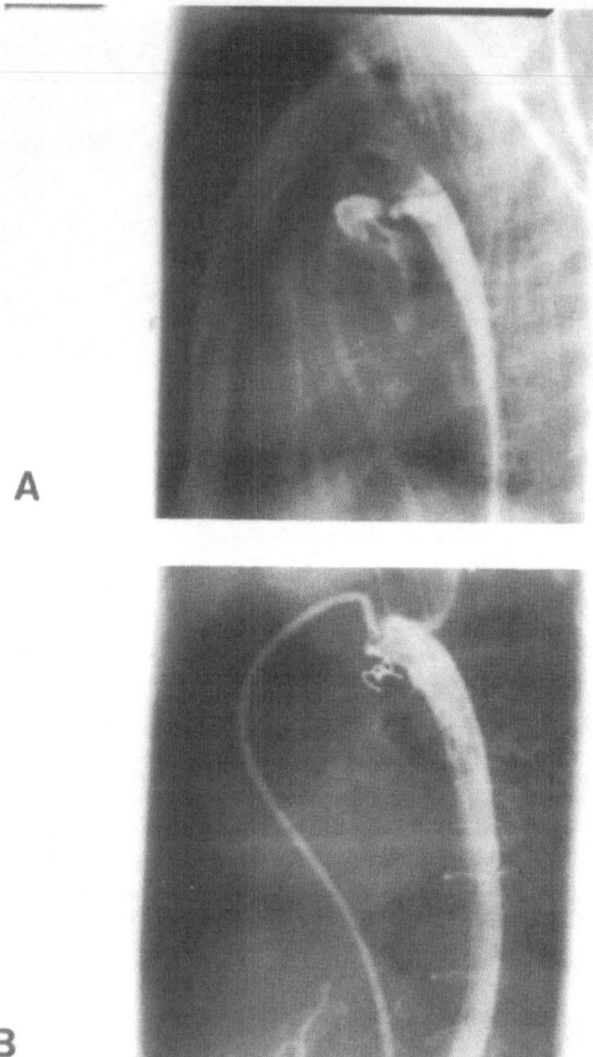

Figure 7. Interventional occlusion of a patent duct in a 1.5 kg preterm infant is shown (lateral view). In this infant with double inlet left ventricle and d-malposition of the great arteries a surgical banding of the main pulmonary artery had been performed for later univentricular repair. After spontaneous reopening (A) of the duct pulmonary congestion occurred. Interventional occlusion of the duct was performed using a platinum-coil (diameter 2 mm)(B), which was applied through a 3F tracker-catheter. The 4F Judkins catheter is positioned in the aortic arch (via femoral vein) to perform angiography during the procedure.

preinterventional imaging echocardiography and magnetic resonance imaging are most commonly used [86]. A patent duct, coronary fistulae and aortopulmonary shunts can be visualized in many small patients sufficiently using echocardiography, whereas imaging of aortopulmonary collaterals is impossible due to the overlying lung tissue. Magnetic resonance imaging can be used to depict the proximal portions of such collaterals but selective angiography is necessary immediately before the intervention to show the precise three dimensional anatomy of the fistula. Of particular importance is the delineation of a stenotic and tortuous segment, which helps to prevent peripheral embolization of the detached coils and to demonstrate adjacent vessels at risk of inadvertent occlusion, such as spinal arteries, cerebral vessels and coronary vessels. Standard coils should only be used if a stenotic distal segment can be demonstrated. However, if retrievable coils are used the risk of embolization is of minor importance, because the stable position of the coil can be controlled and the coil is only released after complete thrombosis of the abnormal vessel has occurred.

If coil embolisation of an abnormal vessel is impossible or hazardous because of its large size and a high flow within the vessel with the risk of coil embolization, implantation of a Rashkind-PDA-Occluder is used as an alternative method [87–89]. Although this device has been developed for occlusion of the patent duct, it is also routinely used to occlude other abnormal vessels. The ultimate decision between coil-embolization and implantation of an umbrella depends on the accurate demonstration of the anatomy of the vascular structure to occlude (Figure 8). Thus, preinterventional noninvasive imaging shows the principal diagnosis and may give preliminary information about the anatomy of the vessel, but definite imaging still requires selective angiography.

Transcatheter occlusion of the patent duct [87–92] by using the Rashkind-PDA occluder requires preinterventional imaging of the duct and differentiation from an aortopulmonary window, or a coronary fistula. Furthermore, associated congenital heart disease (such as coarctation) should be excluded. In most patients, echocardiography fulfils all these needs. However, selection of the correct device requires accurate sizing of the duct for two reasons. First, the small (12 mm) device should not be implanted in ducts larger than 4 mm in diameter, and the larger device (17 mm) not in those larger than 9 mm. Second, the duct has to be larger than the long sheath that is to be used for transcatheter occlusion. Using the standard technique an 8F sheath is required for the 12 mm device and an 11F sheath for the 17 mm device. Using the "frontloading" technique a 6F sheath is required for the 12 mm device and a 8F sheath for the 17 mm device, respectively. Echocardiography is not sufficient for the accurate assessment of the ductal diameter and geometry, so that aortography is still required for the selection of the device. However, a long, tubular duct can be visualized in most instances using echocardiography. In tubular ducts with stenosis at the pulmonary end of the duct coil embolization is an alternative approach to using the Rashkind-

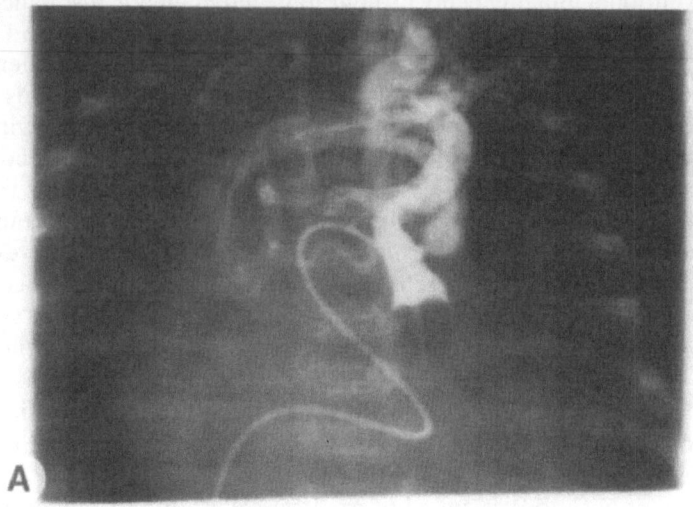

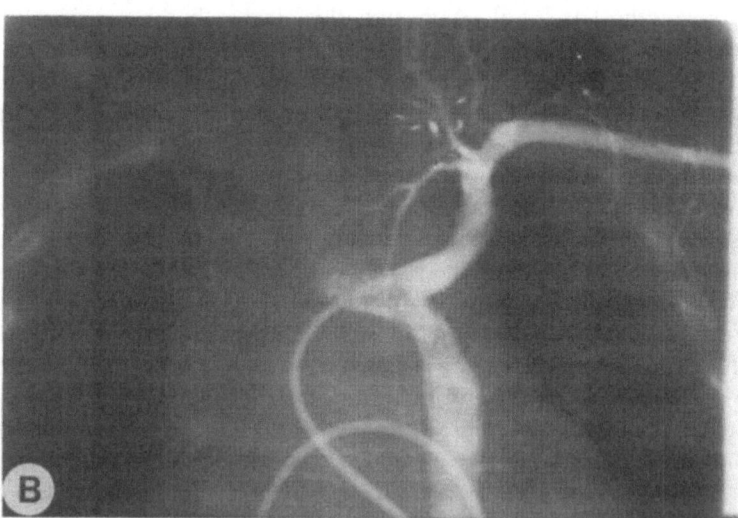

Figure 8. Occlusion of an arteriovenous fistula originating from the left subclavian artery in a 3 weeks old infant with congestive heart failure due volume overload (aortogram, posteroanterior view). The fistula was closed using two umbrellas. While Figure A shows the arteriovenous fistula, which drained into the innominate vein, the result of transcatheter occlusion is shown in Figure B. Two months later the fistula was completely occluded.

PDA-occluder. In any case, both for the selection of the technique (coil or umbrella) and the diameter of the device, angiographic delineation of the duct is essential to achieve adequate depiction and valid measurements.

Closure of intracardiac defects

Atrial septal defect

While angiography is still the best imaging technique for the interventional occlusion of abnormal vascular structures, this is not the case with intracardiac defects. For the preinterventional assessment of atrial septal defects echocardiography is of outstanding importance and superior to angiography. Echocardiography allows the precise assessment of the defect, its dimensions, the position within the atrial septum and its relationship to adjacent structures such as the pulmonary and systemic veins, the eustachian and atrioventricular valves as well as the ascending aorta, which is lying within the interatrial groove. While in small infants (age below 5 years) the atrial septal defect is usually accurately visualized by the transthoracic and subxiphoidal echocardiographic approach, in older children and adults transesophageal imaging is usually superior. Before transcatheter closure of atrial septal defects is performed, "sizing" of the defect is mandatory [12–14, 93–102]. Sizing requires determination of the "stretched" diameter of the defect, which is performed by using a latex-balloon which is inflated within the left atrium and then withdrawn to occlude the defect. Complete occlusion is demonstrated by absence of a left-to-right shunt as assessed by colour-coded-doppler imaging. By slowly decreasing the size of the balloon, the critical diameter, at which left-to-right shunting reoccurs is determined, and the device selected accordingly. Thus, preinterventional imaging of atrial septal defects is usually done by echocardiography with the advantage that it can also be used during invasive sizing. Even the implantation of the device can be elegantly performed using echocardiographic guidance, which shows residual shunting and the relation of the device to the neighbouring structures [12, 93, 94]. Although magnetic resonance imaging can very nicely depict the size of an atrial septal defect in 3 dimensions, it has not been used to guide intervention and has the disadvantage at present of not permitting imaging during intervention.

Endocardial cushion defect

Exact evaluation of the defect and its relation to surrounding structures is of particular importance, if flow reduction in atrioventricular septal defects (primum type atrial septal defect, endocardial cushion defect) is attempted

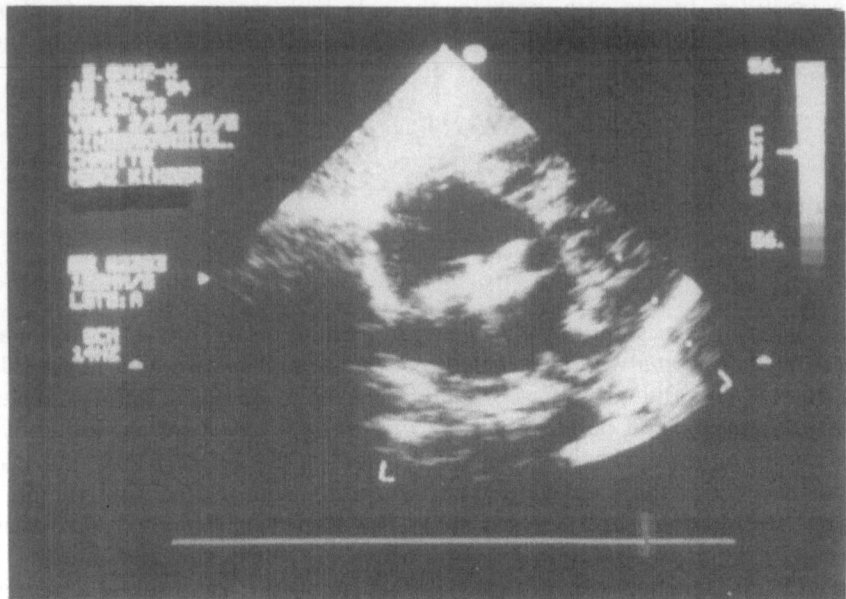

Figure 9. The echocardiogram (subxiphoidal view) of a 3-month-old infant with atrioventricular septal defect is shown. An PDA-occluder has been implanted into the patent foramen ovale. Thus, the primum defect within the atrial septum is partially covered by the umbrella, reducing the left-to-right shunt through the atrial septal defect, thereby redirecting blood flow into the left ventricle.

(Figure 9). Preinterventional imaging has to delineate the residual atrial septum, the foramen ovale or the secundum atrial septal defect and the primum defect. Technically an umbrella is implanted into the foramen ovale, so the basal part of the device overrides the primum defect thereby reducing its size. By reducing the size of the defect flow reduction through the primum defect is achieved and the blood from the pulmonary veins is redirected to the left ventricle, which is of particular importance in patients with hypoplastic left ventricle. Preinterventional imaging has to demonstrate the size of the residual septum and the distance between foramen ovale and the atrioventricular valves accurately, in order to avoid laceration of these valves. Although magnetic resonance imaging has the potential to demonstrate the atrial septal defect accurately, sizing and implantation cannot be performed using this technique, so that echocardiography is the preferred technique.

Ventricular septal defect

Interventional closure of ventricular septal defects is rarely performed in children and adults because no specific device has been developed for this purpose (Figure 10). Most isolated ventricular septal defects are located in close relation to the aortic valve (Figure 11), so that transcatheter closure using an umbrella is often impossible or hazardous [7, 8, 103–106]. In addition to the risk of disturbing the aortic valve by the left sided umbrella, the right sided umbrella has the potential to be caught within chordae of the tricuspid valve, resulting in tricuspidal regurgitation and important mechanical stress to the device. In older patients redundant tricuspid valve tissue is often attached to the defect, resulting in an aneurysm of the membraneous septum, so that interventional closure may be hazardous. Preinterventional imaging has to demonstrate the size of the defect, its relation to the aortic valve leaflets, insertions of the tricuspid valve chordae and has to exclude an aneurysm of the membraneous septum. This is usually achieved by transthoracic echocardiography, although transesophageal echocardiography is superior in adult patients [7, 8, 10, 17]. Tricuspid valve tissue, chordae, and the aortic valve are very thin structures which may also move slightly differently from heartbeat to heartbeat. Although MRI has a spatial resolution of less than 1 mm in plane, averaging of motion over up to 256 heartbeats may result in some blurring of these fine structures. Therefore, magnetic resonance imaging or computerized tomography are only of limited value for the preinterventional assessment of patients with such defects [21, 23, 27–29, 106]. As in atrial septal defects sizing of the ventricular septal defect is critical, because redundant fibrous tissue can make the defect look smaller than its actual size. Thus, the definite preinterventional imaging should consist of selective angiography into the ventricular defect (Figure 11) and additionally in balloon sizing under echocardiographic guidance to assess the balloon diameter which completely occludes the defect as discussed above.

Flow-redirection using stents

Although occlusion of abnormal vessels using coils or umbrellas is the standard interventional approach, flow-redirection using stents is a promising, new technique. To achieve flow-redirection covered stents are under investigation, which occlude the abnormal communication and create a new drainage, the covered stent being comparable to a surgical conduit. Assessment of both, the abnormal communication and the drainage before redirection are critical for this approach. Although abnormal draining veins (for example a left superior vena cava to the left atrium) can be visualized before intervention by colour-coded-echocardiography, contrast- echocardiography and especially magnetic resonance imaging, angiographic demonstration of the anatomy at the time of the intervention is still necessary.

The use of stents for flow redirection as a new concept of univentricular repair is of particular interest. In high-risk patients with tricuspid atresia, mitral atresia or double inlet ventricles, univentricular repair (Fontan-procedure, total cavopulmonary anastomosis) is performed as a staged procedure in most centres. The first stage consists of a hemi-Fontan procedure or

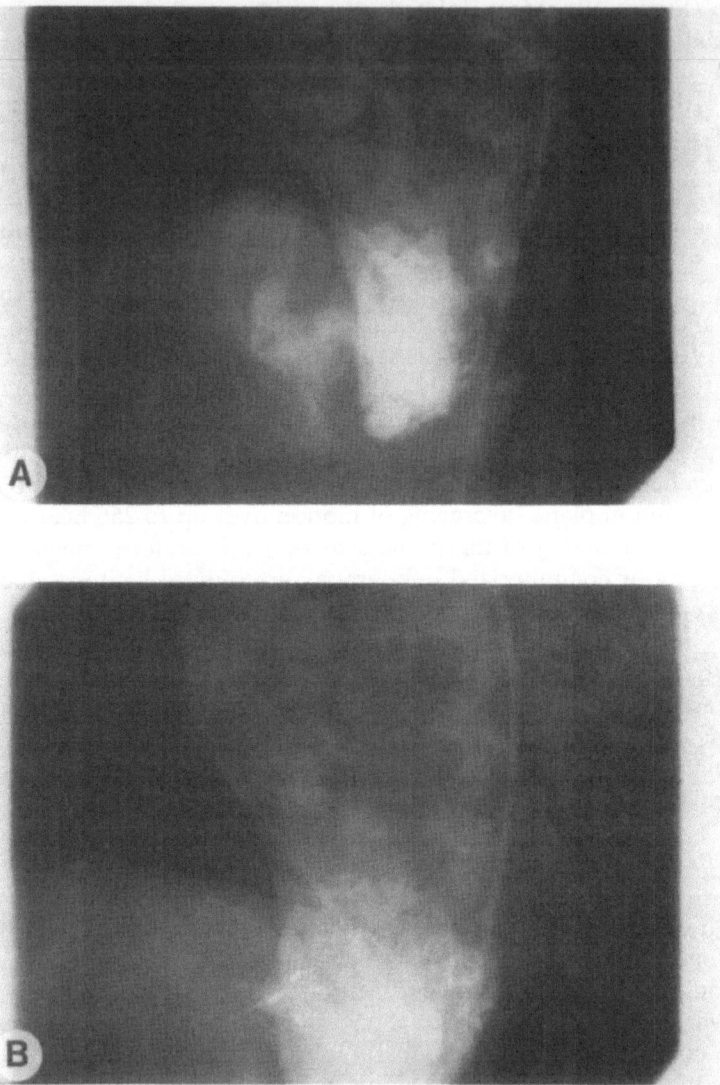

Figure 10. Transcatheter closure of a muscular ventricular septal defect. (A) A left ventricular angiogram is performed in the "four-chamber-view" and reveals a muscular ventricular septal defect. (B) After "sizing" of the defect using an arteriovenous loop from the femoral vein through the ventricular septal defect to the femoral artery transcatheter closure was performed using a Rashkind-PDA-occluder.

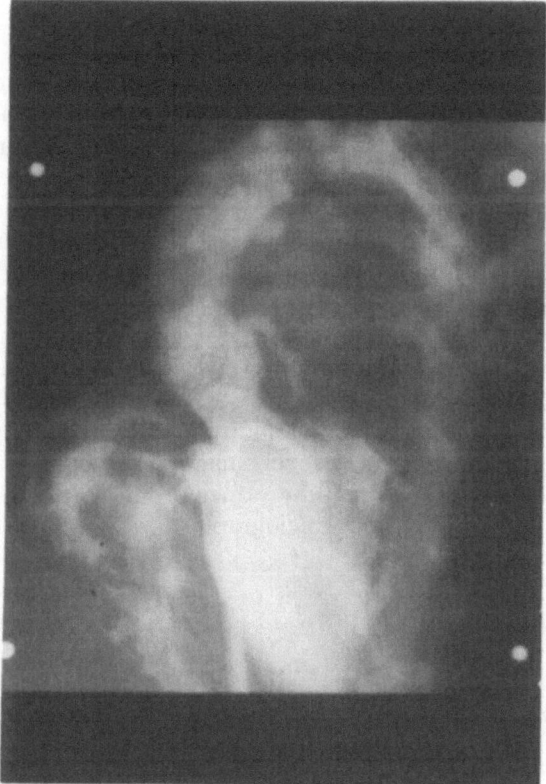

Figure 11. Most ventricular septal defects are located in close relation to the aortic valve. The angiogram (four-chamber view) shows a diagnostic balloon catheter (4F), which was advanced through the defect with the balloon inflated and pulled back to occlude the defect during the angiogram. Thus, the balloon inflated with CO_2 is located in the right ventricle and the ventricular septal defect and its relation to the aortic valve can be demonstrated.

bidirectional Glenn-operation, where the superior vena cava is surgically anastomosed to the right pulmonary artery, while the main pulmonary artery and communication of the superior vena cava with the right atrium are ligated. Thus the blood from the superior vena cava drains passively into the pulmonary artery, while the blood from the inferior vena cava and hepatic veins drains into the systemic ("common") ventricle. As second stage-operation or "completion" of univentricular repair a total cavopulmonary anastomosis is performed, in a way that the blood from the inferior vena cava and hepatic veins also drains passively into the pulmonary artery.

As the risk and postsurgical morbidity are high in patients with risk factors, a new interventional technique to perform completion of univentricular repair was developed at the institution of the author. For this approach as a first stage a hemi-Fontan procedure is performed surgically, however, the communication between superior vena cava and right atrium is not ligated, but strictly narrowed using a band (Figure 12). Interventional completion in the surgically preconditioned patients is performed by balloon dilatation of the narrowed communication between the superior vena cava and the right atrium and insertion of a covered stent as an intracardiac conduit between the superior and inferior vena cava (Figure 12). Thus, a second surgical intervention can be avoided.

Preinterventional imaging has to delineate the exact anatomy of the hepatic veins entering the inferior vena cava, to prevent inadvertent occlusion of hepatic veins by the covered stent. Additionally the length of the stent and the length of the covered part of it have to be evaluated preinterventionally as the length of the stent and the length of its covering have to be selected according to the individual anatomic features. As this technique is rather new, preinterventional angiography is indispensable, including selective injections into the hepatic veins. However, magnetic resonance imaging bears the potential to delineate the anatomy sufficiently to perform this interventional procedure without previous angiography.

Pulmonary atresia

Pulmonary atresia with intact ventricular septum

In some patients the interventional approach consists of several interventions which have to be performed to achieve either an adequate therapy, palliation or – as discussed above – presurgical conditioning. The current interventional approach to pulmonary atresia is an example for a complex intervention, which requires several different techniques [107–110]. The diagnosis of pulmonary atresia with intact ventricular septum is made by echocardiography, which demonstrates the atretic right ventricular outflow tract with the pulmonary arteries perfused retrogradely through a patent duct. The abnormal (retrograde) flow is easily shown by coloured-coded Doppler imaging. The right ventricular cavity is hypoplastic and tricuspid regurgitation is the only "outlet" of the right ventricle. The size of the right ventricle in pulmonary atresia with intact ventricular septum depends on the degree of tricuspid regurgitation.

Preinterventional imaging has to demonstrate the development of the right ventricle, in particular the development of the right ventricular outflow tract. Because the first and most crucial procedure in the interventional therapy of pulmonary atresia is radiofrequency-perforation of the atresia, demonstration of both, an infundibulum and a main pulmonary artery is critical (Figure 13). Although echocardiography is able to demonstrate the right ventricular infundibulum, the echocardiographic visualization of the main pulmonary artery is often inaccurate with either the false positive or false negative

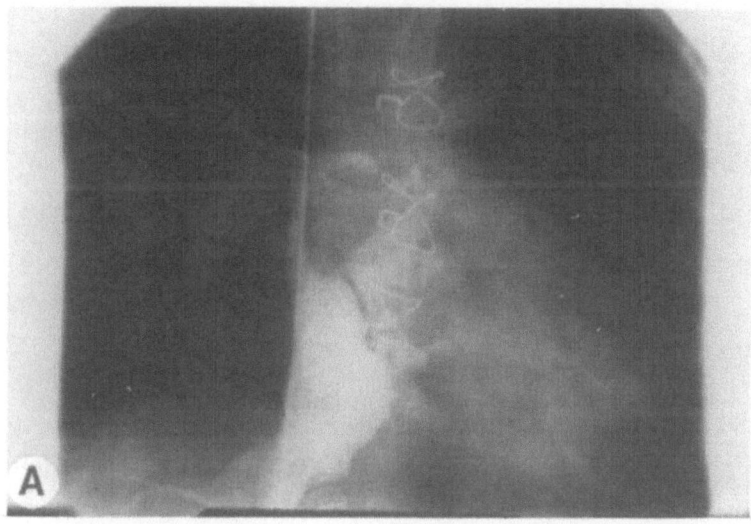

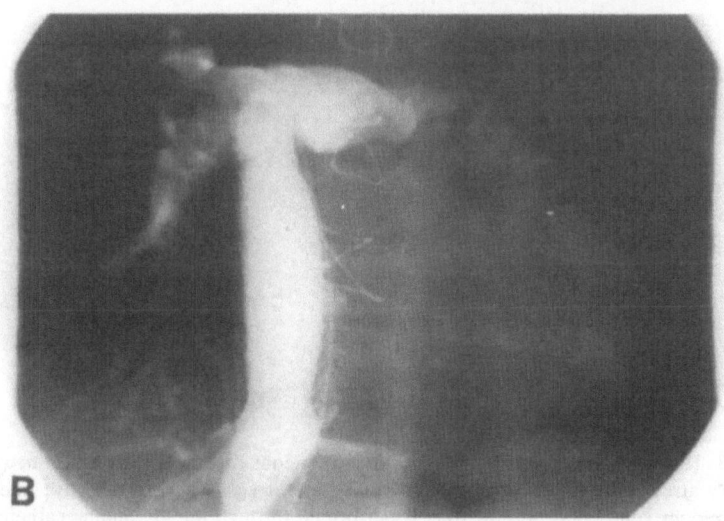

Figure 12. Interventional completion of univentricular repair (Fontan operation) after surgical "preconditioning". (A) For this new technique a hemi-Fontan procedure is performed surgically and the communication between superior vena cava and right atrium is strictly narrowed using a band. (B) Interventional completion is performed by balloon dilatation of the narrowed communication between the superior vena cava and the right atrium and insertion of a covered stent as intracardiac conduit between the superior and inferior vena cava.

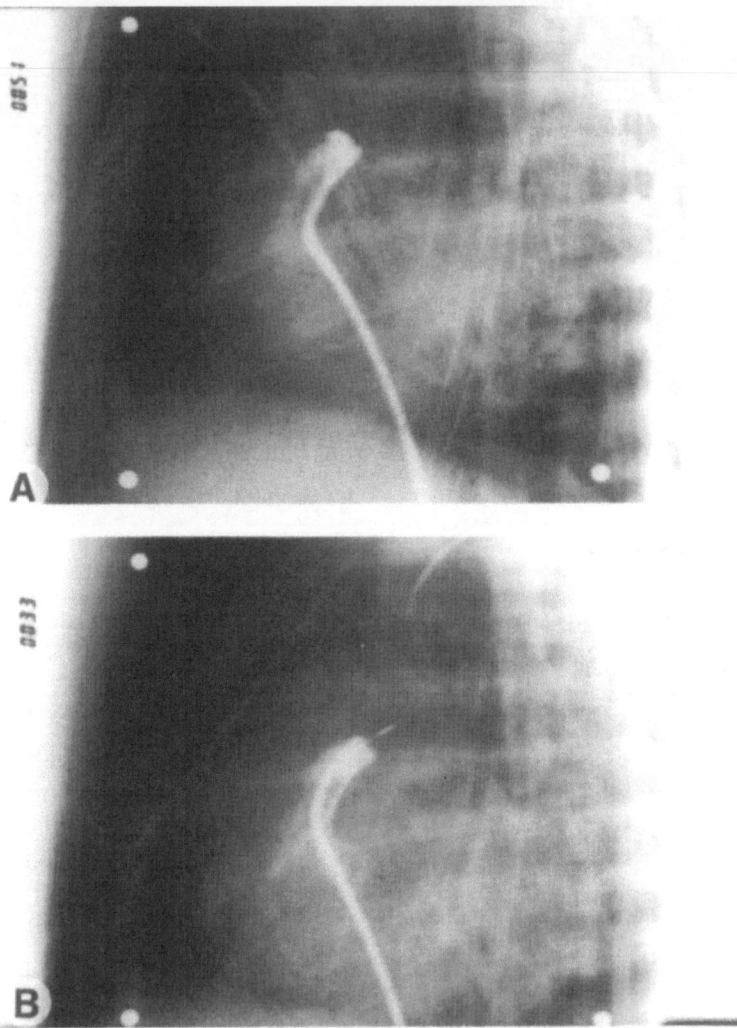

Figure 13. Radiofrequency-perforation of a membraneous atresia is shown in a newborn with pulmonary atresia and intact ventricular septum (lateral view). (A) A selective injection into the atretic right ventricular outflow tract is performed through the 4F guiding catheter. The 2F radiofrequency probe has been advanced to the tip of the guiding catheter and becomes visible (B) after successful perforation of the membraneous atresia. Before perforation was performed the 4F-guiding catheter was repositioned, so that the perforation was performed in the centre of the atretic membrane.

findings of a main pulmonary artery. Because of these discrepancies between the preinterventional echocardiogram and angiographic findings during the intervention, selective angiograms of the atretic right ventricular outflow tract and – if possible – simultaneous angiographic visualization of the pulmonary artery – particularly the main pulmonary artery – are of outstanding importance. Simultaneous angiography of both the infundibulum and the main pulmonary artery demonstrates the exact anatomy of the atresia, which is required for radiofrequency-perforation. The angiographic image can then be used as a road map for the intervention. For the interventional perforation not only the distance between the atretic right ventricular outflow tract and the main pulmonary artery is critical, but also the direction in which the perforation has to be performed. Thus, the three-dimensional relation between both the infundibulum and the main pulmonary artery has to be evaluated to perform perforation in the centre of the atresia. Although 3D-reconstructive imaging techniques using magnetic resonance would be optimal for this purpose, these are not applicable during the intervention. Therefore selective angiography has to be performed during the perforation to assure the correct position of the radiofrequency catheter. After successful perforation balloon dilatation is subsequently performed. The balloon catheter is selected according to the angiographic diameter of the main pulmonary artery, which is usually measured from angiography.

As mentioned above, the right ventricle shows a variable degree of hypoplasia. If echocardiography demonstrates severe hypoplasia of the right ventricle, it has to be assumed that the right ventricle will not be able to maintain pulmonary perfusion. To maintain pulmonary perfusion in these patients the current strategy includes stent-implantation into the patent duct as alternative to surgical creation of an aortopulmonary anastomosis. Preinterventional imaging by echocardiography before stent-implantation has to confirm a stenosis of the duct. However, immediately before stent-implantation selective angiography of the ductal anatomy is performed to select an adequate stent (usually 4 mm diameter).

Rarely, persistent myocardial sinusoids are observed in patients with pulmonary atresia and intact ventricular septum, which are fistulous communications between the right ventricular cavity and the coronary arteries. Stenoses of the coronary arteries are regularly observed, and atresia of the coronary ostia is found in some patients. Thus, coronary perfusion depends in part or even completely on these fistulous communications and a systemic pressure within the right ventricle. Interventional perforation of the atretic right ventricular outflow tract is not indicated in these patients, because the drop in right ventricular pressure would lead to myocardial ischemia or infarction. Although large fistulous communications between the coronary arteries and the right ventricular cavity can be demonstrated using colour-coded-Doppler echocardiography, angiographic demonstration or exclusion of myocardial sinusoids has to be performed in every patient in whom perforation of the atretic pulmonary valve is contemplated. It is also necessary to perform selective angiography of the left coronary artery because this artery neighbours the right ventricular outflow tract.

Pulmonary atresia with ventricular septal defect

Pulmonary atresia with ventricular septal defect is characterized by a normal sized right ventricle. However, the pulmonary arteries in this entity are often extremely hypoplastic. The main pulmonary artery may be completely absent. Additionally, parts of the lungs can be supplied exclusively by aortopulmonary collaterals or by a combination of aortopulmonary collaterals and the pulmonary arteries. A patent duct is often originating abnormally from the mid-aortic arch or a subclavian artery taking a tortuous course from the aortic arch to the pulmonary artery.

MRI is well suited for preinterventional imaging [108–110] of aortopulmonary collaterals, the (hypoplastic) pulmonary artery and the atretic infundibulum. It will also demonstrate the intracardiac anatomy (ventricular septal defect, pulmonary atresia, overriding aorta) and the origin and course of the duct. Nevertheless, before perforation of the atresia is attempted, selective angiography of the infundibulum and the main pulmonary artery is usually performed to provide a road map image for the procedure. However, angiographic demonstration of the main pulmonary artery can be complicated or impossible. When the duct is still patent, angiographic demonstration can be easily performed through the duct (Figure 14). If the duct is closed angiographic demonstration is difficult and either attempted by selective angiography of aortopulmonary collaterals and retrograde filling of the pulmonary artery, or it is attempted by pulmonary "wedge" injections into the pulmonary veins, filling the pulmonary arteries retrogradely. If the pulmonary arteries have to be visualized indirectly and cannot be entered with a catheter, absence of the main pulmonary artery cannot be confirmed, as the main pulmonary artery does not regularly opacify during selective injections of aortopulmonary collaterals or "wedge" angiography. In such a case one has to rely on the information provided by MRI.

While radiofrequency-perforation of pulmonary atresia is impossible in patients without main pulmonary artery, it can be successfully performed in infundibular atresia (Figure 14). However, in this case the perforation is not performed from the right ventricular outflow tract (anterograde) but from the main pulmonary artery, which has to be entered retrogradely. At the time of the intervention, careful selective angiography of the infundibulum (if there is one) and the main pulmonary artery must be performed although preinterventional MRI and echocardiography may already have established to correct diagnosis and most anatomic details.

While the adequate size of the balloon can be derived from the size of the main pulmonary artery in membraneous atresia, this is much more difficult in fibromuscular atresia, because the amount of tissue surrounding the perforation canal is unknown. Even with magnetic resonance imaging or intravascular ultrasound it is impossible to assess the amount of tissue surrounding the atretic zone. Therefore balloon dilatation is initially performed using small balloons and the balloon diameter is increased according to the angiographic findings after dilatation. As overdilatation of the atresia can be hazardous, a stent is implanted to achieve an adequately sized right ventricular outflow tract.

After antegrade pulmonary perfusion is established by creating a right

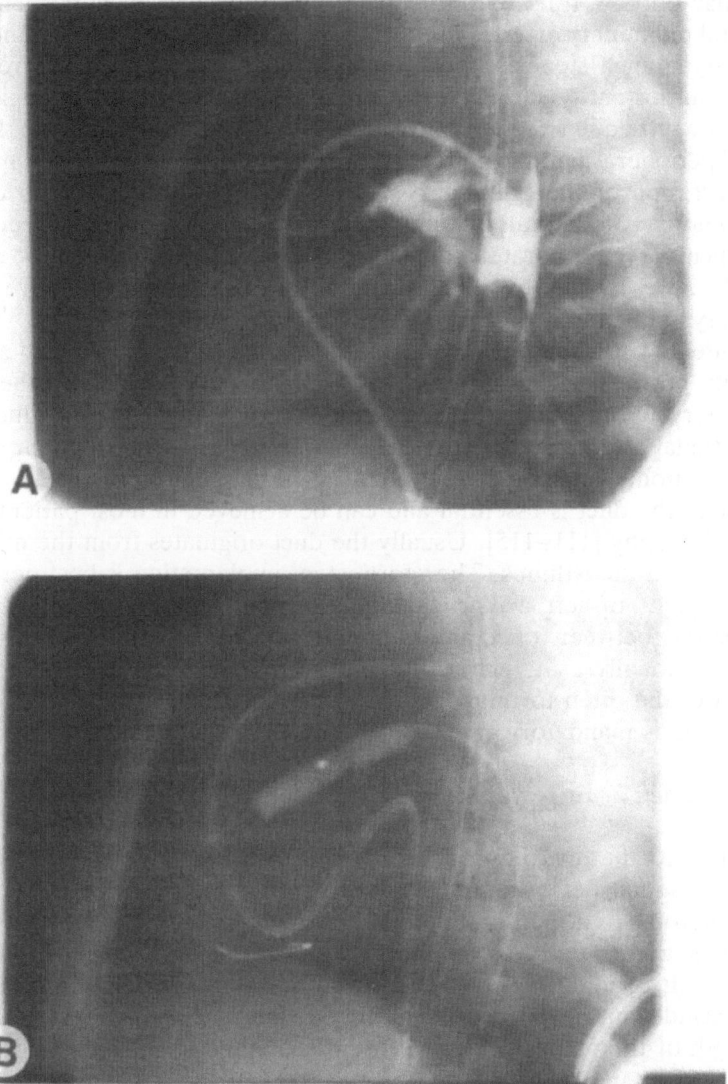

Figure 14. In patients without right ventricular outflow tract, perforation of the atresia cannot be performed antegradely, because no stable position of the catheter can be achieved. Thus, retrograde perforation has to be performed. (A) The anatomy of the pulmonary arteries is depicted by retrograde injection of contrast material through the patent ductus into the main pulmonary artery. (B) In this newborn infant with double inlet ventricle and malposition of the great arteries retrograde perforation with subsequent balloon dilatation and stent-implantation was performed (lateral view).

ventricular outflow tract, careful imaging of the pulmonary branches and peripheral pulmonary arteries for peripheral pulmonic stenosis is mandatory. Pulmonary branch stenosis and peripheral pulmonic stenosis are regularly observed in this entity and need to be relieved either by balloon angioplasty alone or by subsequent stent-implantation into the stenotic segments. Elimination of peripheral pulmonic stenosis is required to achieve adequate antegrade perfusion of the pulmonary vessels, in order to be able to occlude aortopulmonary collaterals without deterioration of pulmonary perfusion. The difficulties of accurately depicting the peripheral pulmonary arteries by MRI and especially by echocardiography were addressed above. Thus, pulmonary angiography is the best technique for this purpose.

In patients with pulmonary atresia and absent main pulmonary artery a continuity between right ventricle and pulmonary artery cannot be established interventionally. In these patients stenting of the patent duct is an interventional alternative to surgical creation of an aortopulmonary shunt. Preinterventional imaging of the right and left pulmonary artery and the anatomy of the duct is essential and can be achieved in most patients using echocardiography [111–115]. Usually the duct originates from the midaortic arch, not from the isthmus. Therefore, stent-implantation is best performed from the right or left axillary artery and not from the femoral vessels. The relation between duct and right/left subclavian artery is established preinterventionally using echocardiography. Nevertheless, angiographic assessment of the often tortuous course of the duct immediately before stent-implantation is mandatory.

Hypoplastic left heart syndrome

In contrast to the anatomy of the arterial duct in pulmonary atresia with ventricular septal defect or tetralogy of Fallot, the duct in hypoplastic left heart syndrome is a continuation of the main pulmonary artery into the descending aorta. Before implanting a stent as a palliative procedure in patients with hypoplastic left heart syndrome a "reversed" coarctation has to be excluded using echocardiography. Additionally the diameter, shape and length of the patent duct have to be evaluated by echocardiography to select an adequate stent [111–115].

Conclusions

Preinterventional catheterization is only very rarely required in children with congenital heart disease. Diagnostic imaging is in most cases successfully performed using echocardiography. The combination of echocardiography and magnetic resonance imaging allows precise evaluation of almost all anatomic features required before the procedure. Using these imaging techniques, it is possible in most patients, to decide whether a surgical or an interventional approach is the optimal therapeutic choice. Thus, diagnostic cardiac catheterization is of decreasing importance for preinterventional imaging. Despite this, selective and supraselective angiographic delineation of specific anatomic features should be performed immediately before and during the interventional procedure. Accurate angiographic imaging is particularly important during complex interventional procedures. While echocardiographic imaging is of increasing importance for preinterventional imaging and imaging during the intervention, magnetic resonance imaging is still restricted to preinterventional imaging. Nevertheless, magnetic resonance imaging has an important role in the preinterventional assessment of older children and adults. Today it is not known whether the development of open magnets will result in a new tool to directly observe and guide interventions in paediatric cardiology.

Acknowledgements

I am thankfully indebted to M. Schneider, J. de Vivie and G. Lorenscheid for their help in preparing and completing the manuscript.

References

1. Burrows PE, Benson LN, Williams WG et al. Iliofemoral arterial complications of balloon angioplasty for systemic obstructions in infants and children. Circulation 1990; 82: 1697–704.
2. Burrows PE, Benson LN, Babyn P, McDonald C. Magnetic resonance imaging of the iliofemoral arteries after balloon dilation angioplasty of aortic arch obstructions in children. Circulation 1994; 90: 915–20.
3. Vermilion RP, Snider AR, Bengur AR, Beekman RH. Doppler evaluation of femoral arteries in children after aortic balloon valvuloplasty or coarctation balloon angioplasty. Pediatr Cardiol 1993; 14: 13–21.
4. Sutherland GR, Stumper OF. Transthoracic versus transesophageal echocardiography in the pediatric patient. Curr Opin Pediatr 1993; 5: 598–605.
5. Skorton DJ, Vandenberg BF. Cardiac ultrasound progress and prospects. Invest Radiol 1993; 28: 19–25.
6. Balzer D, Moorhead S, Saffitz JE et al. Pediatric endomyocardial biopsy performed solely with echocardiographic guidance. J Am Soc Echocardiogr 1993; 6: 510–5.
7. Stumper O, Witsenburg M, Sutherland GR et al. Transesophageal echocardiographic monitoring of interventional cardiac catheterization in children. J Am Coll Cardiol 1991; 18: 1506–20.
8. Van der Velde ME, Sanders SP, Keane JF et al. Transesophageal echocardiographic guidance of transcatheter ventricular septal defect closure. J Am Coll Cardiol 1994; 23: 1660–5.
9. Isner RJ, DiNardo JA. Percutaneous aortic balloon valvuloplasty under transesophageal echocardiographic guidance. J Cardiothorac Vasc Anesth 1994; 8: 81–4.
10. Tee SD, Shiota T, Weintraube R et al. Evaluation of ventricular septal defect by transesophageal echocardiography: Intraoperative assessment. Am Heart J 1994; 127: 585–92.
11. Stevenson JG, Sorensen GK, Gartman DM et al. Transesophageal echocardiography

during repair of congenital cardiac defects: Identification of residual problems necessitating reoperation. J Am Soc Echocardiogr 1993; 6: 356–65.

12. Hellenbrand WE, Fahey JT, McGowan FX et al. Transesophageal echocardiographic guidance of transcatheter closure of atrial septal defect. Am J Cardiol 1990; 66: 207–13.

13. Rao PS, Langhough R. Relationship of echocardiographic, shunt flow, and angiographic size to the stretched diameter of the atrial septal defect. Am Heart J 1991; 122: 505–12.

14. Morimoto K, Matsuzaki M, Tohma Y et al. Diagnosis and quantitative evaluation of secundum-type atrial septal defect by transesophageal Doppler echocardiography. Am J Cardiol 1990; 66: 85–91.

15. Jiang L, Handschumacher MD, Hibberd MG et al. Three-dimensional echocardiographic reconstruction of right ventricular volume: In vitro comparison with two-dimensional methods. J Am Soc Echocardiogr 1994; 7: 150–8.

16. Schwartz SL, Cao QL, Azevedo J, Pandian NG. Simulation of intraoperative visualization of cardiac structures and study of dynamic surgical anatomy with real-time three-dimensional echocardiography. Am J Cardiol 1994; 73: 501–7.

17. Mitchell JD, Weyman AE, King ME, Levine RA. Three-dimensional reconstruction of ventricular septal defects: Validation studies and in vivo feasibility. J Am Coll Cardiol 1994; 23: 201–8.

18. Belohlavek M, Foley DA, Gerber TC et al. Three-dimensional ultrasound imaging of the atrial septum: Normal and pathologic anatomy. J Am Coll Cardiol 1993; 22: 1673–8.

19. Vogel M, Losch S. Dynamic three-dimensional echocardiography with a computed tomography imaging probe: Initial clinical experience with transthoracic application in infants and children with congenital heart defects. Br Heart J 1994; 71: 462–7.

20. Newman B. Imaging of the pediatric cardiovascular system. Curr Opin Radiol 1991; 3: 925–30.

21. Parsons JM, Baker EJ. The use of magnetic resonance imaging in the investigation of infants and children with congenital heart disease: Current status and future prospects. Int J Cardiol 1990; 29: 263–75.

22. Seelos KC, von Smekal A, Steinborn M et al. MR angiography of congenital heart disease: Value of segmented two-dimensional inflow technique and maximum-intensity-projection display. J Magn Reson Imaging 1994; 4: 29–36.

23. Akagi T, Kato H, Kiyomatsu Y et al. Evaluation of arterial, ventricular and atrioventricular septal defects by cine magnetic resonance imaging. Acta Paediatr Jpn 1992; 34: 295–300.

24. Burrows PE, McDonald CE. Magnetic resonance imaging of the pediatric thoracic aorta. Semin Ultrasound CT MR 1993; 14: 129–44.

25. Parsons JM, Baker EJ, Hayes A et al. Magnetic resonance imaging of the great arteries in infants. Int J Cardiol 1990; 28: 73–85.

26. Wong ND, Vo A, Abrahamson D et al. Detection of coronary artery calcium by ultrafast computed tomography and its relation to clinical evidence of coronary artery disease. Am J Cardiol 1994; 73: 223–7.

27. Crochet D, Lefevre M, Grossetete R et al. Comparison of magnetic resonance imaging, echocardiography and catheterization in the diagnosis of congenital heart diseases. Arch Mal Coeur Vaiss 1990; 83: 681–6.

28. McMillan RM. Magnetic resonance imaging vs ultrafast computed tomography for cardiac diagnosis. Int J Cardiac Imaging 1992; 8: 217–27.

29. Schlesinger AE, Hernandez RJ. Congenital heart disease: Applications of computed tomography and magnetic resonance imaging. Semin Ultrasound CT MR 1991; 12: 11–27.

30. Wiles HB. Imaging congenital heart disease. Pediatr Clin North Am 1990; 37: 115–36.

31. Matsumoto AH, Teitelbaum GP, Carvlin MJ et al. Gadolinium enhanced MR imaging of vascular stents. J Comput Assist Tomogr 1990; 14: 357–61.

32. Teitelbaum GP, Raney M, Carvlin MJ et al. Evaluation of ferromagnetism and magnetic resonance imaging artifacts of the Strecker tantalum vascular stent. Cardiovasc Intervent Radiol 1989; 12: 125–7.

33. Girard MJ, Hahn PF, Saini S et al. Wallstent metallic biliary endoprosthesis: MR imaging characteristics. Radiology 1992; 184: 874–6.
34. Vick GW 3d, Rokey R, Huhta JC et al. Nuclear magnetic resonance imaging of the pulmonary arteries, subpulmonary region, and aorticopulmonary shunts: A comparative study with two-dimensional echocardiography and angiography. Am Heart J 1990; 119: 1103–10.
35. Kondo C, Hardy C, Higgins SS et al. Nuclear magnetic resonance imaging of the palliative operation for hypoplastic left heart syndrome. J Am Coll Cardiol 1991; 18: 817–23.
36. Bisset GS. 3-D Magnetic resonance imaging of congenital heart disease in the pediatric patient. Radiol Clin North Am 1991; 29: 279–91.
37. Fawzy ME, v Sinner W, Rifai A et al. Magnetic resonance imaging compared with angiography in the evaluation of intermediate-term result of coarctation balloon angioplasty. Am Heart J 1993; 126: 1380–4.
38. Nyman R, Hallberg M, Sunnegardh J et al. Magnetic resonance imaging and angiography for assessment of coarctation of the aorta. Acta Radiol 1989; 30: 481–5.
39. Stern HC, Locher D, Wallnofer K et al. Noninvasive assessment of coarctation of the aorta: Comparative measurements by two-dimensional echocardiography, magnetic resonance, and angiography. Pediatr Cardiol 1991; 12: 1–5.
40. Teien DE, Wendel H, Bjornebrink J, Ekelund L. Evaluation of anatomical obstruction by Doppler echocardiography and magnetic resonance imaging in patients with coarctation of the aorta. Br Heart J 1993; 69: 352–5.
41. Rashkind WJ, Miller WW. Creation of an atrial septal defect without thoracotomy: A palliative approach to complete transposition of the great arteries. Am J Med Assoc 1966; 196: 173–4.
42. Boutin C, Dyck J, Benson L et al. Balloon atrial septostomy under transesophageal echocardiographic guidance. Pediatr Cardiol 1992; 13: 176–7.
43. Ashfaq M, Houston AB, Gnanapragasam JP et al. Balloon atrial septostomy under echocardiographic control: Six years' experience and evaluation of the practicability of cannulation via the umbilical vein. Br Heart J 1991; 65: 148–51.
44. Beitzke A, Stein JI, Suppan C. Balloon atrial septostomy under two-dimensional echocardiographic control. Int J Cardiol 1991; 30: 33–42.
45. Park SC, Neches WH, Zuberbuhler JR et al. Clinical use of blade atrial septostomy technique Circulation 1978; 58: 600–6.
46. Park SC, Zuberbuhler JR, Neches WH et al. A new atrial septostomy technique. Cathet Cardiovasc Diagn 1975; 1: 195–201.
47. Perry SB, Lang P, Keane JF et al. Creation and maintenance of an adequate interatrial communication in left atrioventricular valve atresia or stenosis. Am J Cardiol 1986; 58: 622–6.
48. Kan JS, White RI Jr, Mitchell SE, Gardner TJ. Percutaneous balloon valvuloplasty: A new method for treating congenital pulmonary valve stenosis. N Engl J Med 1982; 307: 540–2.
49. Kan JS, White RI, Mitchell SE. Percutaneous transluminal balloon valvuloplasty for pulmonary valve stenosis. Circulation 1984; 69: 554–60.
50. Rao PS, Fawzy ME, Solymar L, Mardini MK. Long-term results of balloon pulmonary valvuloplasty of valvar pulmonic stenosis. Am Heart J 1988; 115: 1291–6.
51. Rao PS. How big a balloon and how many balloons for pulmonary valvuloplasty? Am Heart J 1988; 116: 577–80.
52. McCrindle BW. Independent predictors of long-term results after balloon pulmonary valvuloplasty. Valvuloplasty and Angioplasty of Congenital Anomalies Registry Investigators. Circulation 1994; 89: 1751–9.
53. Stanger P, Cassidy SC, Girod DA et al. Balloon pulmonary valvuloplasty: Results of the Valvuloplasty and Angioplasty of Congenital Anomalies Registry. Am J Cardiol 1990; 65: 775–83.

54. Lynch DA, Higgins CB. MR imaging of unilateral pulmonary artery anomalies. J Comput Assist Tomogr 1990; 14: 187–91.
55. Gomes AS, Lois JF, Williams RG. Pulmonary arteries: MR imaging in patients with congenital obstruction of the right ventricular outflow tract. Radiology 1990; 174: 51–7.
56. Hirashi S, Misawa H, Hirota H et al. Noninvasive quantitative evaluation of the morphology of the major pulmonary artera branches in cyanotic congenital heart disease. Circulation 1994; 89: 1306–16.
57. Lock JE, Niemi T, Einzig S et al. Transvenous angioplasty of experimental branch pulmonary artery stenosis in newborn lambs. Circulation 1981; 64: 886–93.
58. Sholler GF, Keane JF, Fellows KE. Balloon dilatation of congenital aortic valve stenosis: Results and influence of technical and morphological features on outcome. Circulation 1988; 78: 351–60.
59. Wren C, Sullivan I, Ball C, Deanfield J. Percutaneous balloon dilatation of aortic valve stenosis in neonates and infants. Br Heart J 1987; 58: 608–12.
60. Hausdorf G, Schneider M, Schirmer KR et al. Anterograde balloon valvuloplasty of aortic stenosis in children. Am J Cardiol 1993; 71: 460–2.
61. Rocchini AP, Beekman RH, Ben-Shachar G et al. Balloon aortic valvuloplasty: Results of the Valvuloplasty and Angioplasty of Congenital Anomalies Registry. Am J Cardiol 1990; 65: 784–9.
62. Witsenburg M, Cromme-Dijkhuis AH, Frohn-Mulder IM, Hess J. Short- and midterm results of balloon valvuloplasty for valvular aortic stenosis in children. Am J Cardiol 1992; 69: 945–50.
63. Hosking MC, Benson LN, Freedom RM. A femoral vein-femoral artery loop technique for aortic dilatation in children. Cathet Cardiovasc Diagn 1991; 23: 253–6.
64. O'Connor BK, Beekman RH, Rocchini AP, Rosenthal A. Intermediate-term effectiveness of balloon valvuloplasty for congenital aortic stenosis. Circulation 1991; 84: 732–8.
65. Leung MP, McKay R, Smith A et al. Critical aortic stenosis in early infancy. Anatomic and echocardiographic substrates of successful open valvotomy. J Thorac Cardiovasc Surg 1991; 101: 526–35.
66. Zeevi B, Keane JF, Castaneda AR et al. Neonatal critical valvar aortic stenosis. A comparison of surgical and balloon dilation therapy. Circulation 1989; 80: 831–9.
67. Rao PS, Chopra PS. Role of balloon angioplasty in the treatment of aortic coarctation. Ann Thorac Surg 1991; 52: 621–31.
68. Huggon IC, Qureshi SA, Baker EJ, Tynan M. Effect of introducing balloon dilatation of native aortic coarctation on overall outcome in infants and children. Am J Cardiol 1994; 73: 799–807.
69. Hellenbrand WE, Alen HD, Golinko RJ et al. Balloon angioplasty for aortic recoarctation: Results of Valvuloplasty and Angioplasty of Congenital Anomalies Registry. Am J Cardiol 1990; 65: 793–7.
70. Tynan M, Finley JP, Fontes V et al. Balloon angioplasty for the treatment of native coarctation: Results of Valvuloplasty and Angioplasty of Congenital Anomalies Registry. Am J Cardiol 1990; 65: 790–2.
71. Harrison JK, Sheikh KH, Davidson CJ et al. Balloon angioplasty of coarctation of the aorta evaluated with intravascular ultrasound imaging. J Am Coll Cardiol 1990; 15: 906–9.
72. Mohiaddin RH, Kilner PJ, Rees S, Longmore DB. Magnetic resonance volume flow and jet velocity mapping in aortic coarctation. J Am Coll Cardiol 1993; 22: 1515–21.
73. Muhler EG, Neuerburg JM, Ruben A et al. Evaluation of aortic coarctation after surgical repair: Role of magnetic resonance imaging and Doppler ultrasound. Br Heart J 1993; 70: 285–90.
74. Mirowitz SA, Lee JK, Gutierrez FR et al. "Pseudocoarctation" of the aorta: Pitfall on cine MR imaging. J Comput Assist Tomogr 1990; 14: 753–5.
75. Grifka RG, Vick GW, O'Laughlin MP et al. Balloon expandable intravascular stents:

Aortic implantation and late further dilation in growing minipigs. Am Heart J 1993; 126: 979–84.

76. Mullins CE, Latson LA, Neches WH et al. Balloon dilation of miscellaneous lesions: Results of Valvuloplasty and Angioplasty of Congenital Anomalies Registry. Am J Cardiol 1990; 65: 802–3.

77. Ichida F, Hashimoto I, Miyazaki A et al. Magnetic resonance imaging: Evaluation of the Blalock-Taussig shunts and anatomy of the pulmonary artery. J Cardiol 1992; 22: 669–78.

78. Vannier MW, Gutierrez FR, Canter CE et al. Evaluation of congenital heart disease by three-dimensional magnetic resonance imaging. J Digit Imaging 1991; 4: 153–8.

79. Canter CE, Gutierrez FR, Mirowitz SA et al. Evaluation of pulmonary arterial morphology in cyanotic congenital heart disease by magnetic resonance imaging. Am Heart J 1989; 118: 347–54.

80. Kan JS, Marvin WJ Jr, Bass JL et al. Balloon angioplasty-branch pulmonary artery stenosis: Results from the Valvuloplasty and Angioplasty of Congenital Anomalies Registry. Am J Cardiol 1990; 65: 798–801.

81. O'Laughlin MP, Perry SB, Lock JE, Mullins CE. Use of endovascular stents in congenital heart disease. Circulation 1991; 83: 1923–39.

82. O'Laughlin MP, Slack MC, Grifka RG et al. Implantation and intermediate-term follow-up of stents in congenital heart disease. Circulation 1993; 8: 605–14.

83. Nakanishi T, Kondoh C, Nishikawa T et al. Intravascular stents for management of pulmonary artery and right ventricular outflow obstruction. Heart Vessels 1994; 9: 40–8.

84. Driscoll DJ, Hesslein PS, Mullins CE. Congenital stenosis of individual treatment veins: Clinical spectrum and unsuccessful treatment by transvenous balloon dilatation. Am J Cardiol 1982; 49: 1767–72.

85. Hosking MC, Alshehri M, Murdison KA et al. Transcatheter management of pulmonary venous pathway obstruction with atrial baffle leak following Mustard and Senning repair. Cathet Cardiovasc Diagn 199; 30: 76–82.

86. Aydogan U, Onursal E, Cantez T et al. Giant congenital coronary artery fistula to left superior vena cava and right atrium with compression of left pulmonary vein simulating cor triatriatum-diagnostic value of magnetic resonance imaging. Eur J Cardiothorac Surg 1994; 8: 97–9.

87. Rashkind WJ, Mullins CE, Hellenbrand WE, Tait MA. Nonsurgical closure of patent ductus arteriosus. Circulation 1987; 75: 583–92.

88. Lock JE, Cockerham JT, Leane JF et al. Transcatheter umbrella closure of congenital heart defects. Circulation 1987; 75: 593–9.

89. Burrows PE, Edwards TC, Benson LN. Transcatheter occlusion of Blalock-Taussig shunts: technical options. J Vasc Intervent Radiol 1993; 4: 673–80.

90. Rao PS, Sideris EB, Haddad J et al. Transcatheter occlusion of patent ductus arteriosus with adjustable buttoned device. Initial clinical experience. Circulation 1993; 88: 1119–26.

91. Ali-Khan MA, Al-Yousef S, Mullins CE, Sawyer W. Experience with 205 procedures of transcatheter closure of ductus arteriosus in 182 patients, with special reference to residual shunts and long-term follow-up. J Thorac Cardiovasc Surg 1992; 104: 1721–7.

92. Musewe NN, Benson LN, Smallhorn JF, Freedom RM. Two-dimensional echocardiographic and color flow Doppler evaluation of ductal occlusion with the Rashkind prosthesis. Circulation 1989; 80: 1706–10.

93. Sideris EB, Sideris SE, Thanopoulos BD et al. Transvenous atrial septal defect occlusion by the buttoned device. Am J Cardiol 1990; 81: 312–8.

94. Rome JJ, Keane JF, Perry StB et al. Double-umbrella closure of atrial defects. Circulation 1990; 82: 751–8.

95. Rao PS, Langhough R, Beekman H et al. Echocardiographic estimation of balloon-stretched diameter of secundum atrial septal defect for transcatheter occlusion. Am Heart J 1992: 124: 172–5.

96. King TD, Thompson SL, Mills NL. Measurement of atrial septal defect during cardiac catheterization: Experimental and clinical results. Am J Cardiol 1978; 41: 537–42.

97. Babic UU, Grujicic S, Djurisic Z et al. Transcatheter closure of atrial septal defects. Lancet 1990; 336: 566–7.
98. Rao PS, Sideris EB, Chopra PS. Catheter closure of atrial septal defect: Successful use in a 3.6 kg infant. Am Heart J 1991; 121: 1826–9.
99. Lock JE, Hellenbrand WE, Latson L et al. Clamshell umbrella closure of atrial septal defects: Initial experience. Circulation 1989; 80: II–592 (Abstr).
100. Schwinger ME, Gindea AJ, Freedberg RS, Kronzon I. The anatomy of the interatrial septum: A transesophageal echocardiographic study. Am Heart J 1990; 119: 1401–5.
101. Bridges ND, Lock JE, Castaneda AR. Baffle fenestration with subsequent transcatheter closure: Modification of the Fontan operation for patients at increased risk. Circulation 1990; 82: 1681–9.
102. Hausdorf G, Schneider M, Hebe J et al. Combined surgical-interventional procedure in congenital heart defects with postoperative, left ventricular dysfunction. Z Kardiol 1992; 81: 276–82.
103. Redington AN, Rigby ML. Novel uses of the Rashkind ductal umbrella in adults and children with congenital heart disease. Br Heart J 1993; 69: 47–51.
104. Lock JE, Block PC, McKay RG et al. Transcatheter closure of ventricular septal defects. Circulation 1988; 78: 361–8.
105. Bridges ND, Perry SB, Keane JF et al. Preoperative transcatheter closure of congenital muscular ventricular septal defects. N Engl J Med 1991; 324: 1312–7.
106. Baker EJ, Ayton V, Smith MA et al. Magnetic resonance imaging at a high field strength of ventricular septal defects in infants. Br Heart J 1989; 62: 305–10.
107. Qureshi SA, Rosenthal E, Tynan M. Transcatheter laser-assisted balloon pulmonary valve dilatation in pulmonic valve atresia. Am J Cardiol 1991; 68: 428–31.
108. Hausdorf G, Schneider M, Lange P. Catheter creation of an open outflow tract in previously atretic right ventricular outflow tract associated with ventricular septal defect. Am J Cardiol 1993; 72: 354–6.
109. Hausdorf G, Schulz-Neick I, Lange PE. Radiofrequency-assisted "reconstruction" of the right ventricular outflow tract in muscular pulmonary atresia with ventricular septal defect. Br Heart J 1993; 69: 343–6.
110. Hausdorf G, Schneider M, Schirmer KR et al. Interventional high frequency perforation and enlargement of the outflow tract of pulmonary atresia. Z Kardiol 1993; 82: 123–30.
111. Abrams SE, Walsh KP. Arterial duct morphology with reference to angioplasty and stenting. Int J Cardiol 1993; 40: 27–33.
112. Gibbs JL, Rothman MT, Rees MR et al. Stenting of the arterial duct: A new approach to palliation for pulmonary atresia. Br Heart J 1992; 67: 240–5.
113. Ruiz CE, Zhang HP, Larsen RL. The role of interventional cardiology in pediatric heart transplantation. J Heart Lung Transplant 1993; 12: 164–7.
114. Gibbs JL, Wren C, Watterson KG et al. Stenting of the arterial duct combined with banding of the pulmonary arteries and atrial septectomy or septostomy: A new approach to palliation for the hypoplastic left syndrome. Br Heart J 1993; 69: 551–5.
115. Rosenthal E, Qureshi SA, Kakadekar AP et al. Comparison of balloon dilatation and stent implantation to maintain patency of the neonatal arterial duct in lambs. Am J Cardiol 1993; 71: 1373–6.

Corresponding Author: Prof. Gerd Hausdorf Charité, Department of Pediatric Cardiology, Humboldt-University Berlin, Schumannstrasse 20-21, D-10117 Berlin, Germany

30. The role of ultrasound in monitoring of interventional cardiac catheterization in patients with congenital heart disease

OLIVER STÜMPER

Introduction

The introduction of cardiac ultrasound techniques in the practice of paediatric cardiology has revolutionized the diagnosis and management of patients with congenital heart disease over the past 15 years. A high proportion of infants and children undergo complete surgical correction of their congenital cardiac lesions without prior cardiac catheterization. Lesions in which diagnostic catheterization is no longer indicated include: anomalous pulmonary venous connections, atrial septal defects, atrioventricular septal defects, the majority of ventricular septal defects, transposition of the great arteries and also hypoplastic left heart syndrome. Thus, over the past decade the total number of diagnostic cardiac catheterizations in children with congenital heart disease has fallen dramatically. At the same time, however, a range of interventional cardiac catheterization procedures have become available and are now firmly established. With these changes about 40% of all cardiac catheterization procedures in children with congenital heart disease are now interventional procedures.

For many years there has been competition between angiography and echocardiography and it is not until recently that there is a close interaction between these two modalities. Consequently, over the past couple of years more centers employ cardiac ultrasound in the monitoring of selected interventional cardiac catheterization procedures [1, 2]. This chapter will try to define the current role of ultrasound monitoring of the wide range of interventional cardiac catheterization in patients with congenital heart disease.

Choice of ultrasound technique

Transthoracic ultrasound techniques are readily available, non-invasive and yield unlimited scan planes together with very good image quality in the majority of infants and young children. However, the use in the cardiac

C.A. Nienaber and U. Sechtem (eds): Imaging and Intervention in Cardiology, 505–520.
© 1996 Kluwer Academic Publishers. Printed in the Netherlands.

catheterization laboratory is limited because of the interference with routine fluoroscopy and also, in particular in young children, with the sterile area. The principal use of transthoracic and subcostal ultrasound in the monitoring of interventional cardiac catheterization is its use in the guidance of balloon atrial septostomy in children with transposition of the great arteries (Rashkind procedure). This monitoring technique has been established in 1982 and provides very good results in the majority of neonates [3]. Only the use of ultrasound monitoring has made this life-saving procedure a bed-side technique in the very ill neonate (Figure 1).

In about 1989 transesophageal ultrasound probes have been developed for use in small children [4, 5]. Initially the image quality of these probes was limited and only transverse axis imaging probes were available. However, over the past four years high quality and high resolution probes have become, available, which allow imaging both in transverse and in longitudinal planes. Multiplane transesophageal probes for use in even small children are under clinical evaluation.

Although transesophageal ultrasound is an invasive technique which requires general anaesthesia in the majority of paediatric patients, the complication rate for such procedures is very low (less than 1%). The most common complications are esophageal bleeding and atrial arrhythmias. In our own experience with more than thousand studies in children we have not experienced a single life-threatening complication. Considering that most interventional cardiac catheterizations in children are performed under general anaesthesia, it is justified to say that the use of transesophageal ultrasound as a monitoring technique does not increase the risk of the procedure.

Because of the above considerations and the interference of transthoracic ultrasound techniques with the routine fluoroscopic monitoring of the interventional procedure, the transesophageal approach is the most commonly used technique in the monitoring of the wide range of interventions currently used in paediatric cardiology. The following paragraphs summarize indications, limitations and the potential contributions of this technique in patient management.

General considerations

As outlined above the use of transesophageal ultrasound monitoring requires that interventional procedures are carried out under general anaesthesia. Ideally the transesophageal probe should be inserted at the beginning of the procedure and a detailed study should be carried out. Following this the probe should be switched off and should be pulled back to a high esophageal position so as not to interfere with the routine angiographic study. When the final decision is taken to proceed with the intervention the probe is then repositioned. Ideally, radiographic imaging planes should be modified so that the transesophageal probe does not project onto the area of interest during

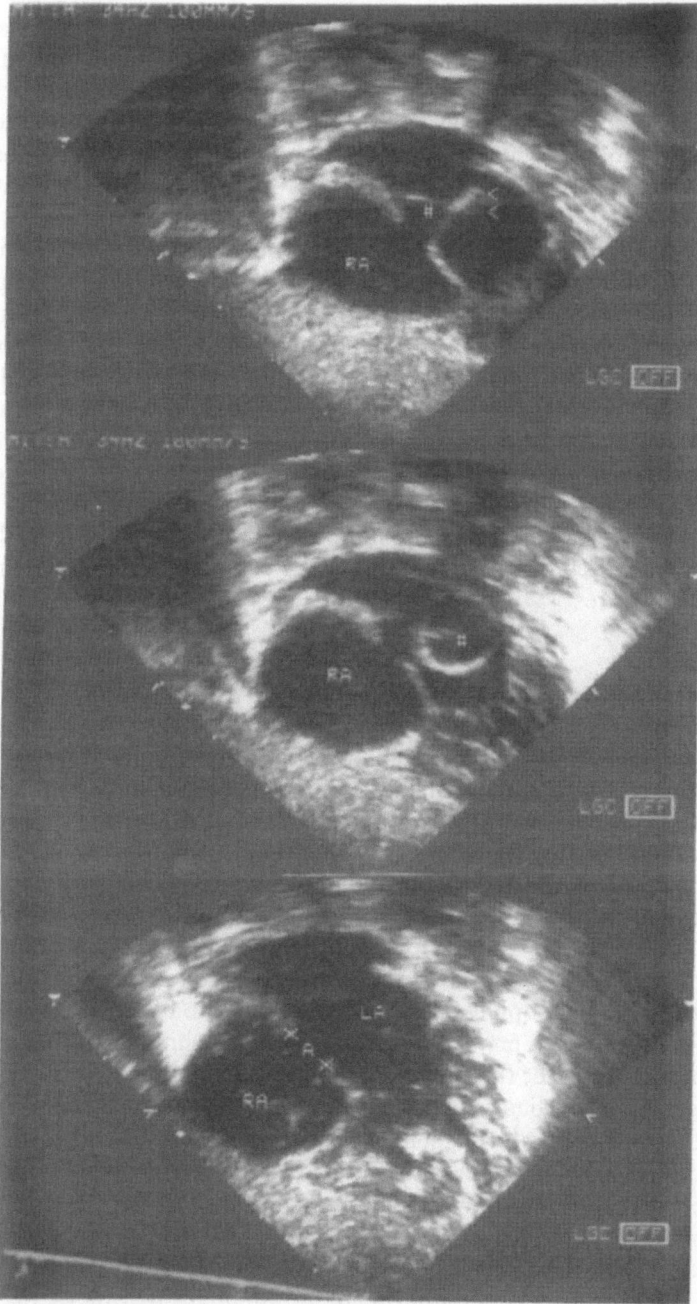

Figure 1. Subcostal ultrasound study in a neonate with transposition of the great arteries undergoing balloon atrial septostomy. Top: The atrial septum is nicely profiled. Note the bulging flap valve of the restrictive foramen ovale (#). The balloon catheter has been advanced to the left atrium and the tip is well away from the mitral valve. Middle: The balloon is fully inflated. Bottom: At the end of the procedure there is a wide atrial communication measuring about 8 mm. On pulsed Doppler studies there was unobstructed bidirectional shunting. Abbreviations: LA = left atrium; RA = right atrium.

fluoroscopy used for catheter manipulation. Only then will it be possible to obtain the maximum value from combining these two imaging modalities.

The screen of the ultrasound machine should be positioned in such a way that both the echocardiographer and the interventionalist can view the screen at all times without difficulties. Ideally a slave monitor should be positioned right next to the videoscreen for fluoroscopy so that the operator can assess both images simultaneously.

In order to obtain the maximal benefit from such studies, there should be an excellent understanding between the echocardiographer and the interventionalist. The echocardiographer has to be aware of the information that is required by the interventionalist at any given stage during the procedure, and has to master the skills to provide this information rapidly. The catheterizer, on the other hand has to have a detailed understanding of transesophageal imaging and Doppler techniques. In particular, the anatomic basis of transesophageal cross-sectional imaging should be fully appreciated by the catheterizer, so as to be able to take advantage of this real-time imaging information during catheter manipulation. This should help to reduce the amount of both screening times and contrast agent requirements during complex procedures.

Atrial septostomy procedures

With the availability of transthoracic ultrasound techniques very good monitoring technique is readily available on most neonatal intensive care units. Thus, there is little need for transesophageal studies during these procedures. Cross-sectional imaging, in most cases, will readily identify the atrial septum and the position of the tip of the balloon catheter prior to inflation. The balloon should not be inflated when the tip is found close to or within the mitral valve apparatus. Colour flow mapping and pulsed wave Doppler rapidly confirms the adequacy of the interatrial communication at the end of the procedure. Transesophageal monitoring has been used by several investigators as an alternative imaging and monitoring technique [6]. However, in the uncomplicated case, the only advantage is the reduced interference with the procedure, in particular when the umbilical venous approach is being used. The use of transesophageal studies should be restricted to those neonates who have unusual atrial anatomies, such as juxtaposed atrial appendages, where a malorientation of the atrial septum often precludes a straightforward passage across the atrial septum [7].

In children older than two months of age, the tissue of the atrial septum markedly thickens and frequently precludes adequate tearing by the balloon septostomy technique. In such cases blade atrial septostomy is the preferred interventional technique [8]. Although good immediate and long-term results together with a low complication rate have been reported, these procedures can be hazardous in less experienced hands. Using transesophageal monitoring during blade atrial septostomies should allow a detailed assessment of the atrial septal morphology, and thus define the most appropriate plane of blade orientation. In addition, malorientation of the blade catheter should be readily identifiable, thus limiting the risk of complications (e.g. perforation of the atrial free wall, pulmonary veins, or the aortic root). Such studies should improve on the safety and efficacy of these procedures. Again, the technique offers precise and immediate documentation of both the morphologic and hemodynamic results. The need for concomitant pressure recordings by means of a second venous catheter, or the need to change the blade septostomy catheter for a diagnostic catheter, would appear to be obviated.

Dilatation of venous obstructions

Obstructions to either the systemic or pulmonary venous return is most commonly found in the postoperative follow-up of patients who underwent either an atrial switch (Mustard or Senning) procedure for transposition of the great arteries, or following surgical correction of total anomalous pulmonary venous connections.

Following Mustard and Senning procedures transesophageal ultrasound has become the imaging technique of first choice in the exclusion of atrial baffle obstruction and baffle leakage [9]. Not surprisingly the technique has also proven to be of major advantage in the selection of patients who may benefit from balloon dilatation and in the monitoring of such procedures [1]. Systemic venous obstructions are most often encountered at the level of the remnant of the atrial septum. Discrete narrowings respond favourably to balloon dilatation whereas long segment and calcific lesions are most likely better treated by stent implantation. Using transesophageal imaging the exact morphology will be documented in detail and the technique can be used with very good results in the monitoring of the positioning of either the balloon catheter or the stent. The immediate haemodynamic changes can be assessed rapidly by a combination of both colour and pulsed wave Doppler. Pulmonary venous obstructions are much rarer lesions after these operations. If balloon angioplasty is considered the addition of transesophageal monitoring should be of particular value if the retrograde approach (via aortic and tricuspid valve) is chosen. During such procedures there is risk of damage of the tricuspid valve apparatus. The use of transesophageal imaging should allow the rapid exclusion of such a catheter malposition, which will be difficult to exclude on fluoroscopy on its own. Again, pulsed wave Doppler studies will provide immediate assessment of haemodynamic result between subsequent inflations. Residual obstruction is readily identified by persistence of continuous turbulent flow patterns throughout the cardiac cycle, whereas a return to phasic flow patterns, with flow velocities approximating zero following atrial contraction, is a good indicator of successful gradient relief.

The initial treatment of pulmonary venous obstruction following repair of total anomalous pulmonary venous obstruction is surgical. In our experience, it is beneficial to create a moderate sized atrial septal defect at the same procedure so as to facilitate subsequent balloon angioplasty which will be needed in the majority of patients. The use of transesophageal ultrasound in the monitoring of balloon dilatations of obstructed pulmonary veins has many advantages. Firstly, all four pulmonary veins will be readily documented on imaging and colour flow mapping studies. This largely facilitates catheter guidance and placement. Secondly, by documenting the exact morphology of the lesion and also the more proximal segments of the pulmonary veins a better insight into the extent of the lesions can be gained. Discrete lesions with dilated proximal pulmonary venous segments will respond favourably to dilatation, whereas long-segment fibrotic lesions without evidence of proximal adequately sized venous segments are unlikely to improve. Changes in morphology and flow patterns can be assessed immediately following dilatation, thereby largely reducing the amount of time and contrast medium used for angiographic and haemodynamic studies. Stent implantation (Figure 2) for recurrent pulmonary venous obstruction has been advocated, however in the experience of most centers reocclusion takes place rapidly and may even be accelerated. Also stent implantation limits future surgical and interventional options.

Balloon valvuloplasty

In the paediatric patient population both balloon dilatation of stenotic pulmonary and aortic valves are firmly established interventional procedures [11, 12]. In contrast, balloon dilatation of stenotic atrioventricular valves (see chapters by Goldstein, Chen and Hausdorf) is rarely performed and is almost exclusively limited to dilatation of post rheumatic lesions. The contribution of transesophageal monitoring in the child undergoing such procedures should be of major benefit, keeping in mind the difficulties and potential risks of transseptal punctures and catheter manipulations in the small patient.

Pulmonary valvuloplasty can be performed with very good success and very low complication rates. However, when transesophageal imaging is used in the monitoring of these procedures it becomes apparent that frequently the balloon catheter will pass through the chordal apparatus of the tricuspid valve [1]. Full balloon inflation with the balloon partially entrapped with the tricuspid valve apparatus can cause chordal rupture and consequently a degree of tricuspid regurgitation post procedure (Figure 3). The course of the balloon catheter and the relationship of the (partially inflated) balloon can be ascertained readily using transesophageal imaging and thus a better position can be chosen prior to full inflation. Using a balloon endhole catheter to place the exchange guidewire largely reduces the risk of a catheter course

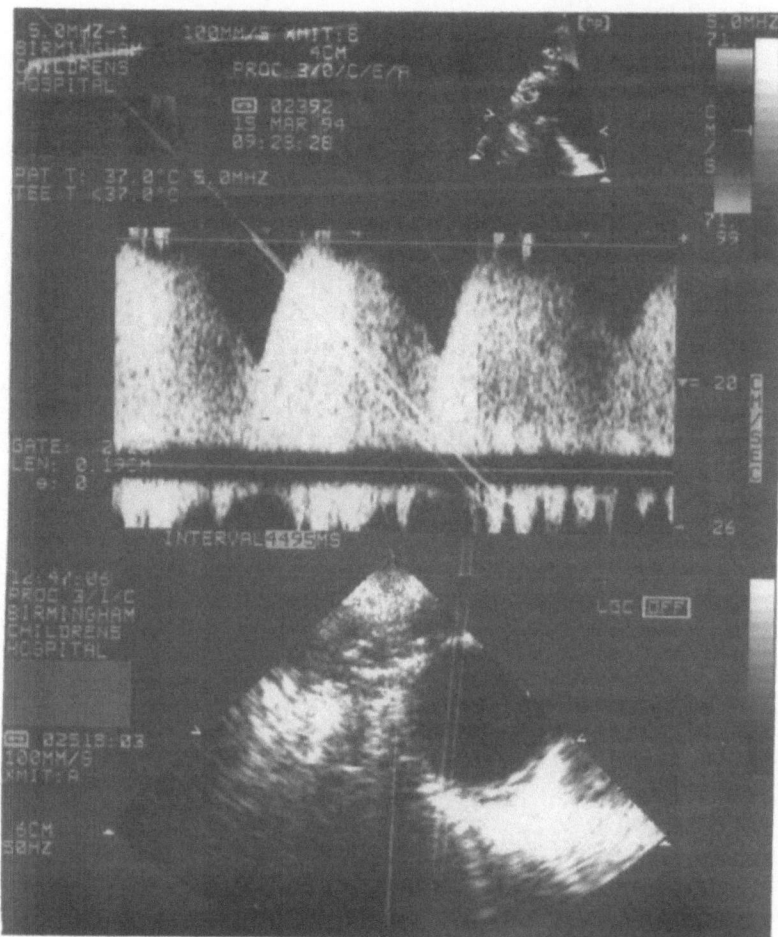

Figure 2. Transesophageal monitoring of stent implantation into the right upper pulmonary vein in child with recurrent venous obstruction following surgical correction of total anomalous venous connection. Top: Pulsed wave Doppler studies confirm the obstructive flow patterns prior to dilatation and stent implantation. Bottom: The stent is implanted within the distal right upper pulmonary vein. Note the characteristic appearance of the meshwork of the stent and the limited expansion within the proximal vein.

through the tricuspid valve apparatus. With respect to the haemodynamic evaluation post procedure, transesophageal Doppler techniques have little to offer, even when biplane technology is being used. The direction of blood flow is almost perpendicular to the Doppler beam irrespective of the imaging plane selected. Therefore, transesophageal studies during pulmonary valvulo-plasty should only be considered in cases where there is an abnormal tricuspid valve (e.g. Ebstein's malformation), or in cases where one would experience

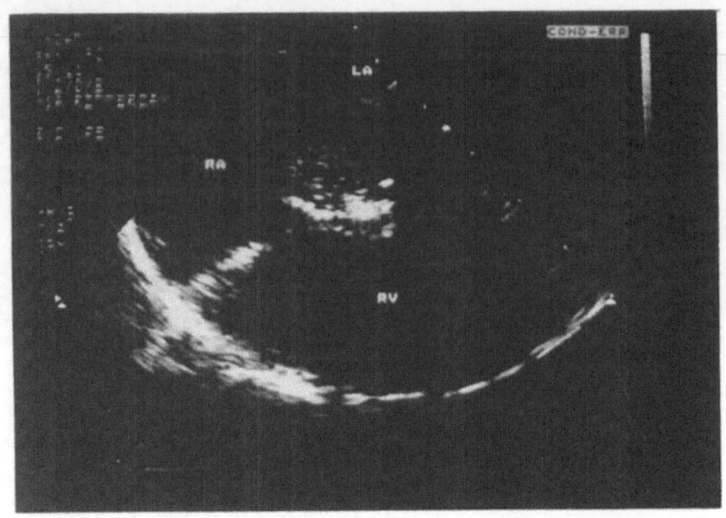

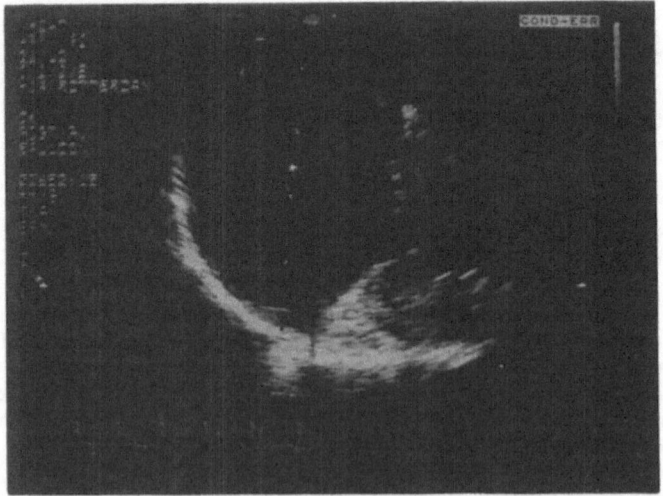

Figure 3. Transesophageal monitoring during pulmonary valvuloplasty in a child. The proximal end of the balloon catheter is seen to cross the plane of the tricuspid valve (A). Following the procedure there is partial chordal rupture of the anterior leaflet of the tricuspid valve (B) giving rise to moderate tricuspid regurgitation. Abbreviations: RV = right ventricle; others as in Figure 1.

difficulties to retrieve the balloon catheter following dilatation. In this latter scenario it is most likely that the balloon catheter is entrapped within the tricuspid valve apparatus.

Aortic valvuloplasty for native or recurrent aortic valve stenosis is a well established procedure in most institutions. The major complication is aortic regurgitation due to cusp laceration or perforation. Transesophageal monitoring during such procedures can significantly add to the safety of this procedure. Using real-time cross-sectional imaging the exact diameter of the aortic root can be assessed most accurately, which is of importance in selecting the appropriate balloon. The course of the exchange guidewire across the stenotic valve can also be ascertained and thereby allowing for the exclusion of cusp perforation. Having inserted the balloon catheter, the course of it relative to mitral valve apparatus should be carefully examined, so as to exclude entrapment within the subvalve apparatus. Finally, colour flow mapping studies are a very sensitive indicator for the occurrence of aortic regurgitation after each inflation. Using transgastric long axis imaging and continuous wave Doppler also the residual gradient can be assessed prior to subsequent inflations.

Balloon angioplasty

The descending aorta can be evaluated in detail using transesophageal imaging, especially when biplane technology is available. However, in cases with native aortic coarctation the intimate anatomical relationship between the descending aorta and the esophagus is frequently distorted and it will only rarely be possible to obtain detailed morphologic information. Angiography is by far the superior imaging technique, in particular in cases where there is tortuous vessel anatomy and collateral vessels. The same limitations hold true in cases with recoarctation, where the fibrous scar tissue further reduces the image quality obtained. The haemodynamic evaluation is limited by the very poor alignment that can be obtained to the direction of blood flow. All these limitations dramatically reduce the potential value which ultrasound monitoring could have on balloon angioplasty of native or recurrent aortic coarctation. The major complication to be excluded following balloon dilatation is the occurrence of aneurysm formation or medial dissection. Intravascular ultrasound studies hold the greatest promise in excluding these complications [13], however, current experience is very limited. Moreover, if balloon sizes are limited to the diameter of the transverse aortic arch, rather than to the diameter of the descending aorta at the level of the diaphragm, the incidence of aneurysm formation is largely reduced from the previously reported incidence.

Balloon angioplasty of branch pulmonary artery stenoses is currently being replaced by transcatheter stent implantation [10], because long-term results of angioplasty have been disappointing. Endovascular stent implantation requires close fluoroscopic control. The addition of ultrasound monitoring will be of benefit in only very few cases. This is primarily because the branch pulmonary arteries are in most cases not accessible by either transthoracic or transesophageal ultrasound because of the interference of the lungs. Intravascular ultrasound may again offer an alternative in these lesions. However, during these procedures it is rather the position of the stent across the stenosis and the relationship to the proximal and distal segments of the pulmonary artery and to any lobar branches, which is of clinical significance, than the change in morphology of the actual stenotic segment. These points are far better assessed by using fluoroscopy and repeat angiography than any of the existing ultrasound modalities. With respect to the haemodynamic evaluation during and after the procedure, the information to be obtained is also of limited value. Changes in the velocity of tricuspid regurgitation jets will document major changes in right ventricular pressure. The comparison of pulmonary venous flow patterns obtained by sampling of the affected and the contralateral lung segment, will give clues to major changes in lung perfusion.

In patients who have undergone a Fontan procedure the systemic venous return enters the pulmonary arteries directly without the use of a pumping chamber. This is most often accomplished by direct (posterior) anastomosis of the right atrium to the pulmonary arteries. Due to the proximity of this area to the esophagus detailed morphologic and haemodynamic information can be obtained by transesophageal imaging [14]. Such studies are indicated to monitor balloon dilatation or stent implantation for two main reasons. Firstly, atrial thrombus formation has to be excluded prior to dilatation and at the end of the procedure. Transesophageal imaging has been shown to be the most sensitive technique [15]. Secondly, comparison of pulmonary venous flow profiles gives a better idea of relative lung perfusion than does angiography in the setting of a Fontan circulation.

Occlusion of left-to-right shunts

Transcatheter occlusion of the patent ductus arteriosus is nowadays the technique of choice in all children beyond infancy. The Rashkind double umbrella device is the most commonly used technique. Fluoroscopy is the ultimate imaging and monitoring technique. The exact shape and the site of the narrowest portion of the duct is readily appreciated during an aortic angiogram in a lateral projection. The device is positioned under fluoroscopic control by observing the relationship of the hinge point and the distal legs relative to the trachea [15]. Routinely procedures can be performed within 30–45 minutes and screening times of around 5 minutes. Thus, there appears to be very limited need for an alternative imaging and monitoring technique. In the few cases we have studied by transesophageal imaging, the presence of the probe has rather interfered with the routine fluoroscopic monitoring.

Also image quality was very limited due to interposition of the left main bronchus between the oesophagus and the area of interest.

Recently the use of double umbrella devices has been extended to the closure of intracardiac shunts, namely atrial and ventricular septal defects. Although these techniques are still under clinical investigation, they hold great future promise in selected patients. From the very start it was appreciated that routine fluoroscopic monitoring is very limited during these procedures. Fluoroscopy can not provide information on intracardiac morphology. Repeat angiography is not feasible because of the large amounts in contrast media required. Thus, not surprisingly, it was only with the advent of real-time transesophageal monitoring that these interventional techniques have become feasible. Hellenbrandt [16] concluded that transesophageal imaging is a prerequisite for a high success rate in atrial septal defect occlusion.

Transesophageal reassessment of the atrial anatomy is crucial for the selection of suitable patients for device occlusion of atrial septal defects. The defect has to have good margins all around (e.g. not too close to either the pulmonary veins or the coronary sinus), should be a single defect (e.g. not fenestration of the atrial septum; Figure 4), and defect size has to be less than 15 mm (in children it is rather the ratio between defect size and total septal length which matters). All this information is readily available from transesophageal imaging and color flow studies [17]. During the procedure

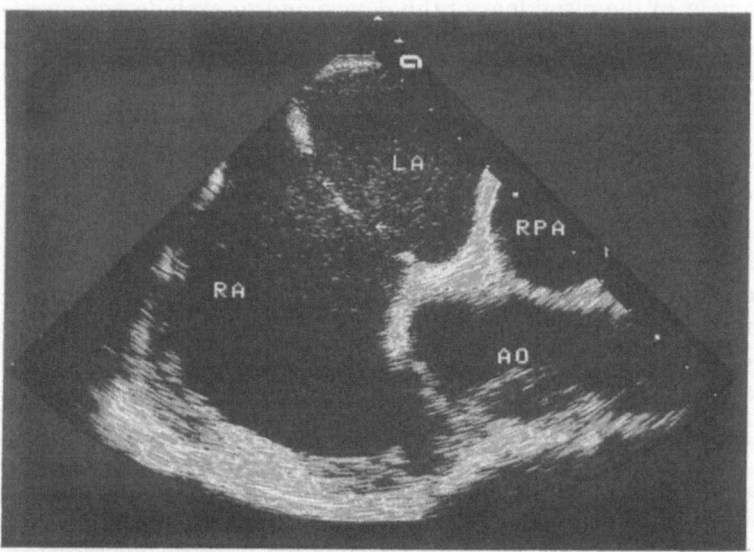

Figure 4. Transesophageal long axis image of the atrial septum in a patient who was scheduled for transcatheter occlusion. the transesophageal study clearly identifies two separate atrial communications (arrows), which precluded occlusion with a single device.

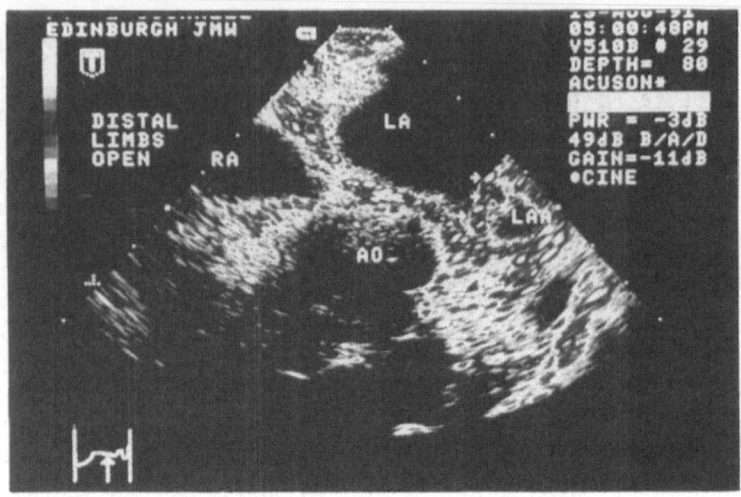

Figure 5. Monitoring of umbrella occlusion of an atrial septal defect. The transesophageal study discloses partial entrapment of the distal limbs of the device within the left atrial appendage.

itself transesophageal imaging should be used continuously to monitor the development of the distal legs of the device and to exclude any interference or entrapment with either the left atrial appendage (Figure 5) or the mitral valve apparatus. Thereafter the long sheath and the delivery system are pulled back simultaneously, so as to allow the distal legs of the device to engage on the left atrial surface of the atrial septum. Scanning from various levels will exclude malpositioning of one or more legs in the majority of cases. Colour flow mapping documents areas of residual shunting. If the device is found to be in an ideal position, the long sheath is pulled back over the delivery system so as to develop the proximal legs. Again the exact position of all the legs of the device relative to the atrial septum should be ascertained on detailed cross-sectional imaging. The long sheath is then advanced over the delivery system so as to oppose the proximal umbrella and the device is released. On demonstration that the knuckle of the delivery system is not entangled within the foam of the umbrella the delivery system is then pulled completely into the long sheath and thereafter both are pulled back to the inferior vena cava. A repeat transesophageal study is performed to document the final result (Figure 6). In our experience it is best to use left anterior oblique projections for concomitant fluoroscopic monitoring. In such a way there will be minimal interference and in particular no superimposition of the image of the transesophageal probe and the device and delivery system.

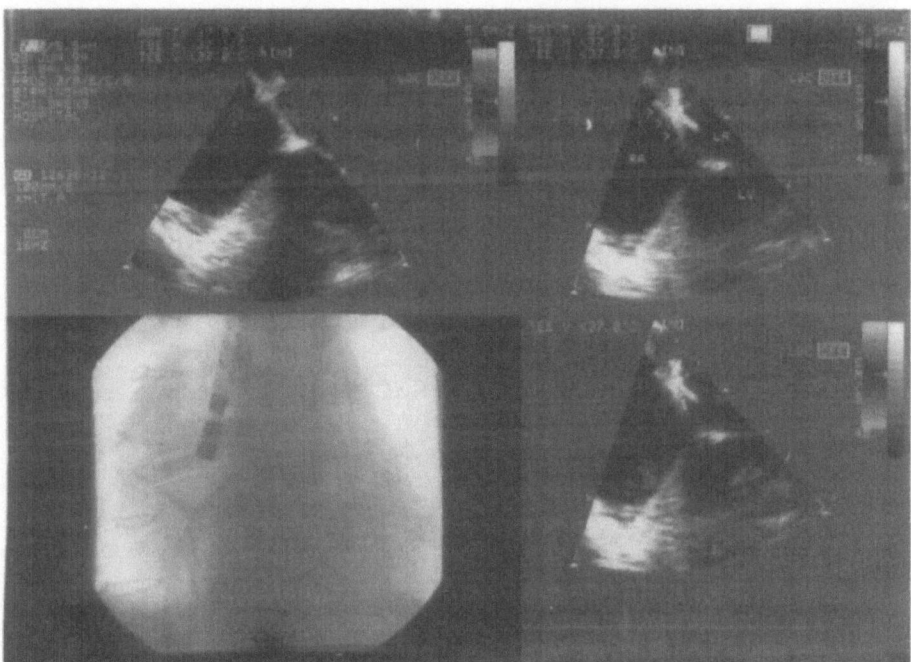

Figure 6. Transesophageal monitoring of umbrella occlusion of an atrial fenestration after Fontan operation. The location of the defect is readily seen on four chamber views (top left). The device is positioned using a combination of fluoroscopy and continuous transesophageal imaging (top right and bottom left). Final colour flow mapping studies excludes residual shunting (bottom right). (For colour plate of this figure see page 541.)

Similarly to the technique used for closure of atrial septal defects, it is now possible to close selected ventricular septal defects. Again, the major contribution of transesophageal imaging lies in the detailed pre-procedure reassessment of the anatomy and in the real-time monitoring of the device placement. However, closure of ventricular septal defects within the perimembranous region is very infrequently attempted, because of the proximity to the atrioventricular valves and their subvalvar apparatus. Thus, the majority of defects are either muscular defects or postoperative residual defects, ideally located around the apical margin of the patch (Figure 7). Placement of the device is largely facilitated using simultaneous fluoroscopy and transesophageal imaging [18]. Limitations of transesophageal technique to visualize the device adequately may however be encountered. These are most commonly related to either the large distance between the esophagus and the area of interest, or to an area of ultrasound masking by a calcified prosthetic patch in postoperative patients.

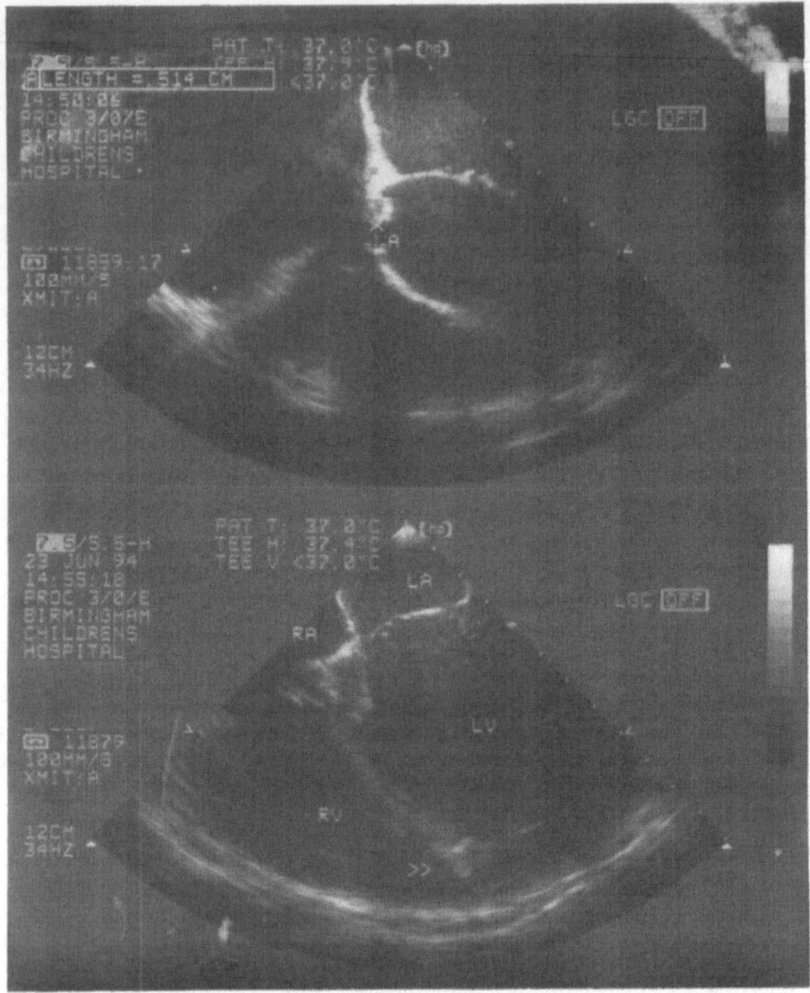

Figure 7. Transesophageal monitoring of transcatheter closure of a residual ventricular septal defect after a Rastelli procedure. Top: There is one defect at the site of the patch close to the crux cordis. The close relationship of the tricuspid valve apparatus to this defect precluded safe occlusion. Bottom: A further defect was documented within the apical muscular septum. This was successfully occluded using a double umbrella device (arrows).

Embolization techniques

Finally a range of embolization techniques, using either coils or detachable balloons, are established in paediatric interventional cardiology. The majority of these procedures, such as embolization of aorto-pulmonary collateral arteries, are performed best using fluoroscopy and angiography alone. The addition of ultrasound techniques would have little if any to offer in these procedures. The same holds true for embolization of pulmonary arterio-venous fistulae and fistulae between the systemic- and the pulmonary venous system. The only indication for transesophageal monitoring would appear to be in patients who undergo embolization of coronary artery fistulae. Such fistulae are readily visualized by transesophageal studies and both the entry and exit sites are well documented, as are the related haemodynamics. Thus, the technique can be used to document reduction in shunt flow after delivery of coils or balloons and can also be used to continuously monitor left ventricular function during the procedure.

References

1. Stümper O, Witsenburg M, Sutherland GR et al. Monitoring of interventional cardiac catheterization by pediatric transesophageal echocardiography. J Am Coll Cardiol 1991; 18: 1504–12.
2. Van der Velde ME, Perry SB, Sanders SP. Transesophageal echocardiography with color Doppler during interventional cardiac catheterization. Echocardiography 1991; 8: 721–30.
3. Allan LD, Leanage R, Wainwright R et al. Balloon atrial septostomy under two-dimensional echocardiographic control. Br Heart J 1982; 47: 41–3.
4. Ritter SB, Hillel Z, Narang J et al. Transesophageal real time Doppler flow imaging in congenital heart disease: Experience with the new pediatric transducer probe. Dyn Cardiovasc Imaging 1989; 2: 92–6.
5. Stümper O, Elzenga NJ, Hess J, Sutherland GR. Transesophageal echocardiography in children with congenital heart disease – an initial experience. J Am Coll Cardiol 1990; 16: 433–41.
6. Kipel G, Arnon R, Ritter S. Transesophageal echocardiographic guidance of balloon atrial septostomy. J Am Soc Echo 1991; 4: 631–5.
7. Stümper O, Rijlaarsdam M, Vargas-Barron J et al. The assessment of juxtaposed atrial appendages by transesophageal echocardiography. Int J Cardiol 1990; 29: 365–71.
8. Plowden JS, Mullins CE, Nihill MR et al. Blade and balloon atrial septostomy: Results and follow-up in 131 patients. J Am Coll Cardiol 1991; 17: 135A (Abstr).
9. Kaulitz R, Stümper O, Geuskens R et al. The comparative values of the precordial and transesophageal approaches in the ultrasound evaluation of atrial baffle function following atrial correction procedures. J Am Coll Cardiol 1990; 16: 686–94.
10. O'Laughlin MP, Perry SB, Lock JE, Mullins CE. Use of endovascular stents in congenital heart disease. Circulation 1991; 83: 1923–39.
11. Stanger P, Cassidy SC, Girod DA et al. Balloon pulmonary valvuloplasty: Results of the valvuloplasty and angioplasty of congenital anomalies registry. Am J Cardiol 1990; 65: 775–83.
12. Rocchini AP, Beekman RH, Ben Shachar G et al. Balloon aortic valvuloplasty: Results of the valvuloplasty and angioplasty of congenital anomalies registry. Am J Cardiol 1990; 65: 784–9.
13. Stümper O, Sutherland GR, Geuskens R et al. Transesophageal echocardiography in the evaluation and management of the Fontan circulation. J Am Coll Cardiol 1991; 17: 1152–60.
14. Fyfe DA, Kline CH, Sade RM, Gillette PC. Transesophageal echocardiography detects thrombus formation not identified by transthoracic echocardiography after the Fontan operation. J Am Coll Cardiol 1991; 18: 1733–7.
15. Magee AG, Stümper O, Burns JE, Godman MJ. Medium-term follow up of residual

shunting and complications after transcatheter occlusion of the ductus arteriosus. Br Heart J 1994: 71: 63–9.

16. Hellenbrand WE, Fahey JT, McGowan FX et al. Transesophageal echocardiographic guidance of transcatheter closure of atrial septal defect. Am J Cardiol 1990; 66: 207–13.

17. Tucillo B, Stümper O, Hess J et al. Transesophageal echocardiographic evaluation of atrial morphology in children with congenital heart disease. Eur Heart J 1992; 13: 223–31.

18. Van der Velde ME, Sanders SP, Keane JF et al. Transesophageal echocardiographic guidance of transcatheter ventricular septal defect closure. J Am Coll Cardiol 1994; 23: 1660–5.

Corresponding Author: Dr Oliver Stümper, Heart Unit, Birmingham Childrens Hospital, Ladywood Middleway, Birmingham B16 8ET, UK

31. Follow-up of patients after transcatheter procedures in congenital heart disease using noninvasive imaging techniques

MICHAEL TYNAN and GUNTER FISCHER

Introduction

Catheter interventions have been in use for the treatment of congenital heart disease since the introduction of balloon atrial septostomy in 1966. However, it has been over the 12 years, following the introduction of balloon valvoplasty, that such procedures have come to comprise a major component of the work of a paediatric cardiology unit. Today in a paediatric cardiology group approximately 50% of cardiac catheterizations will be for interventions. This increase in the numbers of interventional catheterizations has been paralleled by a decrease in diagnostic catheter workload which has been brought about by an increased reliance on and confidence in non invasive diagnostic methods. The views expressed below are the opinions of particular interventional paediatric cardiologists as "consumers" of non invasive investigations and not those of dedicated specialist noninvasive cardiologists.

The mainstay of noninvasive investigation is transthoracic colour Doppler echocardiography and this is as true for the assessment of catheter interventions as it is for primary diagnosis. Other methods include radionuclide angiography, magnetic resonance imaging and transoesophageal echocardiography.

Catheter interventions are new techniques many of which supplant surgical operations of proven efficacy. Careful assessment of the safety and utility of the new methods is mandatory and noninvasive methods are central to this assessment. Early work concerning the effect of balloon valvoplasty relied on follow-up catheterization, today this would be considered clinically undesirable and logistically difficult to achieve. Catheterization is only performed when the screening noninvasive tests suggest the need for a further intervention. It is in this role that they will be discussed and, as interventional cardiologists, we will be considering them from the point of view of consumers of these investigations.

C.A. Nienaber and U. Sechtem (eds): Imaging and Intervention in Cardiology. 521–532.
© 1996 Kluwer Academic Publishers. Printed in the Netherlands.

Noninvasive investigations

Colour Doppler echocardiography

Transthoracic and subcostal echocardiography are the approaches most frequently used in children. Rarely do these views not provide adequate images for assessment. The transoesophageal approach has one major limitation in infants and children, it is so unpleasant that a general anaesthetic is needed. This means that it can only be justified when the information cannot be obtained in some other way and this is rarely the case. Thus transoesophageal echocardiography, although crucial to the performance and acute assessment of the effect of some interventions is of limited value in outpatient follow-up.

Using standard transthoracic and subcostal views morphological information can be obtained from the cross-sectional images, Doppler interrogation provides measurements of the velocity of blood flow from which pressure gradients can be estimated [1] using the modified Bernoulli equation:

$$\Delta P = 4 V max^2,$$

where ΔP is the pressure gradient and Vmax is the maximum velocity measured immediately distal to the obstruction.

Accurate estimation of the true maximal velocity depends on the quality of alignment of the ultrasound beam with the blood flow jet. Overestimation of the gradient compared to catheter measurement is inherent in the technique since the Doppler measurement represents an instantaneous pressure drop whilst the catheter measurement is of peak to peak gradient. However, all the differences between the two techniques cannot be explained by this. The final decision on the quality of the Doppler trace used for the estimation is subjective and may account for some of the apparent inaccuracies encountered. Figure 1 illustrates the relationship between Doppler and catheter estimates of transvalvar gradient in valvar aortic stenosis in our practice. As can be seen there is a wide scatter and the tendency is for higher Doppler gradients to be higher but this is not invariably the case; on occasion the catheter gradient is higher! However, since in general Doppler transvalvar gradients are overestimates compared to those measured at catheter the technique is a safe screening test provided a sufficient margin for error is maintained. Colour flow mapping demonstrates the direction of flow and is easy to use. It is of particular value in the detection of valvar regurgitation which is of value following valvoplasty and also, in the case of the tricuspid valve, for estimating right ventricular systolic pressure. It is also a very sensitive method for detecting persistent shunts after catheter closure procedures e.g. occlusion of persistent arterial duct (persistent ductus arteriosus). Also by its demonstration of the presence of turbulent flow it also facilitates the positioning of the sampling volume for the estimation of maximal velocity

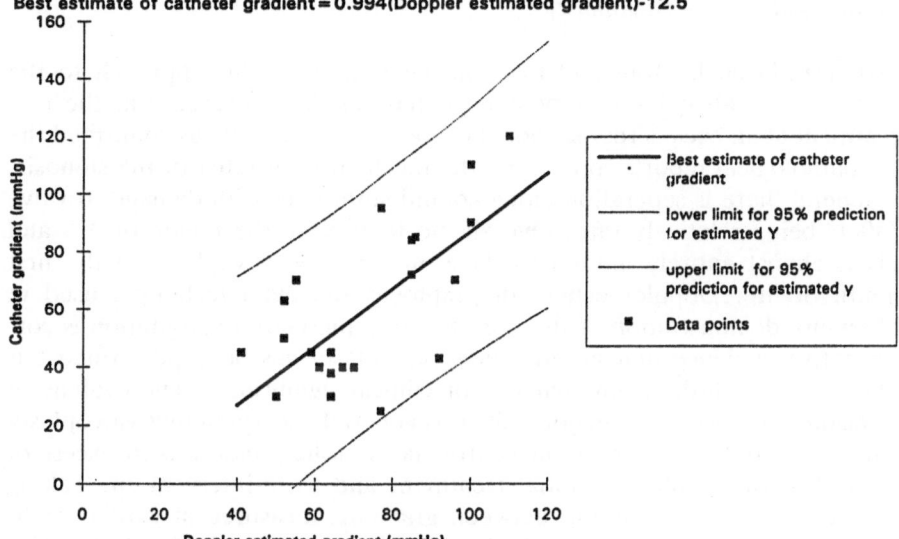

Nomogram for prediction of catheter peak gradient from Doppler derived gradient in aortic stenosis with original data points superimposed

Best estimate of catheter gradient = 0.994(Doppler estimated gradient)-12.5

Figure 1. This figure shows the relationship between the follow-up echocardiographic estimation of peak systolic pressure gradient with that measured at cardiac catheterization.

of flow. However, caution must be exercised when attempting to extract quantitative data from colour flow images.

Magnetic resonance imaging

This is the other major noninvasive imaging method used in this context. Spin echo images give anatomical detail which are the equal of or better than angiography in many situations. It is particularly useful where echocardiography is at its weakest such as visualisation of the aortic arch and descending aorta and the proximal pulmonary artery branches.

Radionuclide angiography

First pass studies can be used to quantitate residual shunts after catheter closure. This is useful since no meaningful quantitation can be made by echocardiography. This methodology will become essential for the assessment of the efficacy of closure of atrial and ventricular septal defects where the objective is to restore haemodynamic "normality" and, thus small residual shunts will be acceptable provided there is no volume overload and that the cardiovascular pressures are normal.

Catheter interventions

Balloon pulmonary valvoplasty

First introduced by Kan and her colleagues in 1982 this approach to the treatment of valvar pulmonary stenosis has supplanted surgery as the first treatment at all ages. Cross-sectional echocardiography [2] has confirmed the few pathological reports concerning the mechanism of relief of the stenosis, in general there is separation along commissural lines with damage to valve leaflets being relatively rare. Overall mortality is in the region of 3% and this is almost entirely limited to those undergoing valvoplasty in the first month of life. Doppler echocardiography is the main technique used in follow-up, demonstration of the presence of pulmonary regurgitation is corroborative evidence that an adequate valvoplasty has been performed but otherwise is of little haemodynamic or clinical significance. The evaluation of residual stenosis is the major task. It is generally accepted that valvoplasty is not indicated unless the right ventricular systolic pressure is in excess of 50 mmHg, this applies to initial treatment and to re-intervention. Taking into account the relationship between gradients measured at cardiac catheterization and those estimated by Doppler interrogation the level of noninvasive gradient should be of the order of 40 to 50 mmHg before reintervention is considered. In the majority of cases the haemodynamic results observed immediately after the valvoplasty persist for at least the intermediate term such that when there is an immediate satisfactory reduction in gradient this is maintained in the majority of patients [3]. Reviewing our own experience over the decade from our first pulmonary valvoplasty in 1983 some 30% of patients have needed a subsequent procedure. The reintervention rates are shown in Figure 2 for the whole group (Figure 2A) and for those in whom the original valvoplasty was performed in the neonatal period (Figure 2B). We can see that those needing valvoplasty in the first month of life have been most at risk for reintervention. This figure also demonstrates that the second procedure has been performed up to a little over two years after the first. During the second 5 year the period of this decade, from 1988 to 1993, there has been a reduction in the need for further procedures in the all age groups so that freedom from reintervention rates are now in the region of 80%. This improvement has been predominantly due to a decrease in the need for early reintervention and reflects a fall in the numbers of failures to perform the initial angioplasty Better guide wires and balloon catheters tailored to infant and paediatric practice account for both the improved success rates and the lower frequency of complications encountered now. Of course this applies to all balloon angioplasty procedures for congenital cardiac defects. Yet still a proportion of patients require further treatment. Thus these data emphasise the need for careful follow-up even in the most established therapeutic procedures both for the management of the

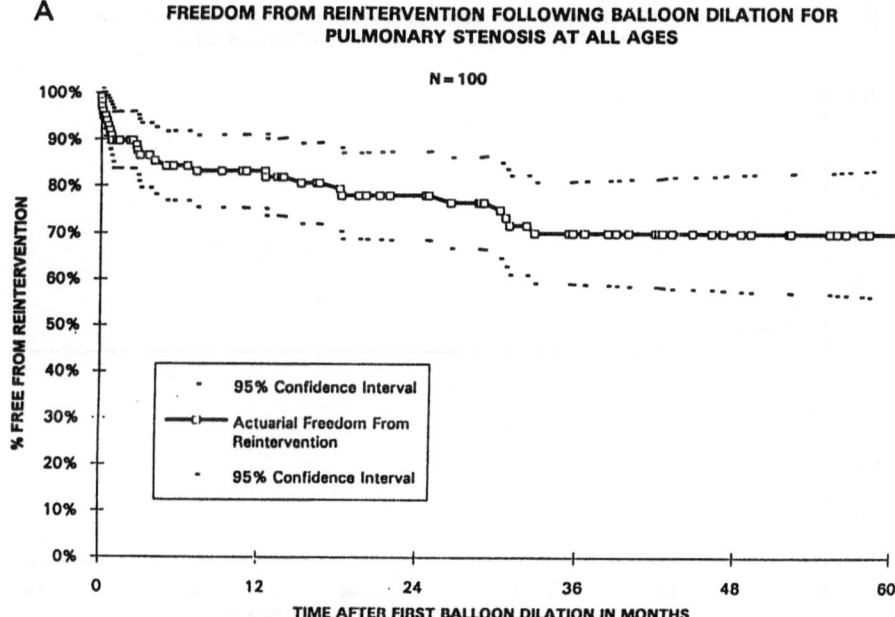

A   FREEDOM FROM REINTERVENTION FOLLOWING BALLOON DILATION FOR
                    PULMONARY STENOSIS AT ALL AGES

Figure 2. Figure 2A shows the reintervention rate for all 100 patients who had balloon pulmonary valvoplasty during the decade 1983 to 1993. Figure 2B shows the reintervention rate for patients under one month of age at the first valvoplasty. As can be seen the reintervention rate is highest in the group of new born babies. In this age group the majority needed a second procedure early in the follow up period due to failure to achieve a valvoplasty. In the older age groups the second procedure was generally performed later and was probably a growth related effect.

individual patient and for the continuing evaluation of the efficacy of the procedure.

Balloon aortic valvoplasty

Balloon aortic valvoplasty has become the first line treatment of valvar aortic stenosis in all children. As with pulmonary stenosis it is safe and effective, mortality and complications are concentrated in those needing treatment early in the first year of life [4]. Unlike pulmonary stenosis the vast majority will need further procedures as life progresses and this is as true of surgery as it is of balloon valvoplasty.

The ultrasound methodology for evaluation of severity of aortic stenosis is similar to that in pulmonary stenosis. However, it is advisable to interrogate from both above and below the valve to ensure that the maximum velocity is found. Thus transducer positions include the suprasternal notch or high

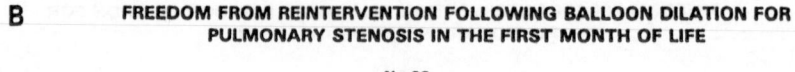

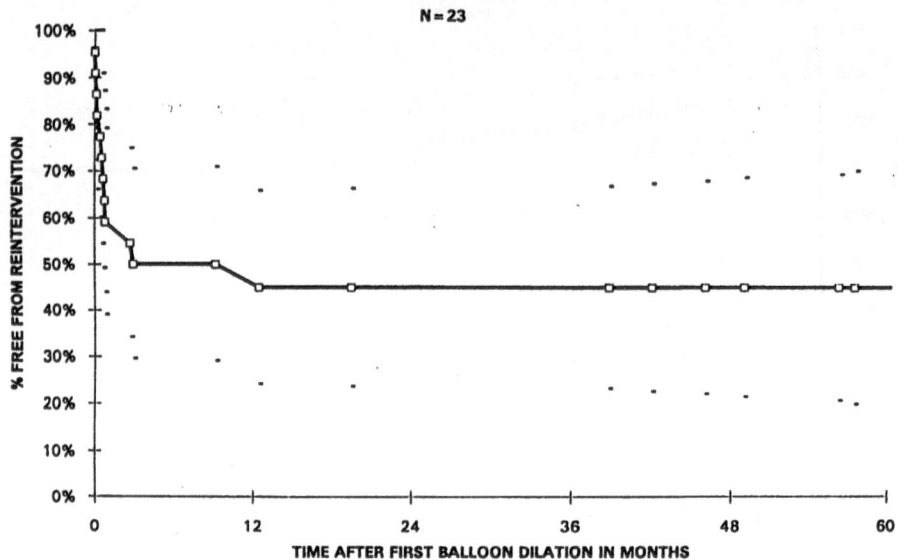

Figure 2. Continued.

right parasternal and an apical position. In the follow-up after balloon valvo-plasty attention is directed both to any residual stenosis but also to the severity of valvar regurgitation. In the later case M-mode measurements of left ventricular size are the best indicators of the need for reintervention. Our guidelines are a left ventricular end systolic dimension of greater than 55 mm in adults and of greater than 29 mm per m^2 BSA in children [5]. If aortic regurgitation is severe enough to need treatment then the patient's own pulmonary valve is used to replace the aortic valve with homograft replacement of the pulmonary valve. This so-called Ross operation, is at present the treatment of choice.

Balloon angioplasty of aortic coarctation and coarctation restenosis

The objective of surgical or catheter treatment of both these entities is relief of stenosis and restoration of normal blood pressure. The ideal result is rarely obtained, at rest there is usually some residual pressure gradient whilst on exercise this is accentuated. We are frequently forced into accepting a less than perfect result and our present criteria for reintervention are a resting upper limb systolic blood pressure above the 95th centile for age with a systolic pressure gradient across the coarctation site of greater than 20 mmHg. Unfortunately the echocardiogram is of little help in making these assessments because the image quality of the descending aorta is poor and the Doppler velocities recorded almost invariably overestimate the pressure gradient. Restenosis is strongly suggested by the finding of continuous flow throughout diastole in the aorta. However, absence of this finding does not exclude it. In this setting MRI is of great value. High quality spin echo images of the descending aorta can be obtained in several projections giving accurate cross-sectional anatomical information. Furthermore, the integrity of the aortic wall at the site of the angioplasty can be assessed [6]. This is important, since aneurysm formation is an inherent risk of balloon angioplasty in both native aortic coarctation and coarctation restenosis [7] (Figure 3). The incidence of this complication is not accurately known but is probably of the order of 10% of cases. As yet, no factors have been found which can be considered causal and therefore avoidable. Certainly, single technical factors such as the relative balloon size do not correlate with aneurysm formation. Since in our hands, the presence of an aneurysm is an absolute indication for surgery, MRI scanning is the essential non invasive method of follow up. Thus magnetic resonance imaging combined with cuff blood pressure measurements in the arms and legs are the best methods of follow up of the treatment of aortic coarctation and coarctation restenosis.

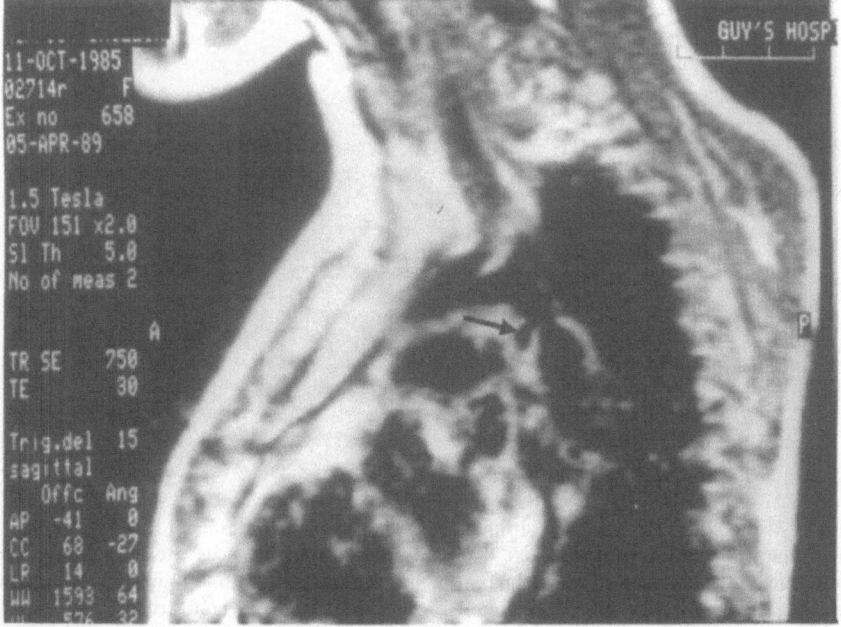

Figure 3. This magnetic resonance spin echo image shows a small aneurysm at the site of balloon dilation for post surgical aortic coarctation restenosis, indicated by the arrow.

Peripheral pulmonary stenosis

In many centres, the unpredictable effects of balloon angioplasty have led to the use of stents for the treatment of branch pulmonary stenosis. Stent implantation results in an immediate predictable improvement in the calibre of the stented vessel and for the short and intermediate term, this improvement is maintained [8]. However, encroachment of neointima within the stent may eventually lead to reoccurrence of stenosis. Following stent implantation, MRI is of little value since the most frequently used stent, the Palmaz, is made of ferro magnetic material and the interference caused would make any images of little value. Colour Doppler echocardiography can establish that the stent is patent and if laminar flow is present it will show this (Figure 4) but when flow is turbulent estimates of pressure gradients across the stented stenosis cannot be relied upon to be accurate. These inaccuracies stem from the difficulty or impossibility of correct alignment of the interrogating beam with the stent flow plus the fact that stenosis and, therefore stents, often extend to generations of pulmonary artery branches which are masked

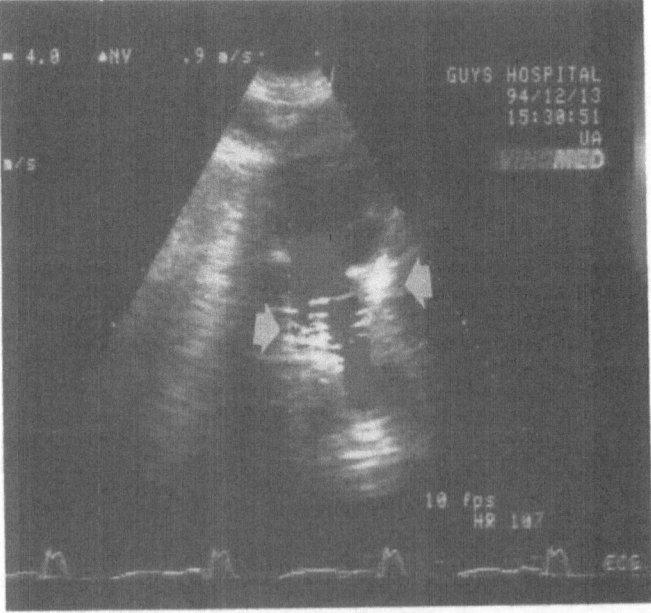

Figure 4. This colour Doppler echocardiogram is from a patient with bilateral pulmonary artery branch stenosis following correction of a common arterial trunk (truncus arteriosus) in the newborn period. At six months of age Palmaz stents were placed in both left and right pulmonary arteries at the same procedure. Both stents are patent and appear unobstructive. At this age alignment with the flow in the left pulmonary artery is satisfactory for velocity estimation but that with the right is less good. In older patients quantitation of velocity is much less reliable. (For colour plate of this figure see **page 542**.)

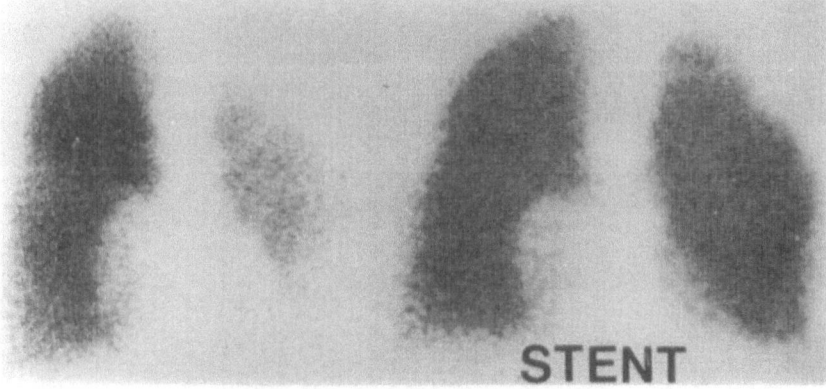

Figure 5. This radionuclide lung perfusion scan shows improvement in blood flow to the left lung following stenting of a stenotic left pulmonary artery.

by lung substance. Inferential information such as an estimate of right ventricular systolic pressure from a tricuspid regurgitant jet can be helpful in excluding a major increase in stenosis following successful stent implantation.

An increase in lung perfusion as determined by pre and post procedure radionuclide perfusion scans is valuable in the assessment of the efficacy of pulmonary arterial balloon dilation or stenting (Figure 5). These scans provide estimates of proportional flow between lungs and lung segments but not absolute volume flow. Their major value is thus predominantly in procedures performed on one pulmonary artery or to a limited number of segments. Pulmonary arterial stenoses are frequently bilateral and proximal in the main branches and for practical reasons, it is recommended that both arteries be stented at the same procedure. In these circumstances perfusion scans must be interpreted with extreme caution.

Occlusion procedures

Many devices have been used in attempts to close intracardiac defects, persistent patency of the arterial duct, arteriovenous fistulas and unwanted surgical shunts. The mainstays of occlusive procedures are implantable thrombogenic coils such as the Gianturco coil, detachable implantable balloons and specialised devices such as the Rashkind double umbrella occluder for persistent patency of the arterial duct. The simplest of these methods is implantation of Gianturco coils for which small, 4 or 5 French, catheters can be used whereas the other techniques require much larger intoducers, 7 up to 11 French. Recently coil embolization has become more versatile, or more complicated, by design modifications such as the introduction of mechanisms for controlling release.

As yet, there is no generally accepted device for septal defect closure

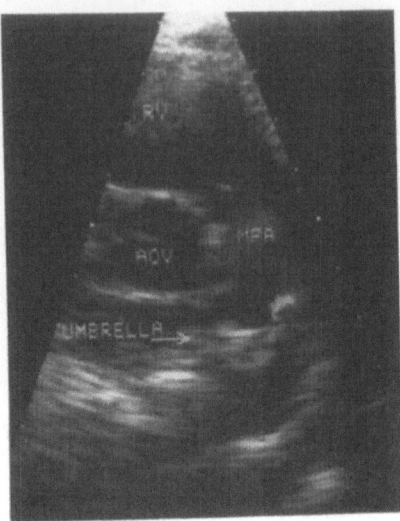

Figure 6. A colour Doppler echocardiogram from a patient with a Rashkind duct occluder in place. The bright echo at the origin of the left pulmonary is from an arm of the occluding umbrella. Adjacent to this can be seen the turbulent "flame" indicating residual flow through the arterial duct. (For colour plate of this figure see **page 542.**)

although many, including the Sideris button device [9], are under evaluation. Structural failure of these devices has been such a problem that fluoroscopy is mandatory for checking their structural integrity and is thus a major non invasive method for studying the safety of use of these devices.

Assessment of success of occlusion procedures is primarily concerned with demonstrating whether or not occlusion has been achieved. In some settings it is important to know that the device is stable in the desired position, this is always good to know, and that it is not encroaching on the lumen of a normal vessel. Doppler echocardiography is capable of answering these questions.

Persistent patency of the arterial duct

Undoubtedly closure of the duct has become the single most commonly performed occlusion procedure in congenital heart disease. The Rashkind double umbrella, originally introduced in the United Stares in the early 1980's [10], has been used in Europe since 1987. Follow up is by colour Doppler echocardiography. Detection of flow from aorta to pulmonary artery indicates a residual shunt and thus incomplete occlusion. It has been found that with this device, only 55% of ducts are occluded immediately after the procedure. By 6 months 75% are and at one year 18% have residual shunts (Figure 6) and after one year closure is unlikely [11]. There is little dispute about these figures but there is dispute about what to do. Some suggest no further action need be taken whilst others, including ourselves, recommend a second procedure to achieve complete closure. Up until recently, the second procedure involved implanting a second Rashkind device which can be difficult and certainly is expensive. Nowadays, simple Gianturco coils are used both for this application and for primary closure of ducts so that resistance to closing even small residual shunts is diminishing. Persistent patency after coil occlusion is less frequent than after implantation of an umbrella. However, this is because residual flow after implantation of a coil leads to immediate delivery of further coils until occlusion is achieved whereas with the umbrella, one is implanted and the result awaited. It is known that when the large, 17 mm, umbrella is used to close a duct in a small child, it can cause left pulmonary artery stenosis [12]. However, to close such a duct with coils may [13] need 4 or 5 coils and this can also cause left pulmonary artery stenosis. Notwithstanding the limitations of Doppler echocardiography in this setting, it is a valuable follow up method for detecting left pulmonary artery stenosis even if the assessment is not absolutely accurate.

Occlusion of other lesions

A variety of communications have been treated by transcatheter occlusion. These include congenital anomalies and iatrogenic lesions [14]. Amongst the congenital anomalies elective occlusion of major aorto-pulmonary collateral arteries in tetralogy of Fallot with pulmonary atresia is the best established. Here the selection and timing is jointly planned with the surgical team. Lesions such as coronary arteriovenous and pulmonary arteriovenous fistulas are best treated by catheter intervention. Iatrogenic communications include Blalock Taussig shunts when these have been incompletely closed at corrective surgery. Usually coil occlusion is satisfactory but since there is often high flow controlled release coils are frequently utilised giving extra security in coil placement. Recently it has become popular amongst surgeons to leave a small interatrial communication when performing the Fontan type of operation when this is considered to have a higher than usual risk. These fenestrations are then closed using a Rashkind double umbrella. In the follow-up of these interventions proof of complete closure is sought using Doppler echocardiography.

The number and type catheter interventions in patients continues to grow. Stents are being used increasingly in unorthodox locations such as the aorta in coarctation restenosis and in the arterial duct in cyanotic newborns [15] instead of surgical shunts. Occlusive devices have already been used in atrial and selected ventricular septal defects and these will, no doubt soon become standard procedures. Equally development and refinement of existing imaging applications such as magnetic resonance gradient echo imaging (which can present cine MRI images and is the basis for flow velocity studies) and three dimensional reconstruction which have the potential of giving more dynamic and spatial information will have a role to play. However, for the foreseeable future the methods in use today will still be the mainstays of the follow up after catheter interventions for congenital heart disease.

References

1. Hatle L, Angelson B. Doppler ultrasound in cardiology, 2nd ed. Lea & Febiger 1985: 24.
2. Robertson M, Benson LN, Smallhorn JS et al. The morphology of the right ventricular outflow tract after percutaneous pulmonary valvotomy: Long term follow up. Br Heart J 1987; 58: 239–44.
3. Mc Crindle BW, Kan JS. Long-term results after balloon pulmonary valvoplasty. Circulation 1991; 83: 1915–22.
4. O'Connor, Beekman, Rocchini AP, Rosenthal A. Intermediate-term effectiveness of balloon valvuloplasty for congenital aortic stenosis: A prospective follow-up study. Circulation 1991; 84: 732–28.
5. Bonow RO, Lakatos E, Maron BJ, Epstein SE. Serial long-term assessment of the natural history of assymptomatic patients with chronic aortic regurgitation and normal left ventricular systolic function. Circulation 1991; 84: 1625–35.
6. Baker EJ, Ayton V, Smith MA et al. Magnetic resonance imaging of coarctation of the aorta in infants: Use of a high field strength. Br Heart J 1989; 62: 97–101.
7. Tynan M, Finlay JP, Fontes V et al. Balloon angioplasty for the treatment of native coarctation: Results of valvoplasty and angioplasty of congenital anomalies registry. Am J Cardiol 1990; 65: 790–2.
8. Laughlin MP, Perry SB, Lock JE, Mullins CE. Use of endovascular stents in congenital heart disease. Circulation 1991; 83: 1923–39.
9. Rao PS, Wilson AD, Levy JM et al. Role of "buttoned" double-disc device in the management of atrial septal defects. Am Heart J 1992; 123: 191–200.
10. Rashkind WJ, Mullins CE, Hellenbrand WE, Tait MA. Nonsurgical closure of patent ductus arteriosus: Clinical application of the Rashkind PDA occluder system. Circulation 1987; 75: 583–92.
11. Report of the European Registry. Transcatheter occlusion of persistent arterial duct. Lancet 1992; 340: 1062–1066.
12. Ottencamp J, Hess J, Talsma MD, Buis-Liem TN. Protrusion of the device: A complication of catheter closure of patent ductus arteriosus. Br Heart J 1992; 68: 301–3.
13. Hijazi ZM, Gegel RL. Results of anterograde transcatheter closure of patent ductus arteriosus using single or multiple Gianturco coils. Am J Cardiol 1994; 74: 925–929.
14. Reidy JF, Jones ODH, Tynan M et al. Embolisation procedures in congenital heart disease. Br Heart J 1985; 54: 184–92.
15. Rosenthal E, Qureshi SA, Tynan M. Percutaneous pulmonary valvotomy and arterial duct stenting in neonates with right ventricular hypoplasia. Am J Cardiol 1994; 74: 304–6.

Corresponding Author: Dr Michael Tynan, Department of Paediatric Cardiology, 11th Floor Guy's Tower-Guy's Hospital, St. Thomas' Street, London SE1 9RT, UK

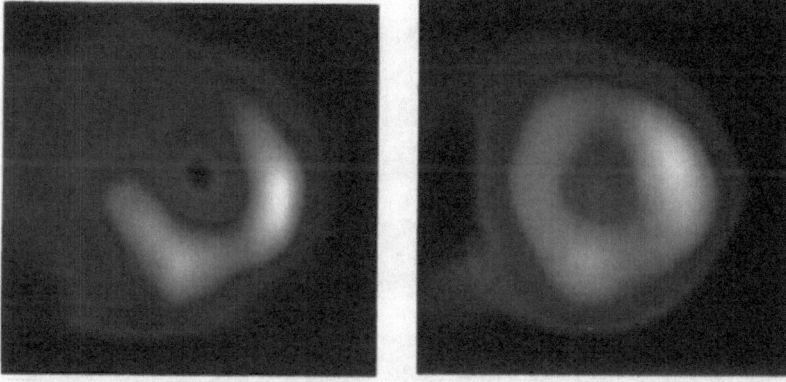

Figure 3B (*Chapter 13*). The MRI abnormality is closely matched by the perfusion defect (left) seen during dipyridamole thallium myocardial perfusion tomography which shows (right) full reversibility. (Reproduced from Pennell et al. with permission [31].)

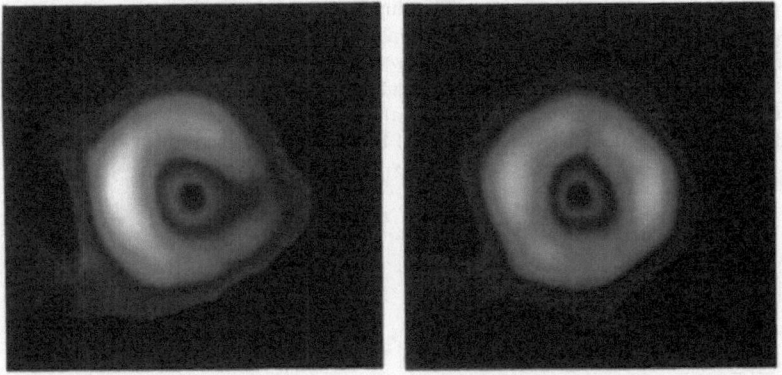

Figure 6B (*Chapter 13*). The reversible perfusion defect seen during dobutamine thallium myocardial perfusion tomography. (Reproduced from Pennell et al. with permission [26].)

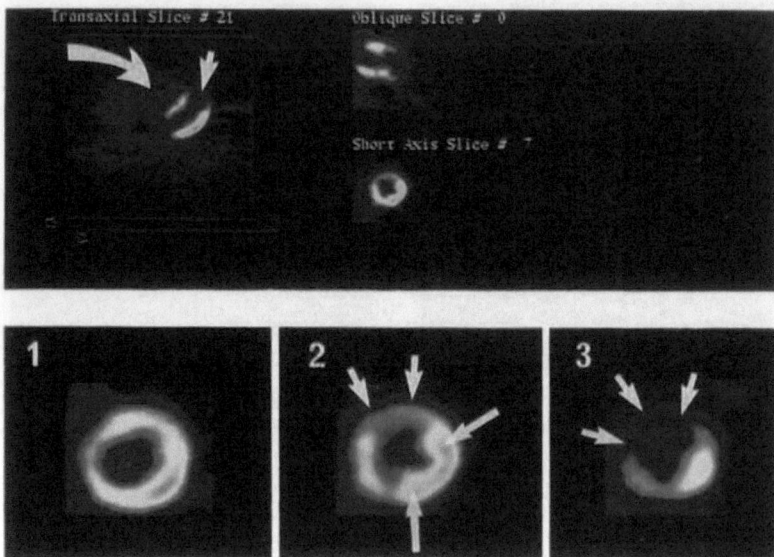

Figure 6B (Chapter 14). FDG-PET images of the same patient. The corresponding transverse image is seen in the upper left of the figure (curved arrow). The region without FDG-uptake (small white arrow) matches exactly the region with severe wall thinning on the diastolic gradient-echo MR image. The basal short axis section is seen in the lower left of the figure (1) and shows normal tracer uptake throughout the myocardium. The somewhat lower uptake of the interventricular septum is due to partial volume effects with the neighbouring aortic root. There is reduced FDG-uptake in the anterior wall (small arrows) of the midventricular section (2) which corresponds exactly to the regional wall thinning in the MR image. Both papillary muscles are visible (longer arrows). In the apical section (3), there is severely reduced FDG-uptake in the anterior wall and the septum (arrows), which fits nicely with the MR image. (Reproduced from: Sechtem U et al. Int J Card Imaging (Suppl 1) 1993; 9: 31–40.)

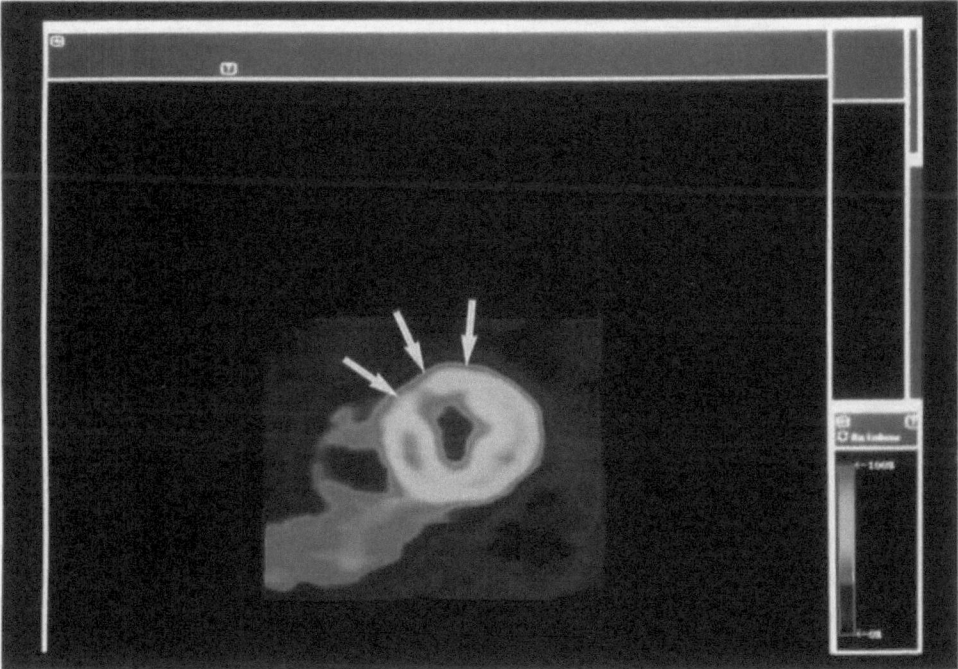

Figure 10B (*Chapter 14*). The corresponding FDG-PET image shows reduced uptake in the anteroseptal region (arrows), but relative uptake is larger than 50%. Therefore, this region is also viable by PET-criteria. The inferior wall shows normal FDG-uptake.

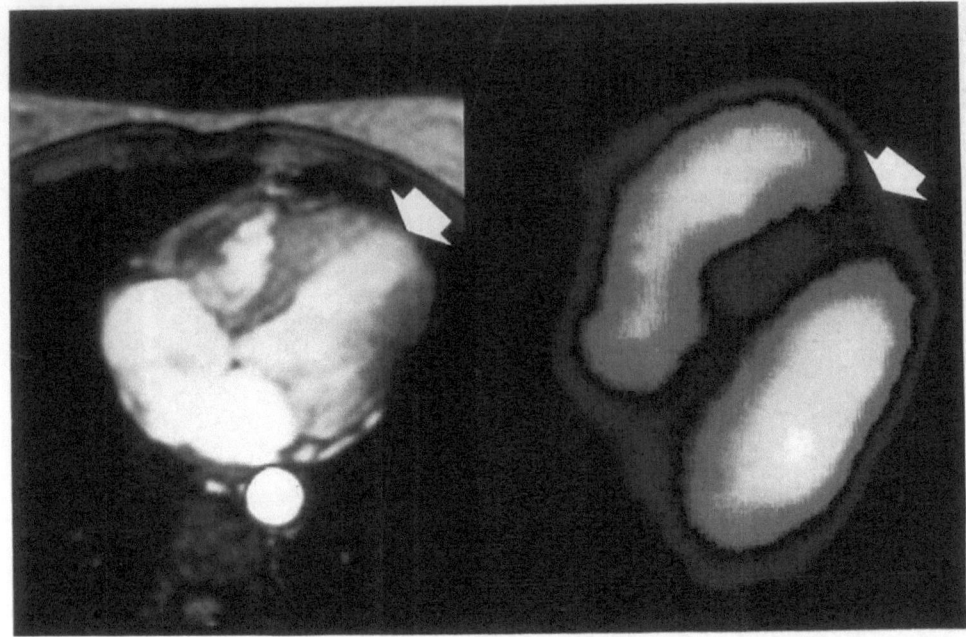

Figure 12 (Chapter 14). Corresponding gradient-echo MR and MIBI-SPECT images. The zone of severe wall thinning seen on the MR image (arrow) corresponds exactly to the region with severely reduced MIBI-uptake (arrow). (Reproduced from: Sechtem U et al. Int J Card Imaging (Suppl 1) 1993; 9: 31–40.)

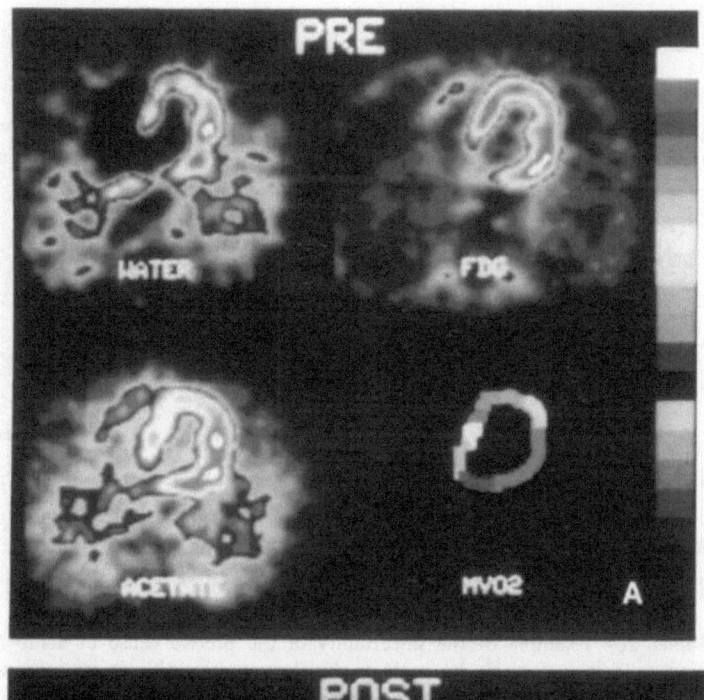

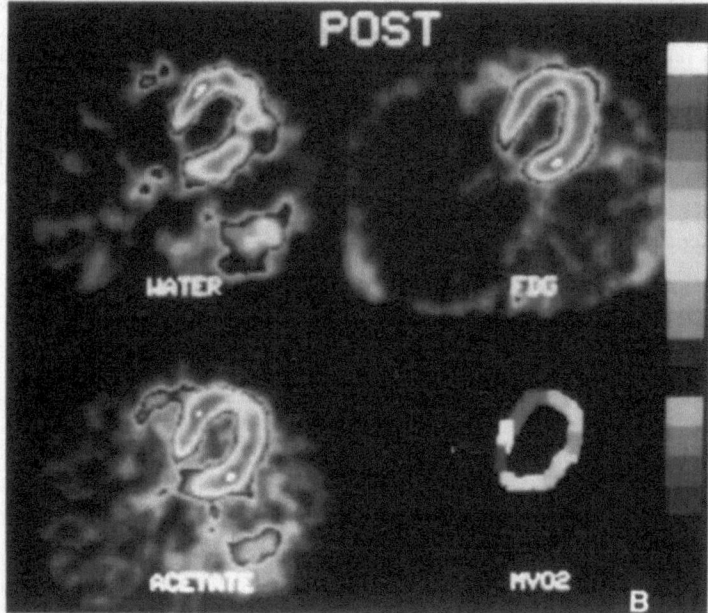

Figure 3 (Chapter 17). Myocardial perfusion, glucose metabolism and acetate uptake in a patient before myocardial revascularization (PRE) with evidence of viable tissue in the anterior left ventricular wall by preserved uptake of FDG whereas flow (O-15 water) is critically reduced. There is also a moderately reduced, but preserved acetate uptake in the perfusion territory of the LAD indicating a reduced Oxygen consumption (MVO_2) in the anterior wall relative to the normal posterolateral wall. (B) After successful revascularization both perfusion and glucose metabolism as well as acetate uptake appear normal.

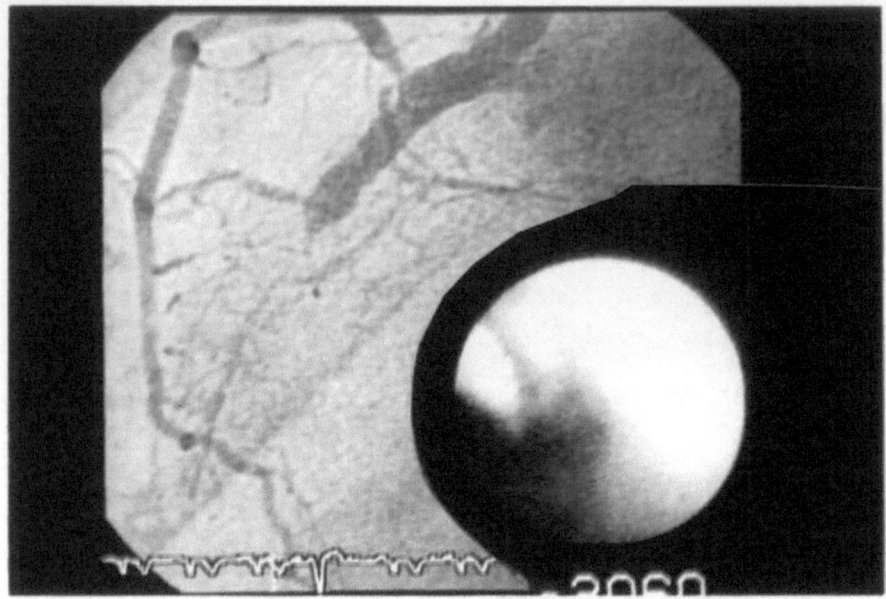

Figure 1 (Chapter 20). Example of the uncertainty of the precise cause of acute coronary occlusion during balloon angioplasty by angiography (left anterior oblique projection), which may be clarified by intracoronary angioscopy. Balloon dilatation of a proximal right coronary artery lesion resulted in the angiographic appearance shown, whereby it is appreciated that although the vessel is now completely occluded, there is no specific sign of the presence of intimal dissection or intracoronary thrombus. Angioscopy performed shortly after occlusion showed complete occlusion of the lumen by a red thrombus (seen here occupying the entire lower left quadrant of the angioscopic field, below the bright white appearance of the guidewire, which has been positioned across the stenosis), with no significant intimal dissection, except for some small superficial intimal disruptions which cannot be appreciated in this still picture and are a characteristic postangioplasty angioscopic feature.

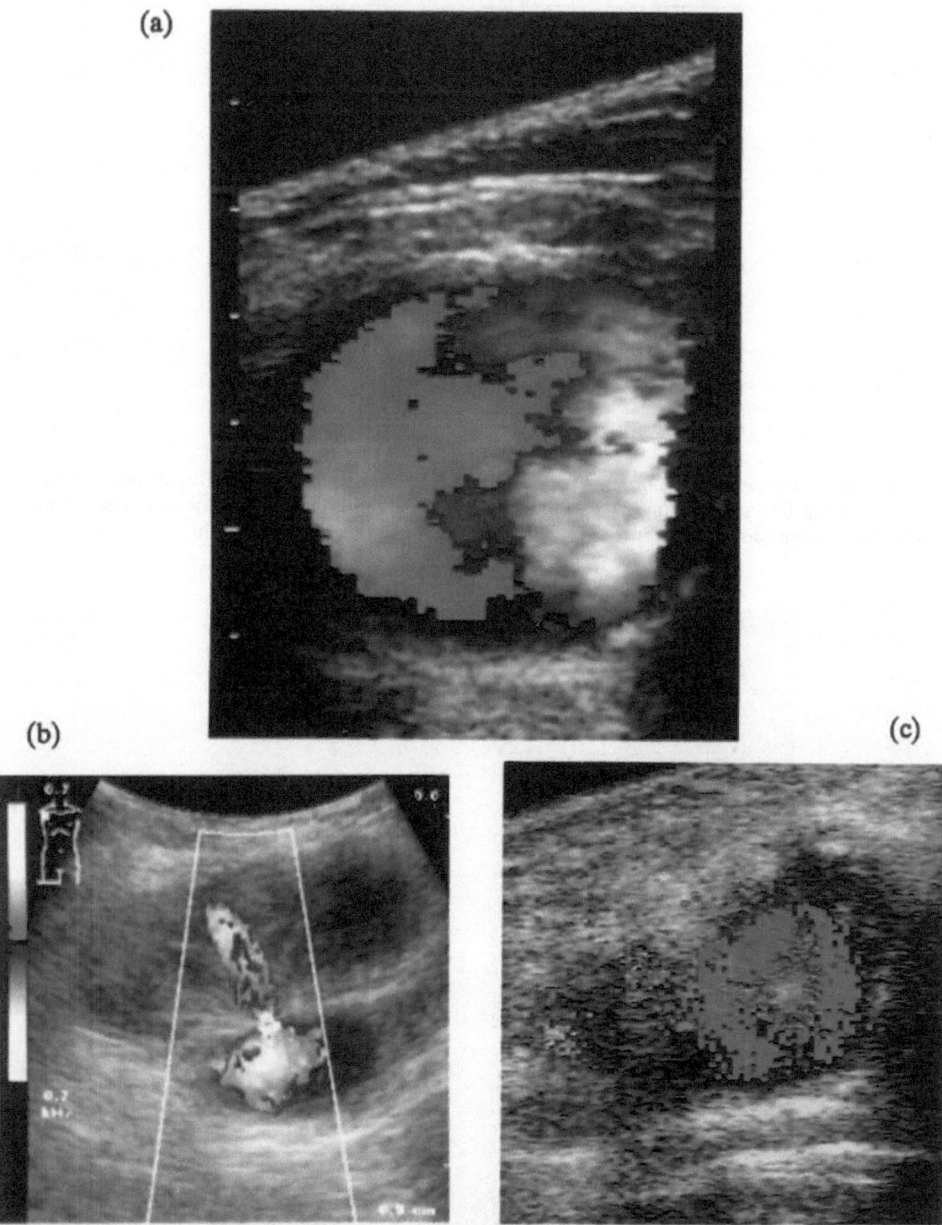

Figure 2 (Chapter 26). CCDS images of pseudoaneurysms of the femoral artery (three different patients). (a) Transverse scan of the right proximal thigh: almost circular flow pattern inside the pseudoaneurysm with red encoding (flow towards the transducer) on the lateral and blue encoding (flow away from the transducer) on the medial site. The feeding artery is displaced medially and not visualized. (b) Almost completely thrombosed large pseudoaneurysm with the feeding artery (dorsal) and the neck of the aneurysm with the defect in the arterial wall (encoding in bright blue). Perfusion is displayed only in the center of the the lesion. (c) Transverse scan of the left proximal thigh: diffuse fresh parially thrombosed pseudoaneurysm lateral to the femoral artery, femoral vein with blue encoding.

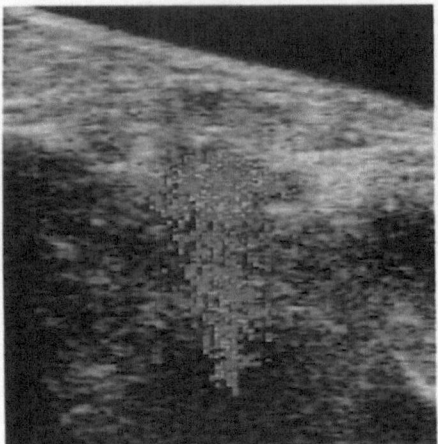

Figure 3A (*Chapter 26*). Arteriovenous fistula of superficial femoral artery: (a) Transverse CCDS images shows typically a fog like mixture of red and blue dots (due to the high blood velocity in the fistula which causes high speed vibration of the soft tissue) which superimpose the artery and vein.

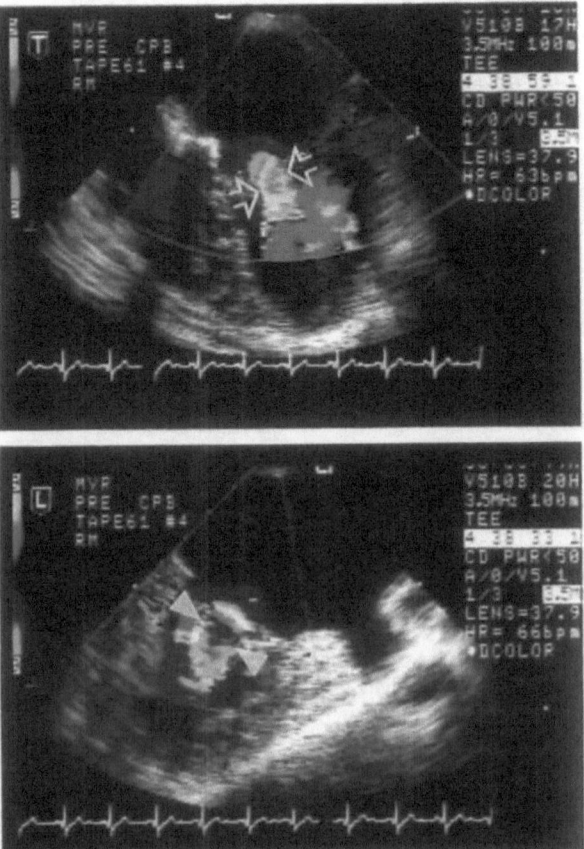

Figure 2 (*Chapter 28*). An example of biplane color Doppler transesophageal echocardiographic (TEE) assessment of severity of mitral stenosis with the use of stenotic jet widths from two orthogonal planes. Note that the stenotic jet width (JW_1, indicated by open arrows) from a TEE horizontal plane at the top is smaller than the jet width (JW_2, indicated by arrow heads) from a vertical TEE plane at the bottom. The mitral valve area is calculated by assuming an oval mitral orifice: $\pi \times JW_1/2 \times JW_2/2$.

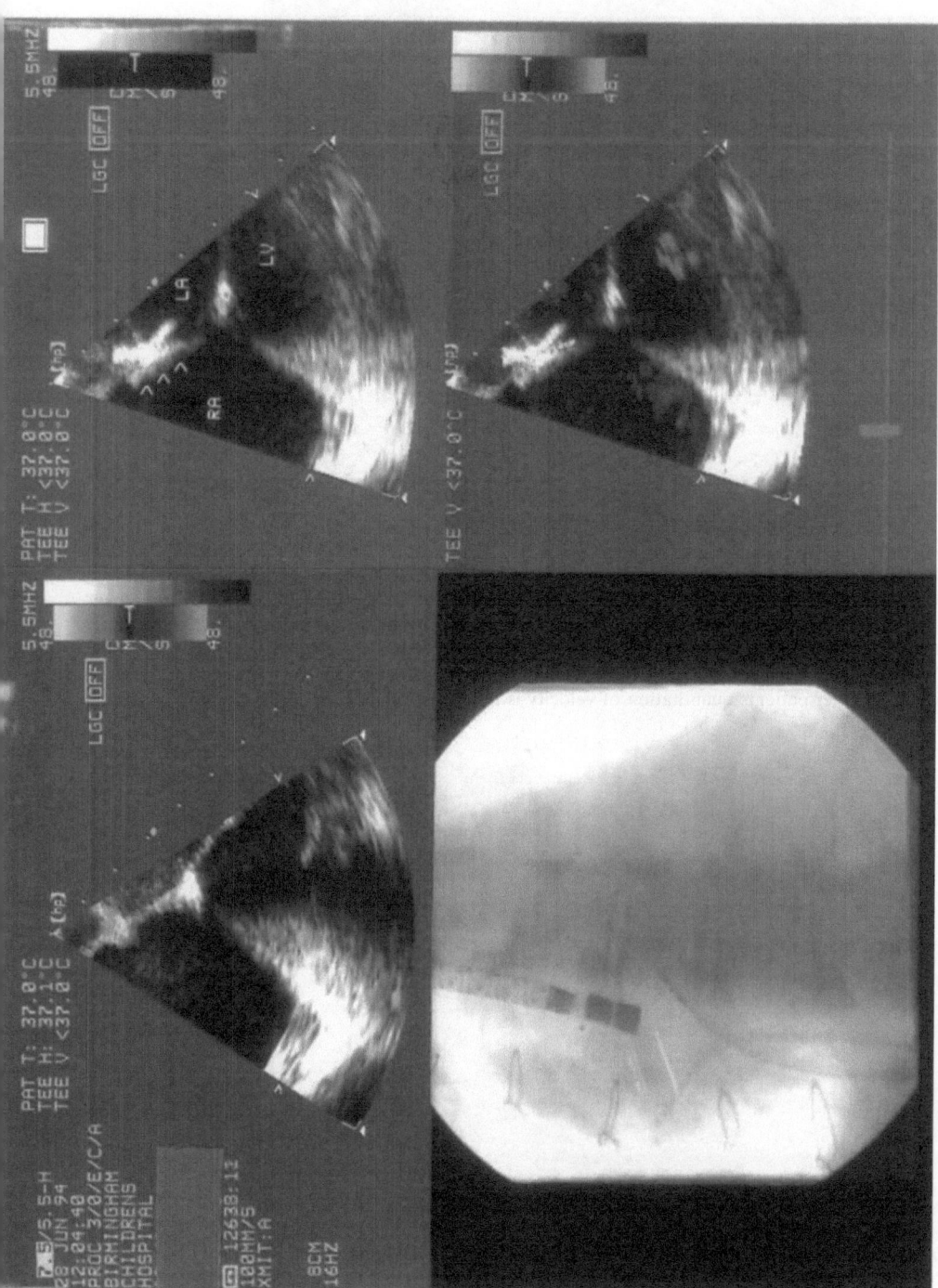

Figure 6 (Chapter 30). Transesophageal monitoring of umbrella occlusion of an atrial fenestration after Fontan operation. The location of the defect is readily seen on four chamber views (top left). The device is positioned using a combination of fluoroscopy and continuous transesophageal imaging (top right and bottom left). Final colour flow mapping studies excludes residual shunting (bottom right).

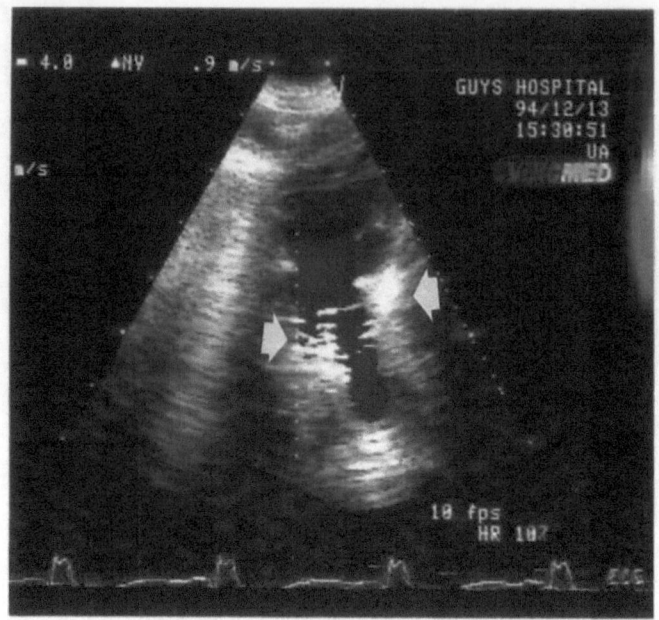

Figure 4 (Chapter 31). This colour Doppler echocardiogram is from a patient with bilateral pulmonary artery branch stenosis following correction of a common arterial trunk (truncus arteriosus) in the new-born period. At six months of age Palmaz stents were placed in both left and right pulmonary arteries at the same procedure. Both stents are patent and appear unobstructive. At this age alignment with the flow in the left pulmonary artery is satisfactory for velocity estimation but that with the right is less good. In older patients quantitation of velocity is much less reliable.

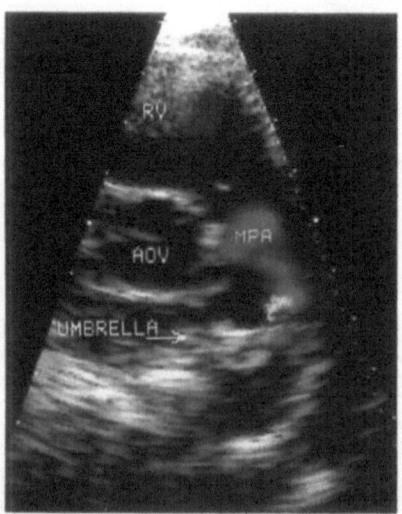

Figure 6 (Chapter 31). A colour Doppler echocardiogram from a patient with a Rashkind duct occluder in place. The bright echo at the origin of the left pulmonary is from an arm of the occluding umbrella. Adjacent to this can be seen the turbulent "flame" indicating residual flow through the arterial duct.

Index

Developments in Cardiovascular Medicine

121. S. Sideman, R. Beyar and A.G. Kleber (eds.): *Cardiac Electrophysiology, Circulation, and Transport.* Proceedings of the 7th Henry Goldberg Workshop (Berne, Switzerland, 1990). 1991   ISBN 0-7923-1145-0
122. D.M. Bers: *Excitation-Contraction Coupling and Cardiac Contractile Force.* 1991
                                                                                ISBN 0-7923-1186-8
123. A.-M. Salmasi and A.N. Nicolaides (eds.): *Occult Atherosclerotic Disease.* Diagnosis, Assessment and Management. 1991   ISBN 0-7923-1188-4
124. J.A.E. Spaan: *Coronary Blood Flow.* Mechanics, Distribution, and Control. 1991
                                                                                ISBN 0-7923-1210-4
125. R.W. Stout (ed.): *Diabetes and Atherosclerosis.* 1991   ISBN 0-7923-1310-0
126. A.G. Herman (ed.): *Antithrombotics.* Pathophysiological Rationale for Pharmacological Interventions. 1991   ISBN 0-7923-1413-1
127. N.H.J. Pijls: *Maximal Myocardial Perfusion as a Measure of the Functional Significance of Coronary Arteriogram.* From a Pathoanatomic to a Pathophysiologic Interpretation of the Coronary Arteriogram. 1991   ISBN 0-7923-1430-1
128. J.H.C. Reiber and E.E. v.d. Wall (eds.): *Cardiovascular Nuclear Medicine and MRI.* Quantitation and Clinical Applications. 1992   ISBN 0-7923-1467-0
129. E. Andries, P. Brugada and R. Stroobrandt (eds.): *How to Face 'the Faces' of Cardiac Pacing.* 1992   ISBN 0-7923-1528-6
130. M. Nagano, S. Mochizuki and N.S. Dhalla (eds.): *Cardiovascular Disease in Diabetes.* 1992   ISBN 0-7923-1554-5
131. P.W. Serruys, B.H. Strauss and S.B. King III (eds.): *Restenosis after Intervention with New Mechanical Devices.* 1992   ISBN 0-7923-1555-3
132. P.J. Walter (ed.): *Quality of Life after Open Heart Surgery.* 1992
                                                                                ISBN 0-7923-1580-4
133. E.E. van der Wall, H. Sochor, A. Righetti and M.G. Niemeyer (eds.): *What's new in Cardiac Imaging?* SPECT, PET and MRI. 1992   ISBN 0-7923-1615-0
134. P. Hanrath, R. Uebis and W. Krebs (eds.): *Cardiovascular Imaging by Ultrasound.* 1992   ISBN 0-7923-1755-6
135. F.H. Messerli (ed.): *Cardiovascular Disease in the Elderly.* 3rd ed. 1992
                                                                                ISBN 0-7923-1859-5
136. J. Hess and G.R. Sutherland (eds.): *Congenital Heart Disease in Adolescents and Adults.* 1992   ISBN 0-7923-1862-5
137. J.H.C. Reiber and P.W. Serruys (eds.): *Advances in Quantitative Coronary Arteriography.* 1993   ISBN 0-7923-1863-3
138. A.-M. Salmasi and A.S. Iskandrian (eds.): *Cardiac Output and Regional Flow in Health and Disease.* 1993   ISBN 0-7923-1911-7
139. J.H. Kingma, N.M. van Hemel and K.I. Lie (eds.): *Atrial Fibrillation, a Treatable Disease?* 1992   ISBN 0-7923-2008-5
140. B. Ostadel and N.S. Dhalla (eds.): *Heart Function in Health and Disease.* Proceedings of the Cardiovascular Program (Prague, Czechoslovakia, 1991). 1992
                                                                                ISBN 0-7923-2052-2
141. D. Noble and Y.E. Earm (eds.): *Ionic Channels and Effect of Taurine on the Heart.* Proceedings of an International Symposium (Seoul, Korea , 1992). 1993
                                                                                ISBN 0-7923-2199-5
142. H.M. Piper and C.J. Preusse (eds.): *Ischemia-reperfusion in Cardiac Surgery.* 1993
                                                                                ISBN 0-7923-2241-X
143. J. Roelandt, E.J. Gussenhoven and N. Bom (eds.): *Intravascular Ultrasound.* 1993
                                                                                ISBN 0-7923-2301-7
144. M.E. Safar and M.F. O'Rourke (eds.): *The Arterial System in Hypertension.* 1993
                                                                                ISBN 0-7923-2343-2
145. P.W. Serruys, D.P. Foley and P.J. de Feyter (eds.): *Quantitative Coronary Angiography in Clinical Practice.* With a Foreword by Spencer B. King III. 1994
                                                                                ISBN 0-7923-2368-8

Developments in Cardiovascular Medicine

Developments in Cardiovascular Medicine

Previous volumes are still available

KLUWER ACADEMIC PUBLISHERS – DORDRECHT / BOSTON / LONDON